Yasser El Miedany
Editor

Comorbidity in Rheumatic Diseases

Springer

Editor
Yasser El Miedany, MD, FRCP
Honorary Senior Clinical Lecturer
King's College London
London, UK

Professor of Rheumatology and Rehabilitation
Ain Shams University
Cairo, Egypt

Consultant Rheumatologist
Department of Rheumatology
Darent Valley Hospital
Dartford, Kent, UK

ISBN 978-3-319-59962-5 ISBN 978-3-319-59963-2 (eBook)
DOI 10.1007/978-3-319-59963-2

Library of Congress Control Number: 2017948206

Printed on acid-free paper

This Springer imprint is published by Springer Nature
The registered company is Springer International Publishing AG
The registered company address is: Gewerbestrasse 11, 6330 Cham, Switzerland

"A true friend is a gift from God"
This book is dedicated to my dear friends whom I have been fortunate enough to meet.
To my dear friends in Egypt, England, the United States, and the Arabian Gulf, many thanks for your support.

Foreword

The practice of rheumatology has been tremendously modified over the past 10–15 years. Fifteen years ago, the relative lack of effective treatments and treatment strategies meant that the rheumatologist was mainly managing the disease and its consequences on the patient's life, sometimes even "running after" the inflammatory process rather than controlling it. Today, thanks to new management strategies, more tight control, and more effective treatments, the prognosis of rheumatic disorders and in particular inflammatory rheumatic disorders has been profoundly improved.

It is in this context of an overall lower disease burden that comorbidities have taken on an increasing importance. Comorbidities are both more frequent and less well screened for in inflammatory rheumatic disorders than in the general population. Comorbidities can be related to the disease process itself, to the consequences of the disease, or to the treatments given for the disease such as glucocorticoids. The responsibility for dealing with these comorbidities is shared between the patient himself or herself, the general practitioner, and the rheumatologist.

It is in this context that the publication of this book is both timely and important. In this book, readers will learn about the prevalence and incidence of comorbidities in different rheumatological diseases and current guidelines and best practice to better screen for these comorbidities, ultimately leading to better care for our patients.

Sorbonne Universités, Pitié Salpêtrière Hospital
Paris, France

Laure Gossec

Preface

This book describes the real-life story of our patients living with arthritis. The story begins when a young healthy person starts to feel joint pain and finds it difficult to do simple things, things that most people take for granted, like sleeping, getting dressed, brushing teeth, or driving. After learning more about arthritis and its treatment, the person may feel overwhelmed or angry. At some point, most people with arthritis realize that the disease is, indeed, a fact of their lives. With this awareness, they may become depressed. As the disease course continues, it becomes clear that, typically, it involves pathology affecting almost all organs of the body, resulting in highly heterogeneous disease patterns, which not only affect the person's physical ability but also self-esteem, roles, relationships, organ fitness, control perceptions, and mood – briefly, life.

Unfortunately, neither the recently published rheumatology textbooks nor the multiauthored books on different rheumatic diseases have dedicated chapters on comorbidity in different rheumatic diseases. Nevertheless, this topic is of interest since associations not only could contribute to the understanding of the pathogenesis of the conditions, but it also gives a warning signal to the clinician to scrutinize some patients for potential risks. As a clinical professor, who has had special interest in getting to know my patients and how to set up treatment plans tailored to their needs, I felt it was time to compile a book focusing on comorbidity in rheumatic diseases with its different patterns, ways of assessment, and management.

The main theme of this book is to deliver a very practical and reader-friendly guide. On one hand, it delivers the science-based evidence and advanced knowledge of comorbidity in different rheumatic diseases; on the other hand, it provides the most recent in this field and examples of recent tools which the readers/researchers can use for their standard practice and clinical trials. With its 19 key chapters, this book is expected to fill an important void in the current literature. It represents what can be considered the best current thinking on comorbidity in different rheumatic diseases. Therefore, *Comorbidity in Rheumatic Diseases* can serve as both excellent introductory and a very good reference, as well as resource for implementation in standard clinical practice and future reading.

This work has been the outcome of the cooperative effort of a large international group of leaders in musculoskeletal medicine and expertise in comorbidity assessment and management. They have done a superb job to produce authoritative chapters including vast amounts of scientific and clinical data to create state-of-the-art descriptions of comorbidity encompassed in different rheumatic diseases. Special thanks to my colleagues and family for their support throughout the whole project, which helped to make this book complete.

Personally, I feel privileged to have compiled this work and am enthusiastic about all that it offers our readers. I hope you too will find this edition a uniquely valuable educational resource.

Meopham, Kent, UK Yasser El Miedany

Contents

Contributors

Ibtisam Al-Hashimi, BDS, MS, PhD Deparment of Surgery, The University of Texas Southwestern Medical Center, Dallas, Texas

Mais Arwani, MD Department of Internal Medicine, Allegheny General Hospital-Allegheny Health Network, Pittsburgh, PA, USA

Maha Azeez Nuffield Department of Orthopaedics, Rheumatology and Musculoskeletal Sciences, University of Oxford, Botnar Research Centre, Oxford, UK

X. Baraliakos, MD Department of Rheumatology, Rheumazentrum Ruhrgebiet, Herne, Germany

J. Braun, MD Department of Rheumatology, Rheumazentrum Ruhrgebiet, Herne, Germany

Isabel Castrejon, MD, PhD Division of Rheumatology, Rush University Medical Center, Chicago, IL, USA

Anna Chapman, MD Department of Dermatology, Lewisham and Greenwich NHS Trust, Queen Elizabeth Hospital, London, UK

Peter T. Chapman, BSc, MD(Otago) FRACP Department of Rheumatology, Immunology and Allergy, Christchurch Hospital, Christchurch, New Zealand

Emanuela Del Giudice, MD Department of Pediatric Immunology and Rheumatology, UMC Utrecht, Wilhelmina Children's Hospital, Utrecht, Netherlands

Department of Paediatrics and Infant Neuropsychiatry, Sapienza University of Rome, Rome, Italy

Sharon Dowell, MBBS Department of Internal Medicine, Division of Rheumatology, Howard University Hospital, Washington, DC, USA

Nadia El Aroussy, MD Department of Rheumatology and Rehabilitation, Ain Shams University, Cairo, Egypt

Yasser El-Miedany, MD, FRCP King's College London, London, UK

Rheumatology and Rehabilitation, Ain Shams University, Cairo, Egypt

Department of Rheumatology, Darent Valley Hospital, Dartford, Kent, UK

James Galloway, MD Department of Rheumatology, King's College London, London, UK

Rajesh Gopalarathinam, MD Department of Internal Medicine, Allegheny General Hospital-Allegheny Health Network, Pittsbutgh, PA, USA

Mohamed Osama Hegazi, MRCP(UK) Al Adan Hospital, Hadiya, Kuwait

Cristina Hernández-Díaz, MD, MCSc Laboratorio de Ultrasonido Musculoesqueletico y Articular, Instituto Nacional de Rehabilitación, Calzada México-Xochimilco, Ciudad de México, Mexico

Meenakshi Jolly, MD, MS Division of Rheumatology, Rush University Medical Center, Chicago, IL, USA

Adham Aboul Fotouh Khalil, MD, MSc New Kasr El Aimi Teaching Hospital, Cairo University, Cairo, Egypt

Sadik A. Khuder, BDS, MPH, PhD Department of Medicine, University of Toledo, Toledo, OH, USA

Uta Kiltz, MD Department of Rheumatology, Rheumazentrum Ruhrgebiet, Herne, Germany

Mihaela Comina Micu, MD Rheumatology Division, Rehabilitation Department, Rehabilitation Clinical Hospital, Cluj-Napoca, Romania

Yair Molad, MD Rheumatology Unit, Rabin Medical Center – Beilinson Hospital, Petach Tikva and Sackler Faculty of Medicine, Tel Aviv, Israel

Anand B. Mutgi, MD, MSc Department of Medicine, University of Toledo, Toledo, OH, USA

Ailda Nika, MD Division of Rheumatology, Rush University Medical Center, Chicago, IL, USA

Elena Nikiphorou, MD Department of Rheumatology, King's College London, London, UK

Deborah Palmer, ANP Department of Rheumatology, North Middlesex University Hospital, London, UK

Mercedes Quinones, MD Department of Internal Medicine, Division of Rheumatology, Howard University Hospital, Washington, DC, USA

Andrew Rutherford, MD Department of Rheumatology, King's College London, London, UK

Winston Sequeira, MD Division of Rheumatology, Rush University Medical Center, Chicago, IL, USA

Tarun S. Sharma, MD Lupus Center of Excellence, West Penn Allegheny Health System, Pittsburgh, PA, USA

Tuulikki Sokka, MD, PhD Department of Rheumatology, Jyväskylä Central Hospital, Jyväskylä, Finland

University of Eastern Finland, Faculty of Health Sciences, Kuopio, Finland

Lisa K. Stamp, MBChB, FRACP, PhD Department of Medicine, University of Otago, Christchurch, New Zealand

J. Steuart Richards, MBBS Medical Service Line, Division of Rheumatology, Veterans Affairs Pittsburgh Healthcare System, Pittsburgh, PA, USA

Joost F. Swart, MD Department of Pediatric Immunology and Rheumatology, UMC Utrecht, Wilhelmina Children's Hospital, Utrecht, The Netherlands

Peter C. Taylor, MA, PhD, FRCP, FRCP Nuffield Department of Orthopaedics, Rheumatology and Musculoskeletal Sciences, University of Oxford, Botnar Research Centre, Oxford, UK

Natasja van Schoor, PhD Department of Epidemiology and Biostatistics, VU University Medical Center, EMGO Institute for Health and Care Research, Amsterdam, The Netherlands

Mary Chester M. Wasko, MD, MSc Division of Rheumatology, Lupus Center of Excellence, West Penn Hospital, Allegheny Health Network, Pittsburgh, PA, USA

Frank A. Wollheim, MD, PhD, FRCP, MACR Institution of Clinical Sciences Lund, Rheumatology, Lund University, Lund, Sweden

N.M. Wulffraat, MD Department of Pediatric Immunology and Rheumatology, UMC Utrecht, Wilhelmina Children's Hospital, Utrecht, The Netherlands

Chapter 1
Comorbidity in Rheumatic Diseases

Rajesh Gopalarathinam, Mais Arwani, Mary Chester M. Wasko, and Tarun S. Sharma

Comorbidity is a condition that coexists along with the disease of interest. Comorbidities could be related to the primary disease, its treatment, or be completely independent. Comorbidities could also be a historic medical condition that is presently active or inactive. The relationship between rheumatic diseases and comorbidities is intriguing in that whereas certain comorbidities occur more frequently in rheumatic diseases, the rheumatic diseases and their treatments could themselves lead to some of these comorbidities. Higher prevalence of comorbidities in rheumatic disease patients compared with those without rheumatic disease could be partly due to a higher inflammatory burden, an overlapping pathophysiology with rheumatic diseases, or increased prevalence as a result of frequent monitoring and screening, and improved survival among these patients. An example of this would be the higher incidence and prevalence of cardiovascular disease (CVD) and traditional cardiovascular (CV) risk factors like dyslipidemia, diabetes and insulin resistance in rheumatoid arthritis (RA), and systemic lupus erythematosus (SLE). Another example would be systemic sclerosis (SSc)-related lung involvement or lupus nephritis where early recognition and management of these disease-related complications has a potential to improve survival. While recent advances have been

R. Gopalarathinam • M. Arwani
Department of Internal Medicine, Allegheny General Hospital-Allegheny Health Network, Pittsburgh, PA, USA

M.C.M. Wasko
Division of Rheumatology, Lupus Center of Excellence, West Penn Hospital, Allegheny Health Network, Pittsburgh, PA, USA

T.S. Sharma (✉)
Lupus Center of Excellence, West Penn Allegheny Health System, Pittsburgh, PA, USA
e-mail: tarun.sharma@ahn.org

Y. El Miedany (ed.), *Comorbidity in Rheumatic Diseases*,
DOI 10.1007/978-3-319-59963-2_1

invaluable to the therapeutic armamentarium of rheumatic diseases, long-term treatment-related risks like infection and malignancy have emerged as concerns. The use of medications like disease-modifying antirheumatic drugs (DMARDs), nonsteroidal anti-inflammatory drugs (NSAIDs), and glucocorticoids for inflammatory arthritis also contribute to comorbidities.

Comorbidities can impact the primary disease in multiple ways. Often they influence the patient's quality of life and prognosis of the primary disease itself. For example, CVD, pulmonary and renal involvement, and infection lead to premature mortality in rheumatic diseases. Comorbidities and the complexity they add in management of the primary disease influence therapeutic decisions on a daily basis. High-risk comorbidities like malignancy, CVD, and infection limit the treatment choices available in rheumatic diseases and thereby adversely affect disease outcomes. On the other hand, comorbidities like osteoporosis need addition of new therapy to prevent fractures and functional limitation. Comorbidities have been known to be managed suboptimally in rheumatic diseases, and the above complexity could be contributing to this.

Some measures of comorbidity utilized in studies include the Charlson comorbidity index. This tool estimates the burden, severity, morbidity and mortality, cost, and hospitalization-related impact of comorbidities [1]. At point of care in clinic, there are no such comprehensive indices, but rather comorbidities are captured mostly via effective history-taking and chart review.

In this introductory chapter, we hope to provide the readers with a broad overview of some of the common and high-impact comorbidities encountered in rheumatic diseases. Subsequent chapters will elaborate on these topics individually in detail.

Cardiovascular Disease in Rheumatic Disease

Epidemiology

CVD-related mortality is known to be high in patients with rheumatic diseases. This has been studied in detail in RA and SLE. While RA has a twofold increased overall mortality, with CVD being the leading cause of death in RA patients [2], SLE has a bimodal peak of mortality – once during younger age due to the disease and its complications and then again while older secondary to atherosclerotic coronary artery disease (CAD) [3]. A meta-analysis of 24 observational studies of CVD-related mortality in patients with RA reported a 50%, 59%, and 52% increased risk of CVD, ischemic heart disease, and cerebrovascular accident (CVA) death, respectively [4]. RA patients are twice as likely to experience unrecognized myocardial infarctions and sudden death [5]. While CVD mortality appears to be declining over recent years in RA, the overall gap between CVD risk in RA and the general population seems to be widening [6, 7]. Women with SLE in age group of 35–44 years are over 50 times more likely to have a myocardial infarction compared to age- and sex-matched controls [8]. SLE patients also have a twofold to tenfold increase in risk of stroke [9]. Accelerated atherosclerosis has also been noted in other rheumatic diseases like vasculitis, psoriatic arthritis (PsA), ankylosing spondylitis (AS), and SSc [10–14]. Patients with PsA and AS have been found to have an increased CV risk [13, 15]. Patients with RA have been found to have twice the risk of developing congestive heart failure (CHF) compared with general population, and this excess risk is not explained by traditional CV risk factors and/or clinical ischemic heart disease [16]. A high proportion of RA patients are reported to have heart failure with preserved ejection fraction (EF ≥ 50%) and less likely to have a history of obesity, hypertension (HTN), or ischemic heart disease compared with non-RA individuals with heart failure [17]. The association between gout and CVD and an estimate of the comorbidity burden has also been elucidated in epidemiological studies [18, 19].

Pathophysiology

Atherosclerosis is known to have a central role in the pathophysiology of CVD in rheumatic diseases. The inflammatory/immunologic response observed in atherosclerosis and RA synovitis is found to be similar [20–22]. Accelerated atherosclerosis and vessel inflammation in the form of vasculitis could have a role in cardiac ischemia [23]. The Feiring Heart Biopsy Study found that inflammatory cell infiltrates in the outer vascular and perivascular layers of the aorta of patients were associated with CAD and infiltrates in the adventitia and media were more common in patients with rheumatic diseases especially in those with a history of smoking and aortic aneurysms [24]. Vascular endothelial cell apoptosis which contributes to vascular dysfunction is seen in SLE and SSc vasculopathy [25, 26].

Risk Factors

Traditional CV risk factors known to increase CVD risk in the general population include increasing age, male gender, smoking, HTN, diabetes, hypercholesterolemia, body composition, and insulin resistance. RA is independently associated with increased CVD after adjusting for traditional CV risk factors [27]. In addition to most traditional CV risk factors, which are more prevalent and deleterious in rheumatic diseases, several other factors including systemic and vascular inflammation and medications like corticosteroids and NSAIDs contribute to increased CV risk. In RA, smoking is known to be more prevalent [28], is a risk factor for development of seropositivity, and is associated with a worse prognosis [29, 30]. Whereas compared with the general population the evidence regarding prevalence of hypertension in RA [28, 31] and AS [13] is mixed, it has been found to be higher in SLE patients [32]. RA is associated with an abnormal lipid pattern especially low HDL levels [33], and while the CVD risk is elevated, the levels of total cholesterol (TC) and LDL are usually low with active disease [34]. Lipid levels in AS and PsA are similarly affected with active disease [13]. Prevalence of diabetes is also found to be higher in some studies of RA [28] and SLE [32]. Insulin resistance is more prevalent in SLE [35] and in RA has been shown to have a direct correlation with disease activity [36, 37]. Low BMI has been reported to have a paradoxical effect on survival in RA with as much as a threefold increase in CVD death [38]. Most NSAIDs and cyclooxygenase-2 (COX-2) inhibitors have been associated with increase CV risk [39]. Corticosteroids increase CV risk due to negative effects on the above risk factors [40], and the increased risk is found to be highest in patients treated with long-term and higher doses (>7.5 mg/day prednisone equivalent) [41]. HTN is a known side effect of cyclosporine and leflunomide [42]. In RA, markers of inflammation such as erythrocyte sedimentation rate (ESR) have been correlated with CV risk [34, 43], and C-reactive protein (CRP) and tumor necrosis factor (TNF)-α levels have been shown to predict CVD and its severity and possibly even have a causal role [44]. Disease activity and severity have been found to correlate with CV events [45, 46]. By the same token, DMARDs such as methotrexate (MTX) and TNF-α inhibitors that lower disease activity have shown to reduce CV risk [47, 48] (Table 1.1).

Assessment and Prediction

The 1998 Framingham Risk Score allows prediction of multivariate coronary heart disease risk in patients [56]. A 2008 version can predict 1-year global risk of CVD and specific CVD end points [57]. A CV risk management guideline from the EULAR taskforce, based on expert consensus opinion, recommends the SCORE algorithm and using a 1.5 multiplication factor when estimating CV risk in patients with RA when a patient meets two or more of the following three criteria: disease duration longer than 10 years, positivity for rheumatoid factor or ACPA, and presence of extra-articular manifestations [58]. Like the Framingham risk score, with this SCORE algorithm, a 10-year risk of incident CV events can be estimated after accounting for gender, age, smoking status, blood pressure, and TC or TC/HDL ratio [59]. In experienced hands, the addition of carotid ultrasonography to detect carotid intimal thickening/plaque could improve cardiovascular risk assessment in patients with RA and PsA [60, 61]. A number of biologic markers for CV risk prediction including genetic, inflammatory, immunologic, and markers of endothelial function have been identified and, although remain to be validated and studied in rheumatic diseases, could have potential role in CV risk prediction models [62].

Table 1.1 Traditional CV risk factors in RA and SLE

CV risk factor	RA	SLE
Smoking	Risk factor for RA and seropositivity, worse RA prognosis; higher prevalence in RA [28–30]	Risk factor for atherosclerosis and vascular events in SLE [49, 50]
Hypertension	Similar prevalence as general population [28]	Higher prevalence than general population [32] and a predictor of mortality and CV events [49, 51]
Dyslipidemia	Low HDL cholesterol (CV protective cholesterol) levels seen [33]	Hypercholesterolemia associated with higher CV events [8, 52]
Diabetes	Possible higher prevalence [28] but inconsistent results in other studies [53, 54]; related to abdominal obesity, disease activity and corticosteroid use [37]	Higher prevalence [32]
Insulin resistance	Higher prevalence [37] and related to RA disease activity [36], abdominal fat [55]	Higher prevalence and related to higher BMI, ESR, TNF-α levels [35]
Body composition	Low BMI associated with threefold increase risk of CVD deaths [38]	Obesity is risk for atherosclerotic vascular events [49]

CV cardiovascular, *RA* rheumatoid arthritis, *SLE* systemic lupus erythematosus, *HDL* high-density lipoprotein, *ESR* erythrocyte sedimentation rate, *TNF* tumor necrosis factor, *CVD* cardiovascular disease, *BMI* body mass index

CV Risk Management

CV risk management in high-risk rheumatic disease patients consists of two main principles – tight control of disease activity, thus reducing systemic inflammatory burden, and minimizing traditional CV risk factors. Tight control of disease activity by early and effective use of DMARDs, such as TNF-α inhibitors and MTX in inflammatory arthritis, has been shown to be independently associated with a lower CV risk [63–69] and has been recommended as part of the treat-to-target principles for management of RA [70]. Hydroxychloroquine has been shown to have pleiotropic beneficial effects, antithrombotic, lipid lowering, and favorable glycemic properties, and may reduce incident CV events in RA [71, 72].

European League Against Rheumatism (EULAR) evidence-based recommendations for cardiovascular risk management in patients with RA and other forms of inflammatory arthritis recommend that patients should be screened for CVD and traditional CV risk factors should be aggressively managed to try to reduce this excess risk [58]. It is conceivable that since CVD risk in RA is similar to that in diabetes, primary prevention and CV risk factor management should be similar to that in diabetes, as others have proposed [27, 31]. Routine CV risk assessment in rheumatic diseases should be strongly considered, along with emphasis on appropriate management of metabolic syndrome, smoking cessation, minimizing use of corticosteroids, and cautious use of NSAIDs. While further research in this area is underway, systematic screening for CV risk via collaboration of care between rheumatologists, cardiologists, and primary care physicians is imperative to achieve optimal management of CVD in rheumatic disease patients.

Infection in Rheumatic Diseases

Infections are a major cause of morbidity and mortality in patients with rheumatic diseases. Although the presence of rheumatic diseases can cause impaired immunity and subsequent infections in the host, the most important risk factor for developing serious infections is the use of immunosuppressive therapy for the treatment of the underlying rheumatic disease [73]. Immunosuppressive drugs such as glucocorticoids induce immunodeficiency at a cellular level and predispose the host to a wide variety of bacterial, viral, fungal, and parasitic infections [74]. The clinical manifestations of infections in rheumatic disease patients are often difficult to appreciate clinically due to diminution of fever and other signs of inflammation by the immunosuppressive therapy. Nonetheless, early diagnosis and treatment is critical to avoid disastrous consequences. This increased risk of infections is due to the fact that various drugs such as traditional DMARDs and glucocorticoids, which are commonly used to treat RA patients, are all associated with immunosuppression [75]. A longitudinal follow-up study on an incidence cohort of 609 RA patients identified advanced age, male sex, increased disease severity, smoking history, leukopenia, presence of extra-articular manifestations of RA, and presence of other comorbid conditions (such as diabetes, chronic lung disease, alcoholism, and dementia) to be strong risk factors associated with an increased infection risk [76]. Among the DMARDs, infection rates appear to be minimal with low-dose MTX [77]. Studies have shown that the use of TNF-α inhibitors is associated with increased risk of serious bacterial infections requiring hospitalization and antibiotic therapy [78, 79]. Results from a meta-analysis of 70 trials that included over 32,000 RA patients showed that there is a small but significant risk (pooled odds ratio [OR], 1.79; 95% confidence interval [CI], 1.17–2.74) of opportunistic infections (for mycobacterial and viral infections) that occurs with biologic drugs without affecting the overall mortality [80]. Patients with RA-associated interstitial lung disease especially those on prednisone >10 mg daily are found to be at higher risk of serious infection in a recent study [81].

Similar to patients with RA, patients with SLE have a greater risk of infection that is related to significant morbidity and mortality. In a large prospective multicenter European study involving 1000 SLE patients over a 10-year follow-up period (from 1990 to 2000), 360 patients (36%) developed infections, and among the 68 patients who died, 25% of the deaths were attributed to infections. Along with active SLE, infections were the most common cause of death (28.9%) among patients in the initial 5-year follow-up [82]. Disease duration, disease activity, leukopenia, nephritis, hypocomplementemia, concomitant use of steroids with cyclophosphamide have been linked in different combinations to an increased risk of infection [83]. A nested case-control study that involved 83 lupus patients to investigate the clinical predictors of infections showed the most frequent bacterial agents involved in causing major infections requiring hospitalization were *Escherichia coli*, *Staphylococcus aureus*, *Mycobacterium tuberculosis*, and *Streptococcus pneumonia* [84]. In this section, we will review the pulmonary, cutaneous, joint, and other site-specific infections related to rheumatic diseases.

Site-Specific Infections

In general, RA patients have an increased incidence of infection compared with the general population [85]. Respiratory tract infections are the most frequent type of infections that occur in RA patients. These can be deadly; lower respiratory tract infections in RA are associated with mortality of almost 22.5% [86]. A dose-related relationship between prednisone use and pneumonia risk has been described [87].

Tuberculosis (TB) deserves a special mention among the pulmonary infections seen in patients with rheumatic diseases. Studies have shown that RA patients have an increased risk of pulmonary tuberculosis, independent of treatment with TNF-α inhibitors [88, 89]. TNF-α plays a crucial role in phagocytosis and killing of mycobacterium tuberculosis by activated macrophages and is also responsible for confining of mycobacteria within granulomas, thereby maintaining a latent state for TB [90]. The use of TNF-α inhibitors is associated with a significant increase in the reactivation of latent TB, resulting in an active TB infection [91, 92]. TNF-α affects both the activation of immune cells and their response to intracellular infection in several different ways, thereby impacting both the innate and adaptive immunity [93]. The British Society for Rheumatology Biologics Register, a large national prospective observational study, reported the rates of TB in RA patients treated with TNF-α inhibitors compared with traditional DMARDs, and investigators concluded that the incidence rate of TB was three to four times higher in RA patients who were treated with infliximab and adalimumab compared to those who received etanercept [94].

In a large, prospective cohort of SLE patients, 25% developed an infection in a 5-year follow-up period with the most common type of infection being pneumonia due to bacterial etiology [95]. Immunosuppressive therapy, particularly corticosteroids, was significantly associated with an increased risk of infection ($P = 0.029$) in this study. Another study demonstrated that the TNF-238A allele and a related haplotype have a strong influence on the risk of developing pneumonia among SLE patients in a large multiethnic cohort [96]. In this study, bacterial pathogens were responsible for 75% of all pneumonia events followed by mycobacteria (12%), fungi (7%), and virus (5%).

Pulmonary infections with other rheumatic diseases such as SSc, Sjögren's syndrome (SS), granulomatosis with polyangiitis, eosinophilic granulomatosis with polyangiitis, Goodpasture's syndrome, and AS may be less common or at least have not been well studied. The clinical manifestations of infectious pulmonary diseases in RA and SLE are often non-specific and similar to the noninfectious complications such as interstitial lung disease, acute lupus pneumonitis, and diffuse alveolar hemorrhage. Therefore, workup should be aggressive to identify the infectious etiology in suspected cases and should include chest X-ray, blood and sputum cultures, and bronchoscopy with bronchoalveolar lavage (BAL) if needed. Patients with suspected pneumonia should always be started on empiric antibiotics, with focused treatment once an infectious organism is identified.

Studies have shown that the incidence of cutaneous infections secondary to bacterial, viral and fungal organisms can occur at an increased rate in patients receiving TNF-α inhibitors [97, 98]. Most skin infections (fungal [dermatomycosis], bacterial [folliculitis, erysipelas], and viral [herpes zoster]) in one large series occurred during active treatment with TNF-α inhibitors [99]. Herpes zoster deserves a special mention among these cutaneous infections seen in patients treated with TNF-α inhibitors. It manifests as a painful dermatomal vesicular rash and occurs due to reactivation of the varicella zoster virus in patients with impaired cellular immunity. A recent study showed that the incidence of herpes zoster is increased in RA patients compared to the general population [100]. The impact of TNF-α inhibitor treatment on risk of herpes zoster infection is controversial, with evidence both supporting and refuting an increased risk with this class of medications [101–104].

Biologic agents have been associated with increased risk of bone and joint infections, mainly septic arthritis. Although rare, a serious infection of the bone and joints is surgical site infection of total joint arthroplasty in patients receiving TNF-α inhibitors [105].

Very few studies have described the incidence of urinary tract infections (UTI) in rheumatic diseases. A retrospective study confirmed the increased rate of UTI among patients with RA (especially elderly females) and attributed the increased risk as a complication to the long-term use of oral steroids [106]. Another study had shown the association of UTI with secondary SS [107].

Chronic hepatitis B and C can be serious comorbid conditions in patients with rheumatic diseases [108]. Reactivation of hepatitis B virus (HBV) leading to serious consequences such as hepatic failure is a well-recognized and frequently occurring complication in HBV infected patients with rheumatic disease undergoing immunosuppressive therapy [109, 110]. Reactivation of HBV infection in patients undergoing immunosuppressive therapy is characterized by an increase in serum HBV-DNA and alanine transaminase (ALT) level [111]. Rheumatic disease patients with hepatitis C virus (HCV) should always be referred to a hepatologist for appropriate antiviral treatment.

Corticosteroids and Risk of Infection

Corticosteroids predispose patients to a wide variety of infections, both mild and serious [112]. In a meta-analysis of 71 clinical trials that compared treatment with steroids and nonsteroids, corticosteroid recipients had a significantly higher rate of infection (12.7%) compared to nonsteroid recipients (8%), with a dose-related increase in risk [113]. The susceptibility to infection may begin within the first few weeks of corticosteroid therapy [114]. Corticosteroids can predispose to opportunistic infections such as listeria, reactivation of pulmonary TB, and pneumocystis jiroveci pneumonia (PJP) [115–117]. Haraoui et al. concluded that although corticosteroids induce remission in RA patients, long-term corticosteroid treatment was not associated with the benefit of sustained remission but rather increased risk for infection [118].

Key Recommendations for Clinical Practice

- For treatment of RA patients with moderate or high disease activity and previous history of serious infections, the American College of Rheumatology (ACR) guidelines conditionally recommend using a combination of traditional DMARDs or abatacept rather than TNF-α inhibitors [119].
- The ACR guidelines recommend screening all patients for pulmonary TB with a tuberculin skin test or an interferon-γ release assay prior to starting TNF-α inhibitors [119]. Latent or active TB warrants referral to a TB specialist for further evaluation and management. In these patients, a minimum of 1 month of antituberculous therapy prior to starting or resuming biologic drug therapy is generally recommended.
- Based on the American Association for the Study of Liver Disease (AASLD) practice guidelines and clinical experience, the ACR guidelines strongly recommend treating RA patients with active HBV infection (who are receiving or have received antiviral treatment) similar to RA patients without HBV infection [119]. Current literature recommends screening of all rheumatic disease patients for HBV infection prior to initiation of biologic DMARDs and hepatology evaluation for antiviral therapy if positive for active infection [120]. During the course of biologic therapy, it is imperative to frequently monitor for viral reactivation in HBV-infected patients and initiate antiviral therapy if necessary [121]. The ACR guidelines conditionally recommend (1) treating RA patients with HCV infection (who are receiving or have received antiviral treatment) similar to RA patients without HCV infection and (2) the use of traditional DMARDs like sulfasalazine and hydroxychloroquine rather than TNF-α inhibitors in RA patients with HCV not requiring or receiving antiviral therapy [119]. Rheumatic disease patients with HCV infection should always be referred to a hepatologist for appropriate antiviral treatment. Currently, there are no strong guidelines suggesting universal screening for HCV prior to starting biologic DMARDs [122], but this testing is advisable.
- Regarding vaccinations, the current ACR guidelines (1) strongly recommend the use of inactivated/killed vaccines (such as pneumococcal vaccine, influenza vaccine, and hepatitis B vaccine) in RA patients receiving biologic therapy, (2) conditionally recommend against the use of live attenuated vaccines (such as zoster

vaccine) in RA patients receiving biologic therapy, and (3) conditionally recommend the use of zoster vaccine in RA patients ≥50 years prior to initiating biologic therapy [119].
- The role of corticosteroids should be limited to bridge therapy to achieve remission when long-term DMARDs or biologic therapy are initiated, with a rapid steroid taper to follow.

Malignancy in Rheumatic Diseases

Increased risk of malignancy has been reported in different rheumatic diseases particularly in RA, SLE, SSc, and idiopathic inflammatory myopathies. This association is partly explained by the presence of common risk factors such as genetics, viruses, and smoking, as these have been implicated in the pathogenesis of both cancers and rheumatic diseases [123, 124].

The inflammatory burden of the autoimmune disease itself and immunological defects associated with rheumatic diseases can play a role in the development of cancers, particularly lymphoproliferative malignancies [125]. The chronic activation of B cells and T cells is a driving force for the development of cancer in rheumatic diseases, especially in primary SS [126] where B cells and autoantibodies are implicated in the disease process and the risk of B-cell lymphoma is increased 40-fold [127].

On the other hand, the immune response can function as an effective extrinsic tumor-suppressor system [128]; when we suppress the immune system with chemotherapeutic agents, we increase the risk of cancer in patients with rheumatic diseases.

Malignancy and Systemic Lupus Erythematous

SLE is associated with increased incidence of different malignancies, particularly hematologic malignancies, more specifically non-Hodgkin lymphoma (NHL) [129]. Aggressive histological subtypes are found to predominate in SLE patients who develop NHL, with the most commonly identified NHL subtype being diffuse large B cell [130].

Lu M et al. conducted a large international SLE cohort, published in 2013, to further study non-lymphoma hematological malignancies in SLE. The most common non-lymphoma hematological malignancies were found to be myeloid types (myelodysplastic syndrome and acute myeloid leukemia) [131]. This contrasts to the general population, where lymphoid types are more common than myeloid non-lymphoma hematological malignancies.

The incidence of certain non-hematologic malignancies has also been found to be elevated in SLE. Observational studies in SLE suggest increased risk of cancer of the vulva, lung, thyroid, and possibly liver, whereas a decreased risk for breast and endometrial and possibly ovarian cancer [132, 133].

Oncogenic viral infections were found to play a role in SLE, an example would be human papillomavirus (HPV)-associated malignant and premalignant conditions. Patients with SLE that were HPV positive were found to be at high risk for anal cancer, vaginal/vulvar cancer, epithelial dysplasia/carcinoma in situ of the uterine cervix, and non-melanoma skin cancer [134].

Malignancy and Rheumatoid Arthritis

Increased risk of lymphomas, leukemia, and myeloma in patients with RA was first reported in 1978 [135]. Subsequently, many studies were conducted to support this linkage. A systematic review of the literature and meta-analysis by Smitten et al. published in 2008 using a Medline search from 1990 to 2007 suggested that RA patients have approximately twofold increase in lymphoma risk (SIR 2.08) with a greater risk of Hodgkin than non-Hodgkin lymphoma. This study also suggests increased risk of lung cancer and decreased risk for colorectal and breast cancer compared with the general population in RA patients [136]. Additional data evaluated using a literature search of relevant observational studies published between 2008 and 2014 conducted by Simon T.A et al. supported previous data of increased risk of lymphoma and lung cancer and decreased risk of colorectal and breast cancer in RA compared with the general population [137]. Others have underscored these associations [138, 139].

Interestingly, a large Danish cohort study published in 2014 included RA patients recruited from a primary care resource and suggested no increased risk of lymphoproliferative or solid cancers during a 4-year follow-up period [140].

Malignancy and Systemic Sclerosis

Increased risk of malignancy in patients with SSc has been observed; however, further studies might be required as data are conflicting. Increased risk of lung and hematologic cancer has been reported [141–143]. A cohort study published in 2006 reported increase in the incidence of esophageal and oropharyngeal cancers [144] (Table 1.2).

A retrospective study conducted in a UK cohort for patients with scleroderma showed increase in frequency of cancers among patients with anti-RNA polymerase III (anti-RNAP) antibody compared with those with anti-Scl-70 antibodies and anti-centromere antibodies (ACAs). The malignancies reported in this study were breast, hematologic, gastrointestinal, and gynecologic [145].

Table 1.2 Rheumatic diseases and associated malignancies

Rheumatic disease	Associated malignancy
SLE	Hematologic malignancies particularly NHL Non-hematologic malignancies: vulva, lung, liver, and thyroid cancer
RA	Hematologic malignancies particularly Hodgkin lymphoma Non-hematologic malignancies: lung and possibly liver and esophageal cancer
SSc	Lung, hematologic, esophageal, and oropharyngeal cancers
Inflammatory myopathies	Ovarian, lung, gastric lymphoma Nasopharyngeal carcinoma in Asian populations
Primary SS	Lymphoproliferative disorders particularly MALT lymphoma

SLE systemic lupus erythematosus, *RA* rheumatoid arthritis, *SSc* systemic sclerosis, *SS* Sjögren's syndrome, *NHL* non-Hodgkin's lymphoma, *MALT* mucosa-associated lymphoid tissue

Malignancy and Inflammatory Myopathies

A linkage between polymyositis (PM) and cancer was first reported in 1916. Since then, several studies have identified this association in both PM and dermatomyositis (DM) [146–148]. A higher incidence of cancer was identified with DM compared with PM [149, 150]. In contrary to the increased risk of malignancy with time in other connective tissue diseases, the risk of malignancy has been found to diminish with time in inflammatory myopathies [151]. Malignancy occurrence has been reported after the diagnosis of PM, whereas it can precede or follow the diagnosis of DM, which leads many to consider DM to be a paraneoplastic syndrome [150].

Given this increased risk of malignancy in DM and PM, many recommend evaluating newly diagnosed patients with DM and PM for the possibility of an underlying malignancy. Some further recommend extensive search for malignancy, particularly with computed tomographic scans, to identify an elusive cancer [152].

Malignancy and Sjögren's Syndrome

It is known that primary SS (pSS) is associated with increased risk of lymphoproliferative disorder. This association was first published in the late 1970s and according to that study, patients with pSS have 40 times higher relative risk of developing lymphoma, particularly NHL, compared to the general population [127]. Subsequent studies published since then have described this association with a relative risk of lymphoma in pSS compared with the general population ranging between 6 and 44 [125]. There is some discrepancy regarding the most common NHL among pSS. Whereas most studies ranked mucosa-associated lymphoid tissue lymphoma (MALTL), a subtype of indolent marginal zone B-cell lymphoma (MZBCL), as the most predominant lymphoma among pSS [153, 154] and high-grade diffuse large

B-cell lymphoma (DLBCL) as the second most common lymphoma subtype of pSS-associated NHL [155, 156], DLBCL was found the most common pSS-associated NHL in others [157, 158]. This discrepancy could be a result of genetic and geographical variations of the recruited patients. The occurrence of MALTL in younger pSS patients compared with the occurrence of DLBCL suggests that DLBCL emerges as an event of gradual transformation from undetected low-grade lymphomas [158].

DMARDs and Malignancy

Both non-biologic and biologic DMARDs have been commonly used in patients with rheumatic diseases. The oncogenic effects of immunosuppression lead many to assess the risk of malignancy associated with the use of both non-biologic and biologic agents in patients with rheumatic diseases. However, the increased risk of malignancies in patients with rheumatic disease and the intensive use of DMARDs in patients with advanced diseases who might already have a higher risk of developing cancer complicated and challenged this assessment [125].

Increased risk of malignancies with cyclophosphamide (CYC) has been reported. Bladder cancer is one of those malignancies and it is thought to be due to CYC metabolites especially acrolein [159]. A higher risk of lymphoma was also suggested in SLE patients treated with CYC and high cumulative dose steroids [160]. Increased incidence of cervical intraepithelial neoplasia in women with SLE treated with intravenous cyclophosphamide and steroid was also reported [161].

Increased risk of lymphoproliferative disorders in patients with rheumatic diseases treated with MTX has been suggested in many reports [162–165]. This increased risk has been especially observed in EBV-positive patients and was further suggested by the remission of lymphoma after stopping MTX therapy [166, 167]. Increased risk of a second non-melanoma skin cancer (NMSC) in RA patients treated with MTX has also been suggested in a retrospective cohort study published in 2016 [168].

With the increased use of TNF-α inhibitors in rheumatic diseases, their associated risk factors such as the possible increased risk of malignancy has been increasingly studied. Suggested data varies among those studies with few studies reporting higher incidence [169, 170] and many finding no association between malignancy and TNF- α inhibitor use [171–175]. Several studies have shown association of melanoma and non-melanoma skin cancer (NMSC) with TNF-α inhibitor use [176–178].

Risk of malignancy has been compared between DMARDs and biologic agents in few studies [179–181]. Based on some of the previous studies [165, 172, 174, 176], ACR published 2015 guidelines for the treatment of RA patients with a past history of treated or untreated malignancy although the level of evidence was considered very low [119]. They conditionally recommended the use of traditional DMARDs over biologics and tofacitinib in patients with previously treated or untreated skin cancer (melanoma or non-melanoma). They also recommended for previously treated lymphoproliferative disorders the use of rituximab over TNF-α inhibitors and combination of traditional DMARDs or abatacept or tocilizumab over TNF-α inhibitors in such patients. For patients with previously treated solid organ malignancy, the conditional recommendation is the same as in patients without history of malignancy. Given low-level evidence and conditional recommendations, further studies might be required to better assess the risk of malignancy associated with the use of TNF-α inhibitors especially for long-term use.

Rheumatic Disease and Osteoporosis

Increased risk of osteoporosis in patients with RA has been reported in many studies [182–185]. This increased risk is attributed to the use of glucocorticoid [182, 184–186] in addition to the disease activity itself including the production of pro-inflammatory cytokines mainly TNF-α, interleukin-1 (IL-1), IL-6, and IL-17, given their role in osteoclast dysfunction and bone homeostasis [187–191].

In addition to blocking local and systemic inflammatory cascades in rheumatic diseases, biologic treatment has also been reported to provide beneficial effects against bone degradation and the development of osteoporosis [189, 192–194].

The ACR 2010 guidelines for prevention and treatment of glucocorticoid-induced osteoporosis (GIOP) elaborate on the risk of developing GIOP, based on FRAX scores, the glucocorticoid dosage, and duration of use [195].

Insulin Resistance and Rheumatic Diseases

The association between RA and insulin resistance (IR) has been reported in many studies [196–200]. This association is attributed to an overlapping pathophysiology of IR and RA, as both are characterized by inflammation. The inflammation in RA is mainly mediated by pro-inflammatory cytokines, TNF-α, and IL-6 which are also found to be overproduced in visceral adipose tissue in patients with IR and lead to impaired insulin receptor signaling [201–203].

IR has been well reported in several RA studies; however, data regarding the association between other rheumatic diseases and diabetes is still controversial, as this association was found in some studies [204–206], though not in others [53, 54].

Glucocorticoids are widely used in rheumatic diseases. Although cumulative glucocorticoids dose was shown to have a negative impact on glucose tolerance state, its role in inducing IR in patients with rheumatic diseases is controversial. Data from many studies consider the use of glucocorticoids, especially long-term use or at high doses, to play a role in inducing IR [207, 208]; however, most data consider the use of low doses [209] and some studies low to medium doses of glucocorticoids not to be associated with glucose metabolism impairment in RA patients as metabolic syndrome is already modified by other processes in RA [210–212]. The use of low doses glucocorticoids might also improve glycemic control through enhanced pancreatic insulin secretion and peripheral insulin sensitivity by its anti-inflammatory effects [201]. Some data suggest that the use of even high dose but for short term is not associated with the deterioration of glucose tolerance [213].

Data from different studies suggests favorable changes in measures of insulin sensitivity with the use of traditional DMARDs [214], such as MTX [215, 216] and hydroxychloroquine [217], mainly by their anti-inflammatory effects. However, the effects of DMARDs on IR might require long-term use as some data suggests no changes in IR with short-term treatment [218]. No clear-cut impact of TNF-α inhibitors on IR has been identified [219–224].

Interstitial Lung Diseases in Rheumatic Diseases

Interstitial lung disease (ILD) represents a diverse group of lung diseases that occur as a frequent and a serious complication associated with significant mortality and morbidity in patients with rheumatic diseases. ILD associated with rheumatic diseases occur commonly in SSc with an incidence of about 45%, followed by PM/DM (20–50%), mixed connective tissue disease (20–60%), RA (20–30%), and less frequently in SS (up to 25%) and SLE (2–8%) [225]. About 25% of all ILD-related deaths are associated with underlying rheumatic diseases [226]. The underlying pathogenesis of ILD is incompletely understood and involves inflammation, fibrosis, or a combination of both under the influence of several pro-inflammatory and pro-fibrotic cytokines [227, 228]. The most common types of ILD associated with rheumatic diseases are non-specific interstitial pneumonia (NSIP) and usual interstitial pneumonia (UIP) followed by lymphocytic interstitial pneumonia (LIP), cryptogenic organizing pneumonia (COP), and less frequently diffuse alveolar damage (DAD) [229]. The distinct histopathological and radiologic patterns in high-resolution computed tomography (HRCT) associated with each type of ILD are highlighted in Table 1.3. Understanding these features is important for diagnosis as well as to predict prognosis among the various types of ILD.

Clinically, ILD manifests as insidious onset and non-specific symptoms such as progressive dyspnea and dry cough. Bronchoalveolar lavage (BAL) can be helpful to rule out infection or malignancy in suspected cases [234]. When the combination of HRCT findings with other investigations does not help in establishing a diagnosis, a lung biopsy is done through bronchoscopy or video-assisted thoracic surgery (VATS). By identifying the specific type of ILD, lung biopsy helps to predict the prognosis and guide treatment [235].

ILD associated with rheumatic diseases are treated with immunosuppressive drugs such as cyclophosphamide, azathioprine, tacrolimus, and mycophenolate mofetil. The Scleroderma Lung Study (SLS) I showed that 1 year of oral cyclophosphamide was effective in improving lung function, dyspnea, and quality of life but

Table 1.3 Rheumatic diseases and associated ILD types

Rheumatic disease	Type of ILD	Histopathologic findings [230]	HRCT findings [225]	Comments
SSc	NSIP	NSIP: uniform appearance with varying proportion of inflammation and fibrosis	Ground glass opacities and reticular markings prominently in the lung bases	ILD is the leading cause of death in SSc patients [225]
PM and DM	NSIP COP is less common	NSIP: as above COP: interstitium has less inflammation and alveolar ducts have inflammatory debris	NSIP: as above COP: ground glass opacities with patchy areas of consolidation	ILD in myositis patients has a strong association with anti-Jo-1 antibodies [225]
MCTD	NSIP	NSIP: as above	NSIP: as above Septal thickening may be seen.	PAH is the most common cause of death [231]
RA	UIP	UIP: patches of marked fibrosis in subplural areas and honeycombing with less inflammation in the interstitium	Overlapping reticular and nodular opacities with honeycombing pattern in the periphery and basilar areas	The 5 year survival rate in RA patients with UIP is less than 50% [225]
Sjögren's syndrome	Most common ILD is NSIP followed by LIP	NSIP: as above	NSIP: as above LIP: cystic pattern with ground glass opacities and nodules mostly in the centrilobular areas	LIP can also be seen in abnormal immune system states such as HIV, dysproteinemia and CVID [232]
SLE	Most common ILD is NSIP. DAD is less common and is seen usually in the setting of acute lupus pneumonitis	DAD: edema with Interstitial inflammation and intra-alveolar hyaline membrane formation [226]	Diffuse ground glass opacities in DAD	ILD presenting as the initial feature of SLE is very rare [233]

ILD interstitial lung disease, *RA* rheumatoid arthritis, *SSc* systemic sclerosis, *SS* Sjögren's syndrome, *SLE* systemic lupus erythematosus, *MCTD* mixed connective tissue disease, *DAH* diffuse alveolar hemorrhage, *NSIP* non-specific interstitial pneumonia, *UIP* usual interstitial pneumonia, *LIP* lymphocytic interstitial pneumonia, *COP* cryptogenic organizing pneumonia, *HIV* human immunodeficiency virus, *CVID* common variable immunodeficiency, *DAD* diffuse alveolar damage with the effects lasting only for 6 months after the drug was stopped [236]. A retrospective study involving a large number of patients with rheumatic disease-associated ILD demonstrated that mycophenolate mofetil is well tolerated with low rate of discontinuation when used either as a second- or third-line steroid-sparing drug in the setting where cyclophosphamide and azathioprine are discontinued because of increased toxicity [88]. There is limited data to suggest the utility of rituximab in the treatment of refractory ILD [237]. Lung transplantation is a treatment option for SSc patients with ILD who fail to respond to immunosuppressive therapy [238].

In general, ILD associated with rheumatic diseases has a more favorable prognosis compared to idiopathic ILD [239]. It is therefore important to evaluate for the presence of an underlying rheumatic disease in all patients with ILD. Among the various types of ILD associated with rheumatic diseases, UIP carries the worst prognosis compared to those with NSIP [240]. A multidisciplinary approach involving a pulmonologist, rheumatologist, pathologist, and radiologist and close monitoring with lung function tests and imaging is required [241].

Anemia in Rheumatic Diseases

Anemia is a frequent comorbidity in patients with systemic rheumatic diseases and is associated with a negative impact on the overall functional status and quality of life of the patients [242]. The etiology of anemia in patients with rheumatic diseases is often multifactorial and commonly related to immune dysregulation leading to alteration in the iron homeostasis [242, 243]. Data suggests that about 50% of RA patients have anemia and the most common type is anemia of chronic disease (ACD) followed by iron deficiency anemia (IDA) [244].

ACD also known as anemia of inflammation occurs in chronic inflammatory disease conditions. The pathophysiology of ACD is complex and incompletely understood. However, it is believed to be mostly immune mediated resulting in iron trapping in the reticuloendothelial system leading to impaired erythropoiesis, blunted erythropoietin response, and reduced red cell survival [245]. Several inflammatory cytokines, particularly TNF- α, IL-1, IL-6, IL-10, interferon gamma and hepcidin (which is an acute phase reactant) play a role in the pathogenesis of ACD [245–247]. The results from a longitudinal study involving 225 RA patients showed that among the 144 patients (64%) who had anemia, 88 patients (77%) had ACD, making it the most frequent cause of anemia in RA [248]. ACD in patients with rheumatic diseases is usually mild, normocytic, and normochromic. Diagnosis of type of anemia is usually by mean corpuscular volume (MCV), plasma iron, total iron-binding capacity, transferrin saturation, transferrin, ferritin, and bone marrow exam (not necessary for diagnosis).

IDA in rheumatic diseases is often caused by chronic blood loss from gastritis or peptic ulcer disease secondary to concomitant use of NSAID, glucocorticoid, and/or aspirin [249–251]. The risk of upper gastrointestinal (UGI) tract bleeding or perforation increases around twofold with the use of oral steroids or low-dose aspirin and increases around fourfold with the use of NSAIDs. However, the risk appears to be more than eightfold higher for concomitant users of both steroids and NSAIDs or aspirin, compared with nonusers of either drug [251]. Iron deficiency anemia can also be seen in associated conditions like inflammatory bowel disease [252] or autoimmune gastritis, celiac disease, or *Helicobacter pylori* infection, all of which can cause decreased iron absorption [253]. Patients with SSc can also develop iron deficiency anemia from chronic UGI bleed secondary to a condition called gastric antral vascular ectasia (GAVE) [254].

Less frequently, megaloblastic anemia can be seen in patients with rheumatic diseases due to deficiency of vitamin B12, folic acid, or secondary to the use of MTX or sulfasalazine [255]. Hemolytic anemia which is a complement-/antibody-mediated destruction of red cells is seen in about 10% SLE patients [256] and in Felty's syndrome (a combination of RA, splenomegaly, and neutropenia) [257]. In patients with adult onset Still's disease, systemic onset juvenile idiopathic arthritis, and SLE, anemia can be caused by hemophagocytic syndrome, a condition that involves widespread activation of macrophages by T-cell-derived cytokines, leading to uncontrolled phagocytosis of red cells by macrophages [258]. Immunosuppressive drugs (such as azathioprine, MTX, mycophenolic acid) can cause anemia in rheumatic disease patients by various mechanisms including suppression of erythropoiesis, reduction of erythrocyte life span, and reactivation of chronic latent infections (such as HBV, HCV, HIV, parvovirus B19, mycobacteria, or intestinal helminths) which in turn can lead to bone marrow suppression, hemolysis, or intestinal bleeding [242].

The management of ACD in inflammatory rheumatic disease patients involves treatment of the underlying disease which often results in improvement of the anemia [259]. Management of IDA involves iron supplementation and treatment of the underlying cause [260, 261]. In patients requiring NSAID treatment, the American College of Gastroenterology (ACG) recommends using alternative therapy or selective COX-2 inhibitors with a proton pump inhibitor depending on the risk for NSAID-related GI complications [262].

Comorbidity Pattern, Effect on Outcomes, and Recommendations for Clinical Practice

Rheumatic diseases are often associated with comorbidities that significantly worsen the prognosis of the primary disease, effectiveness of the treatment, quality of life, frequency of hospitalization, medical costs, and the risk for mortality [263]. While new emerging therapies enable tighter control of disease activity, they are accompanied by potential risk of toxicity especially in an aging rheumatic disease population given the absence of long-term experience and safety data. Patients with higher number of comorbidities are less likely to respond to treatment and often have poor outcomes [264]. A large study by Wolfe et al. involving 11,704 patients with rheumatic diseases showed variations in the pattern comorbidities among rheumatic disease [265]. The study results showed that comorbidities were most common among patients with fibromyalgia followed by patients with SLE compared to RA and non-inflammatory rheumatic disorders. Among the SLE patients, the most frequent comorbidities were hypertension, cataract, depression, CVD, fractures, neurologic, lung, gall bladder, and endocrine disorders. In addition to these findings, the investigators also noticed four major patterns of comorbidities which are (1) those related to aging process, (2) those related to aging but worsened by the presence of the underlying primary rheumatic condition (e.g., CVD would be related to aging but enhanced by the presence of SLE or RA), (3) those being a part of the spectrum of the symptoms related to the primary rheumatic disease, and (4) those that represent life-long characteristics of the underlying disease.

The lack of clear evidence adds to the complexity of managing high-risk comorbidities like malignancy, heart failure, and infection, as these patients are often times excluded from randomized control trials. ACR and EULAR update their recommendations for management of rheumatic diseases every few years taking into account newly accrued evidence. The guidelines mentioned previously in this chapter are developed by expert rheumatologists utilizing advanced guideline development methodologies and after systematically reviewing the literature – they are valuable tools of reference while managing comorbidities in complex rheumatic diseases.

The logical method to address comorbidities would be by raising awareness among providers and patients, regular screening, tight control of rheumatic disease activity while bearing in mind the risks and benefits of treatment choices, and close collaboration between multiple disciplines including the rheumatologist, primary care physicians, and other specialists. Working in partnership with healthcare providers such as nurses and extenders has also shown to facilitate identification of and timely intervention of comorbidities among rheumatic disease patients. Longitudinal data by cohort studies and surveillance registries would also help gain further insight into comorbidities. Subsequent chapters will elaborate on these and other related topics in detail.

References

1. Charlson ME, et al. A new method of classifying prognostic comorbidity in longitudinal studies: development and validation. J Chronic Dis. 1987;40(5):373–83.
2. Wolfe F, et al. The mortality of rheumatoid arthritis. Arthritis Rheum. 1994;37(4):481–94.
3. Urowitz MB, et al. The bimodal mortality pattern of systemic lupus erythematosus. Am J Med. 1976;60(2):221–5.
4. Aviña-Zubieta JA, et al. Risk of cardiovascular mortality in patients with rheumatoid arthritis: a meta-analysis of observational studies. Arthritis Care Res. 2008;59(12):1690–7.
5. Maradit-Kremers H, et al. Increased unrecognized coronary heart disease and sudden deaths in rheumatoid arthritis: a population-based cohort study. Arthritis Rheum. 2005;52(2):402–11.

6. Krishnan E, Lingala VB, Singh G. Declines in mortality from acute myocardial infarction in successive incidence and birth cohorts of patients with rheumatoid arthritis. Circulation. 2004;110(13):1774–9.
7. Gonzalez A, et al. The widening mortality gap between rheumatoid arthritis patients and the general population. Arthritis Rheum. 2007;56(11):3583–7.
8. Manzi S, et al. Age-specific incidence rates of myocardial infarction and angina in women with systemic lupus erythematosus: comparison with the Framingham study. Am J Epidemiol. 1997;145(5):408–15.
9. Mok CC, et al. Incidence and risk factors of thromboembolism in systemic lupus erythematosus: a comparison of three ethnic groups. Arthritis Rheum. 2005;52(9):2774–82.
10. Cohen Tervaert J. Translational mini-review series on immunology of vascular disease: accelerated atherosclerosis in vasculitis. Clin Exp Immunol. 2009;156(3):377–85.
11. Tervaert JWC. Cardiovascular disease due to accelerated atherosclerosis in systemic vasculitides. Best Pract Res Clin Rheumatol. 2013;27(1):33–44.
12. Ogdie A, et al. Risk of major cardiovascular events in patients with psoriatic arthritis, psoriasis and rheumatoid arthritis: a population-based cohort study. Ann Rheum Dis. 2014; annrheumdis-2014-205675.
13. Peters MJ, et al. Cardiovascular risk profile of patients with spondylarthropathies, particularly ankylosing spondylitis and psoriatic arthritis. Semin Arthritis Rheum. 2004;34:585–92.
14. Nussinovitch U, Shoenfeld Y. Atherosclerosis and macrovascular involvement in systemic sclerosis: myth or reality. Autoimmun Rev. 2011;10(5):259–66.
15. Papagoras C, Voulgari P, Drosos A. Atherosclerosis and cardiovascular disease in the spondyloarthritides, particularly ankylosing spondylitis and psoriatic arthritis. Clin Exp Rheumatol. 2012;31(4):612–20.
16. Nicola PJ, et al. The risk of congestive heart failure in rheumatoid arthritis: a population-based study over 46 years. Arthritis Rheum. 2005;52(2):412–20.
17. Davis JM, et al. The presentation and outcome of heart failure in patients with rheumatoid arthritis differs from that in the general population. Arthritis Rheum. 2008;58(9):2603–11.
18. Robinson PC, et al. Hospital admissions associated with gout and their co-morbidities in New Zealand and England 1999–2009. Rheumatology. 2012; kes253.
19. Kuo C-F, et al. Risk of myocardial infarction among patients with gout: a nationwide population-based study. Rheumatology. 2013;52(1):111–7.
20. Winyard PG, et al. Presence of foam cells containing oxidised low density lipoprotein in the synovial membrane from patients with rheumatoid arthritis. Ann Rheum Dis. 1993;52(9):677–80.
21. Pasceri V, Yeh ET. A tale of two diseases atherosclerosis and rheumatoid arthritis. Circulation. 1999;100(21):2124–6.
22. Koenig W, Khuseyinova N. Biomarkers of atherosclerotic plaque instability and rupture. Arterioscler Thromb Vasc Biol. 2007;27(1):15–26.
23. Bacon P, Townend J. Nails in the coffin: increasing evidence for the role of rheumatic disease in the cardiovascular mortality of rheumatoid arthritis. Arthritis Rheum. 2001;44(12):2707–10.
24. Hollan I, et al. Inflammatory rheumatic disease and smoking are predictors of aortic inflammation: a controlled study of biopsy specimens obtained at coronary artery surgery. Arthritis Rheum. 2007;56(6):2072–9.
25. Sgonc R, et al. Endothelial cell apoptosis is a primary pathogenetic event underlying skin lesions in avian and human scleroderma. J Clin Investig. 1996;98(3):785.
26. Van Paassen P, et al. Induction of endothelial cell apoptosis by IgG antibodies from SLE patients with nephropathy. Ann N Y Acad Sci. 2007;1108(1):147–56.
27. Peters MJ, et al. Does rheumatoid arthritis equal diabetes mellitus as an independent risk factor for cardiovascular disease? A prospective study. Arthritis Care Res. 2009;61(11):1571–9.
28. Boyer J-F, et al. Traditional cardiovascular risk factors in rheumatoid arthritis: a meta-analysis. Joint Bone Spine. 2011;78(2):179–83.

29. Masdottir B, et al. Smoking, rheumatoid factor isotypes and severity of rheumatoid arthritis. Rheumatology. 2000;39(11):1202–5.
30. Saevarsdottir S, et al. Patients with early rheumatoid arthritis who smoke are less likely to respond to treatment with methotrexate and tumor necrosis factor inhibitors: observations from the epidemiological investigation of rheumatoid arthritis and the Swedish rheumatology register cohorts. Arthritis Rheum. 2011;63(1):26–36.
31. Van Halm V, et al. Rheumatoid arthritis versus diabetes as a risk factor for cardiovascular disease: a cross-sectional study, the CARRE investigation. Ann Rheum Dis. 2009;68(9):1395–400.
32. Bruce IN, et al. Risk factors for coronary heart disease in women with systemic lupus erythematosus: the Toronto risk factor study. Arthritis Rheum. 2003;48(11):3159–67.
33. Steiner G, Urowitz MB. Lipid profiles in patients with rheumatoid arthritis: mechanisms and the impact of treatment. Semin Arthritis Rheum. 2009;38:372–81.
34. Myasoedova E, et al. Lipid paradox in rheumatoid arthritis: the impact of serum lipid measures and systemic inflammation on the risk of cardiovascular disease. Ann Rheum Dis. 2011;70(3):482–7.
35. Sada K-E, et al. Altered levels of adipocytokines in association with insulin resistance in patients with systemic lupus erythematosus. J Rheumatol. 2006;33(8):1545–52.
36. Chung CP, et al. Inflammation-associated insulin resistance: differential effects in rheumatoid arthritis and systemic lupus erythematosus define potential mechanisms. Arthritis Rheum. 2008;58(7):2105–12.
37. Dessein PH, Joffe BI. Insulin resistance and impaired beta cell function in rheumatoid arthritis. Arthritis Rheum. 2006;54(9):2765–75.
38. Kremers HM, et al. Prognostic importance of low body mass index in relation to cardiovascular mortality in rheumatoid arthritis. Arthritis Rheum. 2004;50(11):3450–7.
39. Bolten WW. Problem of the atherothrombotic potential of non-steroidal anti-inflammatory drugs. Ann Rheum Dis. 2006;65(1):7–13.
40. Panoulas VF, et al. Long-term exposure to medium-dose glucocorticoid therapy associates with hypertension in patients with rheumatoid arthritis. Rheumatology. 2008;47(1):72–5.
41. Wei L, MacDonald TM, Walker BR. Taking glucocorticoids by prescription is associated with subsequent cardiovascular disease. Ann Intern Med. 2004;141(10):764–70.
42. Solomon DH, et al. Immunosuppressive medications and hospitalization for cardiovascular events in patients with rheumatoid arthritis. Arthritis Rheum. 2006;54(12):3790–8.
43. del Rincón I, et al. Association between carotid atherosclerosis and markers of inflammation in rheumatoid arthritis patients and healthy subjects. Arthritis Rheum. 2003;48(7):1833–40.
44. Libby P, Crea F. Clinical implications of inflammation for cardiovascular primary prevention. Eur Heart J. 2010;31(7):777–83.
45. Arts EE, et al. The effect of disease duration and disease activity on the risk of cardiovascular disease in rheumatoid arthritis patients. Ann Rheum Dis. 2014; annrheumdis-2013-204531.
46. Solomon DH, et al. Disease activity in rheumatoid arthritis and the risk of cardiovascular events. Arthritis Rheum. 2015;67(6):1449–55.
47. Barnabe C, Martin BJ, Ghali WA. Systematic review and meta-analysis: anti–tumor necrosis factor α therapy and cardiovascular events in rheumatoid arthritis. Arthritis Care Res. 2011;63(4):522–9.
48. Micha R, et al. Systematic review and meta-analysis of methotrexate use and risk of cardiovascular disease. Am J Cardiol. 2011;108(9):1362–70.
49. Urowitz M, et al. Atherosclerotic vascular events in a multinational inception cohort of systemic lupus erythematosus. Arthritis Care Res. 2010;62(6):881–7.
50. Urowitz MB, Ibañez D, Gladman DD. Atherosclerotic vascular events in a single large lupus cohort: prevalence and risk factors. J Rheumatol. 2007;34(1):70–5.
51. Petri M, et al. Risk factors for coronary artery disease in patients with systemic lupus erythematosus. Am J Med. 1992;93(5):513–9.

52. Fischer LM, et al. Effect of rheumatoid arthritis or systemic lupus erythematosus on the risk of first-time acute myocardial infarction. Am J Cardiol. 2004;93(2):198–200.
53. Simard JF, Mittleman MA. Prevalent rheumatoid arthritis and diabetes among NHANES III participants aged 60 and older. J Rheumatol. 2007;34(3):469–73.
54. Solomon DH, et al. Cardiovascular risk factors in women with and without rheumatoid arthritis. Arthritis Rheum. 2004;50(11):3444–9.
55. Dessein PH, et al. Independent role of conventional cardiovascular risk factors as predictors of C-reactive protein concentrations in rheumatoid arthritis. J Rheumatol. 2007;34(4):681–8.
56. Group EIS, Wilson PW, D'Agostino RB, Levy D, Belanger AM, Silbershatz H, Kannel WB. Prediction of coronary heart disease using risk factor categories. Circulation. 1998;97:1837–47.
57. D'Agostino RB, et al. General cardiovascular risk profile for use in primary care the Framingham heart study. Circulation. 2008;117(6):743–53.
58. Peters M, et al. EULAR evidence-based recommendations for cardiovascular risk management in patients with rheumatoid arthritis and other forms of inflammatory arthritis. Ann Rheum Dis. 2010;69(2):325–31.
59. Conroy R, et al. Estimation of ten-year risk of fatal cardiovascular disease in Europe: the SCORE project. Eur Heart J. 2003;24(11):987–1003.
60. Dessein PH, et al. Traditional and nontraditional cardiovascular risk factors are associated with atherosclerosis in rheumatoid arthritis. J Rheumatol. 2005;32(3):435–42.
61. Eder L, Chandran V, Gladman DD, The Framingham risk score underestimates the extent of subclinical atherosclerosis in patients with psoriatic disease. Ann Rheum Dis. 2013; annrheumdis-2013-203433.
62. Myasoedova E, Gabriel SE. Cardiovascular disease in rheumatoid arthritis: a step forward. Curr Opin Rheumatol. 2010;22(3):342–7.
63. Choi HK, et al. Methotrexate and mortality in patients with rheumatoid arthritis: a prospective study. Lancet. 2002;359(9313):1173–7.
64. Jacobsson LT, et al. Treatment with tumor necrosis factor blockers is associated with a lower incidence of first cardiovascular events in patients with rheumatoid arthritis. J Rheumatol. 2005;32(7):1213–8.
65. Carmona L, et al. All-cause and cause-specific mortality in rheumatoid arthritis are not greater than expected when treated with tumour necrosis factor antagonists. Ann Rheum Dis. 2007;66(7):880–5.
66. Dixon W, et al. Reduction in the incidence of myocardial infarction in patients with rheumatoid arthritis who respond to anti–tumor necrosis factor α therapy: results from the British society for rheumatology biologics register. Arthritis Rheum. 2007;56(9):2905–12.
67. Naranjo A, et al. Cardiovascular disease in patients with rheumatoid arthritis: results from the QUEST-RA study. Arthritis Res Ther. 2008;10(2):1.
68. Symmons D, et al. Longterm mortality outcome in patients with rheumatoid arthritis: early presenters continue to do well. J Rheumatol. 1998;25(6):1072–7.
69. van Halm VP, et al. Disease-modifying antirheumatic drugs are associated with a reduced risk for cardiovascular disease in patients with rheumatoid arthritis: a case control study. Arthritis Res Ther. 2006;8(5):1.
70. Smolen JS, et al. Treating rheumatoid arthritis to target: recommendations of an international task force. Ann Rheum Dis. 2010;69(4):631–7.
71. Sharma TS, et al. Hydroxychloroquine use is associated with decreased incident cardiovascular events in rheumatoid arthritis patients. J Am Heart Assoc. 2016;5(1):e002867.
72. Sharma TS, Joyce E, Wasko MCM. Anti-malarials: are there benefits beyond mild disease? Curr Treatm Opt Rheumatol. 2016;2(1):1–12.
73. Segal BH, Sneller MC. Infectious complications of immunosuppressive therapy in patients with rheumatic diseases. Rheum Dis Clin N Am. 1997;23(2):219–37.
74. Atzeni F, et al. Infections and treatment of patients with rheumatic diseases. Clin Exp Rheumatol. 2008;26(1 Suppl 48):S67–73.

75. Bernatsky S, Hudson M, Suissa S. Anti-rheumatic drug use and risk of serious infections in rheumatoid arthritis. Rheumatology (Oxford). 2007;46(7):1157–60.
76. Doran MF, et al. Predictors of infection in rheumatoid arthritis. Arthritis Rheum. 2002;46(9):2294–300.
77. McLean-Tooke A, et al. Methotrexate, rheumatoid arthritis and infection risk: what is the evidence? Rheumatology (Oxford). 2009;48(8):867–71.
78. Curtis JR, et al. Risk of serious bacterial infections among rheumatoid arthritis patients exposed to tumor necrosis factor alpha antagonists. Arthritis Rheum. 2007;56(4):1125–33.
79. Salliot C, et al. Infections during tumour necrosis factor-α blocker therapy for rheumatic diseases in daily practice: a systematic retrospective study of 709 patients. Rheumatology. 2007;46(2):327–34.
80. Kourbeti IS, Ziakas PD, Mylonakis E. Biologic therapies in rheumatoid arthritis and the risk of opportunistic infections: a meta-analysis. Clin Infect Dis. 2014;58(12):1649–57.
81. Zamora-Legoff JA, et al. Risk of serious infection in patients with rheumatoid arthritis-associated interstitial lung disease. Clin Rheumatol. 2016;29:1–5.
82. Cervera R, et al. Morbidity and mortality in systemic lupus erythematosus during a 10-year period a comparison of early and late manifestations in a cohort of 1,000 patients. Mortality. 2003;82(5):299–308.
83. Bosch X, et al. Infections in systemic lupus erythematosus: a prospective and controlled study of 110 patients. Lupus. 2006;15(9):584–9.
84. Ruiz-Irastorza G, et al. Predictors of major infections in systemic lupus erythematosus. Arthritis Res Ther. 2009;11(4):R109.
85. Doran MF, Crowson CS, Pond GR, O'Fallon WM, Gabriel SE. Frequency of infection in patients with rheumatoid arthritis compared with controls: a population-based study. Arthritis Rheum. 2002;46(9):2287–93.
86. Coyne P, et al. Acute lower respiratory tract infections in patients with rheumatoid arthritis. J Rheumatol. 2007;34(9):1832–6.
87. Wolfe F, Caplan L, Michaud K. Treatment for rheumatoid arthritis and the risk of hospitalization for pneumonia: associations with prednisone, disease-modifying antirheumatic drugs, and anti-tumor necrosis factor therapy. Arthritis Rheum. 2006;54(2):628–34.
88. Fischer A, et al. Mycophenolate mofetil improves lung function in connective tissue disease-associated interstitial lung disease. J Rheumatol. 2013;40(5):640–6.
89. Carmona L, et al. Increased risk of tuberculosis in patients with rheumatoid arthritis. J Rheumatol. 2003;30(7):1436–9.
90. Wajant H, Pfizenmaier K, Scheurich P. Tumor necrosis factor signaling. Cell Death Differ. 2003;10(1):45–65.
91. Winthrop KL, et al. Tuberculosis associated with therapy against tumor necrosis factor α. Arthritis Rheum. 2005;52(10):2968–74.
92. Gómez-Reino JJ, et al. Treatment of rheumatoid arthritis with tumor necrosis factor inhibitors may predispose to significant increase in tuberculosis risk: a multicenter active-surveillance report. Arthritis Rheum. 2003;48(8):2122–7.
93. Harris J, Keane J. How tumour necrosis factor blockers interfere with tuberculosis immunity. Clin Exp Immunol. 2010;161:1–9.
94. Dixon WG, et al. Drug-specific risk of tuberculosis in patients with rheumatoid arthritis treated with anti-TNF therapy: results from the British society for rheumatology biologics register (BSRBR). Ann Rheum Dis. 2010;69(3):522–8.
95. Gladman DD, et al. The nature and outcome of infection in systemic lupus erythematosus. Lupus. 2002;11(4):234–9.
96. Kinder BW, et al. Clinical and genetic risk factors for pneumonia in systemic lupus erythematosus. Arthritis Rheum. 2007;56(8):2679–86.
97. Lee HH, et al. Cutaneous side-effects in patients with rheumatic diseases during application of tumour necrosis factor-alpha antagonists. Br J Dermatol. 2007;156(3):486–91.

98. Dixon WG, et al. Rates of serious infection, including site-specific and bacterial intracellular infection, in rheumatoid arthritis patients receiving anti-tumor necrosis factor therapy: results from the British society for rheumatology biologics register. Arthritis Rheum. 2006;54(8):2368–76.
99. Flendrie M, et al. Dermatological conditions during TNF-alpha-blocking therapy in patients with rheumatoid arthritis: a prospective study. Arthritis Res Ther. 2005;7(3):R666–76.
100. Veetil BMA, et al. Incidence and time trends of herpes zoster in rheumatoid arthritis: a population-based cohort study. Arthritis Care Res. 2013;65(6):854–61.
101. Al S, et al. The risk of herpes zoster in patients with rheumatoid arthritis in the united. Arthritis Rheum. 2007;57:1431–8.
102. Segan J, et al. Risk factors for herpes zoster in rheumatoid arthritis patients: the role of tumor necrosis factor alpha inhibitors. Intern Med J. 2015 Mar;45(3):310–8.
103. Strangfeld A, et al. Risk of herpes zoster in patients with rheumatoid arthritis treated with anti-TNF-alpha agents. JAMA. 2009;301(7):737–44.
104. Winthrop KL, et al. Association between the initiation of anti-tumor necrosis factor therapy and the risk of herpes zoster. JAMA. 2013;309(9):887–95.
105. Gilson M, et al. Risk factors for total joint arthroplasty infection in patients receiving tumor necrosis factor α-blockers: a case-control study. Arthritis Res Ther. 2010;12(4):R145.
106. Puntis D, et al. Urinary tract infections in patients with rheumatoid arthritis. Clin Rheumatol. 2013;32(3):355–60.
107. Tishler M, et al. Increased incidence of urinary tract infection in patients with rheumatoid arthritis and secondary Sjögren's syndrome. Ann Rheum Dis. 1992;51(5):604–6.
108. Vassilopoulos D, Calabrese LH. Management of rheumatic disease with comorbid HBV or HCV infection. Nat Rev Rheumatol. 2012;8(6):348–57.
109. Xuan D, et al. Hepatitis reactivation in patients with rheumatic diseases after immunosuppressive therapy – a report of long-term follow-up of serial cases and literature review. Clin Rheumatol. 2014;33:577–86.
110. Kim YJ, et al. Possible reactivation of potential hepatitis B virus occult infection by tumor necrosis factor-α blocker in the treatment of rheumatic diseases. J Rheumatol. 2010;37(2):346–50.
111. Calabrese LH, Zein NN, Vassilopoulos D. Hepatitis B virus (HBV) reactivation with immunosuppressive therapy in rheumatic diseases: assessment and preventive strategies. Ann Rheum Dis. 2006;65(8):983–9.
112. Lacaille D, et al. Use of nonbiologic disease-modifying antirheumatic drugs and risk of infection in patients with rheumatoid arthritis. Arthritis Rheum. 2008;59(8):1074–81.
113. Stuck AE, Minder CE, Frey FJ. Risk of infectious complications in patients taking glucocorticosteroids. Rev Infect Dis. 1989;11(6):954–63.
114. Fardet L, Petersen I, Nazareth I. Common infections in patients prescribed systemic glucocorticoids in primary care: a population-based cohort study. PLoS Med. 2016;13(5):e1002024.
115. Ward MM, Donald F. Pneumocystis carinii pneumonia in patients with connective tissue diseases: the role of hospital experience in diagnosis and mortality. Arthritis Rheum. 1999;42(4):780–9.
116. Yale SH, Limper AH. Pneumocystis carinii pneumonia in patients without acquired immunodeficiency syndrome: associated illness and prior corticosteroid therapy. Mayo Clin Proc. 1996;71(1):5–13.
117. Sepkowitz KA, et al. Pneumocystis carinii pneumonia among patients without AIDS at a cancer hospital. JAMA. 1992;267(6):832–7.
118. Haraoui B, et al. Use of corticosteroids in patients with rheumatoid arthritis treated with infliximab: treatment implications based on a real-world Canadian population. RMD Open. 2015;1(1):e000078.
119. Singh JA, et al. 2015 American college of rheumatology guideline for the treatment of rheumatoid arthritis. Arthritis Rheum (Hoboken). 2016;68(1):1–26.

120. de Nard F, et al. Risk of hepatitis B virus reactivation in rheumatoid arthritis patients undergoing biologic treatment: extending perspective from old to newer drugs. World J Hepatol. 2015;7(3):344–61.
121. Hwang JP, Lok ASF. Management of patients with hepatitis B who require immunosuppressive therapy. Nat Rev Gastroenterol Hepatol. 2014;11(4):209–19.
122. Calabrese LH, Cacoub PP. For patients with rheumatic disease and hepatitis C infection: the end of interferon. RMD Open. 2015;1:e000008.
123. Szekanecz Z, et al. Malignancies in autoimmune rheumatic diseases – a mini-review. Gerontology. 2011;57(1):3–10.
124. Bojinca V, Janta I. Rheumatic diseases and malignancies. Maedica (Buchar). 2012;7(4):364–71.
125. Turesson C, Matteson EL. Malignancy as a comorbidity in rheumatic diseases. Rheumatology (Oxford). 2013;52(1):5–14.
126. Zintzaras E, Voulgarelis M, Moutsopoulos HM. The risk of lymphoma development in autoimmune diseases: a meta-analysis. Arch Intern Med. 2005;165(20):2337–44.
127. Kassan SS, et al. Increased risk of lymphoma in sicca syndrome. Ann Intern Med. 1978;89(6):888–92.
128. Shankaran V, et al. IFNgamma and lymphocytes prevent primary tumour development and shape tumour immunogenicity. Nature. 2001;410(6832):1107–11.
129. Apor E, et al. Systemic lupus erythematosus is associated with increased incidence of hematologic malignancies: a meta-analysis of prospective cohort studies. Leuk Res. 2014;38(9):1067–71.
130. Bernatsky S, et al. Non-Hodgkin's lymphoma in systemic lupus erythematosus. Ann Rheum Dis. 2005;64(10):1507–9.
131. Lu M, et al. Non-lymphoma hematological malignancies in systemic lupus erythematosus. Oncology. 2013;85(4):235–40.
132. Bernatsky S, et al. Cancer risk in systemic lupus: an updated international multi-centre cohort study. J Autoimmun. 2013;42:130–5.
133. Antonelli A, et al. Thyroid cancer in systemic lupus erythematosus: a case-control study. J Clin Endocrinol Metab. 2010;95(1):314–8.
134. Dreyer L, et al. High incidence of potentially virus-induced malignancies in systemic lupus erythematosus: a long-term followup study in a Danish cohort. Arthritis Rheum. 2011;63(10):3032–7.
135. Isomaki HA, Hakulinen T, Joutsenlahti U. Excess risk of lymphomas, leukemia and myeloma in patients with rheumatoid arthritis. J Chronic Dis. 1978;31(11):691–6.
136. Smitten AL, et al. A meta-analysis of the incidence of malignancy in adult patients with rheumatoid arthritis. Arthritis Res Ther. 2008;10(2):R45.
137. Simon TA, et al. Incidence of malignancy in adult patients with rheumatoid arthritis: a meta-analysis. Arthritis Res Ther. 2015;17:212.
138. Parikh-Patel A, et al. Risk of cancer among rheumatoid arthritis patients in California. Cancer Causes Control. 2009;20(6):1001–10.
139. Khurana R, et al. Risk of development of lung cancer is increased in patients with rheumatoid arthritis: a large case control study in US veterans. J Rheumatol. 2008;35(9):1704–8.
140. Andersen CL, et al. Risk of lymphoma and solid cancer among patients with rheumatoid arthritis in a primary care setting. PLoS One. 2014;9(6):e99388.
141. Rosenthal AK, et al. Scleroderma and malignancy: an epidemiological study. Ann Rheum Dis. 1993;52(7):531–3.
142. Rosenthal AK, et al. Incidence of cancer among patients with systemic sclerosis. Cancer. 1995;76(5):910–4.
143. Onishi A, et al. Cancer incidence in systemic sclerosis: meta-analysis of population-based cohort studies. Arthritis Rheum. 2013;65(7):1913–21.
144. Derk CT, et al. A cohort study of cancer incidence in systemic sclerosis. J Rheumatol. 2006;33(6):1113–6.

145. Moinzadeh P, et al. Association of anti-RNA polymerase III autoantibodies and cancer in scleroderma. Arthritis Res Ther. 2014;16(1):R53.
146. Hill CL, et al. Frequency of specific cancer types in dermatomyositis and polymyositis: a population-based study. Lancet. 2001;357(9250):96–100.
147. Huang YL, et al. Malignancies associated with dermatomyositis and polymyositis in Taiwan: a nationwide population-based study. Br J Dermatol. 2009;161(4):854–60.
148. Stockton D, Doherty VR, Brewster DH. Risk of cancer in patients with dermatomyositis or polymyositis, and follow-up implications: a Scottish population-based cohort study. Br J Cancer. 2001;85(1):41–5.
149. Sigurgeirsson B, et al. Risk of cancer in patients with dermatomyositis or polymyositis. A population-based study. N Engl J Med. 1992;326(6):363–7.
150. Zantos D, Zhang Y, Felson D. The overall and temporal association of cancer with polymyositis and dermatomyositis. J Rheumatol. 1994;21(10):1855–9.
151. Buchbinder R, et al. Incidence of malignant disease in biopsy-proven inflammatory myopathy. A population-based cohort study. Ann Intern Med. 2001;134(12):1087–95.
152. Sparsa A, et al. Routine vs extensive malignancy search for adult dermatomyositis and polymyositis: a study of 40 patients. Arch Dermatol. 2002;138(7):885–90.
153. Papageorgiou A, et al. Predicting the outcome of Sjogren's syndrome-associated non-hodgkin's lymphoma patients. PLoS One. 2015;10(2):e0116189.
154. Voulgarelis M, Moutsopoulos HM. Mucosa-associated lymphoid tissue lymphoma in Sjogren's syndrome: risks, management, and prognosis. Rheum Dis Clin N Am. 2008; 34(4):921–33, viii.
155. Baimpa E, et al. Hematologic manifestations and predictors of lymphoma development in primary Sjogren syndrome: clinical and pathophysiologic aspects. Medicine (Baltimore). 2009;88(5):284–93.
156. Voulgarelis M, et al. Prognosis and outcome of non-Hodgkin lymphoma in primary Sjogren syndrome. Medicine (Baltimore). 2012;91(1):1–9.
157. Theander E, et al. Lymphoma and other malignancies in primary Sjogren's syndrome: a cohort study on cancer incidence and lymphoma predictors. Ann Rheum Dis. 2006;65(6):796–803.
158. Papageorgiou A, Voulgarelis M, Tzioufas AG. Clinical picture, outcome and predictive factors of lymphoma in Sjogren syndrome. Autoimmun Rev. 2015;14(7):641–9.
159. Radis CD, et al. Effects of cyclophosphamide on the development of malignancy and on long-term survival of patients with rheumatoid arthritis. A 20-year followup study. Arthritis Rheum. 1995;38(8):1120–7.
160. Bernatsky S, et al. Lymphoma risk in systemic lupus: effects of disease activity versus treatment. Ann Rheum Dis. 2014;73(1):138–42.
161. Ognenovski VM, et al. Increased incidence of cervical intraepithelial neoplasia in women with systemic lupus erythematosus treated with intravenous cyclophosphamide. J Rheumatol. 2004;31(9):1763–7.
162. Georgescu L, et al. Lymphoma in patients with rheumatoid arthritis: association with the disease state or methotrexate treatment. Semin Arthritis Rheum. 1997;26(6):794–804.
163. Usman AR, Yunus MB. Non-Hodgkin's lymphoma in patients with rheumatoid arthritis treated with low dose methotrexate. J Rheumatol. 1996;23(6):1095–7.
164. Bachman TR, et al. Methotrexate-associated lymphoma in patients with rheumatoid arthritis: report of two cases. Arthritis Rheum. 1996;39(2):325–9.
165. Kameda T, et al. Association of higher methotrexate dose with lymphoproliferative disease onset in rheumatoid arthritis patients. Arthritis Care Res (Hoboken). 2014;66(9):1302–9.
166. Kamel OW, et al. Brief report: reversible lymphomas associated with Epstein-Barr virus occurring during methotrexate therapy for rheumatoid arthritis and dermatomyositis. N Engl J Med. 1993;328(18):1317–21.
167. Miyazaki T, et al. Remission of lymphoma after withdrawal of methotrexate in rheumatoid arthritis: relationship with type of latent Epstein-Barr virus infection. Am J Hematol. 2007;82(12):1106–9.

168. Scott FI, et al. Risk of nonmelanoma skin cancer associated with the use of immunosuppressant and biologic agents in patients with a history of autoimmune disease and nonmelanoma skin cancer. JAMA Dermatol. 2016;152(2):164–72.
169. Bongartz T, et al. Anti-TNF antibody therapy in rheumatoid arthritis and the risk of serious infections and malignancies: systematic review and meta-analysis of rare harmful effects in randomized controlled trials. JAMA. 2006;295(19):2275–85.
170. Bongartz T, et al. Etanercept therapy in rheumatoid arthritis and the risk of malignancies: a systematic review and individual patient data meta-analysis of randomised controlled trials. Ann Rheum Dis. 2009;68(7):1177–83.
171. Askling J, et al. Cancer risk in patients with rheumatoid arthritis treated with anti-tumor necrosis factor alpha therapies: does the risk change with the time since start of treatment? Arthritis Rheum. 2009;60(11):3180–9.
172. Dixon WG, et al. Influence of anti-tumor necrosis factor therapy on cancer incidence in patients with rheumatoid arthritis who have had a prior malignancy: results from the British society for rheumatology biologics register. Arthritis Care Res (Hoboken). 2010;62(6):755–63.
173. Lebrec H, et al. Tumor necrosis factor, tumor necrosis factor inhibition, and cancer risk. Curr Med Res Opin. 2015;31(3):557–74.
174. Raaschou P, Frisell T, Askling J. TNF inhibitor therapy and risk of breast cancer recurrence in patients with rheumatoid arthritis: a nationwide cohort study. Ann Rheum Dis. 2015;74(12):2137–43.
175. Strangfeld A, et al. Risk of incident or recurrent malignancies among patients with rheumatoid arthritis exposed to biologic therapy in the German biologics register RABBIT. Arthritis Res Ther. 2010;12(1):R5.
176. Chakravarty EF, Michaud K, Wolfe F. Skin cancer, rheumatoid arthritis, and tumor necrosis factor inhibitors. J Rheumatol. 2005;32(11):2130–5.
177. Mariette X, et al. Malignancies associated with tumour necrosis factor inhibitors in registries and prospective observational studies: a systematic review and meta-analysis. Ann Rheum Dis. 2011;70(11):1895–904.
178. Wolfe F, Michaud K. Biologic treatment of rheumatoid arthritis and the risk of malignancy: analyses from a large US observational study. Arthritis Rheum. 2007;56(9):2886–95.
179. Mercer LK, et al. Risk of solid cancer in patients exposed to anti-tumour necrosis factor therapy: results from the British society for rheumatology biologics register for rheumatoid arthritis. Ann Rheum Dis. 2015;74(6):1087–93.
180. Setoguchi S, et al. Tumor necrosis factor alpha antagonist use and cancer in patients with rheumatoid arthritis. Arthritis Rheum. 2006;54(9):2757–64.
181. Wu CY, et al. The risk of cancer in patients with rheumatoid arthritis taking tumor necrosis factor antagonists: a nationwide cohort study. Arthritis Res Ther. 2014;16(5):449.
182. Haugeberg G, et al. Bone mineral density and frequency of osteoporosis in female patients with rheumatoid arthritis: results from 394 patients in the Oslo County rheumatoid arthritis register. Arthritis Rheum. 2000;43(3):522–30.
183. Haugeberg G, et al. Reduced bone mineral density in male rheumatoid arthritis patients: frequencies and associations with demographic and disease variables in ninety-four patients in the Oslo County rheumatoid arthritis register. Arthritis Rheum. 2000;43(12):2776–84.
184. Sinigaglia L, et al. A multicenter cross sectional study on bone mineral density in rheumatoid arthritis. Italian study group on bone mass in rheumatoid arthritis. J Rheumatol. 2000;27(11):2582–9.
185. van Staa TP, et al. Clinical assessment of the long-term risk of fracture in patients with rheumatoid arthritis. Arthritis Rheum. 2006;54(10):3104–12.
186. Laan RF, et al. Vertebral osteoporosis in rheumatoid arthritis patients: effect of low dose prednisone therapy. Br J Rheumatol. 1992;31(2):91–6.
187. Cortet B, et al. Factors influencing bone loss in rheumatoid arthritis: a longitudinal study. Clin Exp Rheumatol. 2000;18(6):683–90.

188. Cortet B, et al. Evaluation of bone mineral density in patients with rheumatoid arthritis. Influence of disease activity and glucocorticoid therapy. Rev Rhum Engl Ed. 1997;64(7–9):451–8.
189. Krieckaert CL, et al. Changes in bone mineral density during long-term treatment with adalimumab in patients with rheumatoid arthritis: a cohort study. Rheumatology (Oxford). 2013;52(3):547–53.
190. Rauner M, Hofbauer LC, Aringer M. Local and systemic bone effects of rheumatoid arthritis. Z Rheumatol. 2012;71(10):869–73.
191. Gough AK, et al. Excretion of pyridinium crosslinks correlates with disease activity and appendicular bone loss in early rheumatoid arthritis. Ann Rheum Dis. 1994;53(1):14–7.
192. Korczowska I, Lacki JK, Hrycaj P. Influence of infliximab on cytokines network and markers of bone remodeling in rheumatoid arthritis patients. Yonsei Med J. 2013;54(1):183–8.
193. Vis M, et al. Evaluation of bone mineral density, bone metabolism, osteoprotegerin and receptor activator of the NFkappaB ligand serum levels during treatment with infliximab in patients with rheumatoid arthritis. Ann Rheum Dis. 2006;65(11):1495–9.
194. Dimitroulas T, et al. Biologic therapies and systemic bone loss in rheumatoid arthritis. Autoimmun Rev. 2013;12(10):958–66.
195. Grossman JM, et al. American College of Rheumatology 2010 recommendations for the prevention and treatment of glucocorticoid-induced osteoporosis. Arthritis Care Res. 2010;62(11):1515–26.
196. Svenson KL, et al. Impaired glucose handling in active rheumatoid arthritis: relationship to the secretion of insulin and counter-regulatory hormones. Metabolism. 1987;36(10):940–3.
197. Dessein PH, Stanwix AE, Joffe BI. Cardiovascular risk in rheumatoid arthritis versus osteoarthritis: acute phase response related decreased insulin sensitivity and high-density lipoprotein cholesterol as well as clustering of metabolic syndrome features in rheumatoid arthritis. Arthritis Res. 2002;4(5):R5.
198. Dessein PH, et al. The acute phase response does not fully predict the presence of insulin resistance and dyslipidemia in inflammatory arthritis. J Rheumatol. 2002;29(3):462–6.
199. Chung CP, et al. Prevalence of the metabolic syndrome is increased in rheumatoid arthritis and is associated with coronary atherosclerosis. Atherosclerosis. 2008;196(2):756–63.
200. Giles JT, et al. Insulin resistance in rheumatoid arthritis: disease-related indicators and associations with the presence and progression of subclinical atherosclerosis. Arthritis Rheumatol. 2015;67(3):626–36.
201. Wasko MC, et al. Diabetes mellitus and insulin resistance in patients with rheumatoid arthritis: risk reduction in a chronic inflammatory disease. Arthritis Care Res (Hoboken). 2011;63(4):512–21.
202. Bastard JP, et al. Recent advances in the relationship between obesity, inflammation, and insulin resistance. Eur Cytokine Netw. 2006;17(1):4–12.
203. Popa C, et al. The role of TNF-alpha in chronic inflammatory conditions, intermediary metabolism, and cardiovascular risk. J Lipid Res. 2007;48(4):751–62.
204. Jiang P, Li H, Li X. Diabetes mellitus risk factors in rheumatoid arthritis: a systematic review and meta-analysis. Clin Exp Rheumatol. 2015;33(1):115–21.
205. Dregan A, et al. Chronic inflammatory disorders and risk of type 2 diabetes mellitus, coronary heart disease, and stroke: a population-based cohort study. Circulation. 2014;130(10):837–44.
206. Han C, et al. Cardiovascular disease and risk factors in patients with rheumatoid arthritis, psoriatic arthritis, and ankylosing spondylitis. J Rheumatol. 2006;33(11):2167–72.
207. Dessein PH, et al. Glucocorticoids and insulin sensitivity in rheumatoid arthritis. J Rheumatol. 2004;31(5):867–74.
208. Angelopoulos TP, et al. Steroid-induced diabetes in rheumatologic patients. Clin Exp Rheumatol. 2014;32(1):126–30.
209. Penesova A, et al. Chronic inflammation and low-dose glucocorticoid effects on glucose metabolism in premenopausal females with rheumatoid arthritis free of conventional metabolic risk factors. Physiol Res. 2013;62(1):75–83.

210. Toms TE, et al. Lack of association between glucocorticoid use and presence of the metabolic syndrome in patients with rheumatoid arthritis: a cross-sectional study. Arthritis Res Ther. 2008;10(6):R145.
211. Hoes JN, et al. Glucose tolerance, insulin sensitivity and beta-cell function in patients with rheumatoid arthritis treated with or without low-to-medium dose glucocorticoids. Ann Rheum Dis. 2011;70(11):1887–94.
212. Buttgereit F. Do the treatment with glucocorticoids and/or the disease itself drive the impairment in glucose metabolism in patients with rheumatoid arthritis? Ann Rheum Dis. 2011;70(11):1881–3.
213. den Uyl D, et al. Metabolic effects of high-dose prednisolone treatment in early rheumatoid arthritis: balance between diabetogenic effects and inflammation reduction. Arthritis Rheum. 2012;64(3):639–46.
214. Dessein PH, Joffe BI, Stanwix AE. Effects of disease modifying agents and dietary intervention on insulin resistance and dyslipidemia in inflammatory arthritis: a pilot study. Arthritis Res. 2002;4(6):R12.
215. Zonana-Nacach A, et al. Prevalence and factors associated with metabolic syndrome in patients with rheumatoid arthritis and systemic lupus erythematosus. J Clin Rheumatol. 2008;14(2):74–7.
216. Toms TE, et al. Methotrexate therapy associates with reduced prevalence of the metabolic syndrome in rheumatoid arthritis patients over the age of 60- more than just an anti-inflammatory effect? A cross sectional study. Arthritis Res Ther. 2009;11(4):R110.
217. Wasko MC, et al. Hydroxychloroquine and risk of diabetes in patients with rheumatoid arthritis. JAMA. 2007;298(2):187–93.
218. Solomon DH, et al. Effect of hydroxychloroquine on insulin sensitivity and lipid parameters in rheumatoid arthritis patients without diabetes mellitus: a randomized, blinded crossover trial. Arthritis Care Res (Hoboken). 2014;66(8):1246–51.
219. Kiortsis DN, et al. Effects of infliximab treatment on insulin resistance in patients with rheumatoid arthritis and ankylosing spondylitis. Ann Rheum Dis. 2005;64(5):765–6.
220. Gonzalez-Gay MA, et al. Anti-tumor necrosis factor-alpha blockade improves insulin resistance in patients with rheumatoid arthritis. Clin Exp Rheumatol. 2006;24(1):83–6.
221. Tam LS, et al. Impact of TNF inhibition on insulin resistance and lipids levels in patients with rheumatoid arthritis. Clin Rheumatol. 2007;26(9):1495–8.
222. Chen DY, et al. Significant effects of biologic therapy on lipid profiles and insulin resistance in patients with rheumatoid arthritis. Arthritis Res Ther. 2015;17:52.
223. Rosenvinge A, et al. Insulin resistance in patients with rheumatoid arthritis: effect of anti-TNFalpha therapy. Scand J Rheumatol. 2007;36(2):91–6.
224. Wu JJ, et al. No association between TNF inhibitor and methotrexate therapy versus methotrexate in changes in hemoglobin A1C and fasting glucose among psoriasis, psoriatic arthritis, and rheumatoid arthritis patients. J Drugs Dermatol. 2015;14(2):159–66.
225. Castelino FV, Varga J. Interstitial lung disease in connective tissue diseases: evolving concepts of pathogenesis and management. Arthritis Res Ther. 2010;12(4):213.
226. Schneider F, et al. Pleuropulmonary pathology in patients with rheumatic disease. Arch Pathol Lab Med. 2012;136(10):1242–52.
227. Bagnato G, Harari S. Cellular interactions in the pathogenesis of interstitial lung diseases. Eur Respir Rev. 2015;24(135):102–14.
228. Wells AU, Denton CP. Interstitial lung disease in connective tissue disease – mechanisms and management. Nat Rev Rheumatol. 2014;10(12):728–39.
229. de Lauretis A, Veeraraghavan S, Renzoni E. Review series: aspects of interstitial lung disease: connective tissue disease-associated interstitial lung disease: how does it differ from IPF? How should the clinical approach differ? Chron Respir Dis. 2011;8(1):53–82.
230. Nair A, Walsh SLF, Desai SR. Imaging of pulmonary involvement in rheumatic disease. Rheum Dis Clin N Am. 2015;41(2):167–96.

231. Ngian G-S, et al. Predictors of mortality in connective tissue disease-associated pulmonary arterial hypertension: a cohort study. Arthritis Res Ther. 2012;14(5):R213.
232. Cha S-I, et al. Lymphoid interstitial pneumonia: clinical features, associations and prognosis. Eur Respir J. 2006;28(2):364–9.
233. Mondal S, et al. Interstitial lung disease as presenting feature of SLE. J Case Rep. 2014;4(1):85–7.
234. Meyer KC, Ganesh R. Bronchoalveolar lavage for the evaluation of interstitial lung disease: is it clinically useful? Eur Respir J. 2011;38(4):761–9.
235. Halkos ME, et al. Role of thoracic surgeons in the diagnosis of idiopathic interstitial lung disease. Ann Thorac Surg. 2005;79(6):2172–9.
236. Tashkin DP, et al. Cyclophosphamide versus placebo in scleroderma lung disease. N Engl J Med. 2006;354(25):2655–66.
237. Keir GJ, et al. Rituximab in severe, treatment-refractory interstitial lung disease. Respirology. 2014;19(3):353–9.
238. Schachna L, et al. Lung transplantation in scleroderma compared with idiopathic pulmonary fibrosis and idiopathic pulmonary arterial hypertension. Arthritis Rheum. 2006;54(12):3954–61.
239. Vij R, Strek ME. Diagnosis and treatment of connective tissue disease-associated interstitial lung disease. Chest. 2013;143:814–24.
240. Kim EJ, et al. Usual interstitial pneumonia in rheumatoid arthritis-associated interstitial lung disease. Eur Respir J. 2010;35(6):1322–8.
241. Castelino FV, Goldberg H, Dellaripa PF. The impact of rheumatological evaluation in the management of patients with interstitial lung disease. Rheumatology. 2011;50(3):489–93.
242. Weiss G, Schett G. Anaemia in inflammatory rheumatic diseases. Nat Rev Rheumatol. 2013;9(4):205–15.
243. Baker JF, Ghio AJ. Iron homoeostasis in rheumatic disease. Rheumatology (Oxford). 2009;48(11):1339–44.
244. Remacha AF, et al. Erythroid abnormalities in rheumatoid-arthritis – the role of erythropoietin. J Rheumatol. 1992;19(11):1687–91.
245. Weiss G, Goodnough LT. Anemia of chronic disease. N Engl J Med. 2005;352(10):1011–23.
246. Voulgari PV, et al. Role of cytokines in the pathogenesis of anemia of chronic disease in rheumatoid arthritis. Clin Immunol (Orlando, Fla.). 1999;92(2):153–60.
247. Ferrucci L, et al. Proinflammatory state, hepcidin, and anemia in older persons. Blood. 2010;115(18):3810–6.
248. Peeters HR, et al. Course and characteristics of anaemia in patients with rheumatoid arthritis of recent onset. Ann Rheum Dis. 1996;55(3):162–8.
249. Wolfe F, Hawley DJ. The comparative risk and predictors of adverse gastrointestinal events in rheumatoid arthritis and osteoarthritis: a prospective 13 year study of 2131 patients. J Rheumatol. 2000;27(7):1668–73.
250. Wolfe MM, Lichtenstein DR, Singh G. Gastrointestinal toxicity of nonsteroidal antiinflammatory drugs. N Engl J Med. 1999;340(24):1888–99.
251. García Rodríguez La H-DS. The risk of upper gastrointestinal complications associated with nonsteroidal anti-inflammatory drugs, glucocorticoids, acetaminophen, and combinations of these agents. Arthritis Res. 2001;3(2):98–101.
252. Bergamaschi G, et al. Prevalence and pathogenesis of anemia in inflammatory bowel disease. Influence of anti-tumor necrosis factor- treatment. Haematologica. 2009;95(2):199–205.
253. Hershko C, et al. Role of autoimmune gastritis, Helicobacter pylori and celiac disease in refractory or unexplained iron deficiency anemia. Haematologica. 2005;90(5):585–95.
254. Tian X-P, Zhang X. Gastrointestinal complications of systemic sclerosis. World J Gastroenterol. 2013;19(41):7062–8.
255. Segal R, et al. Anemia, serum vitamin B12, and folic acid in patients with rheumatoid arthritis, psoriatic arthritis, and systemic lupus erythematosus. Rheumatol Int. 2004;24(1):14–9.

256. Bashal F. Hematological disorders in patients with systemic lupus erythematosus. Open Rheumatol J. 2013;7:87–95.
257. Owlia MB, Newman K, Akhtari M. Felty's syndrome, insights and updates. Open Rheumatol J. 2014;8:129–36.
258. Arlet JB, et al. Reactive haemophagocytic syndrome in adult-onset Still's disease: a report of six patients and a review of the literature. Ann Rheum Dis. 2006;65:1596–601.
259. Cullis JO. Diagnosis and management of anaemia of chronic disease: current status. Br J Haematol. 2011;154:289–300.
260. Johnson-Wimbley TD, Graham DY. Diagnosis and management of iron deficiency anemia in the 21st century. Ther Adv Gastroenterol. 2011;4(3):177–84.
261. Powers JM, Buchanan GR. Diagnosis and management of iron deficiency anemia. Hematol Oncol Clin North Am. 2014;28:729–45.
262. Lanza FL, et al. Guidelines for prevention of NSAID-related ulcer complications. Am J Gastroenterol. 2009;104(3):728–38.
263. Elewaut D, Goodson N, Fleischmann R. Should we be morbid about comorbidities in the rheumatic diseases? Rheumatology (Oxford). 2013;52(1):1–2.
264. Ranganath VK, et al. Comorbidities are associated with poorer outcomes in community patients with rheumatoid arthritis. Rheumatology (Oxford). 2013;52(10):1809–17.
265. Wolfe F, et al. Chronic conditions and health problems in rheumatic diseases: comparisons with rheumatoid arthritis, noninflammatory rheumatic disorders, systemic lupus erythematosus, and fibromyalgia. J Rheumatol. 2010;37(2):305–15.

Chapter 2
Impact of Comorbidity

Maha Azeez and Peter C. Taylor

Rheumatic diseases comprise a heterogeneous group of disorders that have in common a varying degree of musculoskeletal involvement. Classification has traditionally been based on pattern recognition with respect to symptoms and signs of disease. However, advances in understanding of the aetiopathogenesis of these disorders and observations of the range of therapeutic responses to targeted therapies implicate particular inflammatory pathways in the clinical presentation in which the expressed tissue tropisms of disease are likely to be dependent on both genetic and environmental factors. Many rheumatic diseases can be considered systemic inflammatory disorders which in some cases, exemplified by rheumatoid arthritis and ankylosing spondylitis, have their predominant manifestations in the peripheral synovial joints and axial skeleton, respectively. But being chronic, systemic inflammatory disorders, involvement of other tissues can occur. And for those clinical phenotypes that share a common immune dysregulation in a major inflammatory pathway, there may be overlapping tissue involvement. For example, inflammatory bowel disease may occur with ankylosing spondylitis; spondylitis may occur with psoriasis, and uveitis may be a feature of a range of rheumatic diseases. Endothelial activation, with accompanying atherosclerosis, is increasingly recognised as a comorbidity across the spectrum of rheumatic disorders. In this chapter we will take an overview of current thinking regarding comorbidities across the range of rheumatic diseases, and subsequent chapters will focus on individual primary rheumatic disorders.

M. Azeez • P.C. Taylor (✉)
Nuffield Department of Orthopaedics, Rheumatology and Musculoskeletal Sciences, University of Oxford, Botnar Research Centre, Oxford, UK
e-mail: peter.taylor@kennedy.ox.ac.uk

Y. El Miedany (ed.), *Comorbidity in Rheumatic Diseases*,
DOI 10.1007/978-3-319-59963-2_2

Comorbidity in Rheumatic Diseases

The management of rheumatic diseases has improved significantly over recent decades with enhanced knowledge of disease pathogenesis, diligent disease activity monitoring and availability of advanced treatment options. With improved disease outcomes and longer survival rates, the impact of comorbidities associated with these conditions and their influence on quality of life and mortality have become apparent. In addition, data from surveillance registries and multinational cohort studies have enabled capturing and recognising the significance of comorbidities associated with rheumatic diseases.

Comorbidity can be defined as the existence or occurrence of any distinct additional entity during the clinical course of a patient who has the index disease under study [1]. Comorbidities can be described in terms of active, past or transient conditions. Chronic inflammation, traditional cardiovascular risk factors, genetics and medications used to treat these conditions all contribute to the increased number of comorbidities observed. Comorbidities commonly encountered in patients with rheumatic diseases are listed in Table 2.1.

It is estimated that the average patient with rheumatoid arthritis (RA) has 1.6 comorbid conditions [2], and the number of conditions increases with age, disease duration and disease activity. The presence of comorbidities has been linked to reduced life expectancy, decreased quality of life, greater functional impairment and decreased quality of life [2, 3]. In addition, comorbidities can impact on disease outcome, patient's self-management and utilisation of healthcare and have a major impact on personal and health system-related costs.

More recently, the concept of multimorbidity has been introduced to describe patients with multiple co-existing diseases and incorporates potential interactions

Table 2.1 Comorbidities in rheumatic diseases

Main comorbidity	Related complication
Cardiovascular	Ischaemic heart disease, hypertension, heart failure, arrhythmias, peripheral vascular disease, deep vein thrombosis and stroke
Lung disease	Interstitial lung disease
Gastrointestinal disease	Peptic ulcers, hepatitis, fatty liver disease, diarrhoea, colitis, perforation
Osteoporosis	Fractures
Oral disease	Periodontitis
Renal disease	Interstitial nephritis, acute/chronic injury
Endocrine	Diabetes, thyroid disease
Infection	Bacterial sepsis
Malignancy	Lymphoma, solid tumours
Depression	Chronic pain syndrome, anxiety
Neurological disorders	Carpal tunnel syndrome, mononeuritis multiplex
Obesity	Metabolic syndrome

between the co-existing diseases and their impact on patients' wellbeing [4]. The multimorbidity model focuses on a more holistic and patient-centred approach, where treatment emphasis is on the patient and effectiveness of treatment is accessed by indices such as quality of life or physical function. Comorbidity is considered with reference to the patient's index disease, with treatment strategies centred on that disease, while the effectiveness of treatment is evaluated by changes in disease-specific indices. The approach to managing patients with comorbidity has to be tailored not only toward the disease of interest but must also incorporate all conditions and aspects that might affect clinical outcomes. There is a pressing need to develop effective and efficient strategies to screen for, prevent and manage comorbidities, in order to provide optimum quality of care for our patients.

Prevalence

The prevalence of comorbidities in patients with rheumatic diseases has been studied in different populations, with comparably high rates being reported. Most of the studies are based on patients with RA. A large international population based, cross-sectional study (COMORA) evaluated prevalence of comorbidities in patients with RA ($n = 3920$) from 17 countries around the world [5]. The most commonly reported comorbidities (past or current) were depression 15%, asthma 7%, cardiovascular events (myocardial infarction, stroke) 6%, solid-organ malignancies 5% and chronic obstructive pulmonary disease 4%. They also reported wide intercountry variability for prevalence of these comorbidities, e.g. prevalence of depression was 2% in Morocco compared to 33% in the USA.

Data from the British Society of Rheumatology Biologics register evaluated 7818 patients with RA initiating biologic therapy [6]. They reported 58% of patients having at least one comorbidity and 25% having more than one, with cardiovascular, respiratory disease and depression being the most frequent comorbid conditions. Another UK-based study evaluated baseline prevalence and cumulative incidence of comorbidity in 1460 patients with RA [3]. Baseline prevalence was 32% for all comorbidities, and 15-year cumulative incidence was 81%, which was associated with mortality and functional decline. Similarly, a Swedish study evaluating patients with early RA (symptoms <12 months) reported 53% of patients to have one or more comorbidity at onset of RA, and 41% had developed a new comorbidity after 5 years of diagnosis [7]. The study also described associations between inflammation and development of a new comorbidity. Similar figures for prevalence of comorbidities in early RA cohorts have been reported in studies from North America (58%) [8], the Netherlands (66%) [9], the UK (31.6%) [3] and Southern Sweden (43%) [10].

The prevalence of comorbidities in spondyloarthritis is also high compared to the general population. Spondyloarthritis (SpA) comprises diseases such as psoriatic arthritis, arthritis related to inflammatory bowel disease, reactive arthritis and ankylosing spondylosis. A large cross-sectional study involving 3984 patients with spondyloarthritis across 22 countries showed the commonest comorbidities to be hypertension (34%), hypercholesterolaemia (27%), osteoporosis (13%) and gastroduodenal ulcer (11%) [11].

There are several factors contributing to the increased frequency of these comorbidities observed in rheumatic conditions. Chronic active inflammation or disease-related organ damage may predispose to the development of comorbidities. In addition, medications used to treat these conditions, especially corticosteroids and other immunosuppressants, can add to the high prevalence observed. Traditional risk factors for cardiovascular disease, such as hypercholesterolaemia and hypertension, are more frequent in this patient population, as well as lifestyle behaviours such as smoking and physical inactivity which can all contribute to the high prevalence of comorbidities observed in patients with rheumatic diseases.

An additional factor which needs to be acknowledged is the close contact which many of these patients with Rheumatic diseases have with healthcare professionals. This may increase their likelihood to be screened for certain comorbidities e.g. osteoporosis, hypertension, hypercholesterolaemia.

Multidimensional Impact of Comorbidity

The simultaneous presence of multiple pathological conditions in the form of comorbidity and multimorbidity is present in all populations of patients with rheumatic disease [12]. Hence, the way we understand the concept of comorbidities associated with rheumatic diseases needs to be adapted. The impact of comorbidities on rheumatic diseases is multidimensional [13], incorporating almost every aspect of patient care, including quality of life, effectiveness of treatment, physical function, work disability, side effects, disease outcome and healthcare utilisation costs. Not all comorbidities have the same effect; CVD, malignancy, infections and respiratory diseases have a significant impact on mortality, whereas depression and fibromyalgia increase the risk of work-related disability [13]. Comorbidities should be considered an umbrella term, which has several facets, significantly impacting upon how we manage our patients (Fig. 2.1).

In contemporary practice, the focus in the management of RA has increasingly emphasised 'treating rheumatoid arthritis to target' [14], where early diagnosis and titration of treatment until low disease activity or remission are achieved, is the primary objective. The role and impact of comorbidities on achieving these targets has received less attention both in the literature and often in the clinic. Furthermore, the management guidelines for rheumatic disease such as those by the European League Against Rheumatism (EULAR) and American College of Rheumatology (ACR) do not comprehensively address the complexity or any trade-off between efficacy and safety issues when treating patients with comorbidities [15].

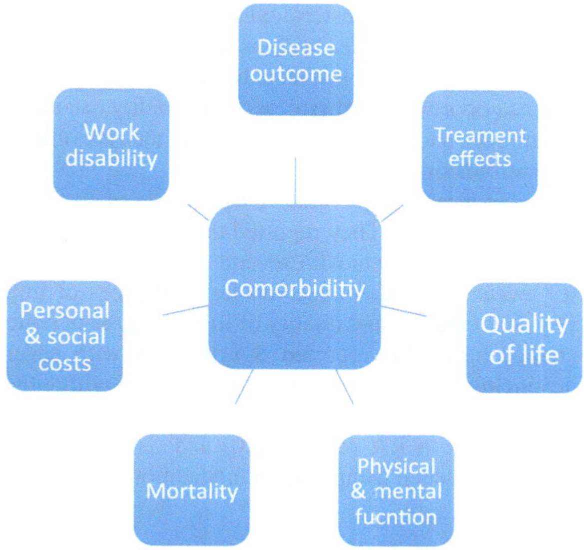

Fig. 2.1 Multidimensional aspects of comorbidity assessment in rheumatic diseases

Rheumatologists involved in caring for patients with rheumatic diseases are in a unique position to take the lead role in coordinating the management of comorbidities, in conjunction with other specialities and primary care colleagues. The multifaceted approach suggested in Fig. 2.1 incorporates treating symptoms and complications of the rheumatic disease in question, while anticipating, observing and managing the effects on other organs and balancing the risk-benefit ratio of a given medication. In order to optimise the recognition and management of comorbidities, the current model of care, where the focus is on the primary diagnosis, needs to be adjusted to incorporate the multiple aspects that affect the conditions being treated. Furthermore, given the impact of comorbidities on overall disease outcome, which is the main means used to evaluate effectiveness and costs of treatments, it is vital to identify and optimally manage comorbidities.

Impact on Prescribing Medications

Recent advances in pharmacotherapy for rheumatic diseases have resulted in markedly improved clinical outcomes, and patients are living longer. Modern treatments are primarily based on modulating or suppressing the immune system; therefore, managing side effects forms a significant part of therapeutic decision-making in these patients. Moreover, the presence of comorbidities adds to the challenge of balancing the risk-benefit ratio associated with any given treatment. Depending on the comorbidity in question, additional treatments may be required or drugs may need to be withdrawn. Even the most commonly prescribed medications such as glucocorticoids or nonsteroidal anti-inflammatory drugs (NSAIDs) can be problematic with comorbidities such as diabetes or renal disease. Some comorbidities are also drug-related, for instance, NSAIDs and peptic ulcer disease and corticosteroids and osteoporosis. Furthermore, comorbidity can affect the ability to tolerate certain treatments, such as bronchiectasis and the risk of infection secondary to either corticosteroids or biologic therapies [16].

A Japanese study evaluated the impact of comorbidity on treatment decisions in a RA cohort [17]. They reported that the use of methotrexate (MXT) and biologics was lower in patients with several comorbidities, despite having high disease activity levels. They also observed lesser degrees of improvement in disease activity, physical function and quality of life measures in patients with comorbidities. Other studies have also reported RA patients with several comorbid conditions and advancing age to be less frequently treated with either MXT or biologics [18, 19]. Another study evaluated the influence of comorbidities on prescribing different medications in RA patients [20] and reported that many comorbidities were not considered when using certain medications.

Financial Impact

The financial burden of comorbidities is a major consideration for healthcare payers across the globe. The chronic nature of these conditions, coupled with an ageing population, makes finding the most cost-effective and efficient healthcare solutions for patients one of the biggest challenges for contemporary healthcare systems. Having a condition such as RA is associated with a significant impact on the cost of care for both patient and society [21–23]. The annual direct healthcare costs of RA in England is estimated to be approximately €780 million per year, and indirect costs related to work disability is up to €6.75 billion per year [24]. Given the high prevalence of comorbidities associated with rheumatic diseases, the influence on the overall cost of healthcare may be even greater [25]. General population studies have highlighted the burden of having multiple chronic conditions on healthcare resources and costs. Similarly, multimorbidity has been associated with increased utilisation of primary care, medications, outpatient specialist services, emergency department presentations and hospitalisations [26]. Similarly, utilisation and cost of medications are also reported to be higher in patients with multiple chronic conditions [27].

Health economic studies are crucial in making decisions with regard to resource allocation, healthcare models and national policies. Trial-based health economics data, which are used to evaluate cost-effectiveness of medical interventions, have to date not adequately assessed the impact of comorbidity on rheumatic diseases. Selection criteria of certain trials may result in underrepresentation of patients with multiple chronic conditions [26] and may not reflect the true impact on health resources and cost.

Impact on Clinical Research

In clinical research studies, the primary outcome is based on disease or patient outcomes. Comorbidities can be a major confounding factor, influencing validity or acting as effect modifiers in studies [28]. Furthermore, patients with multiple comorbidities are often excluded from eligibility to participate in clinical studies. It has been suggested that clinical trial recruitment criteria should mandate characterisation of the participants according to their total morbidity burden and patterns of types of illnesses [12].

Effect of Comorbidity on Mortality

Comorbidities in rheumatic diseases are associated with increased mortality [29]. In general, mortality rates are 1.5–1.6-fold higher in patients with RA than in the general population. The presence of comorbidities is identified as one of the most significant predictors of premature death, more so than shared epitope, rheumatoid factor and erosions [29]. Studies evaluating risks for excess mortality in RA population have identified three factors [30]: (1) RA patients experience more serious comorbid conditions with worse outcomes, (2) RA patients receive suboptimal preventive care for their comorbidities, and (3) systemic inflammation together with immune dysfunction seems to promote and accelerate comorbidity and mortality.

A large prospective study evaluated the association of specific comorbidities with mortality in patients with RA [31]. The reported hazard ratio (HR) was 1.6 (confidence interval [CI] 1.15–2.22) for cardiovascular disease, 1.4 (CI 1.09–1.89) for respiratory conditions, 2 (CI 1.28–3.12) for cancer and 1.35 (CI 1.06–1.72) for depression. The association of depression with mortality has also been shown in other studies [32, 33], as well as being a predictor of myocardial infarction in RA patients [31].

Cardiovascular disease (CVD) is the most common and the most severe comorbidity with the greatest impact on mortality [34]. Mortality rates after a myocardial infarction are significantly higher in patients with RA compared to non-RA populations, with a HR of 1.46 (CI 1.01–2.10) [35]. Similarly, mortality at 1 year following a diagnosis of heart failure was higher in patients with RA compared with non-RA patients, HR 1.89 (CI 1.26–2.84) [35].

The increased risk for CVD comorbidity is partly attributed to traditional risk factors such as hypertension, hyperlipidaemia, diabetes mellitus, smoking, obesity, age and gender. Systemic inflammation, genetic factors and medication have all been linked with increased risk [36]. Epidemiology and pathogenesis of CVD comorbidities in rheumatic diseases have been extensively studied, especially in relation to RA. CVD comorbidity has been described in all rheumatic diseases, with atherosclerosis being the common denominator; however, clinical presentation and pathogenesis of CVD vary between different rheumatic diseases. There are a number of cardiac manifestations observed in patients with rheumatic diseases, the most prevalent being ischaemic cardiovascular disease and others include heart failure, conduction abnormalities and microvascular disease. Despite the advances in treating rheumatic diseases with improved outcomes, the mortality associated with CVD and infections has remained the same [37].

Given the negative impact of comorbidities on mortality, there is a huge need for careful screening, monitoring and treating comorbidities, which could substantially improve outcome and survival of these patients.

Effect of Comorbidity on Physical Function

Physical function is one of the most important predictors of patient outcomes, including mortality, work disability, healthcare resource utilisation as well as personal financial status [38, 39]. Improving or maintaining function is one of the main treatment goals both in terms of efficacy of treatments and patient-reported outcomes. There is strong evidence to suggest an association between comorbidity and increased disability in patients with chronic diseases such as RA. The chronic course of the disease and advancing age also has a negative impact on physical function. The Health Assessment Questionnaire Disability Index (HAQ-DI) is the most widely used tool to assess functional disability [40]. The HAQ score ranges from 0 to 3, where lowest score reflects better function, and is based on assessing function within eight domains (dressing, rising, eating, walking, hygiene, reach, grip and errands). Studies utilising HAQ to measure disability [39, 41] demonstrated that having one comorbidity increases the mean HAQ score by approximately 0.2 and multiple comorbidities increase mean HAQ by approximately 0.8. In addition, evaluation of factors that predict the rate of progression of disability showed that baseline comorbidities such as CVD, diabetes and hypertension as well as number of comorbidities were independently associated with progression of HAQ score [38].

Furthermore, a prospective study involving 380 patients with RA showed physical disability to increase significantly with higher levels of comorbidity, and this effect was independent of disease activity [39]. In this study, comorbidity was measured using Charlson Comorbidity Index (CCI_A) [42], which is a modification of CCI that includes original CCI plus one extra point for each decade of age above 50 years (potential range 0–38). Functional disability was assessed using serial measurements of HAQ over a year. The results showed that with increasing levels of comorbidity (CCI_A 0, 1–2, 3–4, 5–9), the HAQ scores were significantly worse (0.67, 0.80, 1.24, 1.40, respectively; $p < 0.001$). In addition the authors had previously reported increasing level of comorbidity to increase disability within each domain of HAQ [43].

Specific comorbidities can have a different impact on physical and mental function and can have long-term negative outcomes on both. A study evaluated long-term associations between a wide range of comorbidities with physical and mental function in patients with RA [44]. They used both HAQ, (which is disease specific) and physical scale of Medical Outcomes Study Short Form (SF-36) [45], which measures function in general. The results showed circulatory conditions and depression were associated with worse HAQ scores. Respiratory, musculoskeletal conditions, cancer and depression were associated with worse physical function as assessed by SF-36. Respiratory conditions and depression were associated with worse mental functioning. They concluded that SF-36 was better at assessing the full effect of comorbidity on physical function compared to HAQ and recommend combining both scales to identify the whole spectrum of functional disabilities associated with comorbidities. Other studies have also shown a strong association between chronic or even intermittent depression and long-term disability [46]. These studies highlight the need to target specific comorbidities in order to prevent long-term physical and mental disabilities.

Physical function is usually assessed in terms of disease activity, and in theory, with appropriate treatment, physical disability due to high disease activity should be reversible; however, this is not the case for a lot of patients. The data suggests the impact of comorbidity is independent of disease activity and may remain constant throughout the course of disease [39]. This is particularly relevant when assessing treatment responses and setting goals for low disease activity (LDA) or remission in these patients. In chronic diseases, physical function is central in terms of measuring disease outcome, as well as work productivity, healthcare costs and mortality. Given the evidence of high prevalence of comorbidity in populations such as RA and its impact on physical function, the approach to assessing disability in such patients should include the presence of comorbidities. Evidence suggests that improvement in HAQ used in both clinical practice and clinical trials to assess efficacy of treatments may not reflect the multifactorial nature of disability. Furthermore, health economics including cost of treatments and health policy decisions are based on disease outcomes; hence, incorporating all aspects that reflect patient's physical disability including comorbidity is crucial.

Comorbidity and Disease Outcomes

There are several methods used to measure disease outcome in rheumatic disease. These include disease activity indices, radiological changes and measures of physical and mental function, mortality, hospitalisation, work disability, medical costs and quality of life. Comorbid conditions influence such outcomes in different ways [41]. For example, comorbidities such as cardiovascular and pulmonary diseases have the greatest impact on mortality, and work disability is more associated with depression [41].

With advances in treatment for RA, the goal is treat-to-target in order to achieve low disease activity or remission. However, the presence of comorbidities can negatively influence reaching these treatment targets. Several studies have demonstrated presence of comorbidities to be associated with poor disease outcomes. A study from the North American (CORRONA) registry evaluated the impact of comorbidities on achieving remission in RA patients commencing either DMARD or a biologic therapy [47]. Change in clinical disease activity index (CDAI) and CDAI remission were the primary outcomes. The results showed that the patient-reported comorbidities independently correlated with lower CDAI improvement or remission. Similarly, a large multinational cross-sectional study involving 5848 patients with RA showed number of comorbidities to be independently associated with CDAI (odds ratio 0.75; CI 0.68–0.83) [48].

Another study involving 6610 active RA patients treated with adalimumab for 3 months evaluated predictors for achieving disease activity score (DAS28) remission [49]. The odds ratio for achieving DAS28 remission was 0.86 for patients with just one or no comorbidities compared to those who had more than one. Similar results were also observed in etanercept studies, where a number of comorbidities were associated with reduced responses as measured using the Health Assessment Questionnaire Disability Index (HAQ-DI) and CDAI [50]. Furthermore, a study utilising the multimorbidity concept also reported lower rates of remission or low disease activity in 815 RA patients with multiple comorbidities, 1 year after commencing DMARDs [4].

Rheumatic diseases have a significant impact on health-related quality of life (HRQOL), which has been shown to include not only physical aspects but also psychological and social functioning [51]. A Dutch study evaluated the effect of incident comorbidity on HRQOL among 679 RA patients over 2 years. HRQOL was assessed with Dutch version of SF-36, which is a validated self-administered questionnaire used to measure different domains of health status. They reported the effect of comorbidity on HRQOL depended on both types of comorbid condition and the dimension of HRQOL. For instance, cancer was associated with deterioration of physical component of the scale, and gastrointestinal diseases (GI) together with dizziness were associated with worsening of mental component of the scale. Overall, GI diseases, cancer, dizziness with falling and less severe chronic pulmonary conditions and heart complaints resulted in significant changes in HRQOL. They also concluded that summary measures of comorbidity might not reveal the true impact of certain comorbid conditions on HRQOL.

Similar negative effects on quality of life (QOL) have also been reported in RA cohorts in different countries. A UK-based study evaluated the association of comorbidities to QOL in 114 RA patients using the self-administered questionnaire, Euro-QOL (EQ-5D) [52], which is a generic instrument that measures QOL as a single score based on five health domains (mobility, self-care, usual activities, pain/discomfort and anxiety/depression). The EQ-5D single summary score can range from zero (death) to 1.0 (full health). Their results showed EQ-5D scores to be inversely correlated with the overall number of co-existing conditions. Similar low scores of EQ-5D associated with comorbidity in patients with RA have been reported in studies from North America [53], South Korea [54] and Italy [55].

The exact mechanism of comorbidities affecting response to treatment is not fully understood. Disease activity in RA is evaluated using composite indices which include patient global assessment (PGA) and tender joint count, which can be influenced by certain comorbid conditions such as fibromyalgia, OA, back pain and depression [47]. Studies have shown that PGA is a limiting factor for reaching remission [56], and having multiple other conditions associated with their disease can effect patients' perceptions and influence patient-reported outcomes. A cross-sectional and observational study compared patient-reported outcomes in two RA cohorts recruited from the same clinic, one between 1998 and 1999 and the other from 2011 to 2012 [57]. The later cohort showed better functional and work capability but poorer patient-reported general health and higher comorbidities compared to the late 1990s cohort. This unexpected finding may in part reflect expectation bias on the part of patients and also a greater awareness and reporting of comorbidities by rheumatologists.

Current evidence suggests interplay of comorbidities, advancing age, drug-related risks and patient perceptions to have a significant influence on treatment targets and disease outcomes. Therefore, all these factors need to be accounted for or incorporated when setting treat-to-target goals for these patients. One such model of care has been illustrated for RA, incorporating patient remission, structural remission, medication remission and low incidence of comorbidities in addition to disease activity remission (Fig. 2.2) [58].

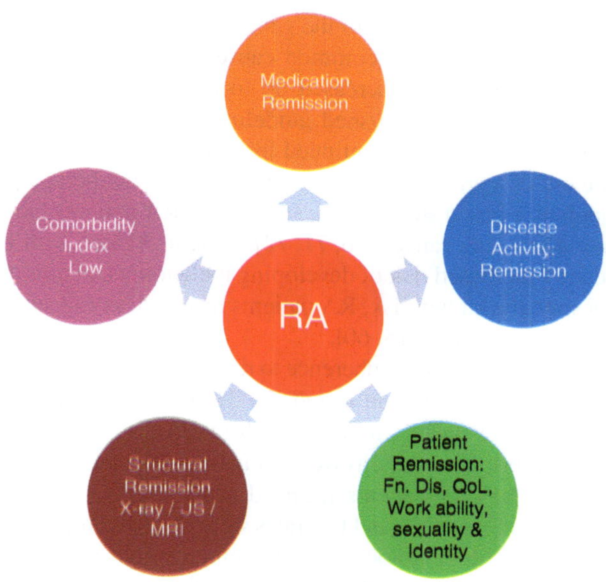

Fig. 2.2 Redefining health outcomes (Reproduced from El Miedany [58], with permission from Springer)

Medical Guidelines and Comorbidities

Recommendations for the management of specific comorbidities associated with rheumatic diseases are lacking. Most of the recommendations are extrapolated from general population studies. Furthermore, recommendations for certain comorbidities can be country specific, dependent on national health policies. Literature on managing comorbidities is focused mainly on CVD, malignancy, infections and osteoporosis. Both NICE [59] and EULAR [14] have published guidelines emphasising the importance of screening patients with RA regularly for associated comorbidities in daily clinical practice. However, uptake or adherence to medical guidelines remains poor [5, 60].

The COMORO study reported high variability not only in the prevalence but also adherence to recommendations for screening, managing and preventing comorbidities among different countries [5]. They reported 9.5% of the total number of patients enrolled in the study did not have their CVD risk optimally managed. Similarly, only 10.3% of patients received influenza and pneumococcal vaccination as per recommendations, and overall screening for malignancies was also low.

EULAR guidelines recommend annual cardiovascular screening for patients with RA [61]. However, evidence shows that management of CVD risk factors is far from ideal [62], with 30–50% patients with RA lacking optimal CVD risk monitoring and management [5]. Similarly, EULAR guidelines recommend influenza and pneumococcal vaccinations in all patients with autoimmune diseases [63], and vaccination uptake rates are suboptimal in RA populations [64, 65].

Patients with RA are at increased risk of developing osteoporosis, with studies reporting double the risk compared to the general population [66]. Glucocorticoid-induced osteoporosis is the most common cause of secondary osteoporosis [67], with risk of vertebral fractures increased up to two to five times, which is dose dependent [68]. EULAR has published guidelines for safe use of glucocorticoids [69, 70]; however, studies report continued high prevalence of osteoporosis in RA patients despite use of aggressive management and biologic therapy [60].

Several population-based studies have shown that RA patients have an increased risk of lymphoma and lung cancer [16, 71, 72]. Patients treated with TNF inhibitors have a significantly increased risk of developing melanoma and non-melanoma skin cancer [71]. Despite the known risk, RA patients receive less cancer screening compared to the general population [5, 60].

Similarly, data has shown poor adherence to recommendations for comorbidities in relation to spondyloarthritis [11]. In a study of 3984 patients with spondyloarthritis across 22 countries, investigators reported high rates of non-compliance to recommendations for monitoring patients, as well as intercountry variability in screening for comorbidities. Only 50% of patients received optimal CVD monitoring, 11–44% patients were screened for cancer, and low rates were observed for vaccination uptake.

These discrepancies observed between recommendations and daily clinical practice with regard to the screening and management of comorbidities can be attributed to several factors. One of the main barriers is the time constraint in a clinical consultation, where the main focus is on the index disease, assessing effectiveness of treatment and managing symptoms and adverse effects. Hence, time can be limited to address other aspects of disease management such as comorbidities. Another factor is the reduced attention on medical prevention in these patients compared to general population [73], as the medical focus is on their rheumatic disease. Data on breast cancer screening (which is more prevalent in rheumatic conditions compared to general population) have shown that mammography is performed less frequently in women with rheumatic diseases [60]. Other contributing factors include unclear role of responsibility between primary and secondary care for screening and managing comorbidities, as well as a lack of awareness among both health professionals and patients on the impact of comorbidities. Furthermore, most of the recommendations on comorbidities (particularly outside of osteoporosis, cardiovascular disease and malignancy, which are addressed in EULAR guidelines) are based on the general population and may not always be relevant to rheumatic diseases. Similarly, global recommendations may not be applicable to some countries depending on local healthcare policies.

Management of Comorbidities

Over the last 20 years, RA disease burden has decreased, owing to the fundamental changes in disease management and novel treatments; however, the level of comorbidities has not changed. Evidence has shown effective management of these comorbidities to be suboptimal [5, 74]. Some of the key points to consider when discussing management of comorbidities are worth highlighting: (1) Who should be responsible for carrying out the screening process? (2) What is the best method for capturing the data? (3) What is the optimal strategy for preventing and managing comorbidities?

One of the main issues raised around managing comorbidities is the question of responsibility, and this varies depending on the set-up of healthcare systems. Evidence show that most rheumatologists agree that it is their responsibility to assess for comorbidities and liaise with another appropriate health professional (general practitioner or other specialists) [75]. In an ideal set-up, the rheumatologist in their daily interactions with the patient would be able to address all issues surrounding the main disease, including disease manifestations, treatment responses and adverse events. In addition to focusing on the main disease, they would identify comorbid conditions, adjust treatments accordingly and promote healthy lifestyle measures. However, the complex nature of some of the cases and the pressures on healthcare systems can make this task challenging at a rheumatology clinic visit.

Recently, EULAR [75] has published points to consider for reporting, screening for and preventing selected comorbidities in chronic inflammatory rheumatic diseases in daily practice. They recommended 15 points to consider and emphasised on three main principles: (1) Comorbidities such as cardiovascular diseases, malignancies, infections, osteoporosis, peptic ulcer and depression should be carefully assessed and managed in patients with chronic inflammatory rheumatic diseases. (2)

All clinicians including health professionals such as nurses, treating general practitioners and rheumatologists and patients through self-administered questionnaires and self-management programmes play a key role in the screening and detection of comorbidities. (3) Comorbidities should be subject to a systematic, standardised periodical review (e.g. at least every 5 years) for those with a chronic inflammatory rheumatic disease. They also provided a detailed practical form that can be used in daily clinical practice, which focused on six selected comorbidities: CVD, malignancies, infections, gastrointestinal diseases, osteoporosis and depression [75].

Rheumatologists in France have aimed to implement these EULAR guidance points to collect and report comorbidities [76]. They also developed management recommendations for selected comorbidities for the treating rheumatologist to use in daily practice, along with a document highlighting collecting and the management of each comorbidity. One of their aims was to provide the rheumatologist a pragmatic guide with specific systemic screening questions but also direct when and which patient requires input from other specialities.

The Canadian Dermatology-Rheumatology initiative has also developed evidence-based recommendations for the management of comorbidities in RA, psoriasis and psoriatic arthritis [77]. They proposed 19 recommendations based around eight common comorbid conditions. The eight focus topics included risk of CVD, effect of treatment on CVD, smoking, weight, malignancies and infections, risk of cancer recurrence or new cancer linked to treatment, osteoporosis and depression. The recommendations centred on diagnosis, management and prevention of comorbidities. Similarly, the Brazilian Society of Rheumatology has also developed recommendations for the management of comorbidities in patients with RA [78]. They included 13 recommendations based on early diagnosis and management of comorbidities, including hypertension, diabetes, metabolic syndrome and atherosclerosis. They also proposed a multidisciplinary approach when managing comorbidities and made drug-specific recommendations for certain comorbidities.

Screening

There are validated screening tools to collect comorbidities. The two main ways to collect the information is to either document them as individual entities (e.g. diabetes, hypertension, etc.) or summarise the comorbidity information into a single score that provides a single parameter for measuring multiple comorbidities, e.g. comorbidity indices and self-administered morbidity questionnaires (this will be discussed in detail in a separate chapter in this book) [79].

Comorbidity indices are useful in predicting outcome, for example, the Charlson Comorbidity Index (CCI) is a validated tool most commonly used to predict 1-year patient mortality [80]. The score is based on 19 predefined comorbidities that were assigned weights 1, 2, 3 and 6, according to the magnitude of the adjusted relative risk associated with each comorbidity [58]. Similarly, FRAX scores in osteoporosis have been successfully applied to predict 10-year probability of a major or hip fracture [81], as well as to guide treatments.

There have been proposals to develop a disease-specific comorbidity scoring system that would be able to predict morbidity, mortality and utilisation of health and cost. As the currently used risk assessment tools such as Framingham Risk Score may not reflect the true CVD risk in patients with rheumatic diseases, one such model has been proposed for RA (RA comorbidity index), which includes parameters such as DAS28 and HAQ scores, steroid therapy, seropositivity, elevated erythrocyte sedimentation rate, age >50 and several cardiovascular diseases [58, 82, 83].

There are several different models of care being used to monitor or screen for comorbidities associated with rheumatic diseases. It is also worth noting the timing of screening for comorbidities; in general population studies, early detection and treatment prevents mortality [84]. For optimal management of comorbidities, patients need to be assessed early and regularly in clinics. The QUEST-RA programme [85] was developed to promote quantitative monitoring of RA patients in daily clinical practice. The assessment included patient self-reported questionnaires incorporating questions on functional and psychological capacity, life style, joint pain and stiffness and work status. This was combined with physician's clinical evaluation, which included disease activity scores, record of extra articular RA features, medication review and past and current comorbidities.

It is worth noting that systemic screening for certain comorbidities may raise concerns regarding anxiety induced by false-positive tests, risk of overtreatment and also the impact on health and financial resources [75]. Furthermore, screening programmes need to be cost-effective, as they have a marked impact on healthcare utilisation and costs. A Canadian study reported routine screening for depression leading to increased treatment rates, but not necessarily reduced impact of depression [75].

Systemic screening is a comprehensive approach to capture comorbidities; however, it can be time-consuming and always not possible to carry out in a busy rheumatology clinic. Some of the suggested models include dedicated systemic yearly review clinics run by rheumatologists or specialist nurses. Use of electronic medical records and screening forms may enhance the impact of screening programmes.

Nurse-led screening programmes have been shown to be effective in managing CVD risk, vaccination uptake and osteoporosis. In a recent study, the impact of nurse-led programme on comorbidity management and patient self-assessment of disease activity was evaluated in 970 patients with RA [60]. In the comorbidity arm, the nurses assessed the patients for comorbidities and reported the results to the rheumatologist and the general practitioner. The number of measures taken per patient was significantly higher in the comorbidity group compared to self-assessment group, 4.54 ± 2.08 versus 2.65 ± 1.57 ($p < 0.001$).

Recently, it has been shown that patient-reported outcome measures (PROMs) are a valuable, efficient and cost-effective method for screening for comorbidities [58]. These measurements can be incorporated into the comorbidity index scores, which will improve capturing all aspects of the disease as well as the comorbidities.

The current knowledge on influence of comorbidities in rheumatic diseases has emphasised the importance of moving away from a disease-orientated model of care to a more multifaceted, goal-orientated approach. One such model of care has been proposed to include comorbidities, patient-reported outcomes, shared decision-making, disease activity measures, early treatment strategies and patient education [58].

Conclusion

Our knowledge on the impact of comorbidity on rheumatic diseases is improving. It is suggested that moving attention away from managing one single disease model to a more holistic approach will likely result in better quality of care for the patients. Consensus recommendations on screening and optimal management of comorbidities require expansion and updating to reflect the more global approach outlined in this chapter. It is likely that increasing focus on pragmatic solutions for managing these patients in a multi-specialty, multidisciplinary clinical setting will enable us to reduce complications related to comorbidities, improve quality of care and reduce mortality and burden on health systems.

Managing comorbidities should incorporate patient education and health promotion as well as coordination with other specialities and primary care. The development and implementation of standardised programmes to detect, manage and prevent comorbidities in daily clinical practice may greatly facilitate the identification of and interventions to reduce the prevalence of comorbidities among patients with RA.

In future, the influence of comorbidities on outcome measures in relation to clinical trials and clinical practice should encourage development of disease-specific outcome measures that account for comorbidity. Moreover, disease-specific risk assessment tools will enhance screening and preventative strategies, as well as target at-risk groups early. Improving adherence to screening for comorbidities can be achieved by implementing efficient, comprehensive and realistic care plans.

Finally, development of new treatment models, which are goal orientated and integrate all aspects that influence outcome, including comorbidities, will enrich the quality of care for patients with rheumatic disease.

Key Points

- Comorbidities are detected more frequently in patients with rheumatic diseases compared to the general population.
- Comorbidities adversely affect quality of life, disability, disease outcome and mortality in patients with rheumatic diseases.
- Evaluation for comorbidity should be a crucial part of disease assessments.
- Management involves screening for comorbidities early, prevention and treatment.
- New models of care incorporating comorbidity assessment and management can be expected to improve outcomes.

References

1. Feinstein AR. The pre-therapeutic classification of co-morbidity in chronic disease. J Chronic Dis. 1970;23:455–68.

2. Gabriel SE, Michaud K. Epidemiological studies in incidence, prevalence, mortality, and comorbidity of the rheumatic diseases. Arthritis Res Ther. 2009;11:229.
3. Norton S, Koduri G, Nikiphorou E, Dixey J, Williams P, Young A. A study of baseline prevalence and cumulative incidence of comorbidity and extra-articular manifestations in RA and their impact on outcome. Rheumatology (Oxford). 2013;52:99–110.
4. Radner H, Yoshida K, Smolen JS, Solomon DH. Multimorbidity and rheumatic conditions-enhancing the concept of comorbidity. Nat Rev Rheumatol. 2014;10:252–6.
5. Dougados M, Soubrier M, Antunez A, et al. Prevalence of comorbidities in rheumatoid arthritis and evaluation of their monitoring: results of an international, cross-sectional study (COMORA). Ann Rheum Dis. 2014;73:62–8.
6. Hyrich KL, Watson KD, Isenberg DA, Symmons DP, Register BSRB. The British society for rheumatology biologics register: 6 years on. Rheumatology (Oxford). 2008;47:1441–3.
7. Innala L, Sjoberg C, Moller B, et al. Co-morbidity in patients with early rheumatoid arthritis – inflammation matters. Arthritis Res Ther. 2016;18:33.
8. Gabriel SE, Crowson CS, O'Fallon WM. Comorbidity in arthritis. J Rheumatol. 1999;26:2475–9.
9. Kroot EJ, van Gestel AM, Swinkels HL, Albers MM, van de Putte LB, van Riel PL. Chronic comorbidity in patients with early rheumatoid arthritis: a descriptive study. J Rheumatol. 2001;28:1511–7.
10. Kapetanovic MC, Lindqvist E, Simonsson M, Geborek P, Saxne T, Eberhardt K. Prevalence and predictive factors of comorbidity in rheumatoid arthritis patients monitored prospectively from disease onset up to 20 years: lack of association between inflammation and cardiovascular disease. Scand J Rheumatol. 2010;39:353–9.
11. Molto A, Etcheto A, van der Heijde D, et al. Prevalence of comorbidities and evaluation of their screening in spondyloarthritis: results of the international cross-sectional ASAS-COMOSPA study. Ann Rheum Dis. 2016;75:1016–23.
12. Starfield B. Threads and yarns: weaving the tapestry of comorbidity. Ann Fam Med. 2006;4:101–3.
13. Sokka T, Puolakka K, Turesson C. Comorbidities of rheumatic disease. In: Watts PGC RA, Denton C, Foster H, Isaacs J, Müller-Ladner U, editors. Oxford textbook of rheumatology. 4th ed. Oxford: Oxford University Press; 2013. p. 1–26.
14. Smolen JS, Landewe R, Breedveld FC, et al. EULAR recommendations for the management of rheumatoid arthritis with synthetic and biological disease-modifying antirheumatic drugs: 2013 update. Ann Rheum Dis. 2014;73:492–509.
15. Aletaha D, Dorner T. Considering comorbidity in managing rheumatic diseases: going where trials cannot go. Arthritis Res Ther. 2011;13:116.
16. Dougados M. Comorbidities in rheumatoid arthritis. Curr Opin Rheumatol. 2016;28:282–8.
17. Nakajima A, Inoue E, Shimizu Y, et al. Presence of comorbidity affects both treatment strategies and outcomes in disease activity, physical function, and quality of life in patients with rheumatoid arthritis. Clin Rheumatol. 2015;34:441–9.
18. Iikuni N, Inoue E, Tanaka E, et al. Low disease activity state with corticosteroid may not represent 'true' low disease activity state in patients with rheumatoid arthritis. Rheumatology (Oxford). 2008;47:519–21.
19. Seto Y, Inoue E, Shidara K, et al. Functional disability can deteriorate despite suppression of disease activity in patients with rheumatoid arthritis: a large observational cohort study. Mod Rheumatol. 2013;23:1179–85.
20. Al-Bishri J, Attar S, Bassuni N, et al. Comorbidity profile among patients with rheumatoid arthritis and the impact on prescriptions trend. Clin Med Insights Arthritis Musculoskelet Disord. 2013;6:11–8.
21. Kalkan A, Hallert E, Bernfort L, Husberg M, Carlsson P. Costs of rheumatoid arthritis during the period 1990–2010: a register-based cost-of-illness study in Sweden. Rheumatology (Oxford). 2014;53:153–60.

22. van Onna M, Boonen A. The challenging interplay between rheumatoid arthritis, ageing and comorbidities. BMC Musculoskelet Disord. 2016;17:184.
23. Cross M, Smith E, Hoy D, et al. The global burden of rheumatoid arthritis: estimates from the global burden of disease 2010 study. Ann Rheum Dis. 2014;73:1316–22.
24. Gavan S, Harrison M, Iglesias C, Barton A, Manca A, Payne K. Economics of stratified medicine in rheumatoid arthritis. Curr Rheumatol Rep. 2014;16:468.
25. Joyce AT, Smith P, Khandker R, Melin JM, Singh A. Hidden cost of rheumatoid arthritis (RA): estimating cost of comorbid cardiovascular disease and depression among patients with RA. J Rheumatol. 2009;36:743–52.
26. McPhail SM. Multimorbidity in chronic disease: impact on health care resources and costs. Risk Manag Healthc Policy. 2016;9:143–56.
27. Hopman P, Heins MJ, Rijken M, Schellevis FG. Health care utilization of patients with multiple chronic diseases in The Netherlands: differences and underlying factors. Eur J Intern Med. 2015;26:190–6.
28. de Groot V, Beckerman H, Lankhorst GJ, Bouter LM. How to measure comorbidity. A critical review of available methods. J Clin Epidemiol. 2003;56:221–9.
29. Sokka T, Abelson B, Pincus T. Mortality in rheumatoid arthritis: 2008 update. Clin Exp Rheumatol. 2008;26:S35–61.
30. Gabriel SE. Cardiovascular morbidity and mortality in rheumatoid arthritis. Am J Med. 2008;121:S9–14.
31. Scherrer JF, Virgo KS, Zeringue A, et al. Depression increases risk of incident myocardial infarction among veterans administration patients with rheumatoid arthritis. Gen Hosp Psychiatry. 2009;31:353–9.
32. Ang DC, Choi H, Kroenke K, Wolfe F. Comorbid depression is an independent risk factor for mortality in patients with rheumatoid arthritis. J Rheumatol. 2005;32:1013–9.
33. van den Hoek J, Boshuizen HC, Roorda LD, et al. Association of somatic comorbidities and comorbid depression with mortality in patients with rheumatoid arthritis: a 14-year prospective cohort study. Arthritis Care Res. 2016;68:1055–60.
34. Avina-Zubieta JA, Thomas J, Sadatsafavi M, Lehman AJ, Lacaille D. Risk of incident cardiovascular events in patients with rheumatoid arthritis: a meta-analysis of observational studies. Ann Rheum Dis. 2012;71:1524–9.
35. Davis JM 3rd, Roger VL, Crowson CS, Kremers HM, Therneau TM, Gabriel SE. The presentation and outcome of heart failure in patients with rheumatoid arthritis differs from that in the general population. Arthritis Rheum. 2008;58:2603–11.
36. Nurmohamed MT, Heslinga M, Kitas GD. Cardiovascular comorbidity in rheumatic diseases. Nat Rev Rheumatol. 2015;11:693–704.
37. Kapetanovic MC, Lindqvist E, Geborek P, Saxne T, Eberhard K. Long-term mortality rate in rheumatoid arthritis patients with disease onset in the 1980s. Scand J Rheumatol. 2011;40:433–8.
38. Michaud K, Wallenstein G, Wolfe F. Treatment and nontreatment predictors of health assessment questionnaire disability progression in rheumatoid arthritis: a longitudinal study of 18,485 patients. Arthritis Care Res. 2011;63:366–72.
39. Radner H, Smolen JS, Aletaha D. Impact of comorbidity on physical function in patients with rheumatoid arthritis. Ann Rheum Dis. 2010;69:536–41.
40. Fries JF, Spitz P, Kraines RG, Holman HR. Measurement of patient outcome in arthritis. Arthritis Rheum. 1980;23:137–45.
41. Michaud K, Wolfe F. Comorbidities in rheumatoid arthritis. Best Pract Res Clin Rheumatol. 2007;21:885–906.
42. Charlson M, Szatrowski TP, Peterson J, Gold J. Validation of a combined comorbidity index. J Clin Epidemiol. 1994;47:1245–51.
43. Radner H, Smolen JS, Aletaha D. Comorbidity affects all domains of physical function and quality of life in patients with rheumatoid arthritis. Rheumatology (Oxford). 2011;50:381–8.

44. van den Hoek J, Roorda LD, Boshuizen HC, Tijhuis GJ, van den Bos GA, Dekker J. Physical and mental functioning in patients with established rheumatoid arthritis over an 11-year followup period: the role of specific comorbidities. J Rheumatol. 2016;43:307–14.
45. Ware JE Jr. SF-36 health survey update. Spine (Phila Pa 1976). 2000;25:3130–9.
46. Morris A, Yelin EH, Panopalis P, Julian L, Katz PP. Long-term patterns of depression and associations with health and function in a panel study of rheumatoid arthritis. J Health Psychol. 2011;16:667–77.
47. Ranganath VK, Maranian P, Elashoff DA, et al. Comorbidities are associated with poorer outcomes in community patients with rheumatoid arthritis. Rheumatology (Oxford). 2013;52:1809–17.
48. Sokka T, Hetland ML, Makinen H, et al. Remission and rheumatoid arthritis: data on patients receiving usual care in twenty-four countries. Arthritis Rheum. 2008;58:2642–51.
49. Burmester GR, Ferraccioli G, Flipo RM, et al. Clinical remission and/or minimal disease activity in patients receiving adalimumab treatment in a multinational, open-label, twelve-week study. Arthritis Rheum. 2008;59:32–41.
50. Martin WJ, Shim M, Paulus HE, et al. Older age at rheumatoid arthritis onset and comorbidities correlate with less health assessment questionnaire-disability index and clinical disease activity index response to etanercept in the RADIUS 2 registry. J Clin Rheumatol. 2014;20:301–5.
51. Rupp I, Boshuizen HC, Jacobi CE, Dinant HJ, van den Bos G. Comorbidity in patients with rheumatoid arthritis: effect on health-related quality of life. J Rheumatol. 2004;31:58–65.
52. Group TE. EuroQol: a new facility for the measurement of health-related quality of life. Health Policy. 1990;16:199–208.
53. Wolfe F, Michaud K, Li T, Katz RS. Chronic conditions and health problems in rheumatic diseases: comparisons with rheumatoid arthritis, noninflammatory rheumatic disorders, systemic lupus erythematosus, and fibromyalgia. J Rheumatol. 2010;37:305–15.
54. Lee TJ, Park BH, Son HK, et al. Cost of illness and quality of life of patients with rheumatoid arthritis in South Korea. Value Health. 2012;15:S43–9.
55. Salaffi F, Carotti M, Ciapetti A, Gasparini S, Grassi W. A comparison of utility measurement using EQ-5D and SF-6D preference-based generic instruments in patients with rheumatoid arthritis. Clin Exp Rheumatol. 2011;29:661–71.
56. Studenic P, Radner H, Smolen JS, Aletaha D. Discrepancies between patients and physicians in their perceptions of rheumatoid arthritis disease activity. Arthritis Rheum. 2012;64:2814–23.
57. Uutela T, Kautiainen H, Jarvenpaa S, Salomaa S, Hakala M, Hakkinen A. Patients with rheumatoid arthritis have better functional and working ability but poorer general health and higher comorbidity rates today than in the late 1990s. Scand J Rheumatol. 2015;44:173–81.
58. El Miedany Y. Co-morbidity index in rheumatoid arthritis: time to think. Clin Rheumatol. 2015;34:1995–2000.
59. National Institute for Health and Clinical Excellence (NICE). The management of rheumatoid arthritis in adults; 2009. Available at: http://www.nice.org.uk/CG79.
60. Dougados M, Soubrier M, Perrodeau E, et al. Impact of a nurse-led programme on comorbidity management and impact of a patient self-assessment of disease activity on the management of rheumatoid arthritis: results of a prospective, multicentre, randomised, controlled trial (COMEDRA). Ann Rheum Dis. 2015;74:1725–33.
61. Peters MJ, Symmons DP, McCarey D, et al. EULAR evidence-based recommendations for cardiovascular risk management in patients with rheumatoid arthritis and other forms of inflammatory arthritis. Ann Rheum Dis. 2010;69:325–31.
62. Primdahl J, Clausen J, Horslev-Petersen K. Results from systematic screening for cardiovascular risk in outpatients with rheumatoid arthritis in accordance with the EULAR recommendations. Ann Rheum Dis. 2013;72:1771–6.
63. van Assen S, Bijl M. Immunization of patients with autoimmune inflammatory rheumatic diseases (the EULAR recommendations). Lupus. 2012;21:162–7.
64. Sowden E, Mitchell WS. An audit of influenza and pneumococcal vaccination in rheumatology outpatients. BMC Musculoskelet Disord. 2007;8:58.

65. Feuchtenberger M, Kleinert S, Schwab S, et al. Vaccination survey in patients with rheumatoid arthritis: a cross-sectional study. Rheumatol Int. 2012;32:1533–9.
66. Haugeberg G, Uhlig T, Falch JA, Halse JI, Kvien TK. Bone mineral density and frequency of osteoporosis in female patients with rheumatoid arthritis: results from 394 patients in the Oslo County rheumatoid arthritis register. Arthritis Rheum. 2000;43:522–30.
67. Briot K, Roux C. Glucocorticoid-induced osteoporosis. RMD Open. 2015;1:e000014.
68. van Staa TP, Geusens P, Bijlsma JW, Leufkens HG, Cooper C. Clinical assessment of the long-term risk of fracture in patients with rheumatoid arthritis. Arthritis Rheum. 2006;54:3104–12.
69. Hoes JN, Jacobs JW, Boers M, et al. EULAR evidence-based recommendations on the management of systemic glucocorticoid therapy in rheumatic diseases. Ann Rheum Dis. 2007;66:1560–7.
70. Duru N, van der Goes MC, Jacobs JW, et al. EULAR evidence-based and consensus-based recommendations on the management of medium to high-dose glucocorticoid therapy in rheumatic diseases. Ann Rheum Dis. 2013;72:1905–13.
71. Gullick NJ, Scott DL. Co-morbidities in established rheumatoid arthritis. Best Pract Res Clin Rheumatol. 2011;25:469–83.
72. Turesson C, Matteson EL. Malignancy as a comorbidity in rheumatic diseases. Rheumatology (Oxford). 2013;52:5–14.
73. Kremers HM, Bidaut-Russell M, Scott CG, Reinalda MS, Zinsmeister AR, Gabriel SE. Preventive medical services among patients with rheumatoid arthritis. J Rheumatol. 2003;30:1940–7.
74. Gossec L, Salejan F, Nataf H, et al. Challenges of cardiovascular risk assessment in the routine rheumatology outpatient setting: an observational study of 110 rheumatoid arthritis patients. Arthritis Care Res. 2013;65:712–7.
75. Baillet A, Gossec L, Carmona L, et al. Points to consider for reporting, screening for and preventing selected comorbidities in chronic inflammatory rheumatic diseases in daily practice: a EULAR initiative. Ann Rheum Dis. 2016;75:965–73.
76. Gossec L, Baillet A, Dadoun S, et al. Collection and management of selected comorbidities and their risk factors in chronic inflammatory rheumatic diseases in daily practice in France. Joint Bone Spine. 2016;83(5):501–9.
77. Roubille C, Richer V, Starnino T, et al. Evidence-based recommendations for the management of comorbidities in rheumatoid arthritis, psoriasis, and psoriatic arthritis: expert opinion of the Canadian dermatology-rheumatology comorbidity initiative. J Rheumatol. 2015;42:1767–80.
78. Pereira IA, Mota LM, Cruz BA, et al. 2012 Brazilian society of rheumatology consensus on the management of comorbidities in patients with rheumatoid arthritis. Rev Bras Reumatol. 2012;52:474–95.
79. Molto A, Dougados M. Comorbidity indices. Clin Exp Rheumatol. 2014;32:S-131–4.
80. Charlson ME, Pompei P, Ales KL, MacKenzie CR. A new method of classifying prognostic comorbidity in longitudinal studies: development and validation. J Chronic Dis. 1987;40:373–83.
81. Kanis JA, Oden A, Johansson H, Borgstrom F, Strom O, McCloskey E. FRAX and its applications to clinical practice. Bone. 2009;44:734–43.
82. El Miedany Y, El Gaafary M, Youssef S, Bahlas S, Ahmed I, Hegazi M. Rheumatoid arthritis comorbidity index: development and validation of a new specific tool for classifying prognostic comorbidity in rheumatoid arthritis patients. Ann Rheum Dis. 2016;75(Suppl2):154.
83. El Miedany Y, El Gaafary M, Youssef S, Bahlas S, Ahmed I, Hegazi M. Psoriatic arthritis comorbidity index: development and validation of a new specific tool for classifying prognostic comorbidity in psoriatic arthritis patients. Ann Rheum Dis. 2016;75(Suppl2):89.
84. Gonzalez A, Maradit Kremers H, Crowson CS, et al. The widening mortality gap between rheumatoid arthritis patients and the general population. Arthritis Rheum. 2007;56:3583–7.
85. Sokka T, Kautiainen H, Toloza S, et al. QUEST-RA: quantitative clinical assessment of patients with rheumatoid arthritis seen in standard rheumatology care in 15 countries. Ann Rheum Dis. 2007;66:1491–6.

Chapter 3
Rheumatoid Arthritis

Andrew Rutherford, Elena Nikiphorou, and James Galloway

There has been an explosion in the available evidence base for managing rheumatoid arthritis in the last 30 years. However, it is notable that the majority of clinical trials have recruited highly selected cohorts of people with active rheumatoid, with patients with multiple comorbidities excluded from study. This is not a criticism of the research, which sets out to test specific hypotheses (e.g. is anti-TNF effective for RA?), but an acknowledgement that such designs limit the external validity of findings: i.e. is the research relevant to the patient I am currently seeing in clinic?

The burden of societal comorbidity has been rising in recent decades, driven by two key factors: (1) increasing population longevity and (2) increased intensity of risk factors (smoking, alcohol, obesity). In rheumatoid arthritis, our patients are not exempted from these factors. Although historically RA was considered a cachectic state, associated with weight loss, this is now the exception. When we look in our clinic waiting rooms, we are perpetually reminded of the western epidemic of 'diabesity'.

Perhaps the most valuable pieces of recent research come from the COMORA study [1]. This is an international cross-sectional study of over four and half thousand patients. The population was representative of a contemporary RA cohort, with an average disease duration of 10 years. The most frequently associated diseases (past or current) were depression, 15%; asthma, 6.6%; cardiovascular events (myocardial infarction, stroke), 6%; solid malignancies (excluding basal cell carcinoma), 4.5%; and chronic obstructive pulmonary disease, 3.5% (Fig. 3.1).

The 'Questionnaires in Standard Monitoring of Patients with Rheumatoid Arthritis' (QUEST-RA) project was another multicentre international study that investigated the prevalence of comorbidities in RA. This showed that individuals

A. Rutherford • E. Nikiphorou • J. Galloway (✉)
Department of Rheumatology, King's College London, London, UK
e-mail: james.galloway@nhs.net

Y. El Miedany (ed.), *Comorbidity in Rheumatic Diseases*,
DOI 10.1007/978-3-319-59963-2_3

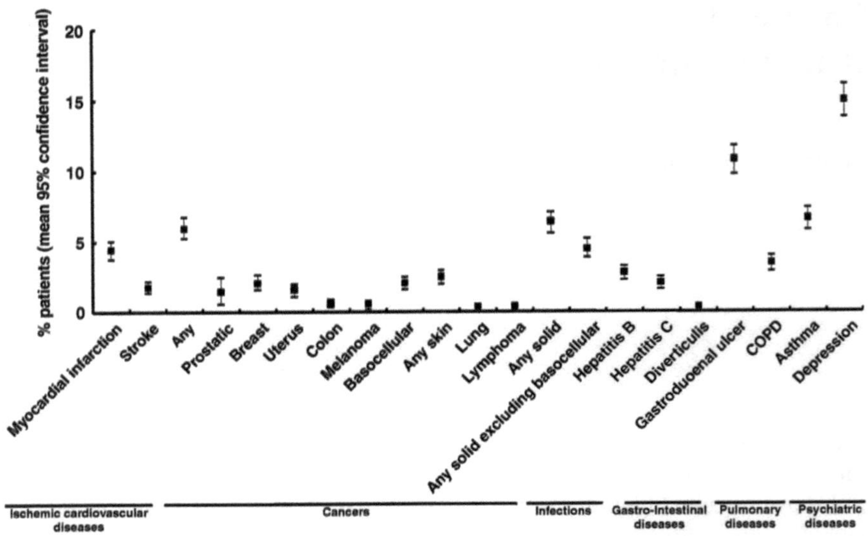

Fig. 3.1 Prevalence of evaluated comorbidities in the 3920 patients with rheumatoid arthritis. *COPD* chronic obstructive pulmonary disease (From Dougados et al. [1], with permission)

with RA had a median of two comorbid conditions with hypertension (31.5%), osteoporosis (17.6%), osteoarthritis (15.5%) and hyperlipidaemia (14.2%) the most prevalent [2]. The prevalence of comorbidities was greatest in countries with a high gross domestic product (GDP) which may represent a surveillance bias.

As a community, we must come up with cohesive strategies to best care for our patients, and part of this requires consideration of where responsibility lies. Is comorbidity management the responsibility of the primary care physician or the rheumatologist? There are two sides to this question: as experts in the field, we are likely to be more cognoscente of potential comorbidities; however, countenancing this, many rheumatologists would feel ill equipped to actively manage many comorbidities: what is the latest evidence base for managing hypertension, asthma and depression? What constitutes appropriate age-related screening for malignancy? Perhaps the pragmatic solution is to acknowledge that the role of the rheumatologist should be primarily in recognition of comorbidity rather than comprehensive disease management. After all, as a specialist community, we are not strangers to multisystem disease; indeed this could be considered to be one of our great strengths within our subspecialty.

The aim of this chapter is to highlight the relationship between RA and the major comorbidities that are encountered, considering prevalence, mechanistic relationships, impacts upon the disease and treatments and finally providing pragmatic strategies for screening and guidance on management.

Cardiovascular Disease

Cardiovascular disease in RA is common and associated with higher morbidity and mortality risk compared to the general population [3]. Data from the QUEST-RA project ($n = 4363$, 48 sites, 15 countries) suggest that the prevalence for lifetime cardiovascular events was 3.2% for myocardial infarction, 1.9% for stroke, and 9.3% for any cardiovascular event [4]. The prevalence for hypertension was 32% and for diabetes 8% [4]. The role of inflammation in the development of heart disease in RA is now better understood, with the recognition that the immune-related and mechanistic pathways of heart disease and RA have many similarities. Therefore, optimal control of the inflammation and metabolic changes in RA is crucial in preventing potentially lethal cardiovascular complications.

Pericardial Disease

Pericardial disease represents the most common autoimmune cardiac involvement in RA, seen in 30–50% of RA patients to some degree. It is often present concurrently with pleuritis, and myocardial and endocardial inflammation may also be seen [5]. Pericardial disease is associated with severely destructive patterns of RA, with nodulosis, other extra-articular manifestations and also male gender [6]. In the majority of cases, pericarditis seems to occur after the onset of arthritis; however, pericarditis can be a presenting symptom in some patients with RA. In these cases, a full workup including screening for autoantibodies is important. In patients with confirmed RA, treatment with NSAIDs, corticosteroids and/or other immunosuppressive drugs is appropriate and if severe, then pericardiectomy may need to be considered. The prognosis of RA patients with pericarditis appears to be impaired, especially in the first year after diagnosis, and is highest in those with constrictive or rapidly progressive effusive pericarditis [7].

Ischaemic Heart Disease

RA is a significant independent risk factor for premature ischaemic heart disease (IHD). Up to 50% of the excess mortality seen in RA is secondary to ischaemic heart disease (IHD) [8], with a 1.5-fold increase in the standardised mortality ratio due to cardiovascular events compared with the general population [9]. This is thought to be partly due to the enhancement of the atherogenic process in RA, with evidence of endothelial dysfunction culminating in increased arterial stiffness, plaque formation and coronary artery calcification [10]. Traditional cardiovascular risk factors alone (smoking, high lipid levels, diabetes, hypertension and BMI) do not seem to explain the presence of atherosclerotic disease, suggesting the implication of RA-related factors in the development of cardiovascular disease in RA. Furthermore, the higher frequency of ischaemic heart disease seen in established compared to early RA supports this concept [11].

Aside from acute coronary syndromes, cardiac ischaemia can result in ventricular arrhythmias, which can subsequently result in sudden cardiac death. Although abnormalities involving the coronary vessels in RA are mainly due to atherosclerosis, coronary vasculitis has been reported in up to 20% of post-mortem studies published in the early 1960s [12], although during life it is rarely diagnosed. Differentiating between cardiac vasculitis and atherosclerosis can be challenging but may be obtained via electron beam CT or through endomyocardial biopsy, and if the former is confirmed, prompt treatment with immunosuppressive drugs should be instituted.

Recent studies suggest that RA-associated inflammation may have a direct effect on lipoproteins such as HDL and also on the endothelial integrity. Effective treatment of RA has been associated with increased lipid levels, particularly total and HDL cholesterol levels. Studies have shown a significant inverse correlation of HDL and total cholesterol levels with disease activity in patients receiving nonbiologic DMARDs. Improvement in disease activity was linearly associated with the total cholesterol/HDL ratio ('atherogenic index'), due primarily to increases in HDL-C levels [13]. A study evaluating the effects of etanercept therapy in RA demonstrated an increase in overall lipid levels but a significant and sustained decrease in the apoB/apoA-I ratio in patients with good or moderate EULAR response [14]. This may have a beneficial effect on the cardiovascular risk in patients with RA. Other studies have shown that amongst RA patients on anti-TNF not receiving lipid-lowering therapy, there were increases in mean and total cholesterol [15]. Other possible roles of TNF-alpha in the development of atherosclerosis include the recruitment of inflammatory cells to the site of injury or the promotion of adverse vascular smooth muscle cell remodelling. TNF-alpha may also act as a proinflammatory factor in plaque rupture [16]. Tocilizumab (IL-6 receptor monoclonal antibody) has been associated with increased levels in total, HDL and LDL cholesterol with a recent study demonstrating an increase in these levels during the first year of tocilizumab treatment but no further increase during extension studies and stable atherogenic index [17]. Despite raised lipid profile levels, the anti-TNF agents and tocilizumab have been associated with potential cardiovascular protective effects including reduced arterial stiffness [18], reduced blood pressure [19], improvement in peripheral insulin sensitivity [20] and improvements in haemoglobin A1C in the case of tocilizumab [21].

Data from the Consortium of Rheumatology Research of North America (CORRONA) registry ($n = 10,156$) showed a reduced cardiovascular risk in anti-TNF users compared to users of nonbiologic DMARDs [22]. In contrast, data from the British Society for Rheumatology Biologics Register (BSRBR) cohort study showed no protective cardiovascular benefits in anti-TNF users compared to nonbiologic DMARD users [23], although an earlier study showed a reduced risk of myocardial infarction amongst anti-TNF patients with established (not early) RA [24].

Use of NSAIDs, COX-2 inhibitors and corticosteroids has also been implicated in ischaemic heart disease in RA, and they should be used with caution. However, prolonged use of treatments such as methotrexate, sulfasalazine, leflunomide, glucocorticoids and anti-TNF agents appears to be associated with a reduced risk of cardiovascular disease [4], through reduction of the inflammation and better control of disease activity.

Cardiomyopathy

RA-related cardiomyopathy is rare, and its aetiology can be challenging to unravel. It is thought to be the result of focal non-specific, diffuse necrotizing or granulomatous myocarditis based on post-mortem evidence [5]. Amyloid deposition has also been implicated as a rare cause of restrictive cardiomyopathy, more frequently associated with male gender and longer disease duration [25]. In these patients, early and intensified immunosuppressive therapy is crucial. Drugs used in RA have also been implicated in the onset of cardiomyopathy, as, for example, with corticosteroids and antimalarial drugs. In particular, antimalarial drug-related cardiotoxicity in the form of restrictive or dilated cardiomyopathy has been described, leading to heart transplantation [26]. Furthermore, corticosteroid exposure, NSAID use and anti-TNF agents could all contribute to ventricular dysfunction and cardiomyopathy, necessitating caution with their use in RA and other rheumatic diseases.

Congestive Cardiac Failure

Emerging evidence suggests that congestive cardiac failure appears to be an important contributor to the excess mortality seen in RA [27]. This is thought to be due to the increased incidence of CCF in RA compared to non-RA patients, rather than the increased mortality associated with CCF [28]. The risk of developing CCF in RA is twice that of developing CCF in non-RA persons, and this is not explained by traditional cardiovascular risk factors and/or clinical ischaemic heart disease [29]. Furthermore, studies have shown that left ventricular systolic dysfunction is three times more common than in the general population and is associated with abnormal electrocardiography, suggesting the latter as a useful means for evaluating these patients [30]. The observation for an increased acute-phase response prior to the new onset of cardiac failure suggests that inflammatory stimuli may be involved in the onset of CCF in RA [31]. Corticosteroids should be used with caution in CCF in RA, balancing the potential side effects with the advantages of corticosteroid use, namely, the reduction in inflammation, lipid-lowering effects and thereby the reduction in the pro-atherogenic effect of inflammation [13]. The use of anti-TNF in RA with cardiovascular disease has been debated due to the observation of an increased mortality in these patients, resulting in specific recommendations for the use of anti-TNF in patients with known CCF.

Valve Disease

Mitral valve insufficiency is the most prevalent valve disease seen in RA (30–80%), followed by aortic valve insufficiency (9–33%) [32]. Mitral valve disease appears to be associated with nodular RA. In a small study of 34 volunteers with RA undergoing transesophageal echocardiography, various different types of valve lesions were seen, with valve nodules and thickening being its distinctive features; others included valve regurgitation and stenotic valve lesions [33]. Even though the numbers were small, valvular heart disease was not found to correlate with duration, activity, severity, pattern of onset and course, extra-articular disease, serology or therapy of RA.

Arrhythmia Including QT Effects of Drugs

Arrhythmia in RA can be secondary to ischaemia, conduction defects as a result infiltration of the AV node or other conducting tissue by mononuclear cells or rheumatoid granulomas or rarely amyloid, vasculitis of the arterial supply to the conductive tissue, haemorrhage into a rheumatoid nodule, extension of an inflammatory lesion from the aortic or mitral valve and congestive cardiac failure [34]. Coronary vasculitis, superimposed coronary thrombosis, myocarditis and pulmonary hypertension further contribute to rhythm disturbances [34]. Infiltration of the atrioventricular (AV) node can cause right bundle branch block in 35% of patients [34]. AV block is usually complete but is rarely seen. If present though, it does not respond to anti-inflammatory and immunosuppressive therapy [34]. Complete heart block (CHB) has been described in 0.1% of RA patients, mainly in females, and appears to be more prevalent in patients with subcutaneous nodules [35]. However, in the small proportion of patients who are anti-Ro/SSA positive, no major conduction disorders were noted [36].

Studies have shown that QT intervals are longer in RA compared to healthy controls, suggesting that QT dispersion may be a useful marker of cardiovascular morbidity and mortality due to complex ventricular arrhythmias in RA [37].

Hypertension

Hypertension in RA is highly prevalent although it is often under-recognised and under-treated [38]. Studies suggest that hypertension associates with subclinical atherosclerosis in RA and is one of the most significant independent predictors of cardiovascular disease. Hypertension in RA seems to be driven, amongst other factors, by inflammation, physical inactivity but also polypharmacy [39]. Drugs implicated in the development or worsening of hypertension in RA include NSAIDs, coxibs, glucocorticoids and some disease-modifying drugs, and cautions should be taken especially if used concurrently and in the presence of underlying cardiovascular disease. Hypertension, including other cardiovascular risk factors such as smoking and hyperlipidaemia, should be specifically targeted for screening and treatment.

Stroke and Peripheral Vascular Disease

RA is associated with an accelerated cerebrovascular (as well as coronary artery) atherosclerosis and is a risk factor for ischaemic stroke [40]. The pathogenic mechanisms driving ischaemic stroke and peripheral vascular disease in RA include, firstly, atherosclerosis as an immune-mediated inflammatory process [41] and secondly by impaired endothelial dysfunction [42]. Furthermore, traditional cardiovascular risk factors are more prevalent in patients with systemic autoimmune diseases like RA, and finally, the higher risk of atherosclerosis and generally cardiovascular risk may be iatrogenic, as, for example, with use of NSAIDs and corticosteroids. Smoking is a common risk factor for RA and stroke, and in addition, the involvement of heart valve structure in RA may lead to atrial fibrillation, a well-documented risk factor for stroke [43].

Thromboembolic Disease

RA, like many other autoimmune-driven diseases, can be considered as a prothrombotic state, with a higher risk for cardiovascular disease and venous thromboembolic events. Based on data from a systematic review and meta-analysis, the pooled risk ratios of deep venous thrombosis, pulmonary embolism and venous thromboembolism in RA patients compared to non-RA persons were 2.08 (95% CI 1.75–2.47), 2.17 (95% CI 2.05–2.31) and 1.96 (95% CI 1.81–2.11), respectively [44].

Increased rheumatoid factor has been shown to be associated with up to a threefold increased long-term risk and up to a ninefold increased 1-year risk of deep venous thrombosis [45].

Respiratory Disease

Respiratory complications are common in rheumatoid arthritis. They can affect any part of the lung including the interstitium, airways and pleura. There is increasing evidence to suggest that the lung is an important site for inflammation induced by external triggers such as smoking which leads to generation of rheumatoid arthritis-specific immunity with secondary targeting of the joints [46]. However, there is also evidence suggesting that hypoxia is an important regulator of angiogenesis and inflammation in RA [47].

Interstitial Lung Disease

In routine clinical practice, the reported incidence of interstitial lung disease is estimated at about 4% [48]. This is likely to be an under-representation as imaging studies using computed tomography have shown that evidence of ILD is present in 15–20% of RA patients [49, 50]. Clinical examination and plain radiographs of the chest are both insensitive at detecting interstitial lung disease. Dawson et al. found that just 11% of patients with radiographically confirmed ILD had abnormalities on clinical examination [49].

Antibody status has long been associated with interstitial lung disease with both rheumatoid factor and anti-citrullinated protein antibodies (ACPA) conveying an increased risk [51]. Meta-analysis has shown that the risk of developing ILD is approximately three times higher in RA patients who are ACPA positive compared with those who are ACPA negative [52].

A British study found that articular disease usually predated the onset of ILD (83% of cases). Lung disease predated joint disease in 10% of cases, and the two conditions occurred simultaneously in 7% of cases [51]. ILD is associated with a threefold increase in mortality rates amongst patients with rheumatoid arthritis though the risk will vary depending on the ILD subtype [53].

Subtypes of ILD

The two most common subtypes of ILD seen in RA are usual interstitial pneumonia (UIP) and non-specific interstitial pneumonia (NSIP) though cryptogenic organising pneumonia is also seen. A multicentre study in the UK found that UIP accounted for 65% of ILD in RA, NSIP 24% and COP 5% [51]. The remaining 6% represented overlap syndromes. Lung biopsy is the gold standard for diagnosis of ILD, but with improved high-resolution CT scanning, this has become less common. There is good correlation between CT appearances and biopsy findings particularly with UIP [54].

Treatment of ILD in RA

Lung biopsies in RA patients show a different histological pattern with increased CD4+ T-cells when compared with idiopathic cases of ILD [55]. As such, treatment of interstitial lung disease in RA with immunosuppressive drugs is usually recommended irrespective of the subtype of ILD detected. This is in contrast to idiopathic pulmonary fibrosis where immunosuppressive therapy has not shown significant benefit. There are no high-quality randomised controlled trials comparing treatments, but azathioprine, cyclophosphamide and rituximab have all been used in patients with RA-associated ILD with varying degrees of success [56].

Treatment Considerations in ILD

The link between methotrexate and interstitial lung disease is controversial. Whilst there is good evidence that methotrexate can cause an acute pneumonitis, its role in the development of ILD is less clear [57]. Historically methotrexate was given to individuals with more severe RA who were more at risk of developing ILD leading to potential channelling bias in observational studies. A meta-analysis of over 1600 patients with psoriasis, psoriatic arthritis and inflammatory bowel disease found no increase in the incidence of lung disease [58]. A larger meta-analysis of RA patients did find an increased incidence of lung disease (RR 1.10, 95% confidence interval 1.02–1.19), though this was driven largely by an increase in the number of respiratory infections as opposed to ILD [57].

There are case reports linking leflunomide with the onset of ILD in RA, but a recent meta-analysis of eight RCTs containing 4579 participants did not show an increased risk of developing any form of lung disease [59]. In this study, there were six cases of pneumonitis reported but all were in the comparator arm [59].

Early RCTs of anti-TNF therapies did not show increased rates of ILD, but they were designed to demonstrate efficacy and were not powered to show a difference in rates of rare events such as ILD. However, there have been over 100 case reports of either incident ILD or worsening of existing ILD in patients commencing TNF inhibitors for the treatment of RA [60]. A large observational study of over 8000 patients found that anti-TNF did not increase the occurrence of ILD when compared with nonbiologic therapies, but this study did not examine the impact of anti-TNF on patients with existing lung disease [61].

Case reports have suggested that rituximab may be associated with the development of interstitial lung disease in patients with RA and lymphoma [62]. The most common presentation was acute/subacute hypoxaemic organising pneumonia starting 2 weeks after the last infusion and resolving with glucocorticoid therapy [62]. Rituximab has also been increasingly used as a potential treatment for ILD associated with RA, though the results have been mixed [63].

Airways Disease

Obstructive airways disease is common in RA affecting between 8% and 32% of patients [64, 65]. Smoking is a potential confounder but does not fully explain the increased risk of airways disease in patients with RA [66]. One study looking only at non-smokers found that patients with RA were significantly more likely to have obstructive spirometry compared with matched controls seen in a rheumatology clinic with degenerative or infective arthritis (16% vs 0%, $P < 0.001$) [67].

Bronchiectasis

Bronchiectasis and rheumatoid arthritis seem to occur together more often than one would expect by chance [68]. One of the earliest studies of bronchiectasis in RA found that it affected 3.1% of individuals compared with 0.3% of controls with osteoarthritis [69]. It also appears to be associated with increased mortality. A British case-control study found that patients with RA-bronchiectasis were 7.3 times more likely to die than the general population, 5.0 times more likely than the RA group and 2.4 times more likely than the bronchiectasis-only group [68].

Pleural Disease

Some degree of pleural disease is common in rheumatoid arthritis, but it is usually asymptomatic. Autopsy studies have shown that up to 70% of RA patients have a small pleural effusion, but only less than 5% of patients will develop symptomatic effusions [70].

Pulmonary Nodules

Rheumatoid nodules are thought to affect up to a third of seropositive patients with RA. Normally they are subcutaneous over extensor surfaces, but in approximately 0.4% of patients, they will occur in the lungs [71]. Pulmonary nodules do not generally cause any symptoms or require specific treatment. Case reports have shown regression with rituximab or tocilizumab.

Malignancy

Cancers and Rheumatoid Arthritis

A number of studies have contrasted the incidence of malignancies in people with rheumatoid arthritis to the general population, using standardised incidence ratios (SIRs). Overall the SIR appears to be increased by around about 30% with lung cancers and non-Hodgkin's lymphomas accounting for the bulk of the excess risk of cancer. Historically, cancers, such as bowel and breast, were reported as occurring at reduced frequency in rheumatoid arthritis, although more contemporary datasets have not confirmed this, perhaps due to historic protection from non-steroidal use, which has declined in recent years.

The excess risks in lung cancer are largely attributed to the shared risk factor of smoking whilst the risks of non-Hodgkin's lymphoma are attributed to the underlying disease process. A large case-control study of over 300 rheumatoid arthritis patients with lymphoma and over 300 rheumatoid arthritis patients without lymphoma found that those with lymphoma were 60-fold more likely to have been in the highest decile of cumulative disease activity [72]. Perhaps the most extreme example of the disease itself, causing lymphoma, comes from the example of Felty's syndrome – triad of seropositive rheumatoid with an enlarged spleen and agranulocytosis. It is now recognised that Felty's syndrome lies on the spectrum of an indolent T-cell large granular lymphoma, which occurs in the setting of long-standing untreated autoimmune disease.

The impact of drugs on cancer risks is less clear. There are some striking examples where drugs have definitely been implicated in cancer formation. For example, methotrexate-associated lymphoproliferative disorder – a condition which develops in people who have usually been on long-standing methotrexate and develop a disease that is clinically and histologically very similar to diffuse large B-cell lymphoma, but which regresses spontaneously (usually within 4 weeks) upon withdrawal of the methotrexate and does not recur. The methotrexate-associated lymphoproliferative diseases are more commonly EBV positive than the general B-cell lymphomas (44% versus 15%) [73]. This pattern of lymphoma however is very rare and looking at immunosuppressive treatments in more general manner, and their risk upon cancer has been less revealing. A significant amount of work has been done to look at biologic therapies and in particular the anti-tumour necrosis factor agents.

Data from numerous pharmacovigilance studies provide us with answers regarding biologic therapies and cancer risk, and indeed the British Society for Rheumatology Biologics Register (BSRBR-RA) was conceived and powered specifically to be able to detect a doubling in the risk of lymphoproliferative disease over 5 years.

Solid Cancers

The evidence regarding solid malignancies with biologic therapies is overwhelmingly reassuring. The data from the UK registry has shown no signal whatsoever of any excess risk of solid malignancies [74]. An important caveat to a number of these registries is that at the time the registries recruited patients there were recommendations in place that individuals with a prior history of malignancy should be excluded from receiving biologic therapy. In light of this, there may have been a selection bias earlier on in the registry removing at-risk individuals from the cohort. In order to address this, additional analyses were also conducted to look at survival after cancer diagnosis in patients enrolled in the register. It could also be argued that blocking the TNF pathway may not predispose people to more frequent incident cancers but might alter the body's ability to control the cancer if it developed, thereby cancer mortality may be different. The data were again reassuring, showing no difference in survival after a cancer diagnosis. This observation was replicated in the Swedish Biologics Register which confirmed any association between survival after a cancer diagnosis and biologic exposure. The Swedish dataset was able to take this one step further by looking at the recurrence rates in people with prior breast cancer who were initiated on an anti-TNF therapy within 5 years of their original tumour diagnosis [75]. A cohort of 120 rheumatoid arthritis individuals were matched to another group of patients without rheumatoid arthritis who had a cancer of similar stage and were never exposed to an anti-TNF therapy. Subsequent follow-up was then looked at to determine whether there was any difference in the rate of occurrence in the RA cohort who subsequently received anti-TNF after their cancer diagnosis (within 5 years of treatment) and demonstrated no difference: a further reassuring observation.

Skin Cancers

The relation between skin cancers and immune suppression is well established in the transplant field. It is known that in the general population approximately 80% of skin cancers are basal cell carcinoma, whilst 20% are squamous cell carcinomas. In the transplant literature, the skin cancer rate has increased by around 300-fold and that the ratio of squamous cell to base cell carcinomas is inverted. In the RA literature, no such excess risk is observed. Pulling the data from across the observational registries that have reported on skin cancers shows the hazard ratio is increased by approximately 30% and that there is no reversal of the ratio of squamous cell carcinomas and basal cell carcinomas – i.e. there appears to be a small but significant increase in the risk of predominantly basal cell skin cancers in patients on anti-TNF therapy. It is hard to know exactly how much this impacts on treatment decision as most basal cell carcinomas can be managed simply with topical therapy, cryotherapy or minor surgical resection. We know from the clinical trials and from the registry data that most people who have a basal cell skin cancer, whilst on anti-TNF therapy, remain on treatment.

Melanoma represents a distinct skin cancer in which there is a specific biological plausible link with anti-TNF therapy: indeed this has been shown that in people with limb melanoma, single limb perfusion with TNF itself can result in tumour regression. For this reason, specific research looking at melanoma has been conducted in countries with higher background rates of melanoma. In the UK, for example, melanoma is an exceptionally rare cancer, and there have simply been too few cases in the registry data to draw any conclusions. In the Scandinavian data in Sweden, the risk of melanoma with anti-TNF therapy has been reported at approximately 50% higher than the background rate [76]. However, a pooled analysis of over 130,000 patients from 11 different registers in Europe with over 500,000 patient years of follow-up did not show a significant link (standardised incidence ratio 1.2, 95% CI 0.99–1.60) [77].

Lymphoma

Lymphoma risk in rheumatoid arthritis has already been established to be increased, and it is associated with disease severity. Given that biologics tend to be administered to those with the most severe disease, there is important confounding that needs to be borne in mind when looking at analysis. However, to date data from the British registries as well as data from European collaboration have shown no signal for the increased risk of lymphoma that can be attributable to the drug [78]. However, all of these analysis come with two important caveats: one, lymphoma is a very rare event and the studies continue to lack robust power to be sure that they have excluded small risk differences; and two, the current duration for most of these studies averages around 5 years and the data thus far cannot exclude more delayed risks of cancer.

To summarise these findings, it would be reasonable to say that the research to date has not shown significant excess risk of cancers with biologics, but it must be emphasised that the data predominantly relate to TNF inhibitors and that for the rarer cancers (melanoma and lymphoma) further research is still needed. It is clear, however, that a prior malignancy in recent years, particularly of solid malignancies such as breast cancer, should not be considered as a contraindication to treatment with an anti-TNF in a patient in whom active rheumatoid is present and treatment is indicated.

Monitoring for Malignancy and Routine Care

It is always important to contextualise comorbidities, both in terms of relative and absolute risk and in the context of rheumatoid arthritis; although the relative risks for a number of cancer have increased, the absolute risk overall remains small, and there is no indication for extending screening beyond what is routinely done in the general population for most patients. For example, in the UK, there is a national breast screening programme for adult females aged between 50 and 73 years of age, bowel screening programme for people aged between 60 and 69 years of age and a cervical screening programme for women aged 25–64 years of age. Signposting patients to these services is important, particularly given the anecdotal reports from patients that they will see their rheumatologist, more often than their primary care practitioner and particularly a year of intensive management where we may be seeing patients three or four times a year; it is vital that they do not miss out on the standard screening interventions that are recommended for the general public.

Management of Patients Who Develop Malignancy During Treatment

Clearly, when someone is commenced on chemotherapy or is about to undergo surgery for the management of cancer, immunosuppression should be interrupted. In addition, many of the chemotherapy regimens are complemented by a biologic immune modulation targeting the cancer (e.g. checkpoint inhibition), and these may be aiming to directly activate the immune system, which can result in exacerbation of underlying autoimmune disease. In general, during active cancer treatment, the current dogma is to use cautious amounts of corticosteroids but avoid targeted immunosuppression. Once the cancer has been treated and cancer-specific immunosuppression is withdrawn, then cautious introduction of standard antirheumatic treatment is indicated. In this setting, most data available support the reintroduction of anti-TNF therapy, particularly in the context of solid malignancies. However, there are clear examples where a cancer subtype might prompt a change of treatment from the rheumatoid perspective – e.g. preferential use of rituximab in people who have had B-cell malignancies or avoidance of TNF pathway drugs in patients with prior melanoma.

Infections

Infections can be a major problem in patients with RA. A UK-based survey found that 7.7% of patients reported an admission to hospital for serious infection in the preceding 12-month period [79]. Many more experienced infections that didn't require hospitalisation with 40% of respondents reporting that they had received at least one course of antibiotics over the same period [79]. An American cohort study found that individuals with RA were approximately 50% more likely than matched non-RA controls to suffer from serious infections (rate ratio 1.53, 95% CI 1.41–1.65) [80].

There are several proposed mechanisms as to why patients with RA are more susceptible to infections but broadly speaking these fall into two categories, first the disease itself and second treatment effects.

Rheumatoid arthritis has long been associated with neutropaenia which may occur due to either to the presence of circulating immune complexes or to a reduced marrow neutrophil reserve [81]. Studies examining T-cell homeostasis have shown premature 'immunological ageing' with RA patients in their 20s and 30s having levels of TREC CD4 + ve T-cells similar to those found in health controls in their 50s and 60s [82].

The strongest predictor of infection in RA patients is a past history of hospitalised infection though increasing age, disability, active disease and drug treatments have all been shown to significantly increase the risk of developing infections [83].

Nonbiologic DMARDs and Infections

Whilst nonbiologic DMARDs have long been linked with an increase in risk of infection, the evidence is less clear cut. A large Canadian observational study containing over 27,000 individuals with 162,000 patient years of follow-up did not find an increased risk of infection in individuals on DMARDs alone (adjusted RR 0.92, 95% CI 0.85–1.0) [84]. A limitation of this study is that it did not differentiate between the type and dose of DMARD being used.

Most studies looking at individual DMARDs are of methotrexate users and have shown contradictory findings. This may be due to variations in the dose used as well as the choice of control and degree of adjustment for potential confounders. A prospective cohort study in the Netherlands found that the risk of infection and antibiotic usage amongst methotrexate users was increased compared with RA controls not on methotrexate [85]. A more recent analysis of methotrexate users in the REAL database in Japan did not find an increased risk of infection compared with individuals using alternative treatments [86]. However, the comparator group in this study was a very heterogeneous group of patients using different synthetic DMARDs and biologics to control their RA.

An early phase 3 trial of leflunomide found that the rate of serious infection was not any higher in those taking leflunomide than those taking either placebo or sulfasalazine [87]. However, this study was powered to assess efficacy and not rarer safety outcomes. Larger-scale registry data have since shown that leflunomide appears to be associated with an increased risk of developing infections in particular pneumonia [88].

Glucocorticoids have long been associated with an increased risk of infection. However, a large meta-analysis of 21 RCTs found no increase in the rate of infection amongst glucocorticoid users (RR 0.97–95% CI, 0.69–1.36) [89]. Small numbers of events and inconsistent reporting of adverse events in the trials meant that a clinically important increase or decrease in infection rates could not be ruled out. Interestingly the same meta-analysis looked at 42 observational studies and found a significant increase in infection rates amongst glucocorticoid users (RR of 1.67–95% CI, 1.49–1.87) [89].

Biologics and Infections

Biologics have revolutionised the treatment of RA but are associated with an increased risk of infection. Registry data from the UK has shown that the risk of infection is approximately 20% higher in anti-TNF users than in similar RA patients treated with DMARDs [90]. The risk appears to be greatest in the first 6–12 months of therapy, and by 3 years, there was no longer an increased risk [90]. The impact of anti-TNF on infection risk is bigger for some infections than others. Soft tissue, skin and joint infections are all seen significantly more frequently in patients treated with anti-TNF than matched controls [91, 92]. In early studies of anti-TNF drugs, there was an increase in the incidence of reactivation of latent TB [93]. However, with better screening techniques for latent TB now available, this risk appears to be falling [94].

A small proportion of infections in patients treated with biologics will be opportunistic infections. Opportunistic infections occur at a rate approximately tenfold higher than the general population though the absolute risk is small affecting approximately 0.1% of biologic-treated RA patients each year [95].

Viral Hepatitis and Rheumatoid Arthritis

Treatment of rheumatoid arthritis in patient with hepatitis B and hepatitis C can present a unique challenge. DMARDs such as leflunomide and methotrexate can cause direct liver injury, whilst other immunosuppressants such as glucocorticoids and biologics alter the host's immune response to the hepatitis infection [96, 97]. In a prospective study of over 500 RA patients with evidence of previous hepatitis B infection, the risk of hepatotoxicity was approx. 3% [96]. The risk was the same in those treated with nonbiologic DMARDs as those treated with biologics (2.6% vs 2.8%, $p = 0.87$). Of those who developed hepatotoxicity, there were no cases of liver failure, hepatic encephalopathy or liver transplant [96].

HIV and Rheumatoid Arthritis

With improving survival in HIV, we are likely to see more patients with coexisting HIV and rheumatoid arthritis. HIV itself can lead to the development of rheumatoid factor and anti-cyclic citrullinated peptide antibodies but usually at low titres of doubtful significance [98]. There is insufficient safety data to recommend use of specific DMARDs in RA patients with HIV [98]. One of the main concerns in HIV patients is the potential for drug interactions. Ritonavir in particular is a potent inhibitor of the cytochrome P450 3A4 and can dramatically increase the serum concentration of drugs cleared by this pathway including methotrexate and glucocorticoids [99]. There are case reports of patients on ritonavir developing cushingoid features following a single intra-articular injection of triamcinolone.

Rheumatoid Vasculitis

Rheumatoid vasculitis is an extra-articular manifestation of the disease and not a comorbidity per se. The incidence appears to be falling with data from the Norfolk Vasculitis Register showing an incidence of 9.1 cases annually per million population between 1988 and 2000 compared with 3.9 cases annually per million population between 2001 and 2010 [100]. This is likely to represent better treatment of RA since the advent of biologics as well as lower rates of smoking. Smoking and extra-articular manifestations such as rheumatoid nodules are strongly associated with the development of rheumatoid vasculitis [101]. Presentation usually occurs in patients with long-standing RA and is unusual in those with a disease duration of less than 5 years. Rheumatoid vasculitis affects small- and medium-sized vessels and most commonly presents in the skin but can affect any organ system [101]. There are no validated diagnostic or classification criteria for rheumatoid vasculitis, and it is a relatively rare entity making high-quality trials of treatments a challenge. An open trial of 45 patients with rheumatoid vasculitis suggested that cyclophosphamide and methylprednisolone were superior to conventional treatment at healing leg ulcers and neuropathy with a lower rate of relapse [102].

Secondary MSK Disease

Osteoporosis

Individuals with rheumatoid arthritis are at increased risk of fractures. A large study of primary care patients in the UK found that the risk of hip and vertebral fractures was doubled in RA patients compared with age- and sex-matched controls [103]. The reason for this increased risk is multifactorial with disease-specific effects on bone mineral density, treatment side effects and an increased risk of falling due to sarcopaenia all playing a role [104]. There is evidence to suggest that effective treatment of RA can help to prevent the loss of bone mineral density [105]. However, larger-scale trials with longer duration are required to assess the impact of treatment on fracture rates.

Osteoarthritis

Secondary osteoarthritis is a problem in many patients with RA. There is evidence that the number and volume of joint erosions correlates positively with the number and volume of osteophytes in patients with RA [106]. Even in an early RA patients, the prevalence of osteoarthritis on baseline hand and feet radiographs is 40–50% [107].

Fibromyalgia

Fibromyalgia is thought to affect approximately 2% of the general population but is seen in approximately 17% of RA patients [108]. This is a major challenge for clinicians as typical disease measures such as DAS28 do not distinguish between active inflammatory arthritis and fibromyalgia. A recent study of RA patients with a DAS28 score above 2.6 found that those with concurrent fibromyalgia had higher disease activity scores, worse disability but significantly less power Doppler and greyscale synovitis on ultrasound [109]. Whilst patients with fibromyalgic RA may show response to treatment, they are much less likely to achieve remission or low disease activity states [110]. Managing patients with persistent physical symptoms in the absence of inflammation is an increasing challenge in RA.

Psychological Comorbidity

Psychological comorbidity is a major problem in RA. With intensive treatment strategies, we are getting better at treating the inflammatory component of RA but we are not seeing the same degree of improvement in quality of life outcomes. A multicentre observational study over 18 years in the UK showed that the average DAS28 had fallen from 5.2 to 3.7 between 1996 and 2014 but HAQ remained unchanged (1.30–1.32) over the same period [111]. This shows that focussing treatment entirely on reducing synovitis is insufficient and a more holistic approach to RA is required addressing biological, psychological and social factors.

Depression

Depression is a common feature in many chronic diseases. A large meta-analysis of 72 studies with over 13,000 participants found that the incidence of major depressive disorders in RA was 16% [112]. The same meta-analysis found significant depressive symptoms present in 38.8% using the Patient Health Questionnaire (PHQ-9) [112]. This compares to the general population where the lifetime incidence of major depressive episodes is reported as 6.7% [113]. The presence of depression in RA is important as it associates with clinical outcomes and the probability of responding to treatment [114]. Secondary analysis of a recent RCT showed that those with baseline depression had higher DAS28 scores at follow-up, and this was driven mainly by the subjective components of the disease activity score (patient global and tender joint count) [114]. There are several potential explanations including lower rates of treatment concordance in patients with depression though there is also evidence to suggest that pro-inflammatory cytokines, including IL-17, may play a role in the development of depression [115].

Depression and anxiety levels will vary over time in response to changes in disease activity and other life events. A study by Norton et al. found that patients could be divided into four distinct groups based on the trajectory of their hospital anxiety and depression scale (HADS) scores [116]. They found that the majority of patients (68%) will have low-stable HADS scores with a small but significant reduction in HADS scores over time. The other three groups were roughly equal in size with

11% experiencing initially low scores but increasing significantly over time, 12% having high scores that remained stable and 9% having initially high scores that improved over time. Unsurprisingly, this study found most rapid changes in psychological distress levels occurred early in the disease course and then tended to stabilise over time.

There is good evidence for both psychotherapy (mainly cognitive behavioural therapy) and anti-depressants for the treatment of major depressive disorders. A large meta-analysis of 30 RCTs found that the degree of improvement from psychotherapy and anti-depressants was similar [117]. Combination treatment with psychotherapy and pharmacotherapy has been shown to be superior to individual therapy with either modality and can be used when one or other modality is insufficient alone [118, 119].

Anxiety

Anxiety is more common in patients with RA than in the general population. An international study looking at HADS scores in RA found that over a third of patients reported significant anxiety with 21.8% reporting depression and anxiety and 13.5% reporting anxiety without depression [120]. Anxiety is associated with worse outcomes including higher levels of arthritis pain and functional disability [114].

Psychosis

Psychosis is relatively rare in rheumatoid arthritis. When it does occur, it is often unrelated or related to therapy for RA rather than the underlying disease. The most common drug class associated with psychosis in RA is corticosteroids, though there are sporadic case reports linking methotrexate and hydroxychloroquine with the onset of psychosis.

Impact of Comorbidities in RA

Comorbidities have a direct impact on outcomes in patients with rheumatoid arthritis. A prospective cohort study of 380 patients from Austria found that physical disability, measured using HAQ, increased with increasing levels of comorbidity [121]. This remained significant even when adjusting for disease activity, gender and disease duration. A sensitivity analysis from the same study found that the physical component score of the SF-36 worsened with increasing comorbidity but the mental component score did not. Data from the CORRONA registry has shown that patients with comorbidities experience smaller responses when starting a new treatment and are less likely to achieve states of remission [122]. Unadjusted analysis from the same study also found that older patients were also significantly less likely to achieve remission states, but this was no longer significant when adjusting for comorbidities suggesting that comorbidity may be the mechanism through which age influences the likelihood of achieving remission.

Assessment and Management of Comorbidities in RA

The EULAR guidelines for the management of rheumatoid arthritis state specifically that rheumatologists are the specialists who should primarily care for RA patients. They recommend that when therapy needs to be adjusted the rheumatologist should not just consider disease activity but should consider factors such as comorbidities. The guidelines implicitly state 'reaching the outcome of low disease activity or remission is not an absolute prerequisite and that it is equally important to account for comorbidities and other contraindications when targeting a good outcome' [123].

In 2016 EULAR produced guidelines for the reporting, screening and prevention of selected comorbidities in chronic inflammatory rheumatic diseases (CIRDs) [124]. These guidelines highlight six comorbidities of particular importance that are more common in individuals with CIRDs and where the management is often suboptimal. These comorbidities were cardiovascular disease, malignancy, infection, peptic ulceration, osteoporosis and depression. Whilst there are not specific guidelines for each individual comorbidity, there are EULAR recommendations for cardiovascular risk management in patients with RA [125]. There are ten recommendations based on three overarching principles. These principles state that (1) clinicians should be aware of the increased risk of CVD in patients with RA, (2) the rheumatologist should ensure CVD risk assessment is done in all patients with RA and (3) the use of NSAIDs and corticosteroids should be in line with existing EULAR recommendations. A key point in these guidelines is the importance of controlling disease activity which will reduce the overall risk of cardiovascular disease. The guidelines suggest an assessment of cardiovascular risk be carried out every 5 years, though in many countries screening will be done more frequently than this as part of an annual review process.

Conclusion

Rheumatoid arthritis remains a lifelong condition without any cure. With increasing life expectancy in the general population being mirrored in the RA population, it is unsurprising that we are seeing an increasing number of patients with multiple comorbidities. This is a major challenge for the clinician as remaining up to date with guidelines for relatively common comorbidities such as hypertension, diabetes and asthma can be difficult. As a rheumatologist, one cannot expect to be an expert in managing each individual condition but should at least be aware of the complex interplay between these comorbidities and the management of RA itself and be able to signpost the patient to the appropriate care.

References

1. Dougados M, Soubrier M, Antunez A, Balint P, Balsa A, Buch MH, et al. Prevalence of comorbidities in rheumatoid arthritis and evaluation of their monitoring: results of an international, cross-sectional study (COMORA). Ann Rheum Dis. 2014;73(1):62–8.
2. Gron KL, Ornbjerg LM, Hetland ML, Aslam F, Khan NA, Jacobs JW, et al. The association of fatigue, comorbidity burden, disease activity, disability and gross domestic product in patients with rheumatoid arthritis. Results from 34 countries participating in the Quest-RA program. Clin Exp Rheumatol. 2014;32(6):869–77.
3. Goodson NJ, Wiles NJ, Lunt M, Barrett EM, Silman AJ, Symmons DP. Mortality in early inflammatory polyarthritis: cardiovascular mortality is increased in seropositive patients. Arthritis Rheum. 2002;46(8):2010–9.
4. Naranjo A, Sokka T, Descalzo MA, Calvo-Alen J, Horslev-Petersen K, Luukkainen RK, et al. Cardiovascular disease in patients with rheumatoid arthritis: results from the QUEST-RA study. Arthritis Res Ther. 2008;10(2):R30.
5. Hurd ER. Extraarticular manifestations of rheumatoid arthritis. Semin Arthritis Rheum. 1979;8(3):151–76.
6. Voskuyl AE, Zwinderman AH, Westedt ML, Vandenbroucke JP, Breedveld FC, Hazes JM. Factors associated with the development of vasculitis in rheumatoid arthritis: results of a case-control study. Ann Rheum Dis. 1996;55(3):190–2.
7. Hara KS, Ballard DJ, Ilstrup DM, Connolly DC, Vollertsen RS. Rheumatoid pericarditis: clinical features and survival. Medicine (Baltimore). 1990;69(2):81–91.
8. Nurmohamed MT, Heslinga M, Kitas GD. Cardiovascular comorbidity in rheumatic diseases. Nat Rev Rheumatol. 2015;11(12):693–704.
9. Avina-Zubieta JA, Choi HK, Sadatsafavi M, Etminan M, Esdaile JM, Lacaille D. Risk of cardiovascular mortality in patients with rheumatoid arthritis: a meta-analysis of observational studies. Arthritis Rheum. 2008;59(12):1690–7.
10. Bartoloni E, Alunno A, Luccioli F, Moscatelli S, Biscontini D, Santoboni G, et al. Atherosclerotic vascular damage and rheumatoid arthritis: a complex but intriguing link. Expert Rev Cardiovasc Ther. 2010;8(9):1309–16.
11. del Rincon I, Freeman GL, Haas RW, O'Leary DH, Escalante A. Relative contribution of cardiovascular risk factors and rheumatoid arthritis clinical manifestations to atherosclerosis. Arthritis Rheum. 2005;52(11):3413–23.
12. Lebowitz WB. The heart in rheumatoid arthritis (rheumatoid disease). A clinical and pathological study of sixty-two cases. Ann Intern Med. 1963;58:102–23.
13. Boers M, Nurmohamed MT, Doelman CJ, Lard LR, Verhoeven AC, Voskuyl AE, et al. Influence of glucocorticoids and disease activity on total and high density lipoprotein cholesterol in patients with rheumatoid arthritis. Ann Rheum Dis. 2003;62(9):842–5.
14. Jamnitski A, Visman IM, Peters MJ, Dijkmans BA, Voskuyl AE, Nurmohamed MT. Beneficial effect of 1-year etanercept treatment on the lipid profile in responding patients with rheumatoid arthritis: the ETRA study. Ann Rheum Dis. 2010;69(11):1929–33.
15. Curtis JR, John A, Baser O. Dyslipidemia and changes in lipid profiles associated with rheumatoid arthritis and initiation of anti-tumor necrosis factor therapy. Arthritis Care Res (Hoboken). 2012;64(9):1282–91.

16. Sarzi-Puttini P, Atzeni F, Shoenfeld Y, Ferraccioli G. TNF-alpha, rheumatoid arthritis, and heart failure: a rheumatological dilemma. Autoimmun Rev. 2005;4(3):153–61.
17. Nishimoto N, Ito K, Takagi N. Safety and efficacy profiles of tocilizumab monotherapy in Japanese patients with rheumatoid arthritis: meta-analysis of six initial trials and five long-term extensions. Mod Rheumatol. 2010;20(3):222–32.
18. Kume K, Amano K, Yamada S, Hatta K, Ohta H, Kuwaba N. Tocilizumab monotherapy reduces arterial stiffness as effectively as etanercept or adalimumab monotherapy in rheumatoid arthritis: an open-label randomized controlled trial. J Rheumatol. 2011;38(10):2169–71.
19. Klarenbeek NB, van der Kooij SM, Huizinga TJ, Goekoop-Ruiterman YP, Hulsmans HM, van Krugten MV, et al. Blood pressure changes in patients with recent-onset rheumatoid arthritis treated with four different treatment strategies: a post hoc analysis from the BeSt trial. Ann Rheum Dis. 2010;69(7):1342–5.
20. Schultz O, Oberhauser F, Saech J, Rubbert-Roth A, Hahn M, Krone W, et al. Effects of inhibition of interleukin-6 signalling on insulin sensitivity and lipoprotein (a) levels in human subjects with rheumatoid diseases. PLoS One. 2010;5(12):e14328.
21. Ogata A, Morishima A, Hirano T, Hishitani Y, Hagihara K, Shima Y, et al. Improvement of HbA1c during treatment with humanised anti-interleukin 6 receptor antibody, tocilizumab. Ann Rheum Dis. 2011;70(6):1164–5.
22. Greenberg JD, Kremer JM, Curtis JR, Hochberg MC, Reed G, Tsao P, et al. Tumour necrosis factor antagonist use and associated risk reduction of cardiovascular events among patients with rheumatoid arthritis. Ann Rheum Dis. 2011;70(4):576–82.
23. Lunt M, Watson KD, Dixon WG, Symmons DP, Hyrich KL. No evidence of association between anti-tumor necrosis factor treatment and mortality in patients with rheumatoid arthritis: results from the British Society for Rheumatology biologics register. Arthritis Rheum. 2010;62(11):3145–53.
24. Dixon WG, Watson KD, Lunt M, Hyrich KL, Silman AJ, Symmons DP. Reduction in the incidence of myocardial infarction in patients with rheumatoid arthritis who respond to anti-tumor necrosis factor alpha therapy: results from the British Society for Rheumatology biologics register. Arthritis Rheum. 2007;56(9):2905–12.
25. Voskuyl AE. The heart and cardiovascular manifestations in rheumatoid arthritis. Rheumatology (Oxford). 2006;45(Suppl 4):iv4–7.
26. Costedoat-Chalumeau N, Hulot JS, Amoura Z, Delcourt A, Maisonobe T, Dorent R, et al. Cardiomyopathy related to antimalarial therapy with illustrative case report. Cardiology. 2007;107(2):73–80.
27. Van Doornum S, McColl G, Wicks IP. Accelerated atherosclerosis: an extraarticular feature of rheumatoid arthritis? Arthritis Rheum. 2002;46(4):862–73.
28. Nicola PJ, Crowson CS, Maradit-Kremers H, Ballman KV, Roger VL, Jacobsen SJ, et al. Contribution of congestive heart failure and ischemic heart disease to excess mortality in rheumatoid arthritis. Arthritis Rheum. 2006;54(1):60–7.
29. Crowson CS, Nicola PJ, Kremers HM, O'Fallon WM, Therneau TM, Jacobsen SJ, et al. How much of the increased incidence of heart failure in rheumatoid arthritis is attributable to traditional cardiovascular risk factors and ischemic heart disease? Arthritis Rheum. 2005;52(10):3039–44.
30. Bhatia GS, Sosin MD, Patel JV, Grindulis KA, Khattak FH, Hughes EA, et al. Left ventricular systolic dysfunction in rheumatoid disease: an unrecognized burden? J Am Coll Cardiol. 2006;47(6):1169–74.
31. Maradit-Kremers H, Nicola PJ, Crowson CS, Ballman KV, Jacobsen SJ, Roger VL, et al. Raised erythrocyte sedimentation rate signals heart failure in patients with rheumatoid arthritis. Ann Rheum Dis. 2007;66(1):76–80.
32. Wislowska M, Sypula S, Kowalik I. Echocardiographic findings and 24-h electrocardiographic Holter monitoring in patients with nodular and non-nodular rheumatoid arthritis. Rheumatol Int. 1999;18(5–6):163–9.

33. Roldan CA, DeLong C, Qualls CR, Crawford MH. Characterization of valvular heart disease in rheumatoid arthritis by transesophageal echocardiography and clinical correlates. Am J Cardiol. 2007;100(3):496–502.
34. Seferovic PM, Ristic AD, Maksimovic R, Simeunovic DS, Ristic GG, Radovanovic G, et al. Cardiac arrhythmias and conduction disturbances in autoimmune rheumatic diseases. Rheumatology (Oxford). 2006;45(Suppl 4):iv39–42.
35. Ahern M, Lever JV, Cosh J. Complete heart block in rheumatoid arthritis. Ann Rheum Dis. 1983;42(4):389–97.
36. Cavazzana I, Franceschini F, Quinzanini M, Manera C, Del Papa N, Maglione W, et al. Anti-Ro/SSA antibodies in rheumatoid arthritis: clinical and immunologic associations. Clin Exp Rheumatol. 2006;24(1):59–64.
37. Goldeli O, Dursun E, Komsuoglu B. Dispersion of ventricular repolarization: a new marker of ventricular arrhythmias in patients with rheumatoid arthritis. J Rheumatol. 1998;25(3):447–50.
38. Panoulas VF, Douglas KM, Milionis HJ, Stavropoulos-Kalinglou A, Nightingale P, Kita MD, et al. Prevalence and associations of hypertension and its control in patients with rheumatoid arthritis. Rheumatology (Oxford). 2007;46(9):1477–82.
39. Panoulas VF, Metsios GS, Pace AV, John H, Treharne GJ, Banks MJ, et al. Hypertension in rheumatoid arthritis. Rheumatology (Oxford). 2008;47(9):1286–98.
40. Kaplan MJ. Cardiovascular disease in rheumatoid arthritis. Curr Opin Rheumatol. 2006;18(3):289–97.
41. Ross R. Atherosclerosis – an inflammatory disease. N Engl J Med. 1999;340(2):115–26.
42. Vaudo G, Marchesi S, Gerli R, Allegrucci R, Giordano A, Siepi D, et al. Endothelial dysfunction in young patients with rheumatoid arthritis and low disease activity. Ann Rheum Dis. 2004;63(1):31–5.
43. Liou TH, Huang SW, Lin JW, Chang YS, Wu CW, Lin HW. Risk of stroke in patients with rheumatism: a nationwide longitudinal population-based study. Sci Rep. 2014;4:5110.
44. Ungprasert P, Srivali N, Spanuchart I, Thongprayoon C, Knight EL. Risk of venous thromboembolism in patients with rheumatoid arthritis: a systematic review and meta-analysis. Clin Rheumatol. 2014;33(3):297–304.
45. Meyer-Olesen CL, Nielsen SF, Nordestgaard BG. Increased rheumatoid factor and deep venous thrombosis: 2 cohort studies of 54628 individuals from the general population. Clin Chem. 2015;61(2):349–59.
46. Chatzidionisyou A, Catrina AI. The lung in rheumatoid arthritis, cause or consequence? Curr Opin Rheumatol. 2016;28(1):76–82.
47. Konisti S, Kiriakidis S, Paleolog EM. Hypoxia – a key regulator of angiogenesis and inflammation in rheumatoid arthritis. Nat Rev Rheumatol. 2012;8(3):153–62.
48. Norton S, Koduri G, Nikiphorou E, Dixey J, Williams P, Young A. A study of baseline prevalence and cumulative incidence of comorbidity and extra-articular manifestations in RA and their impact on outcome. Rheumatology (Oxford). 2013;52(1):99–110.
49. Dawson JK, Fewins HE, Desmond J, Lynch MP, Graham DR. Fibrosing alveolitis in patients with rheumatoid arthritis as assessed by high resolution computed tomography, chest radiography, and pulmonary function tests. Thorax. 2001;56(8):622–7.
50. Wang JX, Du CG. A retrospective study of clinical characteristics of interstitial lung disease associated with rheumatoid arthritis in Chinese patients. Med Sci Monit. 2015;21:708–15.
51. Kelly CA, Saravanan V, Nisar M, Arthanari S, Woodhead FA, Price-Forbes AN, et al. Rheumatoid arthritis-related interstitial lung disease: associations, prognostic factors and physiological and radiological characteristics – a large multicentre UK study. Rheumatology (Oxford). 2014;53(9):1676–82.
52. Zhu J, Zhou Y, Chen X, Li J. A metaanalysis of the increased risk of rheumatoid arthritis-related pulmonary disease as a result of serum anticitrullinated protein antibody positivity. J Rheumatol. 2014;41(7):1282–9.

53. Bongartz T, Nannini C, Medina-Velasquez YF, Achenbach SJ, Crowson CS, Ryu JH, et al. Incidence and mortality of interstitial lung disease in rheumatoid arthritis: a population-based study. Arthritis Rheum. 2010;62(6):1583–91.
54. Mathieson JR, Mayo JR, Staples CA, Muller NL. Chronic diffuse infiltrative lung disease: comparison of diagnostic accuracy of CT and chest radiography. Radiology. 1989;171(1):111–6.
55. Turesson C, Matteson EL, Colby TV, Vuk-Pavlovic Z, Vassallo R, Weyand CM, et al. Increased CD4+ T cell infiltrates in rheumatoid arthritis-associated interstitial pneumonitis compared with idiopathic interstitial pneumonitis. Arthritis Rheum. 2005;52(1):73–9.
56. Kelly C, Saravanan V. Treatment strategies for a rheumatoid arthritis patient with interstitial lung disease. Expert Opin Pharmacother. 2008;9(18):3221–30.
57. Conway R, Low C, Coughlan RJ, O'Donnell MJ, Carey JJ. Methotrexate and lung disease in rheumatoid arthritis: a meta-analysis of randomized controlled trials. Arthritis Rheum (Hoboken). 2014;66(4):803–12.
58. Conway R, Low C, Coughlan RJ, O'Donnell MJ, Carey JJ. Methotrexate use and risk of lung disease in psoriasis, psoriatic arthritis, and inflammatory bowel disease: systematic literature review and meta-analysis of randomised controlled trials. BMJ. 2015;350:h1269.
59. Conway R, Low C, Coughlan RJ, O'Donnell MJ, Carey JJ. Leflunomide use and risk of lung disease in rheumatoid arthritis: a systematic literature review and Metaanalysis of randomized controlled trials. J Rheumatol. 2016;43(5):855–60.
60. Jani M, Hirani N, Matteson EL, Dixon WG. The safety of biologic therapies in RA-associated interstitial lung disease. Nat Rev Rheumatol. 2014;10(5):284–94.
61. Herrinton LJ, Harrold LR, Liu L, Raebel MA, Taharka A, Winthrop KL, et al. Association between anti-TNF-alpha therapy and interstitial lung disease. Pharmacoepidemiol Drug Saf. 2013;22(4):394–402.
62. Liote H, Liote F, Seroussi B, Mayaud C, Cadranel J. Rituximab-induced lung disease: a systematic literature review. Eur Respir J. 2010;35(3):681–7.
63. Keir GJ, Maher TM, Ming D, Abdullah R, de Lauretis A, Wickremasinghe M, et al. Rituximab in severe, treatment-refractory interstitial lung disease. Respirology (Carlton, Vic). 2014;19(3):353–9.
64. Mori S, Koga Y, Sugimoto M. Different risk factors between interstitial lung disease and airway disease in rheumatoid arthritis. Respir Med. 2012;106(11):1591–9.
65. Geddes DM, Webley M, Emerson PA. Airways obstruction in rheumatoid arthritis. Ann Rheum Dis. 1979;38(3):222–5.
66. Wilsher M, Voight L, Milne D, Teh M, Good N, Kolbe J, et al. Prevalence of airway and parenchymal abnormalities in newly diagnosed rheumatoid arthritis. Respir Med. 2012;106(10):1441–6.
67. Vergnenegre A, Pugnere N, Antonini MT, Arnaud M, Melloni B, Treves R, et al. Airway obstruction and rheumatoid arthritis. Eur Respir J. 1997;10(5):1072–8.
68. Swinson DR, Symmons D, Suresh U, Jones M, Booth J. Decreased survival in patients with co-existent rheumatoid arthritis and bronchiectasis. Rheumatology. 1997;36(6):689–91.
69. Walker WC, Wright V. Pulmonary lesions and rheumatoid arthritis. Medicine. 1968;47(6):501–20.
70. Corcoran JP, Ahmad M, Mukherjee R, Redmond KC. Pleuro-pulmonary complications of rheumatoid arthritis. Respir Care. 2014;59(4):e55–e9.
71. Sargin G, Senturk T. Multiple pulmonary rheumatoid nodules. Reumatologia. 2015;53(5):276–8.
72. Baecklund E, Iliadou A, Askling J, Ekbom A, Backlin C, Granath F, et al. Association of chronic inflammation, not its treatment, with increased lymphoma risk in rheumatoid arthritis. Arthritis Rheum. 2006;54(3):692–701.
73. Salloum E, Cooper DL, Howe G, Lacy J, Tallini G, Crouch J, et al. Spontaneous regression of lymphoproliferative disorders in patients treated with methotrexate for rheumatoid arthritis and other rheumatic diseases. J Clin Oncol. 1996;14(6):1943–9.

74. Mercer LK, Lunt M, Low AL, Dixon WG, Watson KD, Symmons DP, et al. Risk of solid cancer in patients exposed to anti-tumour necrosis factor therapy: results from the British Society for Rheumatology biologics register for rheumatoid arthritis. Ann Rheum Dis. 2015;74(6):1087–93.
75. Raaschou P, Frisell T, Askling J. TNF inhibitor therapy and risk of breast cancer recurrence in patients with rheumatoid arthritis: a nationwide cohort study. Ann Rheum Dis. 2015;74(12):2137–43.
76. Raaschou P, Simard JF, Holmqvist M, Askling J. Rheumatoid arthritis, anti-tumour necrosis factor therapy, and risk of malignant melanoma: nationwide population based prospective cohort study from Sweden. BMJ. 2013;346:f1939.
77. Mercer LK, Askling J, Raaschou P, Dixon WG, Dreyer L, Hetland ML, et al. Risk of invasive melanoma in patients with rheumatoid arthritis treated with biologics: results from a collaborative project of 11 European biologic registers. Ann Rheum Dis. 2016;76:386–91.
78. Mercer LK, Galloway JB, Lunt M, Davies R, Low AL, Dixon WG, et al. Risk of lymphoma in patients exposed to antitumour necrosis factor therapy: results from the British Society for Rheumatology biologics register for rheumatoid arthritis. Ann Rheum Dis. 2016;0:1–7.
79. Subesinghe S, Rutherford AI, Ibrahim F, Harris H, Galloway J. A large two-centre study in to rates of influenza and pneumococcal vaccination and infection burden in rheumatoid arthritis in the UK. BMC Musculoskelet Disord. 2016;17:322.
80. Doran MF, Crowson CS, Pond GR, O'Fallon WM, Gabriel SE. Frequency of infection in patients with rheumatoid arthritis compared with controls: a population-based study. Arthritis Rheum. 2002;46(9):2287–93.
81. Bucknall RC, Davis P, Bacon PA, Jones JV. Neutropenia in rheumatoid arthritis: studies on possible contributing factors. Ann Rheum Dis. 1982;41(3):242–7.
82. Koetz K, Bryl E, Spickschen K, O'Fallon WM, Goronzy JJ, Weyand CM. T cell homeostasis in patients with rheumatoid arthritis. Proc Natl Acad Sci U S A. 2000;97(16):9203–8.
83. Au K, Reed G, Curtis JR, Kremer JM, Greenberg JD, Strand V, et al. High disease activity is associated with an increased risk of infection in patients with rheumatoid arthritis. Ann Rheum Dis. 2011;70(5):785–91.
84. Lacaille D, Guh DP, Abrahamowicz M, Anis AH, Esdaile JM. Use of nonbiologic disease-modifying antirheumatic drugs and risk of infection in patients with rheumatoid arthritis. Arthritis Rheum. 2008;59(8):1074–81.
85. van der Veen MJ, van der Heide A, Kruize AA, Bijlsma JW. Infection rate and use of antibiotics in patients with rheumatoid arthritis treated with methotrexate. Ann Rheum Dis. 1994;53(4):224–8.
86. Sakai R, Komano Y, Tanaka M, Nanki T, Koike R, Nakajima A, et al. The REAL database reveals no significant risk of serious infection during treatment with a methotrexate dose of more than 8 mg/week in patients with rheumatoid arthritis. Mod Rheumatol. 2011;21(4):444–8.
87. Smolen JS, Kalden JR, Scott DL, Rozman B, Kvien TK, Larsen A, et al. Efficacy and safety of leflunomide compared with placebo and sulphasalazine in active rheumatoid arthritis: a double-blind, randomised, multicentre trial. European Leflunomide Study Group. Lancet (London). 1999;353(9149):259–66.
88. Wolfe F, Caplan L, Michaud K. Treatment for rheumatoid arthritis and the risk of hospitalization for pneumonia: associations with prednisone, disease-modifying antirheumatic drugs, and anti-tumor necrosis factor therapy. Arthritis Rheum. 2006;54(2):628–34.
89. Dixon WG, Suissa S, Hudson M. The association between systemic glucocorticoid therapy and the risk of infection in patients with rheumatoid arthritis: systematic review and meta-analyses. Arthritis Res Ther. 2011;13(4):R139.
90. Galloway JB, Hyrich KL, Mercer LK, Dixon WG, Fu B, Ustianowski AP, et al. Anti-TNF therapy is associated with an increased risk of serious infections in patients with rheumatoid arthritis especially in the first 6 months of treatment: updated results from the British

society for rheumatology biologics register with special emphasis on risks in the elderly. Rheumatology (Oxford). 2011;50(1):124–31.

91. Galloway JB, Hyrich KL, Mercer LK, Dixon WG, Ustianowski AP, Helbert M, et al. Risk of septic arthritis in patients with rheumatoid arthritis and the effect of anti-TNF therapy: results from the British society for rheumatology biologics register. Ann Rheum Dis. 2011;70(10):1810–4.
92. Galloway JB, Mercer LK, Moseley A, Dixon WG, Ustianowski AP, Helbert M, et al. Risk of skin and soft tissue infections (including shingles) in patients exposed to anti-tumour necrosis factor therapy: results from the British society for rheumatology biologics register. Ann Rheum Dis. 2013;72(2):229–34.
93. Dixon WG, Hyrich KL, Watson KD, Lunt M, Galloway J, Ustianowski A, et al. Drug-specific risk of tuberculosis in patients with rheumatoid arthritis treated with anti-TNF therapy: results from the British society for rheumatology biologics register (BSRBR). Ann Rheum Dis. 2010;69(3):522–8.
94. Cantini F, Niccoli L, Goletti D. Tuberculosis risk in patients treated with non-anti-tumor necrosis factor-alpha (TNF-alpha) targeted biologics and recently licensed TNF-alpha inhibitors: data from clinical trials and national registries. J Rheumatol Suppl. 2014;91:56–64.
95. Salmon-Ceron D, Tubach F, Lortholary O, Chosidow O, Bretagne S, Nicolas N, et al. Drug-specific risk of non-tuberculosis opportunistic infections in patients receiving anti-TNF therapy reported to the 3-year prospective French RATIO registry. Ann Rheum Dis. 2011;70(4):616–23.
96. Burton MJ, Curtis JR, Yang S, Chen L, Singh JA, Mikuls TR, et al. Safety of biologic and non-biologic disease-modifying antirheumatic drug therapy in veterans with rheumatoid arthritis and hepatitis B virus infection: a retrospective cohort study. Arthritis Res Ther. 2015;17:136.
97. Aithal GP. Hepatotoxicity related to antirheumatic drugs. Nat Rev Rheumatol. 2011;7(3):139–50.
98. Cunha BM, Mota LM, Pileggi GS, Safe IP, Lacerda MV. HIV/AIDS and rheumatoid arthritis. Autoimmun Rev. 2015;14(5):396–400.
99. Carroll MB, Fields JH, Clerc PG. Rheumatoid arthritis in patients with HIV: management challenges. Open Access Rheumatol. 2016;8:51–9.
100. Ntatsaki E, Mooney J, DGI S, Watts RA. Systemic rheumatoid vasculitis in the era of modern immunosuppressive therapy. Rheumatology. 2014;53(1):145–52.
101. Makol A, Matteson EL, Warrington KJ. Rheumatoid vasculitis: an update. Curr Opin Rheumatol. 2015;27(1):63–70.
102. Scott DG, Bacon PA. Intravenous cyclophosphamide plus methylprednisolone in treatment of systemic rheumatoid vasculitis. Am J Med. 1984;76(3):377–84.
103. van Staa TP, Geusens P, Bijlsma JW, Leufkens HG, Cooper C. Clinical assessment of the long-term risk of fracture in patients with rheumatoid arthritis. Arthritis Rheum. 2006;54(10):3104–12.
104. Hoes JN, Bultink IE, Lems WF. Management of osteoporosis in rheumatoid arthritis patients. Expert Opin Pharmacother. 2015;16(4):559–71.
105. Krieckaert CL, Nurmohamed MT, Wolbink G, Lems WF. Changes in bone mineral density during long-term treatment with adalimumab in patients with rheumatoid arthritis: a cohort study. Rheumatology (Oxford). 2013;52(3):547–53.
106. Figueiredo CP, Simon D, Englbrecht M, Haschka J, Kleyer A, Bayat S, et al. Quantification and impact of secondary osteoarthritis in patients with anti-Citrullinated protein antibody-positive rheumatoid arthritis. Arthritis Rheumatol. 2016;68(9):2114–21.
107. McWilliams DF, Marshall M, Jayakumar K, Doherty S, Doherty M, Zhang W, et al. Erosive and osteoarthritic structural progression in early rheumatoid arthritis. Rheumatology (Oxford). 2016;55(8):1477–88.
108. Wolfe F, Michaud K. Severe rheumatoid arthritis (RA), worse outcomes, comorbid illness, and sociodemographic disadvantage characterize ra patients with fibromyalgia. J Rheumatol. 2004;31(4):695–700.

109. Mian AN, Chaabo K, Wajed J, Subesinghe S, Gullick NJ, Kirkham B, et al. Rheumatoid arthritis patients with fibromyalgic clinical features have significantly less synovitis as defined by power Doppler ultrasound. BMC Musculoskelet Disord. 2016;17(1):404.
110. Duran J, Combe B, Niu J, Rincheval N, Gaujoux-Viala C, Felson DT. The effect on treatment response of fibromyalgic symptoms in early rheumatoid arthritis patients: results from the ESPOIR cohort. Rheumatology (Oxford). 2015;54(12):2166–70.
111. Mian AN, Ibrahim F, Scott IC, Bahadur S, Filkova M, Pollard L, et al. Changing clinical patterns in rheumatoid arthritis management over two decades: sequential observational studies. BMC Musculoskelet Disord. 2016;17:44.
112. Matcham F, Rayner L, Steer S, Hotopf M. The prevalence of depression in rheumatoid arthritis: a systematic review and meta-analysis. Rheumatology (Oxford). 2013;52(12):2136–48.
113. Waraich P, Goldner EM, Somers JM, Hsu L. Prevalence and incidence studies of mood disorders: a systematic review of the literature. Can J Psychiatry. 2004;49(2):124–38.
114. Matcham F, Norton S, Scott DL, Steer S, Hotopf M. Symptoms of depression and anxiety predict treatment response and long-term physical health outcomes in rheumatoid arthritis: secondary analysis of a randomized controlled trial. Rheumatology (Oxford). 2016;55(2):268–78.
115. Liu Y, Ho RC, Mak A. The role of interleukin (IL)-17 in anxiety and depression of patients with rheumatoid arthritis. Int J Rheum Dis. 2012;15(2):183–7.
116. Norton S, Sacker A, Young A, Done J. Distinct psychological distress trajectories in rheumatoid arthritis: findings from an inception cohort. J Psychosom Res. 2011;71(5):290–5.
117. Cuijpers P, van Straten A, van Oppen P, Andersson G. Are psychological and pharmacologic interventions equally effective in the treatment of adult depressive disorders? A meta-analysis of comparative studies. J Clin Psychiatry. 2008;69(11):1675–85; quiz 839–41.
118. Cuijpers P, Dekker J, Hollon SD, Andersson G. Adding psychotherapy to pharmacotherapy in the treatment of depressive disorders in adults: a meta-analysis. J Clin Psychiatry. 2009;70(9):1219–29.
119. Cuijpers P, van Straten A, Warmerdam L, Andersson G. Psychotherapy versus the combination of psychotherapy and pharmacotherapy in the treatment of depression: a meta-analysis. Depress Anxiety. 2009;26(3):279–88.
120. Covic T, Cumming SR, Pallant JF, Manolios N, Emery P, Conaghan PG, et al. Depression and anxiety in patients with rheumatoid arthritis: prevalence rates based on a comparison of the depression, anxiety and stress scale (DASS) and the hospital, anxiety and depression scale (HADS). BMC Psychiatry. 2012;12:6.
121. Radner H, Smolen JS, Aletaha D. Impact of comorbidity on physical function in patients with rheumatoid arthritis. Ann Rheum Dis. 2010;69(3):536–41.
122. Ranganath VK, Maranian P, Elashoff DA, Woodworth T, Khanna D, Hahn T, et al. Comorbidities are associated with poorer outcomes in community patients with rheumatoid arthritis. Rheumatology. 2013;52:1809–17.
123. Smolen JS, Landewe R, Breedveld FC, Buch M, Burmester G, Dougados M, et al. EULAR recommendations for the management of rheumatoid arthritis with synthetic and biological disease-modifying antirheumatic drugs: 2013 update. Ann Rheum Dis. 2014;73(3):492–509.
124. Baillet A, Gossec L, Carmona L, Wit M, van Eijk-Hustings Y, Bertheussen H, et al. Points to consider for reporting, screening for and preventing selected comorbidities in chronic inflammatory rheumatic diseases in daily practice: a EULAR initiative. Ann Rheum Dis. 2016;75(6):965–73.
125. Agca R, Heslinga SC, Rollefstad S, Heslinga M, McInnes IB, Peters MJL, et al. EULAR recommendations for cardiovascular disease risk management in patients with rheumatoid arthritis and other forms of inflammatory joint disorders: 2015/2016 update. Ann Rheum Dis. 2016;76:17–28.

Chapter 4
Psoriasis

Anna Chapman and Yasser El Miedany

Psoriasis is a chronic, hyper-proliferative, immune-mediated inflammatory skin disease affecting approximately 1–3% of the population worldwide [1–3]. Chronic plaque psoriasis, the most common form of psoriasis vulgaris, is characterised by sharply demarcated erythematous papules and plaques with scales. It has a variable severity, distribution and disease course [3, 4]. Over the past few years, there has been an increasing evidence to substantiate that psoriasis is not just a disorder of the skin but a systemic inflammatory disease [4–8], with systemic manifestations that look similar to, and shared with, other chronic inflammatory conditions, such as rheumatoid arthritis. Being an immune-mediated inflammatory disease, psoriasis has been linked to a wide range of comorbidities [1–5]. Recently, several comorbid conditions have been reported as related to the chronic inflammatory status of psoriasis. The understanding of the pathophysiology of these conditions and their treatments will certainly lead to better management of the disease [3, 5–8]. Figure 4.1 depicts how psoriasis starts with genetic predisposition and environmental triggers causing the known skin disease. It also shows a list of its associated comorbidities. This chapter will give a background to psoriasis, pathophysiology linked to its associated comorbidities and the new concept of "psoriatic march". It will also discuss the scientific evidence for each comorbidity, its therapeutic implications and approaches to screen in standard daily practice.

A. Chapman
Department of Dermatology, Lewisham and Greenwich NHS Trust,
Queen Elizabeth Hospital, London, UK

Y. El Miedany (✉)
King's College, London, UK

Rheumatology and Rehabilitation, Ain Shams University, Cairo, Egypt

Department of Rheumatology, Darent Valley Hospital, Dartford, Kent, UK
e-mail: yasser_elmiedany@yahoo.com

Y. El Miedany (ed.), *Comorbidity in Rheumatic Diseases*,
DOI 10.1007/978-3-319-59963-2_4

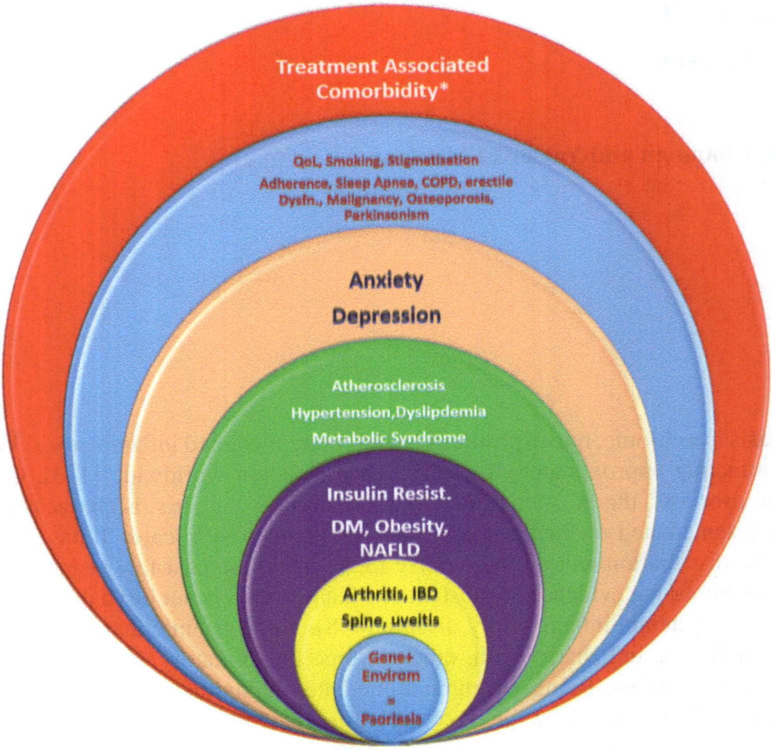

Fig. 4.1 Psoriasis disease and its associated comorbidities: starts with genetic predisposition and environmental triggers. (1) Skin and musculoskeletal disease (arthritis, enthesitis, spondylitis, dactylitis), IBD (inflammatory bowel disease). (2) Systemic inflammation: insulin resistance, DM (diabetes mellitus), obesity, NAFLD (non-alcoholic fatty liver disease); cardiovascular: atherosclerosis, hypertension, dyslipidemia, metabolic syndrome, myocardial infarction, stroke. (3) Psychologic: depression, anxiety, self-helplessness. (4) Quality of life (QoL) and lifestyle. (5) Other comorbidities: sleep apnoea, COPD (chronic obstructive pulmonary disease), malignancy, erectile dysfunction, osteoporosis, parkinsonism, celiac disease. (6) Treatment-associated comorbidities*: dyslipidemia (acitretin and cyclosporine), nephrotoxicity (cyclosporine), hypertension (cyclosporine), hepatotoxicity (methotrexate, leflunomide, and acitretin), skin cancer (PUVA)

Inflammatory Pathway: "The Psoriatic March" from Gene to Clinic

There is growing evidence indicating that psoriasis is more than "skin-deep" and that it is associated with systemic manifestations, similar to other chronic inflammatory diseases, such as rheumatoid arthritis [9]. Of emerging significance is the relationship between cardiovascular disease and severe psoriasis, which may explain the increased mortality in the psoriatic patients. Studying the inflammatory pathway, psoriatic patients revealed a cascade of inflammatory processes, called the

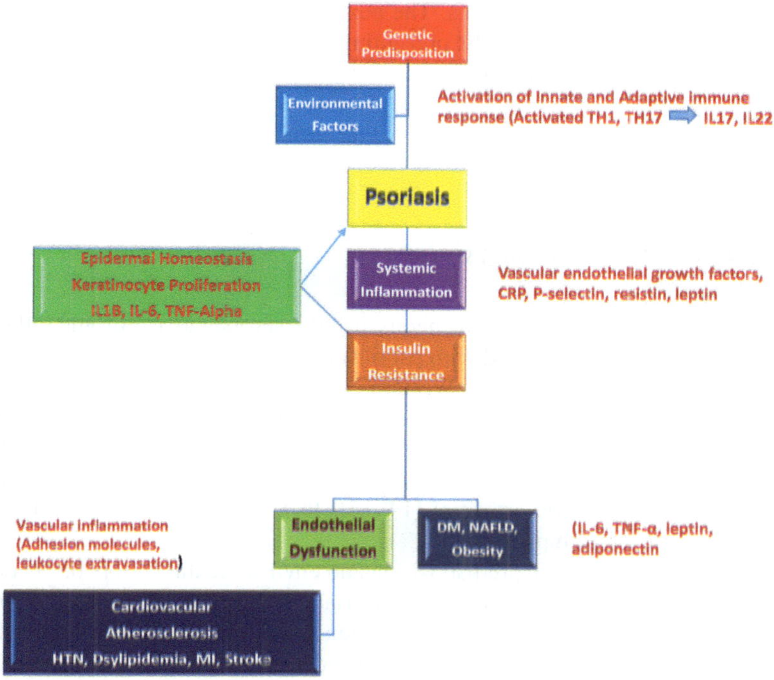

Fig. 4.2 From gene to clinic "The psoriatic march": simplified mechanism of the inflammatory pathway. According to the hypothesis, severe psoriasis is a chronic systemic inflammatory disorder, which increases the inflammatory burden and causes a state of insulin resistance, resulting in endothelial cell dysfunction and atherosclerosis

"psoriatic march", linking the psoriatic skin disease and its associated comorbidities particularly the cardiovascular ones. A recent review outlined a suggested scenario for how the march of psoriasis unfolds from gene to clinic [10]. Genetic factors drive disease-specific processes (step 1), possibly triggered by environmental factors, involving both innate and adaptive immune responses (step 2) and leading to disease expression (step 3); comorbidity would then "likely result from chronic inflammation" (step 4). The chronic inflammatory status will lead to a cascade of systemic inflammatory pathways starting with insulin resistance which in turn lead to type 2 diabetes mellitus as well as endothelial cell dysfunction and consequently atherosclerosis (Fig. 4.2). At the level of coronary, carotid or cerebral arteries, this cascade will result in myocardial infarction or stroke [11].

As shown in Fig. 4.1, psoriasis-associated comorbidities can be classified into those linked to the skin disease such as psoriatic arthritis, inflammatory bowel disease, uveitis and dactylitis or related to the inflammatory process itself. This includes cardiovascular, obesity and metabolic syndrome. It also includes psychological comorbidities, other systemic disorders as well as comorbidities associated with the treatment given to psoriatic patients. The next part of the chapter will discuss each of these comorbidities individually, presenting the science-based evidence and therapeutic implications for each one.

Psoriatic Arthritis

Background and Pathophysiology

Psoriatic arthritis (PsA) is a heterogeneous, usually seronegative, chronic inflammatory spondyloarthritis associated with psoriasis. The prevalence of PsA ranges from 20 to 420 cases per 100,000 in the Western countries [12, 13]. The wide variability in its prevalence rates might be attributed to the existence of five different diagnostic criteria with considerable variations in sensitivity and specificity: (1) Moll and Wright, (2) Bennet, (3) Vasey and Espinoza, (4) Fournié and (5) CASPAR (classification criteria for psoriatic arthritis) [14–18]. PsA prevalence varies from 6% to 42% among patients with psoriasis.

A combination of genetic predisposition and environmental factors has been proposed as a possible etiopathogenesis for psoriatic arthritis. In contrast to psoriasis, which is associated with specific HLA antigens, single nucleotide polymorphisms in the IL-13 gene have been recently associated with specific risk of PsA, without correlation with psoriasis [19, 20].

Environmental factors, including infection (gram-positive bacteria such as *Streptococcus* or retroviruses such as HIV), drugs and joint trauma (particularly in children) and emotional stress, play an important role as a trigger for both skin and joint psoriasis; however, the neuro-immuno-endocrine mechanisms involved in this process still need to be elucidated [19, 21, 22]. From the immunological point of view, changes are observed both in humoral and cellular immunity [23]. Most lymphocytes are of type CD4+, whose CD4+/CD8+ ratio reaches 2:1 in the synovial fluid. CD8+ cells are most commonly found at the enthesis sites [24].

Science-Based Medicine

The peak incidence of PsA occurs between ages 30 and 50 years. Clinically PsA is characterized by joint pain, swelling as well as stiffness, surrounding soft tissue pain mainly in the form of ligament and tendon inflammation (enthesitis and dactylitis), spinal pain and limited range of motion as well as nail changes. The association between synovitis and enthesitis of tendons and ligaments of a single finger/toe is called dactylitis or "sausage digit", and it is identified in 30% of PsA patients [21, 25]. Up to 20% of affected patients suffer from severely destructive and mutilating forms of the disease [26].

In about 75% of the cases, skin affection precedes arthritis, whereas it occurs concomitantly in 10%. In the other 15%, arthritis may precede the skin lesion. A correlation between the type or severity of skin lesions and the presence, type or extent of joint affection is not common [27]. When skin lesions appear after articular affection, eventually after 10–5 years, it is called "PsA sine psoriasis" [28]. Nail changes are seen in up to 90% of individuals with PsA but only in 45% of patients with psoriasis [29, 30]. In 2006, the classification criteria of psoriatic arthritis (CASPAR) study group set up a highly sensitive (91–100%) and specific (97–99%) set of criteria that allow for the diagnosis of PsA even in cases of PsA sine psoriasis and in patients with positive rheumatoid factor [18, 31].

Different tools have been developed to screen patients with psoriasis for their musculoskeletal affection. The Psoriatic Arthritis Screening and Evaluation (PASE) is a screening tool that has been developed to increase detection of PsA by dermatologists. It is a self-administered questionnaire whose score greater than or equal to 47 has a sensitivity of 82% and a specificity of 73% for symptoms of PsA [31]. Multidimensional Patient-Reported Outcome Measures for spondyloarthritis has been published in 2010 [32] to be completed by the patient, and it includes patient self-reported assessment for the painful joints and soft tissue spots, record of the patient's functional ability and quality of life and measure for the patient psoriatic global assessment and psoriatic quality of life (Fig. 4.3).

Radiographic features of peripheral PsA are asymmetric distribution, involvement of the distal interphalangeal joint, periostitis and pencil-in-cup deformity in advanced cases of the disease. Ultrasonography (US) is a reliable method to detect signs of subclinical Achilles tendon enthesopathy and confirm diagnosis in patients with symptoms [33]. A recent study was carried out aiming at identifying the clinical predictors of arthritis in patients with psoriasis and to evaluate the use of musculoskeletal ultrasonography (US) as a predictor for inflammatory structural progression in psoriatic patients [34]. Results revealed that family history of psoriatic arthritis, large BMI (>25), high percentage of psoriatic body surface area and nail involvement were significantly associated with early-onset psoriatic arthritis. Baseline US grayscale score of ≥2, power Doppler score of ≥2, presence of enthesitis, enhanced vascularity at enthesitis, higher enthesitis score (GUESS score was used in that study) and onychopathy, as well as persistent synovitis and enthesitis at 6 months, were predictors of progressive early psoriatic arthritis. On another front, MRI helped in identifying that synovial inflammation in PsA is usually a secondary phenomenon to extra-synovial inflammation (primary affection), which aids to differentiate it from rheumatoid arthritis [35]. Therefore, it can be summarized that "radiography detects more erosions and osteoproliferation, but is less sensitive in the detection of changes in general. Effusions and synovitis are often detected by MRI and US" [36–38].

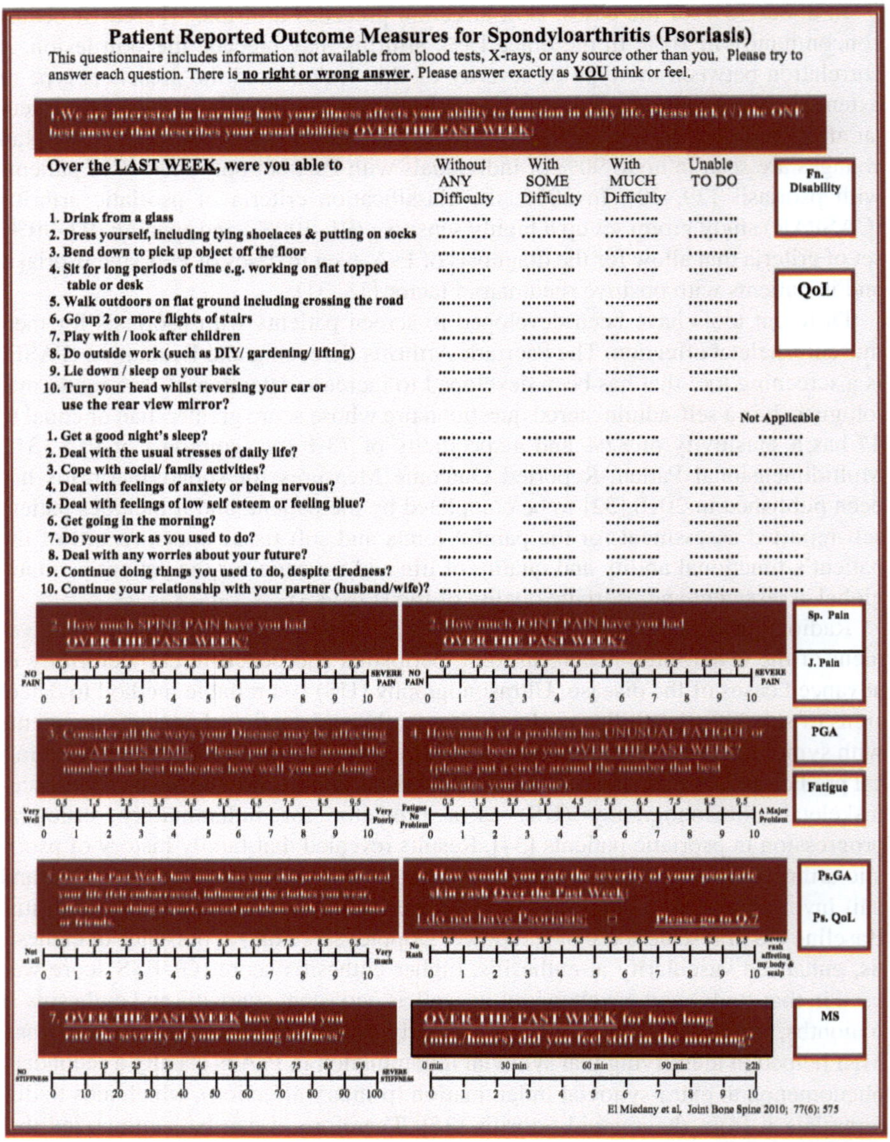

Patient Reported Outcome Measures for Spondyloarthritis (Psoriasis)

This questionnaire includes information not available from blood tests, X-rays, or any source other than you. Please try to answer each question. There is **no right or wrong answer**. Please answer exactly as **YOU** think or feel,

1.We are interested in learning how your illness affects your ability to function in daily life. Please tick (√) the ONE best answer that describes your usual abilities OVER THE PAST WEEK:

Over the LAST WEEK, were you able to	Without ANY Difficulty	With SOME Difficulty	With MUCH Difficulty	Unable TO DO	Not Applicable
1. Drink from a glass	....	....	....	....	
2. Dress yourself, including tying shoelaces & putting on socks	....	....	....	....	
3. Bend down to pick up object off the floor	....	....	....	....	
4. Sit for long periods of time e.g. working on flat topped table or desk	....	....	....	....	
5. Walk outdoors on flat ground including crossing the road	....	....	....	....	
6. Go up 2 or more flights of stairs	....	....	....	....	
7. Play with / look after children	....	....	....	....	
8. Do outside work (such as DIY/ gardening/ lifting)	....	....	....	....	
9. Lie down / sleep on your back	....	....	....	....	
10. Turn your head whilst reversing your car or use the rear view mirror?	....	....	....	....	
1. Get a good night's sleep?	....	....	....	....	....
2. Deal with the usual stresses of daily life?	....	....	....	....	....
3. Cope with social/ family activities?	....	....	....	....	....
4. Deal with feelings of anxiety or being nervous?	....	....	....	....	....
5. Deal with feelings of low self esteem or feeling blue?	....	....	....	....	....
6. Get going in the morning?	....	....	....	....	....
7. Do your work as you used to do?	....	....	....	....	....
8. Deal with any worries about your future?	....	....	....	....	....
9. Continue doing things you used to do, despite tiredness?	....	....	....	....	....
10. Continue your relationship with your partner (husband/wife)?	....	....	....	....	....

Fn. Disability

QoL

2. How much SPINE PAIN have you had OVER THE PAST WEEK?

NO PAIN 0 0.5 1 1.5 2 2.5 3 3.5 4 4.5 5 5.5 6 6.5 7 7.5 8 8.5 9 9.5 10 SEVERE PAIN

2. How much JOINT PAIN have you had OVER THE PAST WEEK?

NO PAIN 0 0.5 1 1.5 2 2.5 3 3.5 4 4.5 5 5.5 6 6.5 7 7.5 8 8.5 9 9.5 10 SEVERE PAIN

Sp. Pain

J. Pain

3. Consider all the ways your Disease may be affecting you AT THIS TIME. Please put a circle around the number that best indicates how well you are doing:

Very Well 0 0.5 1 1.5 2 2.5 3 3.5 4 4.5 5 5.5 6 6.5 7 7.5 8 8.5 9 9.5 10 Very Poorly

4. How much of a problem has UNUSUAL FATIGUE or tiredness been for you OVER THE PAST WEEK? (please put a circle around the number that best indicates your fatigue).

Fatigue No Problem 0 0.5 1 1.5 2 2.5 3 3.5 4 4.5 5 5.5 6 6.5 7 7.5 8 8.5 9 9.5 10 A Major Problem

PGA

Fatigue

5. Over the Past Week, how much has your skin problem affected your life (felt embarrassed, influenced the clothes you wear, affected you doing a sport, caused problems with your partner or friends.

Not at all 0 0.5 1 1.5 2 2.5 3 3.5 4 4.5 5 5.5 6 6.5 7 7.5 8 8.5 9 9.5 10 Very much

6. How would you rate the severity of your psoriatic skin rash Over the Past Week:

I do not have Psoriasis: □ Please go to Q.7

No Rash 0 0.5 1 1.5 2 2.5 3 3.5 4 4.5 5 5.5 6 6.5 7 7.5 8 8.5 9 9.5 10 Severe rash affecting my body & scalp

Ps.GA

Ps. QoL

7. OVER THE PAST WEEK how would you rate the severity of your morning stiffness?

NO STIFFNESS 0 5 10 15 20 25 30 35 40 45 50 55 60 65 70 75 80 85 90 95 100 SEVERE STIFFNESS

OVER THE PAST WEEK for how long (min./hours) did you feel stiff in the morning?

0 min 30 min 60 min 90 min ≥2h

0 1 2 3 4 5 6 7 8 9 10

MS

El Miedany et al, Joint Bone Spine 2010; 77(6): 575

Fig. 4.3 Multidimensional Patient-Reported Outcome Measures for patients with psoriasis/psoriatic arthritis (From El Miedany et al. [32], with permission)

Right	Left
Upper Limb	
Tip of the Shoulder	Tip of the Shoulder
Outer side of the Arm	Outer side of the Arm
Outer/ inner side of the elbow	Outer/ inner side of the elbow
Lower Limb	
Outer Hip Area	Outer Hip Area
Front of the knee	Front of the knee
Back of the ankle	Back of the ankle
Heel	Heel
Jaw	
Jaw (Rt.)	Jaw (Lt.)
Trunk	
Neck	Chest
Upper Back	Abdomen
Lower Back	Other:

Please place(√) at the most painful area(s) over your body which you feel painful TODAY.

Enthesitis score

Please place a (X) in the appropriate box to indicate in which of your joints you feel painful TODAY.

Tender Joints

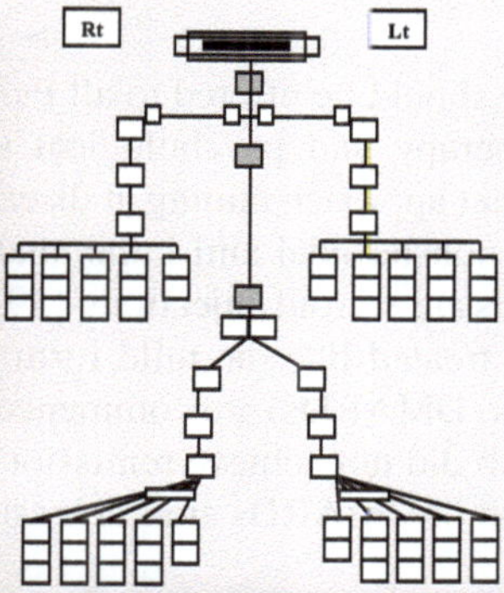

Neck
Shoulder
Shoulder Blade
Elbow
Wrist
Knuckles / Fingers
Low Back
Sacroiliac Joint
Hip
Knee
Ankle
Top Foot
Toes

7. Please tick (√) if you have experienced any of the following OVER THE LAST MONTH:

Fever		Dry Eye		Vertebral Fracture(s)		Cardiovascular Risk Assessment	
Weight gain (> 10 lbs)		Dry Mouth		Weakness/Paralysis of arms or legs		Age > 50 years old	
Weight Loss (> 10 lbs)		Pain in the eye / photophobia		Numbness or tingling		High Blood pressure	
Night Sweat		Headache		Muscle pain, ache or cramps		High Cholesterol	
Loss of appetite		Wheezing in the chest		Problems with thinking/memory		Current Smoker	
Soreness in the mouth		Cough		Absent from work due to spine pain		Ischemic heart Disease	
Genital Ulcers		Blood in your Phlegm		Short plans for having a baby		Stroke	
Skin Rash		Shortness of breath		Sexual relationship Problems		Irregular Heart Beats	
Psoriasis		Heartburn		Problems with erection (for men)		Diabetes Mellitus	
Painful Swollen finger/ toe		Dark or bloody stools		Falls Risk Assessment			
Change color/ thickening of your nail		Feeling Sickly / Nausea		>1 Fall in the last year		Take steroids > 5mg/day	
Inflammatory bowel Disease		Constipation		Problems with your sight		Ulcer or stomach problem	
Heart Valve lesion		Diarrhea		Loss of your balance		Lung Disease	
Problems with hearing		Problems with urination		Change in Gait / Walking Speed		Admitted cos of infection	
Ringing in the ears		> 3 Alcoholic drinks per day		Weakness of your grip strength		Liver Disease	

8. The statements below concern your personal beliefs. Please circle the number that best describes how do you feel about the statement. 0 = Not at all; 10 = Strongly Agree

Pt. Activ.

1. I understand the nature of my condition, the reasons for the symptoms, the course it runs and the consequences if left untreated.	0 1 2 3 4 5 6 7 8 9 10
2. I am aware of the different treatment options available to me and I understand what each of my medications do.	0 1 2 3 4 5 6 7 8 9 10
3. Overall I understand I am in charge of managing my condition and I feel confident I would know when to seek medical advice.	0 1 2 3 4 5 6 7 8 9 10
4. I am aware of my role in my own care, and feel able to stop the disease symptoms from interfering with my everyday activities.	0 1 2 3 4 5 6 7 8 9 10
5. I have the confidence to discuss any questions I may have or raise any concerns regarding my condition or treatment with my Doctor/nurse.	0 1 2 3 4 5 6 7 8 9 10
6. I am confident I am able to take any tablet and/or administer any injection prescribed for me.	0 1 2 3 4 5 6 7 8 9 10
7. I am able to self-manage my condition, ease the symptoms and overcome some of the difficulties associated with my condition.	0 1 2 3 4 5 6 7 8 9 10
8. I feel confident and able to find a solution to any new problem related to my condition	0 1 2 3 4 5 6 7 8 9 10
9. I am able to maintain life style changes like diet and exercise and feel confident I can continue these during difficult times.	0 1 2 3 4 5 6 7 8 9 10
10. I am confident I can find reliable sources of information about my condition and health choices.	0 1 2 3 4 5 6 7 8 9 10

□ I consent to my clinical data being used for research/audit. Signature: Date: / /20

Fig. 4.3 (continued)

Therapeutic Implications

Counseling should be offered to all PsA patients regarding their illness, in addition to physiotherapy and psychological support. Treatment protocols should adopt treat-to-target approach aiming at disease remission. Mild forms of the disease may respond to nonsteroidal anti-inflammatory drugs with or without intra-articular or local soft tissue steroid injections [39]. Moderate to severe forms of PsA should initially be treated like the mild form of the disease; disease-modifying antirheumatic drugs (DMARDs) are commenced in persistent arthritis case [40]. Refractory cases, which did not achieve remission or showed satisfactory response to one or a combination of DMARDs after at least 6 months of use, should be offered biologic therapy.

In a study carried out by Queiro-Silva and coauthors [41], PsA patients were followed up for more than 10 years. Fifty-five percent of the cases had five or more joint deformities. It was suggested that patients with initial presentation of five or more affected joints exhibit worse prognosis in relation to erosion and deformity. On the other hand, male gender, beginning in "early "age, small number of inflamed joints and improved functional class were associated with a higher chance of remission [27].

Wong et al. [42] identified increased rates of mortality among patients with PsA (59% and 65% in women and men, respectively), when compared to the healthy population. Jamnitski et al. [43] found a higher prevalence of risk factors and cardiovascular disease in patients with PsA, when compared with the general population. However, suppression of inflammation and changes in lifestyle have shown positive impact on the patient's mortality as well as morbidity.

Inflammatory Bowel Disease

Background and Pathophysiology

Inflammatory bowel disease, namely, Crohn's disease and ulcerative colitis, have been demonstrated to be significantly higher in patients with psoriasis than in the normal population, suggesting the possibility of a genetic link and share of the chronic inflammation process [44, 45]. Th17 cells in psoriatic skin produce IL-23, which is an essential cytokine for intestinal inflammation [46]. Polymorphisms in IL-23 and IL-12B receptor genes are also thought to play a role in all three disease processes [47–50].

Although individual susceptibility to psoriasis, Crohn's disease and ulcerative colitis has been located in close chromosomal loci, several other genetic loci have also been reported in each of these conditions. In a recent study, seven susceptibility loci shared by psoriasis and Crohn's disease were identified [45]. The susceptibility loci of psoriasis, Crohn's disease and ulcerative colitis all lie in the 6p21 locus, which encompasses the major histocompatibility complex. The IBD3 locus associated with Crohn's disease and ulcerative colitis and the PSORS1 locus of psoriasis lie at the same place as well [46, 51, 52].

Science-Based Medicine

Cohen et al. [45] examined the prevalence of inflammatory bowel disease in 12,502 patients with psoriasis and 24,287 age- and sex-matched control group members. They found a significantly higher prevalence of both Crohn's disease and ulcerative colitis in psoriatic patient group compared to the control group. These associations are biologically plausible, as systemic inflammation and TNF-alpha play an important role in all three diseases.

In a Nurses' Health Study (NHS) of 174,476 women with psoriasis or psoriatic arthritis, psoriasis was associated with an increased risk of developing Crohn's disease during both NHS I (1996–2008) (RR 4.00; 95% CI, 1.72–9.27) and NHS II (1991–2007) (RR 3.76; 95% CI, 1.82–7.74). The risk of Crohn's disease was highest among women with concomitant psoriatic arthritis (RR 6.43; 95% CI, 2.04–20.32) [53].

Other digestive diseases, such as celiac disease, also show a higher prevalence in the psoriasis population. In a case-control study by Birkenfeld et al. [54], the prevalence of celiac disease in patients from Israel with psoriasis was 0.29%, compared to 0.11% in controls ($P < 0.001$). Psoriasis was associated with celiac disease with an OR of 2.73 (95% CI, 1.65–4.53). Wu et al. [55] also found an association between psoriasis and celiac disease, with an OR of 2.2 (95% CI, 1.5–3.2) in a population of 25,341 Southern California Kaiser Permanente psoriatic patients.

Therapeutic Implications

Systemic medication, both DMARDs and biologic therapies, used to stop the inflammatory process and treat moderate to severe psoriasis is also indicated in inflammatory bowel diseases.

Methotrexate is used for treating active Crohn's disease in steroid-dependent patients. TNF-alpha inhibitors such as infliximab, adalimumab as well as golimumab have been employed for severe active Crohn's disease/ulcerative colitis that has not responded to conventional treatment [56].

Paradoxically, TNF-alpha inhibitors have been shown to induce psoriasis in some studies [51, 56–58]. All three TNF-alpha inhibitors that are US Food and Drug Administration approved for psoriasis (infliximab, etanercept and adalimumab) were associated with the induction of psoriasiform lesions, with a mean time of 9.5 months for the appearance of the lesions [57, 58]. It is thought that TNF-alpha inhibitors could favour the recruitment of activated T-cells in the skin of patients genetically predisposed to an enhancement of the chemokine receptor CXCR3 [59].

Certain psoriasis treatments can cause gastrointestinal side effects, and it could be difficult to separate a diagnosis of inflammatory bowel disease from these side effects. Infliximab, adalimumab, ustekinumab, methotrexate, acitretin and cyclosporine have side effects of abdominal pain, diarrhoea, dyspepsia and nausea.

Obesity

Background and Pathophysiology

Noninvasive imaging technique developments enabled the differentiation of two different depots of abdominal fat: (1) subcutaneous abdominal fat (which is the fat located just under the skin) and (2) visceral fat (which is the intra-abdominal excess fat present in the abdominal cavity). Furthermore, it is now recognized that abdominal obesity (central obesity or upper body obesity or android obesity) is the form of obesity most likely to be associated with an altered risk factor profile contributing to an increased cardiovascular disease (CVD) and type 2 diabetes risk, while gynoid obesity (or lower body obesity where fat is located around the buttocks and hips) is seldom associated with metabolic complications [60]. Therefore, intra-abdominal fat is no more considered as a merely inert mass (storing fat (lipids) as a source of energy to meet future needs of the body) but an active metabolic and endocrine organ. The discovery of leptin, a hormone secreted by these adipose cells, transferred that adipose tissue to an active endocrine gland, able to communicate with the brain to participate in the regulation of various body functions. Through its production of other important proteins (adipocytokines), including prothrombotic products such as plasminogen activator inhibitor-1, pro-inflammatory cytokines, such as tumour necrosis factor-α (TNF-alpha), (interleukin-6 (IL-6), renin-angiotensin system proteins, adiponectin and others; adipose tissue actively participates in disease evolution processes which can lead to hypertension, insulin resistance and type 2 diabetes as well as CVD [61]; promoting inflammation, affecting glucose metabolism as well as vascular endothelial biology [62, 63]. Hyperleptinaemia has been also associated with increased common carotid artery intimal media thickness (IMT) and arterial thrombosis. Besides, subcutaneous fat cells (adipocytes) bear Toll-like receptors which behave as a component of innate immunity and allow an immediate response to foreign pathogens and release cytokines [63]. As systemic inflammation continues and with increasing BMI, adiponectin is downregulated, while leptin and resistin are upregulated, which induces insulin resistance and causes endothelial cells to produce adhesion molecules, promoting a hepatic release of both fibrinogen and C-reactive protein and augmenting the procoagulant effects on platelets [2, 62–64]. Hence, obesity is considered a chronic, low-grade inflammatory condition [65].

Several studies have shown that psoriasis may be linked to obesity; however, controversy still exists as to whether obesity is a result or a causative factor of psoriasis [1, 3, 66]. Either way, this strong association makes psoriasis an important healthcare issue.

Science-Based Medicine

A strong and significant association between obesity, increased adiposity and psoriasis has been reported over the past years [67–69]. A recent study showed that increased body mass index (BMI) was a predisposing factor for developing psoriatic arthritis and severe psoriasis [70–73]. Other studies have shown that psoriatic patients have increased levels of leptin, and psoriasis itself is an independent risk factor for hyperleptinaemia [74–78].

The relationship between psoriasis and obesity is hypothesized to be bidirectional, with obesity predisposing patients to psoriasis and psoriasis increasing the risk of obesity [79, 80]. A meta-analysis of 16 observational studies [81] assessed the epidemiological associations between obesity and psoriasis in a population of 2.1 million patients (201,831 of them were patients living with psoriasis). The pooled OR for obesity among patients with mild psoriasis was 1.46 (95% CI, 1.17–1.82) and 2.23 (95% CI, 1.63–3.05) for severe psoriasis. One incidence study found that psoriatic patients have an HR of 1.18 (95% CI, 1.14–1.23) for new-onset obesity. In comparison with the general population, psoriatic patients in that study had a higher prevalence and incidence of obesity. Patients with more severe psoriasis have higher odds of obesity compared to those with mild psoriasis.

Therapeutic Implications

Advice on weight loss and leading healthy, active lifestyles should be given to all patients living with psoriasis. Patients should be counseled should they fail to adopt a reasonable dieting program to lose weight. In a randomized clinical study [71], mild-to-moderate psoriatic patients with body mass index (BMI) in the range of 27–40 kg/m^2 were allocated to either a standard routine dietary guidance group or an intensive weight loss therapy group. After 16 weeks, the dieting patients had a significantly less BMI with a statistical weight loss difference between the two groups of 15.4 kg (95% CI, 12.3–18.5 kg; $P < 0.001$). Dieting patients experienced a greater mean reduction in their PASI score compared to the control group (−2.3 versus 0.3), although this difference was not statistically significant ($P = 0.06$).

Several studies have found that TNF inhibitors such as adalimumab, etanercept and infliximab can cause weight gain [82–86]. The mechanism of weight gain among patients treated with TNF inhibitors is still unclear, although TNF-alpha is known to be involved in body weight homeostasis and is purported to influence appetite by modulating leptin release from adipocytes [87]. On another front, psoriatic patient weights can have cost-effectiveness role as it affects the dosing of IV, and sometimes subcutaneous, biologics. Furthermore, it may be one of the factors in the biologic therapy choice for psoriatic patients. A study revealed that weight-dosed IV biologics (such as infliximab) demonstrated consistent clinical responses in overweight and obese patient populations, while fixed-dosed biologics (such as etanercept) may not [88].

Diabetes Mellitus/Insulin Resistance

Background and Pathophysiology

Type 2 diabetes mellitus (DM) is a metabolic disorder characterized by increased insulin resistance and hyperglycaemia. Th1 cytokines, which have been reported to be overproduced in psoriasis, are thought to promote insulin resistance as well [89–91]. On another front, obesity, which, as mentioned above, is a comorbidity commonly reported in psoriatic patients, is a major risk factor for both type 2 DM and psoriasis [92]. Another possible contributing factor for the association between psoriasis and diabetes is the presence of chronic inflammation that occurs due to secretion of TNF-alpha and other pro-inflammatory cytokines such as IL-1 and IL-6, which precipitate both psoriasis and diabetes.

Science-Based Medicine

Psoriatic patients have been found to be more insulin resistant and to have impaired glucose tolerance and higher fasting insulin levels than healthy subjects [89, 93–95].

Azfar et al. [92] conducted a large cohort study of 108,132 psoriatic patients. After controlling for age, sex, BMI, hypertension and hyperlipidaemia, psoriasis was found to be an independent risk factor for incident type 2 DM (HR 1.14; 95% CI, 1.10–1.18). The risk was greatest in patients with severe disease (HR 1.46; 95% CI, 1.30–1.65).

A large observational study by Brauchli et al. [90] demonstrated an increased risk of incident diabetes mellitus in patients with psoriasis when compared to a psoriasis-free study group. Among 1061 incident cases of diabetes mellitus, 59% had a history of psoriasis. Also, results of that study revealed that the risk was higher for patients with a longer psoriasis disease duration.

Coto-Segura et al. [88] published a recent report involving observational studies assessing the relationship between psoriasis or psoriatic arthritis and type 2 diabetes mellitus; their findings supported the association between psoriasis, psoriatic arthritis and type 2 diabetes mellitus. Another study carried out by Armstrong et al. [94]

demonstrated an increased prevalence and incidence of diabetes among patients living with psoriasis and indicated that this association is stronger among those with severe psoriasis. In another study carried out by Cohen and his colleagues [95], results were in concordance with the previous reports as it showed that the age-adjusted proportion of diabetes was found to be significantly higher in psoriatic patients as compared to the control group, suggestive of an association between psoriasis and diabetes mellitus. This was supported by the findings of a forth study [96] which revealed that the prevalence of type 2 diabetes mellitus in mild and severe psoriasis and in controls in a case-control study of 1835 psoriatic patients was 37.4%, 41% and 16%, respectively ($P < 0.00001$).

Therapeutic Implications

In addition to its role in inflammatory arthritis, TNF has also been reported to mediate insulin resistance [97]. As a result of their higher TNF levels, diabetic patients living with chronic inflammatory conditions such as psoriasis may need higher insulin doses. When anti-TNF therapy is started, insulin sensitivity is thought to improve, and insulin requirements are lowered [98]. There have been multiple case reports of hypoglycaemia associated with etanercept, an anti-TNF treatment, in patients with psoriasis and type 2 diabetes mellitus [99, 100]. Treating dermatologists as well as rheumatologists should be aware that diabetic patients on both anti-TNF and insulin therapy may experience hypoglycaemia.

Thiazolidinediones (e.g. pioglitazone and rosiglitazone) are antidiabetic drugs that improve insulin sensitivity and have anti-inflammatory effects [101, 102]. They activate peroxisome proliferator-activated receptor-gamma, which leads to inhibition of proliferation of psoriatic keratinocytes [103]. A meta-analysis of the efficacy of thiazolidinediones on psoriasis found a significant decrease in mean PASI scores of people on pioglitazone, whereas the improvement on rosiglitazone was not significant [104].

Metabolic Syndrome

Background and Pathophysiology

Metabolic syndrome is a cluster of risk factors for cardiovascular disease, such as hypertension, central obesity, glucose intolerance and dyslipidemia. The National Cholesterol Education Program's Adult Treatment Panel III (NCEP ATP III) published the diagnostic criteria diagnosis of metabolic syndrome [105]. Diagnosis is made when a person has at least three of the following five conditions: (1) Fasting glucose of 100 mg/dL or greater (or receiving drug therapy for hyperglycaemia);

(2) Blood pressure of 130/85 mmHg or higher (or receiving drug therapy for hypertension); (3) Triglycerides of 150 mg/dL or higher (or receiving drug therapy for hypertriglyceridemia); (4) HDL cholesterol (high-density lipoprotein cholesterol) less than 40 mg/dL in men or less than 50 mg/dL in women (or receiving drug therapy for reduced HDL cholesterol); (5) Waist circumference of 102 cm (40 inches) or greater in men or 88 cm (35 inches) or greater in women (if Asian-American, 90 cm (35 inches) or greater in men or 80 cm (32 inches) or greater in women)

The metabolic syndrome is an important driver of adverse cardiovascular outcomes. Metabolic syndrome confers double the risk for coronary artery disease and increases the risks of stroke, fatty liver disease and cancer [106, 107]. The prevalence of metabolic syndrome in the general population has been estimated to be between 15% and 24% [108]. Psoriatic patients have an increased prevalence of metabolic syndrome [109].

The underlying pathophysiology linking psoriasis and metabolic syndrome may involve overlapping inflammatory pathways and genetic predisposition. While the pathophysiology of all metabolic syndrome components has not been clarified fully, metabolic syndrome is considered to be a heterogeneous and a complex disorder, developed on the basis of insulin resistance which, in large part, is a consequence of the increased pro-inflammatory cytokine levels, such as TNF-alpha, which play a central role in psoriasis pathogenesis [64, 110].

Chronic inflammation and dysregulation of cytokines not only promote epidermal hyperplasia in psoriasis but may also antagonize insulin signaling, alter adipokine expression and mediate insulin resistance and obesity [111].

Science-Based Medicine

A meta-analysis of 12 observational studies found a pooled OR of 2.26 for metabolic syndrome among a population of 41,853 patients living with psoriasis. The prevalence of metabolic syndrome ranged from 14% to 40%. A population-based, UK-based, cross-sectional study assessed the prevalence of metabolic syndrome in correlation with psoriatic disease severity. The OR for mild psoriatic patients was 1.22 (95% CI, 1.11–1.35), whereas for severe psoriatic patients, it was 1.98 (95% CI, 1.62–2.43) [67]. A cross-sectional study of a random sample of the US population found that 40% of psoriatic patients had metabolic syndrome, which was almost double the control prevalence of 23% [109].

Therapeutic Implications

Psoriatic patients should be screened and regularly monitored for obesity, hypertension, dyslipidemia and diabetes. Patients with suspected metabolic syndrome should be referred to a specialist for management. Advice regarding lifestyle and medical management are important to avoid any negative cardiovascular consequences.

Cardiovascular

Background and Pathophysiology

Along with other chronic inflammatory systemic diseases, psoriasis, rheumatoid arthritis and systemic lupus erythematosus have been linked to increased cardiovascular disease risk. This has been attributed to the shared inflammatory and pathogenic pathways.

T-Cell Activation

Psoriasis and atherosclerosis share a common pattern of Th1 and Th17 cytokine upregulation, T-cell activation and local as well as systemic expression of adhesion molecules and endothelins [112, 113]. Activated T-cells in the vicinity of inflammation areas produce type 1 cytokines such as interferon (IFN)-alpha, interleukin (IL)-2 and tumour necrosis factor (TNF)-alpha. IFN-alpha inhibits apoptosis, thus contributing to the hyperproliferation of keratinocytes. IL-2 stimulates T-cell proliferation [113, 114].

Tumour Necrosis Factor

TNF-alpha became under focus as an inflammatory cytokine involved in both psoriasis and atherosclerosis pathogenesis. In psoriasis, TNF-alpha activates and increases keratinocyte proliferation. TNF-alpha has also been found to induce neutrophil chemotaxis, macrophage cytokine and chemokine production and superoxide production, which can result in endothelial inflammation and dysfunction [115, 116].

C-Reactive Protein (CRP)

CRP is a marker of systemic inflammation that has been associated with atherosclerosis and cardiovascular disease. Elevated CRP is a result of excess formation of pro-inflammatory cytokines IL-6, IL-1 and TNF-alpha [117].

CRP was also reported to be elevated in association with cardiovascular risk factors such as smoking, obesity and diabetes [118]. Several studies have shown that CRP can be used as a predictor of the adverse cardiovascular event risk in both healthy individuals and those with a previous history of myocardial infarction. Psoriatic patients have been shown to have higher baseline CRP levels than healthy controls in two studies ($P < 0.004$ and $P < 0.001$) [119, 120]. In another work, CRP levels were found to correlate significantly with the disease severity. Patients with mild and severe psoriasis had higher levels of CRP in comparison to controls (mean ± standard deviation: 0.31 ± 0.02 mg/dL versus 0.90 ± 0.27 mg/dL; $P < 0.001$). In concordance, patients with severe psoriasis had higher CRP levels than those with mild psoriasis (mean ± standard deviation: 1.16 ± 0.07 versus 0.63 ± 0.03 mg/dL) [121].

Vascular Endothelial Growth Factor (VEGF)

Another possible mechanism of psoriasis-associated atherosclerosis is the VEGF produced by keratinocytes, which is increased in psoriasis. VEGF is a mitogen for endothelial cells and has been linked to intimal hyperplasia. VEGF is also positively associated with the severity of psoriasis [122–124].

As rapid skin turnover and increased keratinocyte activity occur in psoriasis, folate is consumed excessively in order to methylate DNA, a requirement for the rapidly dividing cells [125]. Patients with psoriasis were reported to have lower folate levels and, subsequently, higher homocysteine levels than normal controls [126]. Hyperhomocysteinaemia is an independent risk factor for cardiovascular, peripheral vascular as well as cerebrovascular diseases [127, 128]. High homocysteine levels are able to damage endothelial cells, promote clot formation, decrease the flexibility of the blood vessels and consequently increase aortic stiffness. Elevated homocysteine may be another pathway of how psoriasis can be linked to the increased risk of cardiovascular disease [125]; however, the data on whether higher homocysteine levels correspond to the severity of psoriasis are conflicting [126, 129, 130].

Science-Based Medicine

The risk of developing cardiovascular disease in patients living with psoriasis has been studied in several publications. In the work carried out by Kimball and co-workers [131], the 10-year risk of coronary heart disease and stroke was assessed in 1591 psoriatic patients and was found to be significantly higher in patients with psoriasis when compared to the general population. The risk was estimated at 28% greater for coronary heart disease and 11.8% greater for stroke. In another study, Gelfand et al. [132] examined the incidence of myocardial infraction among patients with and without psoriasis. They monitored 130,976 psoriatic patients in comparison to 556,995 healthy subjects as a control group. Follow-up period lasted for a mean of 5.4 years. The authors showed that psoriatic patients had a higher incidence of myocardial infarction compared to control patients and that patients identified to have severe psoriasis had the highest rate.

In a Danish study [133] which included 36,765 mild psoriatic patients, 2793 severe psoriatic patients and 4,478,926 other individuals, atrial fibrillation and ischemic stroke incidence rates were increased in the psoriasis population. Atrial fibrillation rates were found to be 3.03 per 1000 observational years for normal controls, 4.67 for mild psoriatic patients and 5.96 for severe psoriatic patients ($P < 0.05$). Ischemic stroke incidence rates were 3.06, 4.54 and 6.82 per 1000 observational years for reference patients, mild psoriatic patients and severe psoriatic patients, respectively ($P < 0.05$).

Increased intima-media thickness (IMT) and carotid plaque are considered to be intermediate risk factors for subclinical atherosclerosis and a predictor of stroke and myocardial infraction [134]. One recent study found a significant association between psoriasis and increased common carotid artery IMT (beta 0.016; CI, 0.004–0.028; $P < 0.008$) after controlling for cardiovascular risk factors. However, carotid plaque's association with psoriasis was not significant (OR 1.12; 95% CI, 0.85–1.47) [135]. Three other case-control studies detected a similar increase in IMT and no significant atherosclerotic plaque difference when psoriatic patients were compared to controls [136–140].

Increased arterial stiffness has also been linked to psoriasis. One study [139] found a significantly higher pulse wave velocity (a marker for arterial stiffness) in psoriatic patients versus normal controls (8.78 ± 1.98 versus 7.78 ± 2.0 m/s; $P < 0.03$) after controlling for cardiovascular risk factors. Another study by Balta et al. [113] reported a pulse wave velocity of 7.63 versus 6.96 ($P < 0.01$) for psoriasis versus control patients. The authors also reported increased levels of CRP in psoriatic patients versus controls (2.54 ± 2.6 versus 1.22 ± 0.94; $P < 0.01$). CRP levels were found to be independently predictive of increased arterial stiffness.

Coronary artery calcification was also reported prevalent in psoriatic patients. In a study by Ludwig et al. [141], there was an increased prevalence (59.4% versus 28.1%, $P < 0.015$) of coronary artery calcification in 32 psoriatic patients compared to controls. Other studies [142, 143] have found that coronary artery calcification scores predict atherosclerotic cardiovascular disease events independently of standard risk factors and CRP levels. A study by Osto et al. [144] found that, in young patients with severe psoriasis and no heart disease, coronary flow rate was reduced, suggesting early coronary microvascular dysfunction. The risk of coronary microvascular dysfunction correlated with Psoriasis Area Severity Index (PASI) scores independently of other cardiovascular risk factors.

Therapeutic Implications

Because cardiovascular disease represents an important comorbidity in psoriasis, screening patients for cardiovascular risk factors, reviewing the current medications, monitoring the risk factors and offering counseling to patients regarding healthy lifestyle habits (diet, exercise and smoking cessation) are important to prevent any serious negative consequences.

In managing skin psoriasis, and its associated musculoskeletal manifestations, disease activity is vital to minimize the cardiovascular risk. Methotrexate is the most common medication used for the treatment of psoriasis. Controlling for the disease activity and inflammatory process was found to decrease the risk of cardiovascular disease in chronic inflammatory diseases [145]. However, long-term methotrexate use was also found to cause hyperhomocysteinaemia, which is an independent risk factor for vascular disease [146]. In a retrospective study of US veterans with psoriasis and rheumatoid arthritis, methotrexate was found to significantly reduce the risk of vascular disease (psoriasis, RR 0.73; 95% CI, 0.55–0.98). When folic acid was taken concurrently with methotrexate to lower homocysteine levels, the incidence of vascular disease in psoriatic patients decreased even further (psoriasis, RR 0.56; 95% CI, 0.39–0.80). In a meta-analysis of 10 studies, methotrexate was associated with a 21% lower risk of total cardiovascular disease ($n = 10$ studies; 95% CI, 0.73–0.87; $P < 0.001$) and an 18% lower risk of myocardial infarction ($n = 5$; 95% CI, 0.71–0.96; $P < 0.01$) [145].

In contrast with disease-modifying drug therapy agents (DMARDs), biologic therapy agents showed even better impact on cardiovascular risk in patients with chronic inflammatory conditions. TNF inhibitors have been associated with a reduced incidence of myocardial infraction to a greater degree than methotrexate [147]. A retrospective cohort study of 8845 psoriatic patients found that treatment with TNF inhibitors resulted in a 55% reduction in myocardial infraction incidence when compared to the topical therapy group ($P < 0.001$) [148]. A literature review of TNF inhibitors in the treatment of psoriasis concluded that TNF inhibitors have beneficial effects on cardiovascular biomarkers (CRP and erythrocyte sedimentation rate [ESR]) and may prevent myocardial infarction. A combination of methotrexate and TNF inhibitors is thought to provide the largest cardioprotective effect. In a study by Piaserico et al. [149], biologics were found to be more effective than traditional treatments (methotrexate, acitretin, cyclosporine and psoralen ultraviolet A [PUVA]) in the elderly population.

Hypertension

Background and Pathophysiology

Although psoriasis and hypertension share common risk factors, such as smoking and obesity, psoriasis has been found to be independently associated with hypertension. The exact mechanistic link underlying the relationship between psoriasis and hypertension is unknown, but there are a number of hypotheses regarding this association.

Renin-Angiotensin System

Alterations to the renin-angiotensin system in psoriasis may contribute to poor blood pressure control. Earlier studies revealed that psoriatic patients tend to have elevated plasma renin activity and elevated angiotensin-converting enzyme (ACE) activity [150–152]. High ACE levels may play a role in altering cytokine regulation of the vascular system. Certain ACE gene polymorphisms have also been associated with increased susceptibility to psoriasis, but these results are controversial [153].

Endothelin

Endothelin-1, which is a potent vasoconstrictor, was also found to be elevated in the serum and psoriatic skin lesions [154]. Increased oxidative stress in psoriatic patients is also hypothesized as a contributing factor causing impairment of the vasodilatory mechanism of the endothelium [155, 156].

Although doing less physical activity was suggested by some investigators as a contributing factor to increased cardiovascular risk in psoriatic patients, psoriasis was found to be independently associated with hypertension even after controlling for physical activity level [81, 89, 90]

Science-Based Medicine

In a meta-analysis of 24 observational studies, the pooled ORs for hypertension among patients with mild and severe psoriasis were 1.30 (95% CI, 1.15–1.47) and 1.49 (95% CI, 1.20–1.86), respectively [81]. In a case-control study of 12,502 psoriatic patients, the prevalence of hypertension was significantly higher in psoriatic patients than in controls (38.8% and 29.1%, respectively, $P < 0.001$) [157]. In a multivariate analysis, hypertension was associated with psoriasis after controlling for other risk factors (OR 1.37; 95% CI, 1.29–1.46). Other studies have reported hypertension prevalence of 40.3%, 32% and 11.55% in severe psoriasis, mild to moderate psoriasis and controls, respectively ($P < 0.00001$) [92]. A cross-sectional UK study reported an OR of 1.03 (95% CI, 1.01–1.06) for hypertension in patients with mild psoriasis [6].

Therapeutic Implications

Given the advanced technology and the fact that every patient can have a blood pressure machine at home, patients living with psoriasis should be encouraged to monitor their blood pressure. The importance of healthy lifestyle habits should also be highlighted by the treating physician whether dermatologist or rheumatologist. Patients who have been diagnosed to have hypertension, and started medical management, should follow up with their primary care provider and adhere to treatment.

Hypertension is a commonly reported side effect of the anti-psoriasis drug cyclosporine. Cyclosporine has been found to significantly increase blood pressure in a dose-dependent fashion. A meta-analysis [158] of 17 trials found that lower doses (1–4 mg/kg/day) increased mean blood pressure by an average of 5 mmHg, and higher doses (10 mg/kg/day) increased mean blood pressure by an average of 11 mmHg. Therefore, care must be taken to monitor patient blood pressure while using cyclosporine to control their psoriatic skin lesions.

Beta-blockers have been reported to exacerbate psoriasis [159]. Beta-blockers reduce intracellular concentrations of calcium, which may lead to an accelerated proliferation of keratinocytes and polymorphonuclear leukocytes [160]. However, a case-control study in the UK did not find a significant association between antihypertensive medications and psoriasis [90].

Dyslipidemia

Background and Pathophysiology

Dyslipidemia is a broad term incorporating abnormalities of plasma lipid levels or composition. Dyslipidemia is a well-known and established cardiovascular risk factor for stroke, coronary artery disease, myocardial infarction as well as cardiovascular mortality [161–164]. Classically, it presents as increased low-density lipoprotein (LDL), very low-density lipoprotein (VLDL) and triglyceride levels and decreased high-density lipoprotein (HDL) levels.

Several mechanisms were suggested regarding the possible link between dyslipidemia and psoriasis. The activation of Th1 cells, autoantibodies recognizing oxidized LDL and psoriasis medications such as oral retinoids and cyclosporine was named as purported mechanisms [165]. Specifically, the cytokines IL-1, IL-6 and TNF-alpha that mediate psoriasis may alter the function of hepatocytes and arterial smooth muscle cells, resulting in altered lipoprotein compositions, enhanced expression of cellular adhesion molecules and increased lipid deposition on arterial walls. These processes ultimately lead to the development of arterial plaques. Cytokines increase the expression of matrix metalloproteinases, causing degradation of the plaque's fibrous cap, which, eventually, may cause rupture of the plaque leading to the formation of life-threatening embolia [166].

Furthermore, IL-1, IL-6 and TNF-alpha are also involved in the inhibition of lipoprotein lipase activity, which results in decreased triglyceride clearance and increased plasma triglyceride levels [167–169]. Some studies suggest that these cytokines may elevate lipid levels by augmenting lipolysis and stimulating hepatic de novo fatty acid synthesis [170, 171].

Psoriasis is associated with an increased production of reactive oxygen species that overwhelm the body's antioxidant capacity [172]. Levels of lipid peroxidation products can indirectly measure the production of reactive oxygen species. Lipid peroxidation markers such as malondialdehyde, oxidized LDL (ox-LDL), thiobarbituric acid and anti-ox-LDL autoantibody were found to be elevated in patients with severe psoriasis compared to those with mild psoriasis [173]. Ox-LDL, which is found in the upper epidermis of psoriatic skin, is also an initiator of inflammation and influences the adhesion and oxidant status of endothelial cells. This mechanism is thought to implicate ox-LDL in early atherogenesis [174].

Science-Based Medicine

A systematic review of 25 cross-sectional and case-control studies found that psoriasis was associated with greater odds of dyslipidemia [175]. Twenty of the twenty-five studies reported a positive association between psoriasis and dyslipidemia, with ORs ranging from 1.04 to 5.55. The three studies that accounted for psoriasis severity found that greater psoriasis severity was associated with a higher prevalence of dyslipidemia, with the ORs for mild and severe psoriasis ranging from 1.10–3.38 to 1.36–5.55, respectively. Multiple measures of dyslipidemia were affected, with studies showing increased triglycerides, LDL, total cholesterol and lipoprotein levels, as well as lowered HDL.

Therapeutic Implications

Treatment with the anti-TNF drugs etanercept, infliximab and adalimumab has been shown to reduce the levels of inflammatory markers (CRP) and lipid peroxidation products while increasing serum antioxidant capacity [176]. These effects are associated with an increase in the level of paraoxonase 1 (PON1), an antioxidant enzyme and anti-inflammatory enzyme associated with HDL. HDL levels also increased after treatment.

Anti-TNF drugs have also been reported to induce structural changes in the HDL protein composition [177]. During inflammation, the HDL protein composition changes so that it is unable to protect LDL from oxidation. Anti-TNF drugs were found to restore HDL's protein composition back to an atheroprotective state in patients with rheumatoid arthritis. However, other studies have found no favourable change in lipid profiles of psoriatic patients with TNF inhibitors [178–182].

Drugs that have an unfavourable effect on lipid profile include retinoids and cyclosporine. Retinoids increase triglyceride levels as well as total, LDL and VLDL cholesterol and decrease HDL levels [183–188]. Cyclosporine has also been linked to hypertriglyceridemia, although the mechanism of this association is unclear. Eighty percent of plasma cyclosporine is bound to VLDL, and cyclosporine is hypothesized to either increase hepatic output of VLDL or interfere with the clearance of VLDL [189].

Statins, which lower LDL and maintain plaque stability, also modulate the inflammatory response and are thus of interest in psoriasis. Statins lower CRP and TNF-alpha levels while downregulating adhesion molecules on leukocytes and endothelial cells and inhibiting major histocompatibility complex II expression and chemokine receptors on Th1 cells [190]. Statins can differ by ninefold in their ability to block nuclear factor kappa B, a transcription factor needed for pro-inflammatory cytokine production [191]. This may explain why there have been conflicting reports on whether statins help or hurt in psoriasis [192, 193]. One small pilot study evaluated the efficacy of simvastatin in treating plaque psoriasis and found a significant reduction in PASI scores of 47.34% [194]. Fibrates, another class of lipid-lowering drugs, may exacerbate psoriasis [195, 196].

Non-alcoholic Fatty Liver Disease (NAFLD)

Background and Pathophysiology

NAFLD is defined as an excessive accumulation of triglycerides in hepatocytes of patients without a history of excessive alcohol consumption [197]. NAFLD is classified according to severity: simple NAFLD only consists of fatty infiltration; NASH (non-alcoholic steatohepatitis) is characterized by fatty infiltration and lobular inflammation; NAFLD with fibrosis or cirrhosis is the most severe stage and can progress to hepatocellular carcinoma. NAFLD is considered the hepatic expression of metabolic syndrome and is also associated with type 2 diabetes mellitus and dyslipidemia [198, 199]. The pathophysiology behind the association of NAFLD with psoriasis is thought to be related to chronic inflammation – pro-inflammatory adipokines and skin-derived cytokines (TNF-alpha, IL-17/IL-23) – which induces the development of insulin resistance, which in turn promotes hepatic lipid accumulation [65, 148].

Science-Based Medicine

The relationship between non-alcoholic fatty liver disease (NAFLD) and psoriasis severity has been established. NAFLD is found to be highly prevalent among psoriatic patients, where it is closely associated with obesity and metabolic syndrome [200–204]. Gisondi et al. [202] have demonstrated a significant association between psoriasis and NAFLD with higher frequency of NAFLD in 130 patients with plaque psoriasis compared to a control group (47% versus 28%). This association was present after controlling for BMI, suggesting that NAFLD is linked to psoriasis independently of obesity. Patients with psoriasis and NAFLD also had higher serum C-reactive protein concentrations and greater severity of psoriasis and revealed a higher frequency of metabolic syndrome than those with psoriasis alone. Miele and co-workers [200] prospectively examined the prevalence and characteristics of NAFLD in 142 patients with psoriasis and found NAFLD in 59.2% of the patients. The study revealed that NAFLD in psoriatic patients was significantly correlated with metabolic syndrome.

Therapeutic Implications

NAFLD should be suspected in psoriatic patients with an associated comorbidity such as metabolic syndrome, obesity, diabetes, dyslipidemia or hypertension. Liver enzyme tests should be ordered if risk factors for NAFLD are present, and the patient should be referred to the appropriate specialist.

Methotrexate is known to be hepatotoxic and has been linked to the development of fatty liver disease, fibrosis and cirrhosis. Patients on methotrexate may develop elevations of serum aspartate aminotransferase and alanine aminotransferase; however, these are usually mild and self-limiting and disappear with dose modification of methotrexate [205, 206]. Methotrexate depletes hepatic folate stores. Although a relationship between hepatic toxicity and folate depletion has not been established, oral folic acid supplements were found to reduce serum transaminase levels in patients on low-dose, long-term methotrexate therapy [206, 207].

In the past, the American Academy of Dermatology and National Psoriasis Foundation recommended that all patients with psoriasis undergo liver biopsies after every 1–1.5 g of cumulative methotrexate [208]. In 2009, these recommendations were updated. However, though histological evaluation of a liver biopsy specimen is currently the gold standard for diagnosing, staging and monitoring liver fibrosis due to any cause, the procedure of liver biopsy carries significant morbidity and mortality and is disliked by patients. The need for liver biopsy is commonly cited as a reason for dissatisfaction with treatment by patients or for discontinuing therapy when biopsy is felt to be necessary [209]. In addition, other limitations include the following: the biopsy technique is subject to sample errors, the samples collected are very small, pathological change may not be evenly distributed and, lastly, the interpretation may vary among histologists depending on level of experience, size of biopsy and use of staging/scoring system.

Given the limitations of liver biopsy, significant effort has been invested in identifying clinically useful and noninvasive markers of liver fibrosis that allow identification and quantification of liver fibrosis [210]. Fibroelastography (achieved using the FibroScan) gives a measure of liver elasticity (and therefore fibrosis) by measuring reflected ultrasound echoes before and during compression of the liver. The degree of displacement is related to the tissue elasticity stiffness. This method has been used to evaluate and track fibrosis in chronic liver disease [211] and, as indicated in recent systematic review and economic analysis by the NHS Centre for Evidence-based Purchasing, may have clinical utility for the detection and monitoring of fibrosis due to other causes.

Serum biomarkers of liver fibrosis focus on indirect markers of liver function or direct markers of extracellular matrix components or the enzymes involved in their turnover. Indirect markers of liver function include aspartate aminotransferase (AST), alanine aminotransferase (ALT), c-glutamyl transpeptidase (c-GT), hyaluronic acid, apolipoprotein A1, bilirubin, alpha-2-macroglobulin, haptoglobin, cholesterol, homeostasis model assessment of insulin resistance, platelets and prothrombin time [212]. Direct markers of liver function include collagen IV, collagen VI, tissue inhibitor of metalloproteases-1 (TIMP-1), laminin, human cartilage glycoprotein-39 (YKL-40), tenascin, undulin, matrix metalloproteinase-2 (MMP-2) and procollagen III propeptide (P3NP) [213]. Some of these biomarkers have been combined to improve clinical utility (e.g. the European Enhanced Liver Fibrosis (ELF) panel which combines hyaluronic acid, TIMP-1 and P3NP measurements).

For the last 5–10 years, serial measurement of procollagen III (P3NP) has become a standard practice for monitoring liver fibrosis in patients on methotrexate, with elevated levels indicating the need for treatment cessation and/or consideration of liver biopsy. Continually raised P3NP concentrations were found to be associated with fibrosis in 78–100% of cases but were seen in 15–18% of subjects with a normal liver on biopsy. Current guidelines on the use of methotrexate in psoriasis suggest P3NP measurements be carried out annually and trimonthly after a raised value. P3NP is a sensitive indicator of hepatic fibrosis but may be raised in other conditions, particularly active connective tissue disease [214].

A liver biopsy should be considered if (1) there are three P3NP levels above 4.2 ug/L or (2) two levels above 8.0 ug/L over a 12-month period. A liver biopsy should also be considered if the pretreatment level is above 8.0 ug/L, whereas withdrawing methotrexate should be considered if three samples are >10.0 μg/L in a 12-month period [215].

Malignancy

Background and Pathophysiology

The chronic, inflammatory state induced by psoriasis has been purported to initiate the development of certain neoplastic diseases. As psoriasis is an immune-mediated disease, its pathophysiology has been linked to an increased risk of lymphoma [216]. This association has been reported in other Th1-mediated diseases, such as rheumatoid arthritis [217, 218]. Patients with more severe psoriasis may also be receiving treatment with PUVA therapy, which has been associated with malignancies [219]. A higher prevalence of alcohol or cigarette abuse, risk factors for cancer, has also been reported in psoriatic patients [220, 221].

Science-Based Medicine

The relationship between psoriasis and increased cancer risk is still debated. A large population-based study found an association between duration and severity of psoriasis and specific cancers. Patients with a long duration of psoriasis were at an increased risk of colorectal, bladder, kidney, pancreatic and lymphohematopoietic cancers. Patients with more severe psoriasis who were receiving oral therapy were also at an increased risk of developing cancer (OR 10.17; 95% CI, 3.24–31.94). An analysis of patients without oral treatment (azathioprine, cyclosporine, methotrexate, acitretin, hydroxyurea, mycophenolate mofetil or UV/PUVA therapy) yielded adjusted ORs of 1.59 (95% CI, 1.01–2.50) for patients with psoriasis of under 2-year duration and 2.12 (95% CI, 1.45–3.10) for those with psoriasis of greater than 2-year duration for lymphohematopoietic cancers [219].

A recently reported meta-analysis of epidemiological studies [222], including 1080 articles, indicated that there may be an increased risk of some solid cancers, such as lung cancer, in psoriatic patients, particularly smokers and alcohol users; however, the large heterogeneity between these studies regarding study population and follow-up constituted the limitation of that report. A cohort study of 7061 Taiwanese psoriatic patients found that psoriatic patients were more likely to develop non-melanoma skin cancer and lymphoma. Patients who had never received systemic therapy were also more likely to develop non-melanoma skin cancer and lymphoma, suggesting that psoriasis could be an independent risk factor for these malignancies [223].

Therapeutic Implications

Systemic treatments such as PUVA and cyclosporine have been linked to increased risk of cancer. The PUVA follow-up study [224], which tracked 1380 psoriatic patients for 30 years, found a dose-dependent increase in the risk of squamous cell carcinoma (SCC) and a moderate increase in the risk of basal cell carcinoma after PUVA therapy. More than one-half of patients who received 350 or more PUVA treatments developed squamous cell carcinoma, and a significant risk was noted after 150 treatments. The risk of malignant melanoma also increased about 15 years after initiation of PUVA treatment, especially among patients who underwent more than 250 treatments [225]. Therefore, physicians should weigh the benefits and risks for each patient, taking into account their baseline risk for skin cancer and the number of PUVA treatments needed [224]. The PUVA follow-up study also found an increased incidence of lymphoma in patients who were taking high doses of methotrexate in addition to receiving PUVA therapy (incidence rate ratio 4.39; 95% CI, 1.59–12.06). Patients who were on PUVA therapy only had rates of lymphoma comparable to those of the general population (incidence rate ratio 0.85; 95% CI, 0.37–1.67) [226].

A cohort study of 1252 severe psoriatic patients [227] found that low-dose cyclosporine (2.7–3.1 mg/kg/day) was associated with a sixfold increase in the risk of squamous cell carcinoma within a 5-year follow-up. Patients at greatest risk were those who were treated with cyclosporine for more than 2 years or previously exposed to PUVA, immunosuppressants or methotrexate. Cyclosporine should not be used together with phototherapy, before or after PUVA or in patients with a history of squamous cell carcinoma or melanoma [228].

Some meta-analyses and observational studies have found that TNF-alpha inhibitors are associated with an increased risk of malignancy in rheumatoid arthritis patients, although the evidence is conflicting [229–231]. In concordance with rheumatoid arthritis patients who are usually on concomitant systemic immunosuppressants, this could be also the case in psoriatic patients who are usually treated with combination therapy. However, it is unclear if safety data from rheumatoid arthritis studies can be generalized to psoriasis. One meta-analysis of data from 20 randomized clinical trials of adult patients with plaque psoriasis and psoriatic arthritis treated with anti-TNF-alpha agents did not find a statistically significant increase in the risk of malignancies [232].

Anxiety and Depression

Background and Pathophysiology

Psoriasis is a physically, socially and psychologically disabling disease that negatively impacts quality of life [233–238]. Psoriasis impairs ability to carry out activities of daily living which require the use of hands, walking, sitting and standing for long periods of time. Its negative impact extends also to include work performance, sexual activities and sleep [233, 234]. The visibility of psoriatic lesions can often result in feelings of embarrassment, social withdrawal and lack of self-esteem. Psoriatic patients reported significantly higher degrees of depression and more body cathexis problems. In addition, the risk for developing psoriasis increased significantly in patients with moderate and severe depression [234, 236].

Increased levels of pro-inflammatory cytokines such as IL-1, TNF-alpha and IFN-gamma that are seen in psoriasis are purported to act as neuromodulators and may mediate depressive disorders [239].

Administration of pro-inflammatory cytokines in cancer and hepatitis C therapies, and other chronic inflammatory diseases such as rheumatoid arthritis, has been associated with depression. Researchers have generally found higher levels of depression in patients with a greater percentage of their skin affected by psoriasis [240]. Higher rates of suicidal ideation that correlate with higher self-ratings of disease severity have also been reported [241].

Science-Based Medicine

Depression and anxiety are important psychological comorbidities of psoriasis. Krueger and co-workers [242] assessed patients' perspectives on the impact of psoriasis using a self-administered questionnaire to be completed by the patients living with psoriasis. Seventy-nine percent of the patients reported that psoriasis had a negative impact on their lives, and 40% felt frustrated with the ineffectiveness of their current therapies.

Using the Psoriasis Life Stress Inventory, Gupta and Gupta [243] surveyed 217 patients with a range of psoriasis severity. The most commonly reported stressor was due to disfigurement. Over one-half of patients reported feeling self-conscious around strangers. In another study by Gupta et al. [244], 26% of patients noted that they had experienced an episode in which people "made a conscious effort not to touch them" in the previous month. Another study [245] found that 83% of patients with moderate to severe psoriasis felt they "often" or "always" needed to hide their psoriasis. Seventy-four percent reported that their self-confidence was "often" or "always" affected by their psoriasis, and 83% would "often" or "always" avoid social activities such as swimming.

Analysis of the Psoriasis Life Stress Inventory revealed that psoriatic patients experienced stress from anticipating the reaction and avoidance of others and stress from fear of being evaluated exclusively on the basis of their skin. Psoriatic patients also had significantly higher levels of experiences of stigmatization compared to other dermatology patients [245].

Therapeutic Implications

Physicians should screen their patients for anxiety and depression and explore patients' perceptions of their disease. Various psychosocial interventions have been demonstrated to help patients. In a large study, pharmacotherapy plus a 6-week program of cognitive behavioural therapy led to significantly greater decreases in psoriasis severity, self-reported disability and psychological distress than pharmacotherapy only [239]. These improvements were maintained for more than 6 months after the completion of cognitive behavioural therapy. Effective treatment for psoriasis should involve a multidimensional approach that integrates psychosocial well-being and patients' perceptions of their disease [246].

Osteoporosis

Background and Pathophysiology

Several mechanisms may be implicated as a possible cause for the association between psoriasis and osteoporosis, such as systemic inflammation, anti-psoriatic drug intake and joint dysfunction (attributed to PsA). It is suggested that chronic inflammation associated with psoriasis and psoriatic arthritis affects bone metabolism and may lead to an imbalance between bone resorption and bone formation. Earlier studies [247, 248] revealed that, similar to rheumatoid arthritis, inflammatory cytokines and pro-inflammatory proteins are able to induce bone mineral loss. Both TNF-alpha and IL-6 act by stimulating bone reabsorption. Elevated levels of these cytokines are found in menopausal women and in children with idiopathic osteoporosis.

Science-Based Medicine

Millard et al. [248] observed no statistically significant difference between the Z-score of lumbar vertebrae of individuals with and without psoriasis. However, among psoriatic patients, those with arthropathy showed lower bone density. Hofbauer et al. [249] reported that one-third of PsA patients had low bone density, and osteoporosis was about six times more frequent in men. These findings are in concordance to another subsequent study [250], which identified increased prevalence of osteoporosis in both genders. This, however, was statistically significant only for men. Bone mass loss in PsA still seems to be related to the duration of the disease, its severity (measured by PASI) and the number of joints affected. In a study which included post-/menopausal women, Pedreira et al. [251] observed similarity in bone density among healthy controls, individuals with psoriasis and individuals with PsA. However, osteoporotic fractures were more common in patients with psoriasis and PsA. It is clear, therefore, that the data in the literature are controversial; this might explain why some authors still advocate that there is no association between psoriasis and osteoporosis [252]. In a recently published review, Ogdie and colleagues [253] cited studies showing that the prevalence of osteoporosis in patients with psoriatic arthritis was higher than previously thought and comparable to that in patients with rheumatoid arthritis and ankylosing spondylitis. The authors urged a "high index of suspicion" for osteoporosis in patients with psoriatic arthritis "as complications of undertreated osteoporosis can be devastating". Therefore, it is advised that psoriatic disease patients, especially those with a long history of the disease, should get screened for bone loss.

Uveitis

Although psoriasis is associated with intraocular inflammatory disease, especially uveitis, only few studies have assessed the ophthalmic pathologies that accompany vulgar psoriasis. Its prevalence has been estimated around 2% in patients with cutaneous psoriasis. Most of the published research emphasized its higher prevalence in males and patients with late disease onset [254].

Uveitis has been reported in association with pustular psoriasis, PsA (especially axial PsA) and HLA-B27. Uveitis associated with psoriasis is generally insidious and, if left untreated, often leads to complications such as hypopyon, posterior synechiae and retinal vasculitis. Thus, although this ophthalmologic manifestation is not as frequent as others, it represents a significant problem due to its potential complications [254]. It is recommended, therefore, that physicians pay attention to ocular symptoms and perform routine eye examination for these patients [255]. Urgent ophthalmologic consultation and treatment are highly recommended once the patient is diagnosed of inflammatory eye problems.

Chronic Obstructive Pulmonary Disease (COPD)

Dreiher et al. [256] compared 12,502 psoriatic patients with 24,287 healthy controls, in terms of the presence of COPD, and demonstrated a higher prevalence of COPD in patients with psoriasis. A multivariate logistic regression model demonstrated that psoriasis was significantly associated with COPD, after controlling for confounders including age, sex, socioeconomic status, smoking and obesity. In concordance, another recently performed study from Taiwan [257] reported similar results showing that psoriatic patients were at a greater risk of developing COPD with significantly lower COPD-free survival rates than the comparison cohort.

Obstructive Sleep Apnoea Syndrome (OSAS)

Keeping in mind that psoriasis is associated with obesity and CVD, it is likely that psoriasis can be related to obstructive sleep apnoea syndrome (OSAS). Recent studies have reported that the frequency of OSAS was found to be higher in psoriatic patients in contrast to the normal population. Karaca et al. [258] demonstrated OSAS in 54.5% of patients living with psoriasis. They also reported higher Psoriasis Area Severity Index (PASI) in the OSAS group than in the non-OSAS group. Papadavid et al. [259] explored the association between OSAS and psoriasis in their study and found that psoriatic patients with OSAS presented more frequently with snoring and had lower sleep quality compared with those without OSAS. They also reported that OSAS was associated with increased BMI and hypertension in psoriatic patients.

Erectile Dysfunction

Current evidence suggests that there is a higher prevalence of sexual dysfunction in individuals with psoriasis and, as expected, those with genital lesions suffer an even greater negative impact. Psoriasis has a deleterious impact on the overall quality of life and, in particular, on the sexual life of individuals, although there is no consensus whether it constitutes an independent risk factor for erectile dysfunction [260]. Its association is probably due to incipient pelvic atherosclerosis, and it is, thus, an early predictor of cardiovascular disease that is notably frequent in patients with psoriasis [261]. Depression does not seem to have an additional negative impact on the sexual dysfunction of men living with psoriasis. Decreased libido and erectile dysfunction have been reported during the use of methotrexate. Retinoids have been also linked to sexual dysfunctions both in humans and in animals. At present, it is recommended that the cardiovascular risk of patients with documented erectile dysfunction should be evaluated more carefully [262].

Parkinson's Disease

Recently, it was observed that patients with psoriasis are more likely to develop Parkinson's disease. However, the influence of psoriasis severity, lifestyle habits and individual factors on the risk of developing the disease has not yet been established [263].

Comorbidities Related to Lifestyle and Treatments

Patients with psoriasis have a higher frequency of smoking and drinking habits, which also contribute to an increased risk of cardiovascular disease [264–267]. Smoking habits are strongly associated with pustular forms of psoriasis. The risk of developing the disease is 70% higher in smokers compared to non-smokers [261, 262]. The effect of tobacco would only be nullified after 20 years of abstinence. The prevalence of psoriasis is increased among patients who abuse alcohol, and alcohol consumption is associated with increased risk of hepatic steatosis, cirrhosis, depression and anxiety, as well as less response to psoriasis treatments. Studies have associated alcohol consumption with worsening of psoriasis [268, 269].

In concordance, the classical systemic drugs used in the treatment of psoriasis may worsen comorbidities in these patients and often disable their use [210, 270]. Cyclosporine is nephrotoxic and may cause hypertension and dyslipidemia. Conditions associated with obesity (such as NAFLD) are contraindications to the use of methotrexate. Diabetics, alcoholics and obese patients have a higher risk of developing liver fibrosis. On the other hand, some drugs used to treat these conditions have a recognized potential to worsen psoriasis. Flare-up of psoriatic skin rash has been reported in patients starting their biologic therapy [271]. Therefore, care should be given when biologic therapy is commenced for psoriatic patient. Baseline PASI score is important to document any flare-up of the condition.

Recommendations for Comorbidity Screening in Psoriasis

As comorbidities represent a cornerstone in the management of patients living with psoriasis, it is important to screen patients for comorbid risk factors and refer patients to the appropriate specialists if any risk was suspected. Recent surveys indicated that most physicians are unaware of the connection between psoriasis and cardiovascular disease [272, 273], or simply they do not include comorbidity risk assessment in their day-to-day practice. Treating healthcare professional should also ask psoriatic patients about any management they may have taken in relation to a current comorbidity. For example, sleep quality is usually disturbed in patients with psoriasis due to itching and problems with depression and mood status. Therefore, evaluation and treatment of psoriasis must include psychosomatic approaches. In concordance, in clinical practice, psoriatic patients receiving medication(s) for associated cardiovascular disease could influence the course of their psoriasis therapy; hence, medication history is vital for setting the patient's management plan.

Though highly documented and assessed in clinical research, little has been done regarding practical approaches to ensure screening psoriatic patients in the standard daily practice. Clearly there is a need to establish recommendations for psoriatic patients for early detection of comorbidities. The American Heart Association recommends screening for CV risk factors in psoriatic patients as early as age 20. At the age of 40, the following risk factors need to be screened every 2 years: pulse, blood pressure (target <120/80), body mass index <25 kg/m^2, waist circumference < 35 inches for women and <40 inches for men, total cholesterol <200 mg/dL, HDL cholesterol = or >50 mg/dL, LDL < 100 mg/dL and fasting blood glucose <100 mg/dL. Smoking cessation, moderating alcohol intake and exercising three times a week for 30 min have also been recommended [274].

When dealing with a psoriatic patient especially before choosing a systemic therapy, it is important to make a checklist to detect comorbidities and lifestyle factors (e.g. smoking habits and alcoholism), to make a clinical examination (body weight, height, BMI, waist circumference) and an ophthalmologic examination and to assess the severity of psoriasis (PASI and DLQI). Recent published Patient-Reported Outcome Measures (PROMs) [32] include screening for comorbidities as part of the standard monitoring of the patient condition. Electronic PROMs [275] offered another step forward giving the patients the opportunity to monitor their own comorbidity(ies). Adopting a patient-centred approach in the diagnosis and monitoring of comorbidities is vital on the long-term outcomes. Earlier study [276] revealed that by the sharing the patient his/her disease activity parameters scores as well as comorbidities, led to the patients became more adherent to their medications, less likely to stop their disease-modifying drug/biologic therapy for side effects and made less contact to the secondary as well as primary care. A new psoriatic comorbidity index was recently published [277] which will be discussed later in further details in a separate chapter in this book.

Therapeutic Considerations

Therapeutic decision should be discussed with the patient, taking into account his/her comorbidities and lifestyle. Regardless of the treatment chosen, it is important to remember that, since emotional stress is a triggering and exacerbating factor for psoriasis, activities such as yoga, meditation and relaxation exercises are recommended. Patients should not only receive individualized drug therapy but also nutritional guidance [278, 279]. General recommendations include a hypocaloric diet with low-glycaemic index foods and rich in polyunsaturated fatty acids. Some studies have shown benefit in the adoption of a vegetarian diet rich in omega-3, vitamin C, flavonoids, carotenoids and tocopherols. Gluten should only be removed from the diet of positive anti-gliadin/transglutaminase antibodies subjects, especially if symptomatic. Supplementation of specific nutrients should be evaluated case by case. A shared decision-making approach is vital to ensure good treatment outcomes as well as adherence to therapy. A recent publication [280] revealed that improved patients' understanding of the disease enabled them to have better communication with their treating clinician as well as the ability to make an informed decision.

In conclusion, there is growing evidence supporting the significant relation between psoriasis and associated comorbidities. The concept of psoriasis as a systemic inflammatory disorder provides the pathophysiologic link with many of these and highlights psoriasis as a paradigmatic disorder. Affected patients show higher mortality and hospitalization rates, which highlights the importance of having a multidisciplinary approach in the assessment and management of these patients. The integral approach of psoriasis should include the identification of comorbidity risk particularly cardiovascular risk factors and metabolic diseases, the adaptation of medical therapy to manage the existing comorbidities as well as the valuation of existing psychological/psychiatric disorders. This will enable the treating physician achieve a long-term control of the disease and improve the cumulative quality of life. Early and aggressive treat-to-target approach of severe psoriasis, PsA and associated comorbidities may have a positive impact on the patients' status, his/her well-being and probably the longevity of patients.

References

1. Henseler T, Christophers E. Disease concomittance in psoriasis. J Am Acad Dermatol. 1995;32(6):982–6.
2. Reich K. The concept of psoriasis as a systemic inflammation: implications for disease management. J Eur Acad Dermatol Venereol. 2012;26(Suppl 2):3–11.
3. Gottlieb AB, et al. Psoriasis comorbidities. J Dermatol Treat. 2008;19(1):5–21.
4. Cohen AD, et al. Association between psoriasis and the metabolic syndrome. Dermatology. 2008;216(2):152–5.
5. Langan SM, et al. Prevalence of metabolic syndrome in patients with psoriasis: a population-based study in the United Kingdom. J Invest Dermatol. 2012;132(3 Pt 1):556–62.
6. Neimann AL, et al. Prevalence of cardiovascular risk factors in patients with psoriasis. J Am Acad Dermatol. 2006;55(5):829–35.
7. Takahashi H, Iizuka H. Psoriasis and metabolic syndrome. J Dermatol. 2012;39(3):212–8.
8. Nijsten T, Wakkee M. Complexity of the association between psoriasis and comorbidities. J Invest Dermatol. 2009;129(7):1601–3.
9. Nestle FO, Kaplan DH, Barker J. NEJM. 2009;361:496–509.
10. Griffiths CE, Barker JN. Lancet. 2007;370:263–71.
11. Boehncke W, Boehncke S, Tobin A, Kirby B. The 'psoriatic march': a concept of how severe psoriasis may drive cardiovascular comorbidity. Exp Dermatol. 2011;20:303–7.
12. Hukuda S, Minami M, Saito T, Mitsui H, Matsui N, Komatsubara Y, et al. Spondyloarthropathies in Japan: nationwide questionnaire survey performed by the Japan Ankylosing Spondylitis Society. J Rheumatol. 2001;28:554–9.
13. Ruderman EM, Tambar S. Psoriatic arthritis: prevalence, diagnosis, and review of therapy for the dermatologist. Dermatol Clin. 2004;22:477–86.
14. Moll JM, Wright V. Psoriatic arthritis. Semin Arthritis Rheum. 1973;3:55–78.
15. Bennet RM. Psoriatic arthritis. In: DJ MC, editor. Arthritis and related conditions. Philadelphia: Lea & Febiger; 1979. p. 645.
16. Vasey FB, Espinoza LR. Psoriatic arthropathy. In: Calin A, editor. Spondyloarthropathies. Orlando: Grune & Stratton, Inc.; 1984. p. 151–85.
17. Fournié B, Crognier L, Arnaud C, Zabraniecki L, Lascaux-Lefebvre V, Marc V, et al. Proposed classification criteria of psoriatic arthritis. A preliminary study in 260 patients. Rev Rhum Engl Ed. 1999;66:446–56.

18. Taylor W, Gladman D, Helliwell P, Marchesoni A, Mease P, Mielants H, et al. Classification criteria for psoriatic arthritis. Development of new criteria from a large international study. Arthritis Rheum. 2006;54:2665–73.
19. Gladman DD, Farewell VT, Kopciuk KA, Cook RJ. HLA markers and progression in psoriatic arthritis. J Rheumatol. 1998;25:730–3.
20. Bowes J, Eyre S, Flynn E, Ho P, Salah S, Warren RB, et al. Evidence to support IL- 13 as a risk locus for psoriatic arthritis but not psoriasis vulgaris. Ann Rheum Dis. 2011;70:1016–9.
21. Mease P, Goffe BS. Diagnosis and treatment of psoriatic arthritis. J Am Acad Dermatol. 2005;52:1–19. Finzi AF, Gibelli E. Psoriatic arthritis. Int J Dermatol 1991;30:1–7.
22. Zhang C, Zhu KJ, Zheng HF, Cui Y, Zhou FS, Chen YL, et al. The effect of overweight and obesity on psoriasis patients in Chinese Han population: a hospital-based study. J Eur Acad Dermatol Venereol. 2011;25:87–91.
23. Gottlieb A, Korman NJ, Gordon KB, Feldman SR, Lebwohl M, Koo JY, et al. Guidelines of care for the management of psoriasis and psoriatic arthritis: section 2. Psoriatic arthritis: overview and guidelines of care for treatment with an emphasis on the biologics. J Am Acad Dermatol. 2008;58:851–64.
24. Gladman DD, Brockbank J. Psoriatic arthritis. Expert Opin Investig Drugs. 2000;9:1511–22.
25. Gladman DD, Antoni C, Mease P, Clegg DO, Nash P. Psoriatic arthritis: epidemiology, clinical features, course, and outcome. Ann Rheum Dis. 2005;64:ii14–7.
26. Espinoza LR, Cuellar ML. Psoriatic arthritis and spondylitis: a clinical approach. In: Calin A, Taurog JD, editors. Spondylarthritides. Oxford: Oxford University Press; 1998. p. 97–111.
27. Torre Alonso JC, Rodriguez Perez A, Arribas Castrillo JM, Ballina Garcia J, Riestra Noriega JL, Lopez LC. Psoriatic arthritis (PA): a clinical, immunological and radiological study of 180 patients. Br J Rheumatol. 1991;30:245–50.
28. Slobodin G, Rosner I, Rozenbaum M, Boulman N, Kessel A, Toubi E. Psoriatic arthropathy: where now? Isr Med Assoc J. 2009;11:430–4.
29. Menter A, Gottlieb A, Feldman SR, Van Voorhees AS, Leonardi CL, Gordon KB, et al. Guidelines of care for the management of psoriasis and psoriatic arthritis: section 1. Overview of psoriasis and guidelines of care for the treatment of psoriasis with biologics. J Am Acad Dermatol. 2008;58:826–50.
30. Kyle S, Chandler D, Griffiths CE, Helliwell P, Lewis J, McInnes I, et al. Guideline for anti-TNF-alpha therapy in psoriatic arthritis. Rheumatology (Oxford). 2005;44:390–7.
31. Husni ME, Meyer KH, Cohen DS, Mody E, Qureshi AA. The PASE questionnaire: pilot-testing a psoriatic arthritis screening and evaluation tool. J Am Acad Dermatol. 2007;57:581–7.
32. El Miedany Y, El Gaafary M, Youssef S, Palmer D. Towards a multidimensional patient reported outcome measures assessment: development and validation of a questionnaire for patients with ankylosing spondylitis/spondyloarthritis. Joint Bone Spine. 2010;77(6):575–81.
33. De Simone C, Guerriero C, Giampetruzzi AR, Costantini M, Di Gregorio F, Amerio P. Achilles tendinitis in psoriasis: clinical and sonographic findings. J Am Acad Dermatol. 2003;49:217–22.
34. El Miedany Y, El Gaafary M, Youssef S, Ahmed I, Nasr A. Tailored approach to early psoriatic arthritis patients: clinical and ultrasonographic predictors for structural joint damage. Clin Rheumatol. 2015;34(2):307–13.
35. Schwenzer NF, Kötter I, Henes JC, Schraml C, Fritz J, Claussen CD, et al. The role of dynamic contrast-enhanced MRI in the differential diagnosis of psoriatic and rheumatoid arthritis. AJR Am J Roentgenol. 2010;194:715–20.
36. De Oliveira M, Rocha B, Duarte G. Psoriasis: classical and emerging comorbidities. An Bras Dermatol. 2015;90(1):09–20.
37. Gladman DD, Christopher R. Clinical manifestations and diagnosis of psoriatic arthritis. Uptodate.com [Internet]. 2010; 18.1. Available from: http://www.uptodate.com/contents/clinical-manifestations-and-diagnosisof-psoriatic-arthritis
38. Nash P, Clegg DO. Psoriatic arthritis therapy: NSAIDs and traditional DMARDs. Ann Rheum Dis. 2005;64:ii74–7.

39. Gelfand JM, Kimball AB, Mostow EN, Chiou CF, Patel V, Xia HA, et al. Patient-reported outcomes and health-care resource utilization in patients with psoriasis treated with etanercept: continuous versus interrupted treatment. Value Health. 2008;11:400–7.
40. Rodgers M, Epstein D, Bojke L, Yang H, Craig D, Fonseca T, et al. Etanercept, infliximab and adalimumab for the treatment of psoriatic arthritis: a systematic review and economic evaluation. Health Technol Assess. 2011;15:i–xxi.
41. Queiro-Silva R, Torre-Alonso JC, Tinturé-Eguren T, López-Lagunas I. A polyarticular onset predicts erosive and deforming disease in psoriatic arthritis. Ann Rheum Dis. 2003;62:68–70.
42. Wong K, Gladman DD, Husted J, Long JA, Farewell VT. Mortality studies in psoriatic arthritis: results from a single outpatient clinic. I. Causes and risk of death. Arthritis Rheum. 1997;40:1868–72.
43. Jamnitski A, Symmons D, Peters MJ, Sattar N, McInnes I, Nurmohamed MT. Cardiovascular comorbidities in patients with psoriatic arthritis: a systematic review. Ann Rheum Dis. 2013;72:211–6.
44. Ellinghaus D, Ellinghaus E, Nair RP, Stuart PE, Esko T, Metspalu A, et al. Combined analysis of genome-wide association studies for Crohn disease and psoriasis identifies seven shared susceptibility loci. Am J Hum Genet. 2012;90:636–47.
45. Cohen AD, et al. Psoriasis associated with ulcerative colitis and Chron's disease. J Eur Acad Dermatol Venereol. 2009;23:561–5.
46. Tesmer LA, Lundy SK, Sarkar S, Fox DA. Th17 cells in human disease. Immunol Rev. 2008;223:87–113.
47. Wolf N, Quaranta M, Prescott NJ, et al. Psoriasis is associated with pleiotropic susceptibility loci identified in type II diabetes and Crohn disease. J Med Genet. 2008;45(2):114–6.
48. Capon F, Di Meglio P, Szaub J, et al. Sequence variants in the genes for the interleukin-23 receptor (IL23R) and its ligand (IL12B) confer protection against psoriasis. Hum Genet. 2007;122(2):201–6.
49. Cargill M, Schrodi SJ, Chang M, et al. A large-scale genetic association study confirms IL12B and leads to the identification of IL23R as psoriasis-risk genes. Am J Hum Genet. 2007;80(2):273–90.
50. Nair RP, Ruether A, Stuart PE, et al. Polymorphisms of the IL12B and IL23R genes are associated with psoriasis. J Invest Dermatol. 2008;128(7):1653–61.
51. Aslanidis S, Pyrpasopoulou A, Douma S, Triantafyllou A. Tumor necrosis factor-a antagonist-induced psoriasis: yet another paradox in medicine. Clin Rheumatol. 2008;27(3):377–80.
52. Ahmad T, Marshall SE, Jewell D. Genetics of inflammatory bowel disease: the role of the HLA complex. World J Gastroenterol. 2006;12(23):3628–35.
53. Li WQ, Han JL, Chan AT, Qureshi AA. Psoriasis, psoriatic arthritis and increased risk of incident Crohn's disease in US women. Ann Rheum Dis. 2013;72(7):1200–5.
54. Birkenfeld S, Dreiher J, Weitzman D, Cohen AD. Coeliac disease associated with psoriasis. Br J Dermatol. 2009;161(6):1331–4.
55. Wu JJ, Nguyen TU, Poon KY, Herrinton LJ. The association of psoriasis with autoimmune diseases. J Am Acad Dermatol. 2012;67(5):924–30.
56. Angelucci E, Cocco A, Viscido A, Vernia P, Caprilli R. Another paradox in Crohn's disease: new onset of psoriasis in a patient receiving tumor necrosis factor-alpha antagonist. Inflamm Bowel Dis. 2007;13(8):1059–61.
57. Severs GA, Lawlor TH, Purcell SM, Adler DJ, Thompson R. Cutaneous adverse reaction to infliximab: report of psoriasis developing in 3 patients. Cutis. 2007;80(3):231–7.
58. Wollina U, Hansel G, Koch A, Schönlebe J, Köstler E, Haroske G. Tumor necrosis factor-alpha inhibitor-induced psoriasis or psoriasiform exanthemata: first 120 cases from the literature including a series of six new patients. Am J Clin Dermatol. 2008;9(1):1–14.
59. Aeberli D, Seitz M, Jüni P, Villiger PM. Increase of peripheral CXCR3 positive T lymphocytes upon treatment of RA patients with TNF-alpha inhibitors. Rheumatology (Oxford). 2005;44(2):172–5.

60. Vague J. Sexual differentiation, a factor affecting the forms of obesity. Presse Méd. 1947;30:339–40.
61. Flier JS. Obesity wars: molecular progress confronts an expanding epidemic. Cell. 2004;116:337–50.
62. Kershaw EE, Flier JS. Adipose tissue as an endocrine organ. J Clin Endocrinol Metab. 2004;89(6):2548–56.
63. Coppack SW. Pro-inflammatory cytokines and adipose tissue. Proc Nutr Soc. 2001;60(3):349–56.
64. Cohen AD, et al. Psoriasis and metabolic syndrome. Acta Derm Venereol. 2007;87(6):506–9.
65. Monteiro R, Azevedo I. Chronic inflammation in obesity and the metabolic syndrome. Mediators Inflamm. 2010;2010:Pii 289645–55. doi:10.1155/2010/289645.
66. Nisa N, Qazi MA. Prevalence of metabolic syndrome in patients with psoriasis. Indian J Dermatol Venereol Leprol. 2010;76(6):662–5.
67. Gisondi P, et al. Prevalence of metabolic syndrome in patients with psoriasis: a hospital-based case-control study. Br J Dermatol. 2007;157(1):68–73.
68. Sommer DM, et al. Increased prevalence of the metabolic syndrome in patients with moderate to severe psoriasis. Arch Dermatol Res. 2006;298(7):321–8.
69. Ross R, Aru J, Freeman J, Hudson R, Janssen I. Abdominal adiposity and insulin resistance in obese men. Am J Physiol Endocrinol Metab. 2002;282:E657–63.
70. Carrascosa JM, et al. Body mass index in patients with moderate-to-severe psoriasis in Spain and its impact as an independent risk factor for therapy withdrawal: results of the Biobaderm registry. J Eur Acad Dermatol Venereol. 2013;15 doi:10.1111/jdv.12208.
71. Jensen P, et al. Effect of weight loss on the severity of psoriasis: a randomized clinical study. JAMA Dermatol. 2013;149(7):795–801.
72. Herron MD, et al. Impact of obesity and smoking on psoriasis presentation and management. Arch Dermatol. 2005;141(12):1527–34.
73. Sterry W, et al. Obesity in psoriasis: the metabolic, clinical and therapeutic implications. Report of an interdisciplinary conference and review. Br J Dermatol. 2007;157(4):649–55.
74. Wang Y, Chen J, Zhao Y, Geng L, Song F, Chen H-D. Psoriasis is associated with increased levels of serum leptin. Br J Dermatol. 2008;158(5):1134–5.
75. Chen YJ, Wu CY, Shen JL, et al. Psoriasis independently associated with hyperleptinemia contributing to metabolic syndrome. Arch Dermatol. 2008;144(12):1571–5.
76. Takahashi H, Tsuji H, Takahashi I, Hashimoto Y, Ishida-Yamamoto A, Iizuka H. Plasma adiponectin and leptin levels in Japanese patients with psoriasis. Br J Dermatol. 2008;159(5):1207–8.
77. Coimbra S, Oliveira H, Reis F, et al. Circulating adipokine levels in Portuguese patients with psoriasis vulgaris according to body mass index, severity and therapy. J Eur Acad Dermatol Venereol. 2010;24(12):1386–94.
78. Zhu KJ, Zhang C, Li M, Zhu CY, Shi G, Fan YM. Leptin levels in patients with psoriasis: a meta-analysis. Clin Exp Dermatol. 2013;38(5):478–83.
79. Matarese G, Moschos S, Mantzoros CS. Leptin in immunology. J Immunol. 2005;174(6):3137–42.
80. Carrascosa JM, Rocamora V, Fernandez-Torres RM, et al. Obesity and psoriasis: inflammatory nature of obesity, relationship between psoriasis and obesity, and therapeutic implications. Actas Dermosifiliogr. 2014;105(1):31–44.
81. Armstrong AW, Harskamp CT, Armstrong EJ. The association between psoriasis and obesity: a systematic review and meta-analysis of observational studies. Nutr Diabetes. 2012;2:e54.
82. Florin V, Cottencin AC, Delaporte E, Staumont-Sallé D. Body weight increment in patients treated with infliximab for plaque psoriasis. J Eur Acad Dermatol Venereol. 2013;27(2):e186–90.
83. Renzo LD, Saraceno R, Schipani C, et al. Prospective assessment of body weight and body composition changes in patients with psoriasis receiving anti-TNF-α treatment. Dermatol Ther. 2011;24(4):446–51.

84. Prignano F, Ricceri F, Pescitelli L, et al. Comparison of body weight and clinical-parameter changes following the treatment of plaque psoriasis with biological therapies. Curr Med Res Opin. 2009;25(9):2311–6.
85. Saraceno R, Schipani C, Mazzotta A, et al. Effect of anti-tumor necrosis factor-alpha therapies on body mass index in patients with psoriasis. Pharmacol Res. 2008;57(4):290–5.
86. Gisondi P, Cotena C, Tessari G, Girolomoni G. Anti-tumour necrosis factor-alpha therapy increases body weight in patients with chronic plaque psoriasis: a retrospective cohort study. J Eur Acad Dermatol Venereol. 2008;22(3):341–4.
87. Kirchgessner TG, Uysal KT, Wiesbrock SM, Marino MW, Hotamisligil GS. Tumor necrosis factor-alpha contributes to obesity-related hyperleptinemia by regulating leptin release from adipocytes. J Clin Invest. 1997;100(11):2777–82.
88. Clark L, Lebwohl M. The effect of weight on the efficacy of biologic therapy in patients with psoriasis. J Am Acad Dermatol. 2008;58(3):443–6.
89. Qureshi AA, Choi HK, Setty AR, Curhan GC. Psoriasis and the risk of diabetes and hypertension: a prospective study of US female nurses. Arch Dermatol. 2009;145(4):379–82.
90. Brauchli YB, Jick SS, Meier CR. Psoriasis and the risk of incident diabetes mellitus: a population-based study. Br J Dermatol. 2008;159(6):1331–7.
91. Wellen KE, Hotamisligil GS. Inflammation, stress, and diabetes. J Clin Invest. 2005;115(5):1111–9.
92. Azfar RS, Seminara NM, Shin DB, Troxel AB, Margolis DJ, Gelfand JM. Increased risk of diabetes mellitus and likelihood of receiving diabetes mellitus treatment in patients with psoriasis. Arch Dermatol. 2012;148(9):995–1000.
93. Coto-Segura P, et al. Psoriasis, psoriatic arthritis and type 2 diabetes mellitus: a systematic review and meta-analysis. Br J Dermatol. 2013; doi:10.1111/bjd.12473.
94. Armstrong AW, et al. Psoriasis and the risk of diabetes mellitus: a systematic review and meta-analysis. JAMA Dermatol. 2013;149:84–91.
95. Cohen AD, et al. Psoriasis and diabetes: a population-based crosssectional study. J Eur Acad Dermatol Venereol. 2008;22:585–9.31.
96. Al-Mutairi N, Al-Farag S, Al-Mutairi A, Al-Shiltawy M. Comorbidities associated with psoriasis: an experience from the Middle East. J Dermatol. 2010;37(2):146–55.
97. Marra M, Campanati A, Testa R, et al. Effect of etanercept on insulin sensitivity in nine patients with psoriasis. Int J Immunopathol Pharmacol. 2007;20(4):731–6.
98. Farrokhi F, Taylor HC, McBride NM. Etanercept-induced hypoglycemia and improved glycemic control in a patient with type 2 diabetes. Endocr Pract. 2011;17(2):306–7.
99. Wambier CG, Foss-Freitas MC, Paschoal RS, et al. Severe hypoglycemia after initiation of anti-tumor necrosis factor therapy with etanercept in a patient with generalized pustular psoriasis and type 2 diabetes mellitus. J Am Acad Dermatol. 2009;60(5):883–5.
100. Cheung D, Bryer-Ash M. Persistent hypoglycemia in a patient with diabetes taking etanercept for the treatment of psoriasis. J Am Acad Dermatol. 2009;60(6):1032–6.
101. Morikang E, Benson SC, Kurtz TW, Pershadsingh HA. Effects of thiazolidinediones on growth and differentiation of human aorta and coronary myocytes. Am J Hypertens. 1997;10(4 Pt 1):440–6.
102. Ricote M, Li AC, Willson TM, Kelly CJ, Glass CK. The peroxisome proliferator-activated receptor-gamma is a negative regulator of macrophage activation. Nature. 1998; 391(6662):79–82.
103. Ellis CN, Varani J, Fisher GJ, et al. Troglitazone improves psoriasis and normalizes models of proliferative skin disease: ligands for peroxisome proliferator-activated receptor-gamma inhibit keratinocyte proliferation. Arch Dermatol. 2000;136(5):609–16.
104. Malhotra A, Shafiq N, Rajagopalan S, Dogra S, Malhotra S. Thiazolidinediones for plaque psoriasis: a systematic review and meta-analysis. Evid Based Med. 2012;17(6):171–6.
105. Ford ES, Giles WH, Dietz WH. Prevalence of the metabolic syndrome among US adults: findings from the third National Health and nutrition examination survey. JAMA. 2002;287(3):356–9.

106. Lakka HM, et al. The metabolic syndrome and total and cardiovascular disease mortality in middle- aged men. JAMA. 2002;288(21):2709–16.
107. Meigs JB, et al. Body mass index, metabolic syndrome, and risk of type 2 diabetes or cardiovascular disease. J Clin Endocrinol Metab. 2006;91(8):2906–12.
108. Hu G, Qiao Q, Tuomilehto J, et al. Prevalence of the metabolic syndrome and its relation to all-cause and cardiovascular mortality in nondiabetic European men and women. Arch Intern Med. 2004;164(10):1066–76.
109. Armstrong AW, Harskamp CT, Armstrong EJ. Psoriasis and metabolic syndrome: a systematic review and meta-analysis of observational studies. J Am Acad Dermatol. 2013;68(4):654–62.
110. Singh G, Aneja S. Cardiovascular comorbidity in psoriasis. Indian J Dermatol. 2011;56(5):553–6.
111. Gelfand JM, Yeung H. Metabolic syndrome in patients with psoriatic disease. J Rheumatol Suppl. 2012;89:24–8.
112. Mehta NN, Yu Y, Pinnelas R, et al. Attributable risk estimate of severe psoriasis on major cardiovascular events. Am J Med. 2011;124(8):775.e1–6.
113. Balta I, Balta S, Demirkol S, et al. Aortic arterial stiffness is a moderate predictor of cardiovascular disease in patients with psoriasis vulgaris. Angiology. 2014;65(1):74–8.
114. Späh F. Inflammation in atherosclerosis and psoriasis: common pathogenic mechanisms and the potential for an integrated treatment approach. Br J Dermatol. 2008;159(Suppl 2):10–7.
115. Yildiz M. Arterial distensibility in chronic inflammatory rheumatic disorders. Open Cardiovasc Med J. 2010;4:83–8.
116. Costa L, Caso F, D'Elia L, et al. Psoriatic arthritis is associated with increased arterial stiffness in the absence of known cardiovascular risk factors: a case control study. Clin Rheumatol. 2012;31(4):711–5.
117. Chodorowska G, Wojnowska D, Juszkiewicz-Borowiec M. C-reactive protein and alpha2-macroglobulin plasma activity in medium-severe and severe psoriasis. J Eur Acad Dermatol Venereol. 2004;18(2):180–3.
118. Koenig W, Sund M, Fröhlich M, et al. C-reactive protein, a sensitive marker of inflammation, predicts future risk of coronary heart disease in initially healthy middle-aged men: results from the MONICA (monitoring trends and determinants in cardiovascular disease) Augsburg Cohort study, 1984 to 1992. Circulation. 1999;99(2):237–42.
119. Vanizor Kural B, Orem A, Cims¸it G, Uydu HA, Yandi YE, Alver A. Plasma homocysteine and its relationships with atherothrombotic markers in psoriatic patients. Clin Chim Acta. 2003;332(1–2):23–30.
120. Vanizor Kural B, Orem A, Cims¸it G, Yandi YE, Calapoglu M. Evaluation of the atherogenic tendency of lipids and lipoprotein content and their relationships with oxidant-antioxidant system in patients with psoriasis. Clin Chim Acta. 2003;328(1–2):71–82.
121. Rocha-Pereira P, Santos-Silva A, Rebelo I, Figueiredo A, Quintanilha A, Teixeira F. The inflammatory response in mild and in severe psoriasis. Br J Dermatol. 2004;150(5):917–28.
122. Bhushan M, McLaughlin B, Weiss JB, Griffiths CE. Levels of endothelial cell stimulating angiogenesis factor and vascular endothelial growth factor are elevated in psoriasis. Br J Dermatol. 1999;141(6):1054–60.
123. Nofal A, Al-Makhzangy I, Attwa E, Nassar A, Abdalmoati A. Vascular endothelial growth factor in psoriasis: an indicator of disease severity and control. J Eur Acad Dermatol Venereol. 2009;23(7):803–6.
124. Bhardwaj S, Roy H, Heikura T, Ylä-Herttuala S. VEGF-A, VEGF-D and VEGF-D(DeltaNDeltaC) induced intimal hyperplasia in carotid arteries. Eur J Clin Investig. 2005;35(11):669–76.
125. McDonald I, Connolly M, Tobin AM. A review of psoriasis, a known risk factor for cardiovascular disease and its impact on folate and homocysteine metabolism. J Nutr Metab. 2012;2012:965385.
126. Brazzelli V, Grasso V, Fornara L, et al. Homocysteine, vitamin B12 and folic acid levels in psoriatic patients and correlation with disease severity. Int J Immunopathol Pharmacol. 2010;23(3):911–6.

127. Duell PB, Malinow MR. Homocyst(e)ine: an important risk factor for atherosclerotic vascular disease. Curr Opin Lipidol. 1997;8(1):28–34.
128. El-Khairy L, Ueland PM, Refsum H, Graham IM, Vollset SE. European concerted action project. Plasma total cysteine as a risk factor for vascular disease: the European concerted action project. Circulation. 2001;103(21):2544–9.
129. Malerba M, Gisondi P, Radaeli A, Sala R, Calzavara Pinton PG, Girolomoni G. Plasma homocysteine and folate levels in patients with chronic plaque psoriasis. Br J Dermatol. 2006;155(6):1165–9.
130. Richetta AG, Mattozzi C, Macaluso L, et al. Homocysteine plasmatic status in patients with psoriasis. Eur J Dermatol. 2011;21(4):621–3.
131. Kimball AB, et al. Coronary heart disease and stroke risk in patients with psoriasis: retrospective analysis. Am J Med. 2010;123:350–7.
132. Gelfland JM, et al. Risk of myocardial infarction in patients with psoriasis. JAMA. 2006;296(14):1735–41.
133. Ahlehoff O, Gislason GH, Jørgensen CH, et al. Psoriasis and risk of atrial fibrillation and ischaemic stroke: a Danish Nationwide Cohort study. Eur Heart J. 2012;33(16):2054–64.
134. Lorenz MW, Markus HS, Bots ML, Rosvall M, Sitzer M. Prediction of clinical cardiovascular events with carotid intima-media thickness: a systematic review and meta-analysis. Circulation. 2007;115(4):459–67.
135. Troitzsch P, Paulista Markus MR, Dörr M, et al. Psoriasis is associated with increased intima-media thickness – the Study of Health in Pomerania (SHIP). Atherosclerosis. 2012;225(2):486–90.
136. Balci DD, Balci A, Karazincir S, et al. Increased carotid artery intima-media thickness and impaired endothelial function in psoriasis. J Eur Acad Dermatol Venereol. 2009;23(1):1–6.
137. Enany B, El Zohiery AK, Elhilaly R, Badr T. Carotid intima-media thickness and serum leptin in psoriasis. Herz. 2012;37(5):527–33.
138. El-Mongy S, Fathy H, Abdelaziz A, et al. Subclinical atherosclerosis in patients with chronic psoriasis: a potential association. J Eur Acad Dermatol Venereol. 2010;24(6):661–6.
139. Gisondi P, Fantin F, Del Giglio M, et al. Chronic plaque psoriasis is associated with increased arterial stiffness. Dermatology. 2009;218(2):110–3.
140. Yiu KH, Yeung CK, Zhao CT, et al. Prevalence and extent of subclinical atherosclerosis in patients with psoriasis. J Intern Med. 2013;273(3):273–82.
141. Ludwig RJ, Herzog C, Rostock A, et al. Psoriasis: a possible risk factor for development of coronary artery calcification. Br J Dermatol. 2007;156(2):271–6.
142. Arad Y, Goodman KJ, Roth M, Newstein D, Guerci AD. Coronary calcification, coronary disease risk factors, C-reactive protein, and atherosclerotic cardiovascular disease events: the St Francis heart study. J Am Coll Cardiol. 2005;46(1):158–65.
143. Arad Y, Spadaro LA, Roth M, Newstein D, Guerci AD. Treatment of asymptomatic adults with elevated coronary calcium scores with atorvastatin, vitamin C, and vitamin E: the St Francis heart study randomized clinical trial. J Am Coll Cardiol. 2005;46(1):166–72.
144. Osto E, Piaserico S, Maddalozzo A, et al. Impaired coronary flow reserve in young patients affected by severe psoriasis. Atherosclerosis. 2012;221(1):113–7.
145. Micha R, Imamura F, Wyler von Ballmoos M, et al. Systematic review and meta-analysis of methotrexate use and risk of cardiovascular disease. Am J Cardiol. 2011;108(9):1362–70.
146. Prodanovich S, Ma F, Taylor JR, Pezon C, Fasihi T, Kirsner RS. Methotrexate reduces incidence of vascular diseases in veterans with psoriasis or rheumatoid arthritis. J Am Acad Dermatol. 2005;52(2):262–7.
147. Famenini S, Sako EY, Wu JJ. Effect of treating psoriasis on cardiovascular co-morbidities: focus on TNF inhibitors. Am J Clin Dermatol. 2014;15(1):45–50.
148. Wu JJ, Poon KY. Association of gender, tumor necrosis factor inhibitor therapy, and myocardial infarction risk in patients with psoriasis. J Am Acad Dermatol. 2013;69(4):650–1.
149. Piaserico S, Conti A, Console FL, et al. Efficacy and safety of systemic treatments for psoriasis in elderly patients. Acta Derm Venereol. 2014;94(3):293–7. doi:10.2340/00015555-1719.

150. Huskic´ J, Alendar F. Tissue angiotensin-converting enzyme in patients with various clinical forms of psoriasis. Bosn J Basic Med Sci. 2007;7(2):103–6.
151. Ena P, Madeddu P, Glorioso N, Cerimele D, Rappelli A. High prevalence of cardiovascular diseases and enhanced activity of the renin-angiotensin system in psoriatic patients. Acta Cardiol. 1985;40(2):199–205.
152. Ryder KW, Epinette WW, Jay SJ, Ransburg RC, Glick MR. Serum angiotensin converting enzyme activity in patients with psoriasis. Clin Chim Acta. 1985;153(2):143–6.
153. Liu T, Han Y, Lu L. Angiotensin-converting enzyme gene polymorphisms and the risk of psoriasis: a meta-analysis. Clin Exp Dermatol. 2013;38(4):352–8. quiz 359
154. Armstrong AW, Harskamp CT, Armstrong EJ. The association between psoriasis and hypertension: a systematic review and meta-analysis of observational studies. J Hypertens. 2013;31(3):433–42. discussion 442–443
155. Sowers JR. Hypertension, angiotensin II, and oxidative stress. N Engl J Med. 2002;346(25):1999–2001.
156. Armstrong AW, Voyles SV, Armstrong EJ, Fuller EN, Rutledge JC. Angiogenesis and oxidative stress: common mechanisms linking psoriasis with atherosclerosis. J Dermatol Sci. 2011;63(1):1–9.
157. Cohen AD, Weitzman D, Dreiher J. Psoriasis and hypertension: a case-control study. Acta Derm Venereol. 2010;90(1):23–6.
158. Robert N, Wong GW, Wright JM. Effect of cyclosporine on blood pressure. Cochrane Database Syst Rev. 2010;(1):CD007893.
159. Waqar S, Sarkar PK. Exacerbation of psoriasis with beta-blocker therapy. CMAJ. 2009;181(1–2):60.
160. O'Brien M, Koo J. The mechanism of lithium and beta-blocking agents in inducing and exacerbating psoriasis. J Drugs Dermatol. 2006;5(5):426–32.
161. Wilson PW. Established risk factors and coronary artery disease: the Framingham study. Am J Hypertens. 1994;7(7 Pt 2):7S–12S.
162. Genest JJ Jr, Martin-Munley SS, McNamara JR, et al. Familial lipoprotein disorders in patients with premature coronary artery disease. Circulation. 1992;85(6):2025–33.
163. Manninen V, Tenkanen L, Koskinen P, et al. Joint effects of serum triglyceride and LDL cholesterol and HDL cholesterol concentrations on coronary heart disease risk in the Helsinki heart study. Implications for treatment. Circulation. 1992;85(1):37–45.
164. Miller M, Seidler A, Moalemi A, Pearson TA. Normal triglyceride levels and coronary artery disease events: the Baltimore coronary observational long-term study. J Am Coll Cardiol. 1998;31(6):1252–7.
165. Libby P. Inflammation in atherosclerosis. Nature. 2002;420(6917):868–74.
166. Ribatti D, Levi-Schaffer F, Kovanen PT. Inflammatory angiogenesis in atherogenesis – a double-edged sword. Ann Med. 2008;40(8):606–21.
167. Feingold KR, Marshall M, Gulli R, Moser AH, Grunfeld C. Effect of endotoxin and cytokines on lipoprotein lipase activity in mice. Arterioscler Thromb. 1994;14(11):1866–72.
168. Greenberg AS, Nordan RP, McIntosh J, Calvo JC, Scow RO, Jablons D. Interleukin 6 reduces lipoprotein lipase activity in adipose tissue of mice in vivo and in 3T3-L1 adipocytes: a possible role for interleukin 6 in cancer cachexia. Cancer Res. 1992;52(15):4113–6.
169. Beutler BA, Cerami A. Recombinant interleukin 1 suppresses lipoprotein lipase activity in 3T3-L1 cells. J Immunol. 1985;135(6):3969–71.
170. Feingold KR, Grunfeld C. Role of cytokines in inducing hyperlipidemia. Diabetes. 1992;41(Suppl 2):97–101.
171. Memon RA, Grunfeld C, Moser AH, Feingold KR. Tumor necrosis factor mediates the effects of endotoxin on cholesterol and triglyceride metabolism in mice. Endocrinology. 1993;132(5):2246–53.
172. Rashmi R, Rao KSJ, Basavaraj KH. A comprehensive review of biomarkers in psoriasis. Clin Exp Dermatol. 2009;34(6):658–63.

173. Rocha-Pereira P, Santos-Silva A, Rebelo I, Figueiredo A, Quintanilha A, Teixeira F. Dislipidemia and oxidative stress in mild and in severe psoriasis as a risk for cardiovascular disease. Clin Chim Acta. 2001;303(1–2):33–9.
174. Tekin NS, Tekin IO, Barut F, Sipahi EY. Accumulation of oxidized low-density lipoprotein in psoriatic skin and changes of plasma lipid levels in psoriatic patients. Mediat Inflamm. 2007;2007:78454.
175. Ma C, Harskamp CT, Armstrong EJ, Armstrong AW. The association between psoriasis and dyslipidaemia: a systematic review. Br J Dermatol. 2013;168(3):486–95.
176. Bacchetti T, Campanati A, Ferretti G, Simonetti O, Liberati G, Offidani AM. Oxidative stress and psoriasis: the effect of antitumour necrosis factor-α inhibitor treatment. Br J Dermatol. 2013;168(5):984–9.
177. Jamnitski A, Levels JH, van den Oever IA, Nurmohamed MT. Highdensity lipoprotein profiling changes in patients with rheumatoid arthritis treated with tumor necrosis factor inhibitors: a cohort study. J Rheumatol. 2013;40(6):825–30.
178. Vis M, Nurmohamed MT, Wolbink G, et al. Short term effects of infliximab on the lipid profile in patients with rheumatoid arthritis. J Rheumatol. 2005;32(2):252–5.
179. Kiortsis DN, Mavridis AK, Filippatos TD, Vasakos S, Nikas SN, Drosos AA. Effects of infliximab treatment on lipoprotein profile in patients with rheumatoid arthritis and ankylosing spondylitis. J Rheumatol. 2006;33(5):921–3.
180. Tam LS, Tomlinson B, Chu TT, Li TK, Li EK. Impact of TNF inhibition on insulin resistance and lipids levels in patients with rheumatoid arthritis. Clin Rheumatol. 2007;26(9):1495–8.
181. Mathieu S, Dubost JJ, Tournadre A, Malochet-Guinamand S, Ristori JM, Soubrier M. Effects of 14 weeks of TNF alpha blockade treatment on lipid profile in ankylosing spondylitis. Joint Bone Spine. 2010;77(1):50–2.
182. Lestre S, Diamantino F, Veloso L, Fidalgo A, Ferreira A. Effects of etanercept treatment on lipid profile in patients with moderate-tosevere chronic plaque psoriasis: a retrospective cohort study. Eur J Dermatol. 2011;21(6):916–20.
183. Corbetta S, Angioni R, Cattaneo A, Beck-Peccoz P, Spada A. Effects of retinoid therapy on insulin sensitivity, lipid profile and circulating adipocytokines. Eur J Endocrinol. 2006;154(1):83–6. doi:10.1530/ eje.1.02057.
184. Gupta AK, Goldfarb MT, Ellis CN, Voorhees JJ. Side-effect profile of acitretin therapy in psoriasis. J Am Acad Dermatol. 1989;20(6):1088–93.
185. Vahlquist A, Törmä H. Retinoids and keratinization. Current concepts. Int J Dermatol. 1988;27(2):81–95.
186. Ellis CN, Kang S, Vinik AI, Grekin RC, Cunningham WJ, Voorhees JJ. Glucose and insulin responses are improved in patients with psoriasis during therapy with etretinate. Arch Dermatol. 1987;123(4):471–5.
187. Zech LA, Gross EG, Peck GL, Brewer HB. Changes in plasma cholesterol and triglyceride levels after treatment with oral isotretinoin. A prospective study. Arch Dermatol. 1983;119(12):987–93.
188. Mantel-Teeuwisse AK, Kloosterman JM, Maitland-van der Zee AH, Klungel OH, Porsius AJ, de Boer A. Drug-induced lipid changes: a review of the unintended effects of some commonly used drugs on serum lipid levels. Drug Saf. 2001;24(6):443–56.
189. Grossman RM, Delaney RJ, Brinton EA, Carter DM, Gottlieb AB. Hypertriglyceridemia in patients with psoriasis treated with cyclosporine. J Am Acad Dermatol. 1991;25(4):648–51.
190. Rajpara AN, Goldner R, Gaspari A. Psoriasis: can statins play a dual role? Dermatol Online J. 2010;16(2):2.
191. Hilgendorff A, Muth H, Parviz B, et al. Statins differ in their ability to block NF-kappaB activation in human blood monocytes. Int J Clin Pharmacol Ther. 2003;41(9):397–401.
192. Brauchli YB, Jick SS, Meier CR. Statin use and risk of first-time psoriasis diagnosis. J Am Acad Dermatol. 2011;65(1):77–83.
193. Jacobi TC, Highet A. A clinical dilemma while treating hypercholesterolaemia in psoriasis. Br J Dermatol. 2003;149(6):1305–6.

194. Shirinsky IV, Shirinsky VS. Efficacy of simvastatin in plaque psoriasis: a pilot study. J Am Acad Dermatol. 2007;57(3):529–31.
195. Fisher DA, Elias PM, LeBoit PL. Exacerbation of psoriasis by the hypolipidemic agent, gemfibrozil. Arch Dermatol. 1988;124(6):854–5.
196. Milavec-Puretic´ V, Mance M, Ceovic´ R, Lipozencˇic´ J. Drug induced psoriasis. Acta Dermatovenerol Croat. 2011;19(1):39–42.
197. McCullough AJ. Pathophysiology of nonalcoholic steatohepatitis. J Clin Gastroenterol. 2006;40(Suppl 1):S17–29.
198. Kotronen A, Yki-Järvinen H. Fatty liver: a novel component of the metabolic syndrome. Arterioscler Thromb Vasc Biol. 2008;28(1):27–38.
199. Marchesini G, Bugianesi E, Forlani G, et al. Nonalcoholic fatty liver, steatohepatitis, and the metabolic syndrome. Hepatology. 2003;37(4):917–23.
200. Miele L, et al. Prevalence, characteristics and severity of non-alcoholic fatty liver disease in patients with chronic plaque psoriasis. J Hepatol. 2009;51(4):778–86.
201. Madanagobalane S, Anandan S. The increased prevalence of non-alcoholic fatty liver disease in psoriatic patients: a study from South India. Australas J Dermatol. 2012;53(3):190–7.
202. Gisondi P, et al. Non-alcoholic fatty liver disease in patients with chronic plaque psoriasis. J Hepatol. 2009;51(4):758–64.
203. Wenk KS, et al. Psoriasis and nonalcoholic fatty liver disease. J Eur Acad Dermatol Venereol. 2011;25:383–91.
204. Cassano N, et al. Alcohol, psoriasis, liver disease and anti-psoriasis drugs. Int J Dermatol. 2011;50:1323–31.
205. Weinblatt ME, Coblyn JS, Fox DA, et al. Efficacy of low-dose methotrexate in rheumatoid arthritis. N Engl J Med. 1985;312(13):818–22.
206. Leonard PA, Clegg DO, Carson CC, Cannon GW, Egger MJ, Ward JR. Low dose pulse methotrexate in rheumatoid arthritis: an 8-year experience with hepatotoxicity. Clin Rheumatol. 1987;6(4):575–82.
207. Prey S, Paul C. Effect of folic or folinic acid supplementation on methotrexate-associated safety and efficacy in inflammatory disease: a systematic review. Br J Dermatol. 2009;160(3):622–8.
208. van Ede AE, Laan RF, Rood MJ, et al. Effect of folic or folinic acid supplementation on the toxicity and efficacy of methotrexate in rheumatoid arthritis: a forty-eight week, multicenter, randomized, double-blind, placebo-controlled study. Arthritis Rheum. 2001;44(7):1515–24.
209. Salonen SH. EUROPSO psoriasis patient survey: first results from 17 990 association members with psoriasis. J Eur Acad Dermatol Venereol. 2003;17(S1):36–46.
210. Barker J, Horn EJ, Lebwohl M, Warren RB, Nast A, Rosenberg W, et al. Assessment and management of methotrexate hepatotoxicity in psoriasis patients: report from a consensus conference to evaluate current practice and identify key questions toward optimizing methotrexate use in the clinic. J Eur Acad Dermatol Venereol. 2011;25(7):758–64.
211. Tsochatzis EA, Gurusamy KS, Ntaoula S, Cholongitas E, Davidson BR, Burroughs AK. Elastography for the diagnosis of severity of fibrosis in chronic liver disease: a meta-analysis of diagnostic accuracy. J Hepatol. 2011;54(4):650–9.
212. Cole JA, Emerton DP, Mackenzie A, Lawinski CP, Clinch PJ, Weston JDW, et al. Evidence review: ultrasound elastography. Centre for Evidence-Based Purchasing. 2009;CEP08052:1–41.
213. Miller MH, Ferguson MA, Dillon JF. Systematic review of performance of non-invasive biomarkers in the evaluation of non-alcoholic fatty liver disease. Liver Int. 2011;31(4):461–73.
214. Boffa MJ, Smith A, Chalmers R, Mitchell D, Rowan B, Warnes TW, et al. Serum type III procollagen aminopeptide for assessing liver damage in methotrexate-treated psoriatic patients. Br J Dermatol. 1996;135(4):538–44.
215. Rivera R, Vanaclocha F. Nonalcoholic fatty liver disease and psoriasis. Actas Dermotosifiliogr. 2010;101:657–8.

216. Hannuksela-Svahn A, Pukkala E, Läärä E, Poikolainen K, Karvonen J. Psoriasis, its treatment, and cancer in a cohort of Finnish patients. J Invest Dermatol. 2000;114(3):587–90.
217. Gridley G, McLaughlin JK, Ekbom A, et al. Incidence of cancer among patients with rheumatoid arthritis. J Natl Cancer Inst. 1993;85(4):307–11.
218. Ekström K, Hjalgrim H, Brandt L, et al. Risk of malignant lymphomas in patients with rheumatoid arthritis and in their first-degree relatives. Arthritis Rheum. 2003;48(4):963–70.
219. Brauchli YB, Jick SS, Miret M, Meier CR. Psoriasis and risk of incident cancer: an inception cohort study with a nested case-control analysis. J Invest Dermatol. 2009;129(11):2604–12.
220. Hayes J, Koo J. Psoriasis: depression, anxiety, smoking, and drinking habits. Dermatol Ther. 2010;23(2):174–80.
221. Gerdes S, Zahl VA, Weichenthal M, Mrowietz U. Smoking and alcohol intake in severely affected patients with psoriasis in Germany. Dermatology. 2010;220(1):38–43.
222. Lee MS, Lin RY, Chang YT, Lai MS. The risk of developing nonmelanoma skin cancer, lymphoma and melanoma in patients with psoriasis in Taiwan: a 10-year, population-based cohort study. Int J Dermatol. 2012;51(12):1454–60.
223. Pouplard C, et al. Risk of cancer in psoriasis: a systematic review and metaanalysis of epidemiological studies. J Eur Acad Dermatol. 2013;27(Suppl 3):36–46.
224. Stern RS, PUVA Follow-Up Study. The risk of squamous cell and basal cell cancer associated with psoralen and ultraviolet a therapy: a 30-year prospective study. J Am Acad Dermatol. 2012;66(4):553–62.
225. Stern RS, Nichols KT, Väkevä LH. Malignant melanoma in patients treated for psoriasis with methoxsalen (psoralen) and ultraviolet a radiation (PUVA). The PUVA follow-up study. N Engl J Med. 1997;336(15):1041–5.
226. Stern RS. Lymphoma risk in psoriasis: results of the PUVA follow-up study. Arch Dermatol. 2006;142(9):1132–5.
227. Paul CF, Ho VC, McGeown C, et al. Risk of malignancies in psoriasis patients treated with cyclosporine: a 5 y cohort study. J Invest Dermatol. 2003;120(2):211–6.
228. Colombo MD, Cassano N, Bellia G, Vena GA. Cyclosporine regimens in plaque psoriasis: an overview with special emphasis on dose, duration, and old and new treatment approaches. ScientificWorld Journal. 2013;2013:805705.
229. Bongartz T, Sutton AJ, Sweeting MJ, Buchan I, Matteson EL, Montori V. Anti-TNF antibody therapy in rheumatoid arthritis and the risk of serious infections and malignancies: systematic review and meta-analysis of rare harmful effects in randomized controlled trials. JAMA. 2006;295(19):2275–85.
230. Bongartz T, Warren FC, Mines D, Matteson EL, Abrams KR, Sutton AJ. Etanercept therapy in rheumatoid arthritis and the risk of malignancies: a systematic review and individual patient data metaanalysis of randomised controlled trials. Ann Rheum Dis. 2009;68(7):1177–83.
231. Leombruno JP, Einarson TR, Keystone EC. The safety of anti-tumour necrosis factor treatments in rheumatoid arthritis: meta and exposureadjusted pooled analyses of serious adverse events. Ann Rheum Dis. 2009;68(7):1136–45.
232. Dommasch ED, Abuabara K, Shin DB, Nguyen J, Troxel AB, Gelfand JM. The risk of infection and malignancy with tumor necrosis factor antagonists in adult patients with psoriatic disease: a systematic review and meta-analysis of randomized controlled trials. J Am Acad Dermatol. 2011;64(6):1035–50.
233. Ginsburg IH, Link BG. Psychosocial consequnences of rejection and stigma feelings in psoriasis patients. Int J Dermatol. 1993;32(8):587–91.
234. Devrimci-Ozguven H, et al. The depression, anxiety, life satisfaction and affective expression levels in psoriasis patients. J Eur Acad Dermatol Venereol. 2000;14(4):267–71.
235. Esposito M, et al. An Italian study on psoriasis and depression. Dermatology. 2006;212(2):123–7.
236. Kilic A, et al. Temperament and character profile of patients with psoriasis. J Eur Acad Dermatol Venereol. 2008;22(5):537–42.

237. Sampogna F, et al. Living with psoriasis: prevalence of shame, anger, worry, and problems in daily activities and social life. Acta Derm Venereol. 2012;92:299–303.
238. Dominguez PL, et al. Depression and the risk of psoriasis in US women. J Eur Acad Dermatol Venereol. 2013;27:1163–7.
239. Schiepers OJG, Wichers MC, Maes M. Cytokines and major depression. Prog Neuro-Psychopharmacol Biol Psychiatry. 2005;29(2):201–17.
240. Scharloo M, Kaptein AA, Weinman J, Bergman W, Vermeer BJ, Rooijmans HG. Patients' illness perceptions and coping as predictors of functional status in psoriasis: a 1-year follow-up. Br J Dermatol. 2000;142(5):899–907.
241. Gupta MA, Gupta AK. Depression and suicidal ideation in dermatology patients with acne, alopecia areata, atopic dermatitis and psoriasis. Br J Dermatol. 1998;139(5):846–50.
242. Krueger G, et al. The impact of psoriasis on quality of life: results of a 1998 National Psoriasis Foundation patient-membership survey. Arch Dermatol. 2001;137(3):280–4.
243. Gupta MA, Gupta AK. The psoriasis life stress inventory: a preliminary index of psoriasis-related stress. Acta Derm Venereol. 1995;75(3):240–3.
244. Gupta MA, Gupta AK, Watteel GN. Perceived deprivation of social touch in psoriasis is associated with greater psychologic morbidity: an index of the stigma experience in dermatologic disorders. Cutis. 1998;61(6):339–42.
245. Fortune DG, Main CJ, O'Sullivan TM, Griffiths CE. Assessing illnessrelated stress in psoriasis: the psychometric properties of the psoriasis life stress inventory. J Psychosom Res. 1997;42(5):467–75.
246. Fortune DG, Richards HL, Kirby B, Bowcock S, Main CJ, Griffiths CE. A cognitive-behavioural symptom management programme as an adjunct in psoriasis therapy. Br J Dermatol. 2002;146(3):458–65.
247. Kastelan D, Kastelan M, Massari LP, Korsic M. Possible association of psoriasis and reduced bone mineral density due to increased TNF-alpha and IL-6 concentrations. Med Hypotheses. 2006;67:1403–5.
248. Millard TP, Antoniades L, Evans AV, Smith HR, Spector TD, Barker JN. Bone mine-ral density of patients with chronic plaque psoriasis. Clin Exp Dermatol. 2001;26:446–8.
249. Hofbauer LC, Schoppet M, Christ M, Teichmann J, Lange U. Tumour necrosis factor-related apoptosis-inducing ligand and osteoprotegerin serum levels in psoriatic arthritis. Rheumatology (Oxford). 2006;45:1218–22.
250. Attia EA, Khafagy A, Abdel-Raheem S, Fathi S, Saad AA. Assessment of osteoporosis in psoriasis with and without arthritis: correlation with disease severity. Int J Dermatol. 2011;50:30–5.
251. Pedreira PG, Pinheiro MM, Szejnfeld VL. Bone mineral density and body composition in postmenopausal women with psoriasis and psoriatic arthritis. Arthritis Res Ther. 2011;13:R16.
252. D'Epiro S, Marocco C, Salvi M, et al. Psoriasis and bone mineral density: implications for long term patients. J Dermatol. 2014;41:783–7.
253. Ogdie A, Schwartzman S, Eder L, et al. Comprehensive treatment of psoriatic arthritis: managing comorbidities and extraarticular manifestations. J Rheumatol. 2014;41:2315–22.
254. Fraga NA, Oliveira MF, Follador I, Rocha BO, Rêgo VR. Psoriasis and uveitis: a literature review. An Bras Dermatol. 2012;87:877.
255. Oliveira MFSP, Rocha BO, Boeira VLSV, Fraga NAA Follador I, et al. Ophthalmic manifestations in psoriatic patients in a Brazilian referral center. 3rd World Psoriasis & Psoriatic Arthritis Conference 2012, Stockholm. New York, Springer Healthcare, 2012. 2. S24–S25.
256. Dreiher J, et al. Psoriasis and chronic obstructive pulmonary disease: a case-control study. Br J Dermatol. 2008;159(4):956–60.
257. Chiang YY, Lin HW. Association between psoriasis and chronic obstructive pulmonary disease: a population-based study in Taiwan. J Eur Acad Dermatol Venereol. 2012;26(1):59–65.
258. Karaca S, et al. Might psoriasis be a risk factor for obstructive sleep apnea syndrome. Sleep Breath. 2013;17(1):27580.

259. Papadavid E, et al. Sleep apnea as a comorbidity in obese psoriasis patients: a cross-sectional study. Do psoriasis characteristics and metabolic parameters play a role? J Eur Acad Dermatol Venereol. 2013;27(7):820–6.
260. Reynolds OD. Erectile dysfunction in etretinate treatment. Arch Dermatol. 1991;127:425–6.
261. Wylie G, Evans CD, Gupta G. Reduced libido and erectile dysfunction: rarely reported side-effects of methotrexate. Clin Exp Dermatol. 2009;34:e234.
262. Rossi M, Pellegrino M. Acitretin-associated erectile dysfunction: a case report. Cases J. 2009;2:210.
263. Sheu JJ, Wang KH, Lin HC, Huang CC. Psoriasis is associated with an increased risk of parkinsonism: a population-based 5-year follow-up study. J Am Acad Dermatol. 2013;68:992–9.
264. Higgins E. Alcohol, smoking and psoriasis. Clin Exp Dermatol. 2000;25:107–10.
265. Poikolainen K, Reunala T, Karvonen J, Lauharanta J, Kärkkäinen P. Alcohol intake: a risk factor for psoriasis in young and middle aged men? BMJ. 1990;300:780–3.
266. Poikolainen K, Karvonen J, Pukkala E. Excess mortality related to alcohol and smoking among hospital-treated patients with psoriasis. Arch Dermatol. 1999;135:1490–3.
267. Naldi L, Chatenoud L, Linder D, Belloni Fortina A, Peserico A, Virgili AR, et al. Cigarette smoking, body mass index, and stressful life events as risk factors for psoriasis: results from an Italian case-control study. J Invest Dermatol. 2005;125:61–7.
268. Fortes C, Mastroeni S, Leffondré K, Sampogna F, Melchi F, Mazzotti E, et al. Relationship between smoking and the clinical severity of psoriasis. Arch Dermatol. 2005;141:1580–4.
269. Wolk K, Mallbris L, Larsson P, Rosenblad A, Vingård E, Ståhle M. Excessive body. Weight and smoking associates with a high risk of onset of plaque psoriasis. Acta Derm Venereol. 2009;89:492–7.
270. Gupta MA, Schork NJ, Gupta AK, Kirkby S, Ellis CN. Suicidal ideation in psoriasis. Int J Dermatol. 1993;32:188–90.
271. Park B, Lim H, Kim B, Lee W, Kim D, Lee S. Repeated paradoxical aggravation of preexisting psoriasis during infliximab treatment for Crohn's disease. Ann Dermatol. 2009;21(1):60–2.
272. Kimball AB, Wu Y. Cardiovascular disease and classic cardiovascular risk factors in patients with psoriasis. Int J Dermatol. 2009;48(11):1147–56.
273. Parsi KK, Brezinski EA, Lin TC, Li CS, Armstrong AW. Are patients with psoriasis being screened for cardiovascular risk factors? A study of screening practices and awareness among primary care physicians and cardiologists. J Am Acad Dermatol. 2012;67(3):357–62.
274. Kimball A, Gladman D, Gelfand J, et al. National Psoriasis Foundation clinical consensus on psoriasis co-morbidities and recommendations for screening. J Am Acad Dermatol. 2008;58(6):1031–42.
275. El Miedany Y, El Gaafary M, Youssef S, Bahlas S, Almedany S, Ahmed I, Palmer D. Toward electronic health recording: evaluation of electronic patient-reported outcome measures system for remote monitoring of early rheumatoid arthritis. J Rheumatol. 2016;43(12):2106–12.
276. El Miedany Y, El Gaafary M, Palmer D. Assessment of the utility of visual feedback in the treatment of early rheumatoid arthritis patients: a pilot study. Rheumatol Int. 2012;32(10):3061–8.
277. El Miedany Y, El Gaafary M, Youssef S, Bahlas S, Hegazi M. Psoriatic arthritis comorbidity index: development and validation of a new specific tool for classifying prognostic comorbidity in psoriasis and psoriatic arthritis patients. Rheumatol Orthop Med. 2017;2(2):1–7. doi:10.15761/ROM.1000117.
278. Basavaraj KH, Navya MA, Rashmi R. Stress and quality of life in psoriasis: an update. Int J Dermatol. 2011;50:783–92.
279. Duarte GV, Follador I, Cavalheiro CM, Silva TS, Oliveira MF. Psoriasis and obesity: literature review and recommendations for management. An Bras Dermatol. 2010;85:355–60.
280. El Miedany Y, El Gaafary M, Sayed S, Palmer D, Ahmed I. Implementing shared decision making in clinical practice: outcomes of a new shared decision making aid for chronic inflammatory arthritis patients. J Pat Care. 2016;2:2–7.

Chapter 5
Ankylosing Spondylitis

U. Kiltz, X. Baraliakos, and J. Braun

Introduction

Patients with spondyloarthritis (SpA) constitute a heterogeneous group of inflammatory rheumatic diseases with specific clinical characteristics such as inflammation and ankylosis of the axial skeleton and peripheral manifestations such as arthritis, dactylitis, or enthesitis [1]. Patients with axSpA often have extra-articular symptoms such as anterior uveitis, psoriasis, and chronic inflammatory bowel disease (IBD) [2]. These are disease manifestations of SpA rather than comorbidities. The term "SpA" serves as an umbrella term which includes related diseases such as axial SpA (axSpA) and peripheral SpA (pSpA) including reactive arthritis and psoriatic arthritis (PsA). The term axSpA refers to patients with predominant axial manifestations who may or may not have structural changes on sacroiliac joint (SIJ) radiographs. According to the current classification criteria, patients who do not (yet) have radiographic changes in the SIJ have to show inflammatory activity as visualized by magnetic resonance imaging (MRI) or just carry the HLA-B27 antigen [3]. On this basis, axSpA patients are classified as having ankylosing spondylitis (AS) or non-radiographic axSpA (nr-axSpA) [3, 4]. However, since this cutoff is artificial and the technique unreliable, the terminology should not be used for a clinical diagnosis [5]. Finally, AS and PsA are the best studied subtypes, and most research, especially related to comorbidities, has been performed in these two subgroups.

In the field of SpA, it is especially important to differentiate disease manifestations such as psoriasis or IBD from comorbidities of SpA such as cardiovascular diseases. The basis for this differentiation is the concept of SpA which has both a clinical and a genetic basis [6]. The presence of HLA-B27 seems to be a major factor for the development of disease manifestations such as uveitis or (much rarer)

U. Kiltz (✉) • X. Baraliakos • J. Braun
Department of Rheumatology, Rheumazentrum Ruhrgebiet, Herne, Germany
e-mail: Uta.kiltz@elisabethgruppe.de

Y. El Miedany (ed.), *Comorbidity in Rheumatic Diseases*,
DOI 10.1007/978-3-319-59963-2_5

aortitis in AS [7–10]. AS, psoriasis, and IBD often coexist in the same patient and in their families. The genetic associations between axial SpA and psoriasis or IBD which are not very strong are driven by a variety of different genes [11]. Overall, AS, psoriasis, and IBD seem to share similar pathogenic mechanisms of aberrant intracellular antigen processing or elimination of intracellular bacteria and cytokine production, especially in the IL-17-IL-23 pathway.

This chapter will mainly focus on comorbidities in patients with AS such as osteoporosis or cardiovascular disease (CVD). The risk to develop comorbidities is higher for patients with AS than for the general population – in particular with regard to common disorders such as CVD and osteoporosis [12–14]. Development of comorbidities might be attributed to high disease activity, resulting in various diseases such as amyloidosis. During the past 10 years, knowledge about the prevalence of comorbidities has clearly increased. The data presented in this review are mainly taken from population-based studies and prospective cohorts [12, 13, 15–20]. Data on comorbidities in patients with SpA are mainly available for AS patients, while data for patients with nr-axSpA are scarce. As a matter of fact, until 2015, no data about comorbidities have been published for patients with axSpA. However, in 2015, results of three observational trials have been published [19–21]. Only one study has recently reported on the prevalence of comorbidities in patients with SpA, including patients with axial and peripheral manifestations of SpA (COMOSPA cohort) [18]. Here we review the knowledge about comorbidities in patients with AS in due consideration of current results of comorbidities in axSpA patients.

Comorbidities: General Aspects

There is a huge variety of possible diseases which may occur as comorbidities in patients with AS. Similar to other inflammatory rheumatic diseases, cardiovascular diseases associated with coronary heart disease and myocardial infarction and bone loss associated with osteoporosis and fractures occur rather frequently in AS. Malignancies and infectious diseases need of course to be carefully looked at since clinical implications are important. Reports about renal, pulmonary, or gastrointestinal involvement are scarce, although clinical reasoning would assume an increased prevalence. In a nationwide population-based study including 11,701 patients with AS and 58,505 matching controls from Taiwan, the most prevalent comorbidities in patients with AS were hypertension (16.4%), peptic ulcers (13.9%), and headache (10.2%) [15].

The increased risk to develop comorbidities can be explained by various factors such as systemic inflammation, treatment (side) effects, and coincidence of other conditions. None of the effects has been shown to have a causal effect on the occurrence of comorbidities. Very limited number of studies assessed long-term safety for treatment options. Our knowledge about treatment effects is based almost solely on cohorts receiving tumor necrosis factor inhibitor (TNFi) medications.

Mortality

Increased mortality has been reported in patients with AS because of direct factors such as radium-224 therapy or indirect factors such as cancer and cardiovascular mortality [22, 23]. As in the general population, cardiovascular disease is the leading cause of death in patients with AS (see discussion of data below). Some investigator found that compared to the general population, mortality in AS patients is increased due to alcohol abuse and injury or suicide cause [22]. In any case, data consistently show that increased mortality is mainly based on high disease activity [24]. In a case-control study from Sweden, the crude mortality among patients with AS was 14.5% [24]. The standardized mortality rate (SMR) in this cohort of 677 AS patients was increased by 1.61 (95% C.I. 1.29–1.93). Of note, the SRM was significantly increased among male patients compared with female patients (1.63 vs 1.38, $p < 0.001$). The most frequent cause of death (40.0%) is CVD, followed by malignant (26.8%) and infectious (23.2%) diseases. Factors independently associated with reduced survival were diagnostic delay (Odds ratio (OR) 1.05), increased levels of C-reactive protein (OR 2.68), work disability (OR 3.65), and, of major interest, not or infrequently using nonsteroidal anti-inflammatory drugs (NSAIDs) (OR 4.35). Male gender and higher age independently predicted mortality in another AS pooled cohort study from Sweden with 8600 AS patients and 40.460 age-matched, sex-matched and county-matched general population comparators identified from the National Patient Register and the census register [16]. Statistically significant predictors for death in this cohort were lower level of education, general comorbidities (diabetes, infections, CVD, pulmonary and malignant diseases), and previous hip replacement surgery.

Comorbidities: Specific Aspects

Cardiovascular Disease

Excess mortality has been demonstrated in patients with AS related to an increased risk of CVD [25, 26]. Assessment of CVD was done in respect to ischemic heart disease, myocardial infarction, and/or stroke. Preliminary evidence suggests that subclinical atherosclerosis and arterial stiffness are more prevalent in patients with AS compared with controls. Disease duration as well as known contributing factors for atherosclerosis (e.g. age, BMI) were identified as a determinant of aortic stiffness indices in AS patients from a Dutch cohort [25], which showed that AS patients had a greater intima-media thickness (IMT) (0.62 ± 0.09 mm vs 0.57 ± 0.09 mm in controls; $p = 0.02$) compared to controls, a difference that remained after adjustment for traditional CV risk factors. However, no relationship was found between large-vessel properties and higher Bath AS disease indices or C-reactive protein values. Similar results were found in a Spanish AS cohort, comprising of patients without clinically evident CVD in which disease duration (OR 1.39; 95% confidence intervals (CI) 1.01–1.92; $p = 0.05$) and level of ESR at baseline (OR 1.18; 95% CI, 1.04–1.33; $p = 0.01$) were found to be the best predictor for carotid plaques without clinically evident cardiovascular disease in patients with AS. In addition, increased risk of CVD might be attributed to enhanced inflammatory activity of the arterial wall. Some evidence for this hypothesis comes from a small case-control study in which the level of carotid arterial wall inflammation in patients with AS using 18F-fluorodeoxyglucose (18F-FDG) positron emission tomography with CT was compared with healthy controls [27]. Patients with AS had a 20% increase in arterial wall 18F-FDG uptake compared with controls which was to change when receiving atorvastatin. Three months of atorvastatin 40 mg daily significantly lowered low-density lipoprotein cholesterol (baseline 3.55 ± 1.15 mmol/L, −53%) and CRP (baseline 5.0 (1.5–9.3) mg/L, −58%) with a concomitant decrease of carotid arterial wall inflammation (maximum target-to-background ratio from 1.90 ± 0.30 to 1.67 ± 0.27; $p = 0.009$). In AS patients, CVD and their risk factors were more common in patients compared to matched controls which could be shown in a US database that contains fully adjudicated medical service and prescription drug claims [28]. The prevalence ratios of ischemic heart disease (1.2), atherosclerosis (1.5), peripheral vascular disease 1.6), congestive heart failure (1.8), cerebrovascular disease (1.7), type II diabetes (1.2), hyperlipidemia (1.2), and hypertension (1.3) were all higher in patients than controls. The COMOSPA trial, comprising the whole spectrum of SpA, showed a global prevalence of ischemic heart disease of 2.7% (95% CI 2.2–3.2) and stroke of 1.3% (95% CI 0.9–1.7). The prevalence for any CVD (i.e., ischemic heart disease or stroke) in this cohort was higher in Northern European countries and the USA compared to Africa and Asia [18].

Various explanations might be found for the differences between reported risks: characteristics of the patient group (especially disease duration), inclusion of prevalent and incident patients, and possibility to adjust for a wide range of confounders, including the use of NSAIDs. Several factors, i.e., smoking, altered lipid profile, hypertension, increased fibrinogen level, enhanced number of platelets, and hypercoagulability, might explain the enhanced cardiovascular risk with impaired endothelial function in AS [25, 29, 30]. The excess risk is probably multifactorial, being related both to chronic systemic inflammation and to high prevalence of conventional cardiovascular risk factors. Furthermore, there is accumulating evidence for an etiological role of inflammation in the AS-related cardiac manifestations [31].

CV Risk Factors

When talking about CVD, the prevalence of CV risk factors has to be taken into account. The most prevalent CV risk factor was hypertension with 33.5% (95% CI 32.0–35.0), followed by smoking (29.3% (95% CI 27.9–30.7)), and hypercholesterolemia (27.3% (95% CI 25.9–28.7)) in the COMOSPA cohort [18]. A meta-analysis by Mathieu et al. ($n = 1214$ for patients and $n = 1000$ for controls) showed that AS patients were characterized by a higher weighted mean IMT and higher risk of metabolic syndrome and that in AS patients, a significant decrease in triglycerides, total cholesterol, and high-density lipoprotein (HDL) cholesterol were measured [26, 32].

A more prevalent atherogenic lipid profile in patients with AS, than in the general population, might be a possible explanation for increased CV mortality. The association between disease activity and lipid profile has been explored in 55 patients with AS [33]. In this Dutch cohort, an increase in disease activity was associated with decreases in lipid levels. The decrease in HDL levels tended to be almost twice as large as the decrease in total cholesterol levels, resulting in a more atherogenic lipid profile. Hence, effective treatment of disease activity in patients with AS may lower the CV risk by improving the lipid profile (see Influence of Therapy on CVD below).

Impairment in microvascular function might have a causal relationship as well. Inflammation in AS may cause microvascular dysfunction which has been linked to several risk factors for CVD. Impairment in microvascular function was detected in patients with AS by showing impaired endothelium-dependent vasodilatation and capillary recruitment in a case-control study from the Netherlands [34]. Following TNFi treatment, microvascular function improved significantly for endothelium-dependent vasodilatation ($p = 0.03$) and capillary recruitment ($p = 0.006$).

CVD

Ischemic Heart Disease, Myocardial Infarction, and Left Ventricular Dysfunction An increased risk of ischemic heart disease in AS patients was shown to be present in a population-based cohort study using data from the British Clinical Practice Research Datalink (1987–2012) [13]. At baseline, 4.3% of the patients had ischemic heart disease compared with 3.4% of the controls. After exclusion of preexisting ischemic heart disease, the incidence rate ratios were 1.18 population-based cohort trial (95% CI 0.96–1.46) for ischemic heart disease. Compared with controls, the age-gender-adjusted hazard ratio (HR) for developing ischemic heart disease was 1.20 (95% CI 0.97–1.48). It is important to notice that in discussion about CV risk, the risk of concomitant medications is sometimes neglected or cannot be addressed adequately because of methodological issues. This crucial point can be seen in the study by Essers et al. where NSAIDs use interfere with risk of ischemic heart disease [13]. In female patients, the risk of developing ischemic heart disease was increased (HR 1.88, 95% CI 1.22–2.90), but after adjustment for all possible risk factors, only a nonsignificant trend was found (HR 1.31, 95% CI 0.83–2.08). In particular, NSAID use explained this change (HR IHD adjusted for age-gender-NSAID use 1.57, 95% CI 0.99–2.48). However, a meta-analysis (seven longitudinal studies with AS patients) did not show a difference in incidence of ischemic heart disease between AS patients and controls (2.2 vs 2.3%) [26].

A cohort study from a Swedish heart clinic showed that prevalence of SpA is higher in patients with their first coronary artery bypass grafting (CABG population) compared to the general population [35]. SpA was found to be a stronger independent predictor of early CABG than traditional CV risk factors [adjusted beta −6.2, $p < 0.001$, 95% confidence interval (CI) −9.5 to −2.8].

The results about myocardial infarction (MI) are conflicting, primarily because of small sample sizes and lack of adjustment for concomitant medication (e.g., NSAIDs). The abovementioned population-based cohort study from the UK reported a prevalence of 1.8% of acute MI in AS patients compared with 1.4% of the controls at baseline [13]. The age-gender-adjusted HR for developing acute MI was 0.91 (95% CI 0.65–1.28). A meta-analysis in 2011 revealed a nonsignificant increase in MI resulting in a risk ratio of 1.88 (95% CI 0.83, 4.28 [26]), whereas the meta-analysis published in 2015 revealed a significant increase in MI [OR = 1.60 (95% CI: 1.32–1.93)] in AS patients [32].

Since the increased mortality in AS patients is largely due to CVD, a systematic review investigated if diastolic left ventricular (LV) dysfunction, which serves as a precursor to chronic heart failure, was present in patients with AS [36]. An increased prevalence rate of diastolic LV dysfunction was reaffirmed in patients with AS by reporting a worse E/A ratio (ratio of the early (E) to late (A) ventricular filling velocities) [mean difference −0.13 m/s (95% CI: −0.19 to −0.07)], a prolonged deceleration time [mean difference 13.90 ms (95% CI: 6.03–21.78)], and a prolonged mean isovolumetric relaxation time [mean difference 8.06 ms (95% CI: 3.23–12.89)]. The increased prevalence rate was reported to be higher compared to controls in respect to E/A ratio (9% vs 0%), deceleration time (30% vs 12%), and isovolumetric relaxation time (45% vs 18%), all values suggestive of diastolic LV dysfunction.

Stroke The risk of stroke seems to be increased in patients with AS, although conflicting results have been published in this field [37–40]. A meta-analysis in 2011 did not show a difference in incidence of strokes (AS patients, 2.2% (95% CI 1.3%, 3.4%), controls, 2.3% (95% CI 2.0%, 2.7%) [26]), whereas the same authors reported in 2015 a significant increase in stroke (OR = 1.50 (95% CI: 1.39–1.62)) in AS patients [32]. A population-based matched-cohort study from Taiwan, comprising 1,479 AS patients and a comparison cohort of 5,916 subjects without AS, found HR for subsequent stroke among patients with AS of 2.3 (95% CI 1.9–2.8) [38]. A population-based, age- and sex-matched longitudinal follow-up study from China found an increased HR of ischemic stroke for the AS group at 1.98 (95% CI, 1.20–3.29; $p = 0.0079$) [39]. After controlling for demographic and comorbid medical disorders, the adjusted HR was still significant at 1.93 (95% CI, 1.16–3.20; $p = 0.0110$). However, a retrospective cohort study using routine data from the UK did not show an increase in the MI or CVD/stroke rates in patients with AS compared to those without AS, despite higher rates of hypertension, which may be related to NSAID use [37].

Heart Conduction and Aortic Valve Problems

Apart from CVD, heart conduction disturbances and aortic and valve disease have been recognized as being associated with AS [7, 41, 42]. Conduction disturbances may explain the CV burden, as they are independently associated with cardiac disease. However, almost no robust data are available on this topic. A small observational study from the Netherlands ($n = 131$) reported the occurrence of intraventricular conduction disturbances, particularly in patients with long-standing disease [42]. A first-degree atrioventricular (AV) block was found in six patients (4.6%). One (0.8%) patient suffered from a complete right bundle branch block, and one (0.8%) patient had a left anterior hemiblock. A prolonged QRS interval was observed in 38 (29.2%) patients, including those with a complete or incomplete bundle branch block. In multivariate analyses, disease duration remained independently associated with intraventricular conduction disturbances. Elevated SMR for atrioventricular block (3.97, 95% CI 1.90–7.30) was also statistically significant in a cohort study from Sweden [12]. The absolute rate difference (observed minus expected) was high for atrioventricular block (354 per 100,000 person-years).

Compared with the general population, patients with AS are at increased risk for aortic valvular heart disease 1.58 (95% CI 1.31–1.91) and for non-aortic valvular heart disease 1.58 (95% CI 1.43–1.74) which was shown in a Canadian AS cohort (8,616 individuals diagnosed over the period 1996–2006) [43].

Influence of Therapy on CVD

There is some evidence that therapeutic agents such as TNFi that downregulate the acute phase response also have an effect in reducing CV complications in rheumatoid arthritis (RA) as well as in AS.

Changes in lipid levels occur in AS patients when receiving TNFi treatment [44, 45]. In a recent trial, increase in total cholesterol (+4.6%), low-density lipoprotein cholesterol (+4.3%), and HDL (+3.7%) could be seen after treatment with TNFi over a period of 52 weeks [44]. Changes were most evident in patients with substantial reduction in inflammatory levels. Improvement of lipid levels was demonstrated in another cohort of AS patients receiving 12 weeks of etanercept treatment [45]. CRP levels decreased significantly, whereas total cholesterol, HDL, and apolipoprotein A levels increased significantly. This resulted in a better total cholesterol/HDL ratio (from 3.9 to 3.7) (although the difference was not statistically significant) and an improved Apo B:Apo A-I ratio, which decreased by 7.5% over time ($p = 0.008$). However, change of the atherogenic index could not be confirmed in another study including 34 AS patients who started TNFi treatment [46].

Whether subclinical atherosclerosis of the carotid artery in patients with AS was reduced after anti-inflammatory treatment with TNFi was investigated in a prospective observational cohort study [47]. After a median 4.9 years of follow-up, IMT did not change significantly (paired t test +0.011 mm, $p = 0.561$) in those who continued the use of TNF inhibitors, while IMT increased substantially (+0.057 mm, $p = 0.069$) in those who did not continue their use of TNFi. The effect of TNFi was mainly mediated by a subsequent decrease in AS disease activity. The use of TNF inhibitors might stabilize or slow down the progression of subclinical atherosclerosis in AS patients, reflecting a decreased CV risk in these patients.

Improvement of premature arterial stiffening and IMT progression following treatment of TNFi has been shown in a small cohort of RA, AS, and PsA patients as well [48]. After 1 year of treatment with TNFi, aortic pulse wave velocity was improved in the treatment group, but not in the control group (−0.54 ± 0.79 m/s vs. 0.06 ± 0.61 m/s, respectively; $p = 0.004$). In multivariable analyses, TNFi therapy over time was associated with improved aortic pulse wave velocity and reduced IMT progression. However, these promising results could not be confirmed in two other trials with a TNFi treatment period of 24 and 52 weeks, respectively [49, 50]. Whether TNFi administration results in reduced prevalence of CVD in patients with AS still has to be confirmed.

Osteoporosis

Rate of osteoporotic fractures is clearly increased in patients with AS, and many reports about bone loss, osteoporosis, and vertebral fractures (VFs) have been published over the last decades [14, 20, 51–56]. Decreased bone mineral density (BMD) is a common complication of AS, with a prevalence range of 19–62% [55, 57]. The inflammatory osteitis and diffuse ossification of advanced AS creates a fused spine that is susceptible to VF. VF in AS are common but are often not diagnosed. Although many case reports and small series have been published on patients with AS suffering VF, solid data on clinical outcome are rare, especially about the magnitude of the risk of fracturing.

In the COMOSPA cohort, osteoporosis was the most frequent comorbidity, with a prevalence of 13.4% (95% CI 12.3–14.4). However, the prevalence of VF and proximal hip fractures was very low (2% and 0.2%, respectively) [18]. In an AS cohort from Sweden, a rate of 21% for osteoporosis and 44% for osteopenia according to the World Health Organization (WHO) criteria was diagnosed in patients ≥50 years [14]. In this cohort, VFs were diagnosed in 24 patients (12%) but were previously noted clinically in only 3 of the 24. VFs are associated with advanced age, long-standing disease, impaired back mobility, syndesmophyte formation, and lower BMD in both the central and peripheral skeleton. BMD in the femoral neck, total hip, and estimated BMD showed the strongest association with VF.

In a primary care-based nested case-control study, including 231,778 patients with fracture and 231,778 age- and sex-matched controls, the prevalence of AS was 0.18% in patients with fracture and 0.15% in controls [53]. Patients with AS had an increased risk of clinical vertebral fracture (OR 3.26; 95% CI 1.51–7.02), whereas the risk of fractures of the forearm and hip did not have an increased risk (OR 1.21; 95% CI 0.87–1.69 and OR 0.77; 95% CI 0.43–1.37, respectively).

Significant bone loss was also demonstrated in a cohort from South Korea [52]. BMD levels of the lumbar spine and femur in patients were significantly reduced compared with those of age-matched controls [52]. In a Dutch cohort, more than 10% of patients with SpA showed moderate to severe VFs before the age of 40 years [20]. Almost half of the AS patients had multiple vertebral fractures. Among patients with vertebral fractures, 15.2% had a history of trauma with acute back pain ($p < 0.001$ vs no vertebral fractures). Most fractures were localized in the cervical spine and resulted from low-energy impact. Delayed diagnosis often occurred due to patient- and doctor-related factors.

Reports about the outcome of surgical interventions in patients with vertebral fractures showed a high risk of developing neurological defects (10 out of 20 AS patients) and a high risk of diagnostic delay since the initial radiological study was negative for a spinal fracture in 12 patients [58]. The overall mortality within 3 months after injury was reported as 17.7% in AS patients [54].

Interestingly, a significant increase in BMD can be achieved in AS patients receiving TNFi [59]. In a small study from France, treatment with TNFi was associated with an increase of BMD, which results from a decrease of bone resorption [60]. Although treatment with TNFi decreases inflammation and has shown to be effective in increasing BMD, no reduced risk to develop VF were seen in a prospective longitudinal observational cohort study [56]. In 49 patients with AS, the effects of etanercept on BMD and VFs were studied. During this time, hip BMD increased by 2.2% ($p = 0.014$) and lumbar spine BMD by 7.0% ($p < 0.001$). Despite TNFi, the number of patients with VFs more than doubled (from 6 to 15 patients, $p = 0.003$). Thus, the favorable bone-preserving effect is accompanied by unfavorable outcomes on VFs and radiological damage.

Malignancies

Although increased mortality rates have been seen in patients with AS, malignancies do not seem to be responsible for an excess mortality in SpA [61–64]. Historically, most of the data about malignancies have been published focusing on the development of lymphoma. Almost no data are available on solid malignancies which are more common in the general population than lymphomas. No overall increase in cancer risk was found (standardized incidence ratio (SIR) 1.05, 95% CI 0.94–1.17) [64]. Rectal cancer was less common (SIR 0.41, 95% CI 0.15–0.89), while unspecified kidney cancer was more common (SIR 5.90, 95% CI 1.61–15.1). Risks for colon, renal parenchymal, and renal pelvic cancer were not significantly increased. The findings about solid tumors were confirmed recently by analyzing the Danish and Swedish biologics register [62]. In this cohort the site-specific cancer risk ratio was for prostate 0.5 (95% CI 0.3–0.8), for lung 0.6 (95% CI 0.3–1.3), for colorectal 1.0 (95% CI 0.5–2.0), for breast 1.3 (95% CI 0.9–2.0), for lymphoma 0.8 (95% CI 0.4–1.8), and for melanoma 1.4 (95% CI 0.7–2.6).

Results from population-based case-control study in Sweden did not show an increased risk of lymphoma in AS patients [61]. This was supported by the findings of the Swedish National Patient Register and the Swedish Biologics Register ARTIS [63]. For AS patients, the HR of having lymphoma vs the general population was 0.9 (95% CI: 0.5–1.6) [63]. The numbers and incidence of lymphoma were not different in TNFi-exposed vs TNFi-naive AS and PsA patients, although the numbers of lymphomas were small. In the absence of radiation or radium-224 therapy, and regardless of the other treatments used, the evidence does not support an increased rate of lymphoma or other malignancies compared to the general population [65, 66].

In the COMOSPA cohort, overall prevalence for any type of cancer was estimated at 3.0% (95% CI 2.46–3.52), and the most prevalent cancer was cervical cancer (1.2% (95% CI 0.3–1.7)) [18]. Prevalence of basocellular carcinoma and melanoma were 0.8% (95% CI 0.6–1.2) and 0.7% (95% CI 0.4–1.0), respectively [18].

There is no increased risk of malignancies among axSpA patients treated with TNFi [19, 67, 68]. In patients with SpA, treatment with TNFi was not associated with increased risks of cancer, neither overall nor for the six most common cancer types [62].

The most prevalent risk factor for cancer was family history of breast cancer (15.0% (95% CI 13.1–16.9)), followed by family history of colon cancer (8.0% (95% CI 7.2–8.9)) in the COMOSPA cohort [18].

Infections

No increased risk of infections has ever been demonstrated in SpA, except in some patients concomitantly treated with immunosuppressive drugs such as corticosteroids and/or TNFi [69]. However, most of the studies showed no increased long-term risk of infections (especially serious infections) in axSpA patients under TNFi therapy [21]. A post hoc analysis of trials in AS patients treated with etanercept showed a nonsignificant trend toward serious infections [70]. Rate ratios of serious infections during the double-blind studies were 2.19 (95% CI 0.22–107.79) with no reports about opportunistic infections.

In the discussion about an increased risk of infections in patients with SpA regardless of their current treatment, one has to notice the huge variety of the incidence of infections worldwide. The COMOSPA trial found an overall prevalence of 3.5% (95% CI 2.9–4.0) of hepatitis B infection, with the highest prevalence observed in China and Turkey (12%), and of 1.2% (95% CI 0.9–1.6) of hepatitis C infection, with the highest prevalence in Egypt (4%) and Turkey (5%) [18]. In contrast, the prevalence of hepatitis is around 1% in Western European countries. The prevalence of active tuberculosis (TB) in this cohort was 2.5% (95% CI 2.0–3.0), ranging from 0% in most countries to 9% in South Korea [18].

However, the increased risk of tuberculosis and hepatitis B reactivation while receiving TNFi medications should be taken into account. It has been consistently reported that patients who receive TNFi for RA or AS have higher rates of active TB and other infections than RA or AS patients not receiving these medications. Despite the higher rates of TB in the general population, incidence rates of TB while receiving TNFi have been studied less extensively in Asia and Africa-Middle East regions [71]. Data from Korea about TB incidence rates of patients with AS receiving TNFi medication showed conflicting results [72, 73]. In a cohort from Korea with AS and RA, the TB incidence rate ratios for TNFi-treated vs TNFi-untreated patients were 4.87 for AS (95% CI, 1.50–15.39; $p < 0.001$) and 3.61 for RA (95% CI, 1.38–8.07; $p < 0.001$) [73]. Another cohort from Korea identified no statistically significant difference (risk ratio 0.53; 95% CI 0.144–1.913) in relative risks of TB infections between the TNFi-exposed AS cohort and the TNFi-naive AS cohort [72]. However, implementation of systematic screening strategies to detect patients with latent TB before the start of TNFi medications yields to have a low rate of active TB in TNFi-treated patients [74].

However, clinical guidelines regarding antiviral prophylaxis for HBV surface antigen (HBsAg) carriers starting TNFi are not yet fully established, even in endemic regions of HBV infection. One retrospective study from China found that in AS patients, the HBsAg prevalence with 25.4% is statistically higher than those of other rheumatic conditions or healthy controls ($p < 0.05$) [75]. The prevalence of HBsAg is higher in HLA-B27-positive compared to HLA-B27-negative AS patients (26.68 vs 14.49%, $p < 0.05$). Therefore, hepatitis reactivation can occur in patients receiving TNFi and has been described for patients with AS [76].

Gastrointestinal Disease

Data of gastrointestinal disease manifestation – one can speculate about gastritis or colitis – in AS patients apart from concomitant NSAID medication did almost not exist. Frequency of peptic ulcer disease has been reported with a prevalence of 10.7% (95% CI 9.7–11.7), ranging from 1% in Morocco to 47% in Egypt in the COMOSPA study [18]. Since peptic ulcer disease is multifactorial, no causal relationship can be established on this data.

NSAIDs play a crucial role in the management of AS and should be considered as the main factor in association with peptic ulcer disease in AS patients [77]. Safety data regarding the use of NSAIDs in AS patients are rather limited. However, most of the traditional risk factors for peptic ulcer disease like old age or concomitant medications with glucocorticoids does not apply for patients with AS. Therefore, serious adverse events can be expected to occur in ~1% of patients per year if patients are treated with a full dose of an NSAID taking into account the relatively young age and the low comorbidity in AS patients. In a national register-based cohort study on patients with AS in Sweden, serious adverse events related to non-selective NSAIDs, etoricoxib, and celecoxib were similar and in the range of what would be expected in a group of SpA patients [78]. Patients unexposed to NSAIDs had considerably more baseline comorbidities and increased risk for congestive heart failure, reflecting a selection of patients being prescribed NSAIDs in clinical practice. In a recent noninterventional prospective study of European patients treated with NSAIDs for rheumatic diseases including AS, the investigator could show that the incidence (per 100 person-years) was 18.5 per 100 person-years for uncomplicated GI events and 0.7 per 100 person-years for complicated GI events [79]. It also shows adherence to guidelines for gastroprotection is generally low with a 28% of patients with regular proton pump inhibitor use at enrolment, with strong variation by practice and country.

Renal Disease

Data about renal comorbidities associated with SpA have been reported rarely. The most frequently reported renal disease is secondary renal amyloidosis (62%) (5%) [80]. One 20-year-old study assessed the frequency and clinical significance of amyloid deposits in abdominal fat by investigating 137 patients with AS and a disease duration of more than 5 years [81]. Abdominal subcutaneous fat aspiration was positive in 7% of the patients who developed in 50% over the following years a clinical manifest amyloidosis.

In a recent publication, Maksymowych et al. report age- and sex-specific risks of renal complications in a population-based cohort of AS subjects in Québec, Canada, between 1996 and 2006, relative to the general population [82]. Renal complications were diagnosed among 3.4% of men and 2.1% of women with AS compared with 2.0% and 1.6% of persons without AS, respectively. The magnitude of the risk of renal complications was highest among younger individuals and decreased with advancing age.

One recent report based on a prospective population-based nationwide cohort study reported an increased risk of nephrolithiasis in patients with AS [83]. The adjusted HR of nephrolithiasis in AS patients was given as 2.1 (95% CI 1.8–2.4). Predictors of nephrolithiasis within the AS group included prior diagnosis of inflammatory bowel disease (IBD) (HR 2.3; 95% CI 1.7–3.3), prior diagnosis of nephrolithiasis (HR 16.4; 95% CI 11.5–23.4), and patients receiving TNFi (HR 1.6; 95% CI 1.2–2.1).

Depression

Psychological status had close interaction with disease activity and quality of life in patients with AS. Although depression has been frequently reported in observational studies, epidemiological data about the potential increase in risk are lacking. One recent study compares the rate of doctor-diagnosed depression in a well-defined Swedish cohort of AS (n = 1738) patients to the general population seeking care [17]. The observed depression rate was 10% in the AS cohort (n = 172). This was higher compared to the expected age- and sex-specific rate of 6% in the general population. The standardized estimate of depression-rate ratio was 1.81 (95% CI 1.44–2.24) in women men and 1.49 (95% CI 1.20–1.89) in men. Thus, the rate of doctor-diagnosed depression was increased by about 80% in female and by 50% in male AS patients during a 13-year observation period. However, a case-control study from Turkey could not confirm higher depression scores in patients with AS when compared to age-, sex- and education-matched healthy controls [84]. Higher depression and/ or anxiety scores (measured by Hospital Anxiety and Depression Scale (HADS)) indicated poorer functional outcome and quality of life in this study.

Most of the literature regarding depression is based on observational cohorts investigating association between disease status and presence of depression, fatigue, and sleep disturbances [85–87]. Reports about psychological variables often report depression, anxiety, and fatigue coincidentally [88, 89]. In a Turkish cohort it was found that the contribution of depression on fatigue was 12% [89]. Even though disease activity had a considerable effect on fatigue, the effects of psychological factors, especially depression, should be taken into consideration in the management of AS.

Conflicting evidence exists whether exercise might be beneficial in reducing symptoms of depression. Exercise was proven to be beneficial in reducing self-reported depression scores in a randomized-controlled trial with an exercise group compared to patients with no active exercise (waiting-list group) over a period of 8 weeks from Korea [85]. In contrast, one parallel-group study from a Turkish rehabilitation center showed no differences in self-reported depression scores after 6 weeks of group-based exercise program or home-based exercise program [86].

Significant time effect for self-reported depression scores were observed over 6 weeks in one trial from Turkey in AS patients who started treatment with infliximab [90].

Points to Consider for Daily Care in Patients with AS

Since AS is associated with an increased risk of various comorbidities, risk management is an important issue to consider in daily care of patients. EULAR recommends thinking about reporting, screening for, and preventing comorbidities to improve the management of comorbidities in patients with chronic inflammatory rheumatic diseases [91]. In patients with AS, this recommendation is especially valid for CV risk management because of the body of evidence.

Almost all reports about risk management in rheumatology have been published for CV risk management in inflammatory arthritides, with some reports focusing on AS patients. CV risk management includes identification and treatment of CV risk factors. However, whether and to what extent this is done in daily clinical practice is unknown. In patients with RA, it has been shown that CV risk factors were less frequently identified and managed by rheumatologists in comparison with general practitioners (GP) [92]. When managed in primary care, GPs assessed CV risk factors less frequently in RA than in diabetes. Another report from the Netherlands assessed whether CV risk assessment was managed in accordance with national guidelines [93]. The authors report that of the 138 AS assessed patients, 51 patients had an indication for CV risk treatment of which 42 patients (82%) received some form of CV risk medication. However, 39 (76%) of the 51 patients were treated inadequately due to failure to reach treatment targets for hypertension or hypercholesterolemia or due to total lack of CV risk medication. Obviously, there is a clear need for improvement of risk management in AS, and this should be a joint effort from the rheumatologist and the GP. Special attention should be paid to a systematic, standardized periodical review (e.g., at least every 5 years) for those with a chronic inflammatory rheumatic disease [91].

EULAR published in 2010 recommendations for CV risk management in patients with RA and other forms of inflammatory arthritis [94]. In here, risk assessment, considerations about treatment effects, as well as adherence to national guidelines in preventing and treating comorbidities is addressed. The authors underpin that adequate control of disease activity is necessary to lower the CV risk.

Strategies to adequately address risk assessment and management of the other comorbidities are scarce (infections) or do not exist (e.g., osteoporosis, malignancies). Screening for TB is a requirement before starting TNFi treatment which is documented in the license of these compounds, and adequate treatment strategies in case of either active TB or latent TB have been recommended [95]. Prevention strategies for patients with hepatitis have not been systematically implemented although antiviral prophylaxis helped preventing HBV reactivation in HBsAg carriers starting TNFi.

Conclusion

Comorbidities are an important contributor to the burden of disease in patients with AS – not only because of its influence on management and treatment decisions. Systematic assessment of comorbidities is essential to prevent excess morbidity and mortality. If modifiable risk factors are identified, treatment should be adjusted accordingly.

While osteoporosis and CVD are more frequently observed in patients with AS in comparison to the general population, robust data about higher prevalence regarding malignancies and renal and gastrointestinal disorders are scarce. The increased risk for infections is mainly associated with immunosuppressive drugs. Higher prevalence rates are probably multifactorial, being related both to chronic systemic inflammation and to high prevalence of conventional risk factors. Although comorbidities do occur very frequent in AS patients, comorbidities are suboptimally prevented, screened for, and managed. Nevertheless, CV risk management (CV-RM) could be an effective method to reduce CV mortality and morbidity in AS patients.

References

1. Dougados M, Baeten D. Spondyloarthritis. Lancet. 2011;377(9783):2127–37.
2. Stolwijk C, et al. The epidemiology of extra-articular manifestations in ankylosing spondylitis: a population-based matched cohort study. Ann Rheum Dis. 2015;74(7):1373–8.
3. Rudwaleit M, et al. The development of assessment of SpondyloArthritis international society classification criteria for axial spondyloarthritis (part II): validation and final selection. Ann Rheum Dis. 2009;68(6):777–83.
4. van der Linden S, Valkenburg HA, Cats A. Evaluation of diagnostic criteria for ankylosing spondylitis. A proposal for modification of the New York criteria. Arthritis Rheum. 1984;27(4):361–8.
5. Braun J, Baraliakos X, Kiltz U. Non-radiographic axial spondyloarthritis: a classification or a diagnosis? Clin Exp Rheumatol. 2016;34(1 Suppl 95):S5–6.
6. Brown MA, Kenna T, Wordsworth BP. Genetics of ankylosing spondylitis – insights into pathogenesis. Nat Rev Rheumatol. 2016;12(2):81–91.
7. Roldan CA, et al. Aortic root disease and valve disease associated with ankylosing spondylitis. J Am Coll Cardiol. 1998;32(5):1397–404.
8. Looi JL, et al. Valvulitis and aortitis associated with ankylosing spondylitis: early detection and monitoring response to therapy using cardiac magnetic resonance imaging. Int J Rheum Dis. 2011;14(4):e56–8.
9. Accorinti M, et al. Clinical features and prognosis of HLA B27-associated acute anterior uveitis in an Italian patient population. Ocul Immunol Inflamm. 2010;18(2):91–6.
10. Robinson PC, et al. The genetic associations of acute anterior uveitis and their overlap with the genetics of ankylosing spondylitis. Genes Immun. 2016;17(1):46–51.
11. Chandran V, Rahman P. Update on the genetics of spondyloarthritis – ankylosing spondylitis and psoriatic arthritis. Best Pract Res Clin Rheumatol. 2010;24(5):579–88.
12. Bremander A, et al. Population-based estimates of common comorbidities and cardiovascular disease in ankylosing spondylitis. Arthritis Care Res (Hoboken). 2011;63(4):550–6.
13. Essers I, et al. Ankylosing spondylitis and risk of ischaemic heart disease: a population-based cohort study. Ann Rheum Dis. 2016;75(1):203–9.
14. Klingberg E, et al. Osteoporosis in ankylosing spondylitis – prevalence, risk factors and methods of assessment. Arthritis Res Ther. 2012;14(3):R108.
15. Kang JH, Chen YH, Lin HC. Comorbidity profiles among patients with ankylosing spondylitis: a nationwide population-based study. Ann Rheum Dis. 2010;69(6):1165–8.
16. Exarchou S, et al. Mortality in ankylosing spondylitis: results from a nationwide population-based study. Ann Rheum Dis. 2016;75(8):1466–72.
17. Meesters JJ, et al. The risk for depression in patients with ankylosing spondylitis: a population-based cohort study. Arthritis Res Ther. 2014;16(5):418.
18. Molto A, Etcheto A, van der Heijde D, et al. Prevalence of comorbidities and evaluation of their screening in spondyloarthritis: results of the international cross-sectional ASAS-COMOSPA study. Ann Rheum Dis. 2016;75(6):1016–23.
19. Westhovens I, et al. Anti-TNF therapy and malignancy in spondyloarthritis in the Leuven spondyloarthritis biologics cohort (BIOSPAR). Clin Exp Rheumatol. 2014;32(1):71–6.
20. Geusens P, et al. The prevalence of vertebral fractures in spondyloarthritis: relation to disease characteristics, bone mineral density, syndesmophytes and history of back pain and trauma. Arthritis Res Ther. 2015;17:294.
21. Wallis D, et al. Tumour necrosis factor inhibitor therapy and infection risk in axial spondyloarthritis: results from a longitudinal observational cohort. Rheumatology (Oxford). 2015; 54(1):152–6.
22. Prati C, et al. Mortality in spondylarthritis. Joint Bone Spine. 2011;78(5):466–70.
23. Zochling J, Braun J. Mortality in rheumatoid arthritis and ankylosing spondylitis. Clin Exp Rheumatol. 2009;27(4 Suppl 55):S127–30.

24. Bakland G, Gran JT, Nossent JC. Increased mortality in ankylosing spondylitis is related to disease activity. Ann Rheum Dis. 2011;70(11):1921–5.
25. Peters MJ, et al. Signs of accelerated preclinical atherosclerosis in patients with ankylosing spondylitis. J Rheumatol. 2010;37(1):161–6.
26. Mathieu S, et al. Cardiovascular profile in ankylosing spondylitis: a systematic review and meta-analysis. Arthritis Care Res (Hoboken). 2011;63(4):557–63.
27. van der Valk FM, Bernelot Moens SJ, Verweij SL, et al. Increased arterial wall inflammation in patients with ankylosing spondylitis is reduced by statin therapy. Ann Rheum Dis. 2016;75(10):1848–51.
28. Han C, et al. Cardiovascular disease and risk factors in patients with rheumatoid arthritis, psoriatic arthritis, and ankylosing spondylitis. J Rheumatol. 2006;33(11):2167–72.
29. Peters MJ, et al. Cardiovascular risk profile of patients with spondylarthropathies, particularly ankylosing spondylitis and psoriatic arthritis. Semin Arthritis Rheum. 2004;34(3):585–92.
30. Sari I, et al. Impaired endothelial function in patients with ankylosing spondylitis. Rheumatology (Oxford). 2006;45(3):283–6.
31. Nurmohamed MT, van der Horst-Bruinsma I, Maksymowych WP. Cardiovascular and cerebrovascular diseases in ankylosing spondylitis: current insights. Curr Rheumatol Rep. 2012;14(5):415–21.
32. Mathieu S, Pereira B, Soubrier M. Cardiovascular events in ankylosing spondylitis: an updated meta-analysis. Semin Arthritis Rheum. 2015;44(5):551–5.
33. van Halm VP, et al. Increased disease activity is associated with a deteriorated lipid profile in patients with ankylosing spondylitis. Ann Rheum Dis. 2006;65(11):1473–7.
34. van Eijk IC, et al. Microvascular function is impaired in ankylosing spondylitis and improves after tumour necrosis factor alpha blockade. Ann Rheum Dis. 2009;68(3):362–6.
35. Hollan I, et al. Spondyloarthritis: a strong predictor of early coronary artery bypass grafting. Scand J Rheumatol. 2008;37(1):18–22.
36. Heslinga SC, et al. Diastolic left ventricular dysfunction in ankylosing spondylitis – a systematic review and meta-analysis. Semin Arthritis Rheum. 2014;44(1):14–9.
37. Brophy S, et al. No increased rate of acute myocardial infarction or stroke among patients with ankylosing spondylitis-a retrospective cohort study using routine data. Semin Arthritis Rheum. 2012;42(2):140–5.
38. Keller JJ, et al. Increased risk of stroke among patients with ankylosing spondylitis: a population-based matched-cohort study. Rheumatol Int. 2014;34(2):255–63.
39. Lin CW, et al. Increased risk of ischemic stroke in young patients with ankylosing spondylitis: a population-based longitudinal follow-up study. PLoS One. 2014;9(4):e94027.
40. Peters MJ, et al. Ankylosing spondylitis: a risk factor for myocardial infarction? Ann Rheum Dis. 2010;69(3):579–81.
41. Acar G, et al. Assessment of atrial electromechanical coupling characteristics in patients with ankylosing spondylitis. Echocardiography. 2009;26(5):549–57.
42. Dik VK, et al. The relationship between disease-related characteristics and conduction disturbances in ankylosing spondylitis. Scand J Rheumatol. 2010;39(1):38–41.
43. Szabo SM, et al. Increased risk of cardiovascular and cerebrovascular diseases in individuals with ankylosing spondylitis: a population-based study. Arthritis Rheum. 2011;63(11):3294–304.
44. Heslinga SC, et al. Reduction of inflammation drives lipid changes in ankylosing spondylitis. J Rheumatol. 2015;42(10):1842–5.
45. van Eijk IC, et al. Improvement of lipid profile is accompanied by atheroprotective alterations in high-density lipoprotein composition upon tumor necrosis factor blockade: a prospective cohort study in ankylosing spondylitis. Arthritis Rheum. 2009;60(5):1324–30.
46. Mathieu S, et al. Effects of 14 weeks of TNF alpha blockade treatment on lipid profile in ankylosing spondylitis. Joint Bone Spine. 2010;77(1):50–2.
47. van Sijl AM, et al. Tumour necrosis factor blocking agents and progression of subclinical atherosclerosis in patients with ankylosing spondylitis. Ann Rheum Dis. 2015;74(1):119–23.

48. Angel K, et al. Effect of 1-year anti-TNF-alpha therapy on aortic stiffness, carotid atherosclerosis, and calprotectin in inflammatory arthropathies: a controlled study. Am J Hypertens. 2012;25(6):644–50.
49. Mathieu S, et al. No significant changes in arterial stiffness in patients with ankylosing spondylitis after tumour necrosis factor alpha blockade treatment for 6 and 12 months. Rheumatology (Oxford). 2013;52(1):204–9.
50. Capkin E, et al. Anti-TNF-alpha therapy may not improve arterial stiffness in patients with AS: a 24-week follow-up. Rheumatology (Oxford). 2012;51(5):910–4.
51. Klingberg E, et al. Vertebral fractures in ankylosing spondylitis are associated with lower bone mineral density in both central and peripheral skeleton. J Rheumatol. 2012;39(10):1987–95.
52. Jun JB, et al. Femoral bone mineral density is associated with vertebral fractures in patients with ankylosing spondylitis: a cross-sectional study. J Rheumatol. 2006;33(8):1637–41.
53. Vosse D, et al. Ankylosing spondylitis and the risk of fracture: results from a large primary care-based nested case-control study. Ann Rheum Dis. 2009;68(12):1839–42.
54. Westerveld LA, Verlaan JJ, Oner FC. Spinal fractures in patients with ankylosing spinal disorders: a systematic review of the literature on treatment, neurological status and complications. Eur Spine J. 2009;18(2):145–56.
55. van der Weijden MA, et al. High prevalence of low bone mineral density in patients within 10 years of onset of ankylosing spondylitis: a systematic review. Clin Rheumatol. 2012;31(11):1529–35.
56. van der Weijden MA, et al. Etanercept increases bone mineral density in ankylosing spondylitis, but does not prevent vertebral fractures: results of a prospective observational cohort study. J Rheumatol. 2016;43(4):758–64.
57. Karberg K, et al. Bone loss is detected more frequently in patients with ankylosing spondylitis with syndesmophytes. J Rheumatol. 2005;32(7):1290–8.
58. Sapkas G, et al. Surgical outcome after spinal fractures in patients with ankylosing spondylitis. BMC Musculoskelet Disord. 2009;10:96.
59. Briot K, et al. Prospective assessment of body weight, body composition, and bone density changes in patients with spondyloarthropathy receiving anti-tumor necrosis factor-alpha treatment. J Rheumatol. 2008;35(5):855–61.
60. Briot K, et al. Body weight, body composition, and bone turnover changes in patients with spondyloarthropathy receiving anti-tumour necrosis factor {alpha} treatment. Ann Rheum Dis. 2005;64(8):1137–40.
61. Askling J, et al. Risk for malignant lymphoma in ankylosing spondylitis: a nationwide Swedish case-control study. Ann Rheum Dis. 2006;65(9):1184–7.
62. Hellgren K, et al. Cancer risk in patients with spondyloarthritis treated with TNF inhibitors: a collaborative study from the ARTIS and DANBIO registers. Ann Rheum Dis. 2017; 76(1):105–11.
63. Hellgren K, Dreyer L, Arkema EV, et al. Ankylosing spondylitis, psoriatic arthritis, and risk of malignant lymphoma: a cohort study based on nationwide prospectively recorded data from Sweden. Arthritis Rheumatol. 2014;66(5):1282–90.
64. Feltelius N, Ekbom A, Blomqvist P. Cancer incidence among patients with ankylosing spondylitis in Sweden 1965-95: a population based cohort study. Ann Rheum Dis. 2003;62(12):1185–8.
65. Brown WM, Doll R. Mortality from cancer and other causes after radiotherapy for ankylosing spondylitis. Br Med J. 1965;2(5474):1327–32.
66. Wick RR, et al. Increased risk of myeloid leukaemia in patients with ankylosing spondylitis following treatment with radium-224. Rheumatology (Oxford). 2008;47(6):855–9.
67. Carmona L, et al. Cancer in patients with rheumatic diseases exposed to TNF antagonists. Semin Arthritis Rheum. 2011;41(1):71–80.
68. Dreyer L, et al. Incidences of overall and site specific cancers in TNFalpha inhibitor treated patients with rheumatoid arthritis and other arthritides – a follow-up study from the DANBIO registry. Ann Rheum Dis. 2013;72(1):79–82.

69. Fouque-Aubert A, et al. Serious infections in patients with ankylosing spondylitis with and without TNF blockers: a systematic review and meta-analysis of randomised placebo-controlled trials. Ann Rheum Dis. 2010;69(10):1756–61.
70. van der Heijde D, et al. Rates of serious infections, opportunistic infections, inflammatory bowel disease, and malignancies in subjects receiving etanercept vs. controls from clinical trials in ankylosing spondylitis: a pooled analysis. Scand J Rheumatol. 2014;43(1):49–53.
71. Hammoudeh M, et al. Safety of tumor necrosis factor inhibitors use for rheumatoid arthritis and ankylosing spondylitis in Africa, the Middle East, and Asia: focus on severe infections and tuberculosis. Clin Rheumatol. 2013;32(3):293–300.
72. Kim EM, et al. Incidence of tuberculosis among korean patients with ankylosing spondylitis who are taking tumor necrosis factor blockers. J Rheumatol. 2011;38(10):2218–23.
73. Kim HW, et al. Comparison of tuberculosis incidence in ankylosing spondylitis and rheumatoid arthritis during tumor necrosis factor inhibitor treatment in an intermediate burden area. Clin Rheumatol. 2014;33(9):1307–12.
74. Hsia EC, et al. Comprehensive tuberculosis screening program in patients with inflammatory arthritides treated with golimumab, a human anti-tumor necrosis factor antibody, in phase III clinical trials. Arthritis Care Res (Hoboken). 2013;65(2):309–13.
75. Zheng B, et al. Prevalence of hepatitis B surface antigen in patients with ankylosing spondylitis and its association with HLA-B27: a retrospective study from south China. Rheumatol Int. 2012;32(7):2011–6.
76. Ryu HH, et al. Hepatitis B virus reactivation in rheumatoid arthritis and ankylosing spondylitis patients treated with anti-TNFalpha agents: a retrospective analysis of 49 cases. Clin Rheumatol. 2012;31(6):931–6.
77. Song IH, et al. Benefits and risks of ankylosing spondylitis treatment with nonsteroidal antiinflammatory drugs. Arthritis Rheum. 2008;58(4):929–38.
78. Kristensen LE, et al. Safety of Etoricoxib, celecoxib, and nonselective nonsteroidal Anti-inflammatory drugs in ankylosing spondylitis and other Spondyloarthritis patients: a Swedish National Population-Based Cohort Study. Arthritis Care Res (Hoboken). 2015; 67(8):1137–49.
79. Lanas A, Boers M, Nuevo J. Gastrointestinal events in at-risk patients starting non-steroidal anti-inflammatory drugs (NSAIDs) for rheumatic diseases: the EVIDENCE study of European routine practice. Ann Rheum Dis. 2015;74(4):675–81.
80. Strobel ES, Fritschka E. Renal diseases in ankylosing spondylitis: review of the literature illustrated by case reports. Clin Rheumatol. 1998;17(6):524–30.
81. Gratacos J, et al. Secondary amyloidosis in ankylosing spondylitis. A systematic survey of 137 patients using abdominal fat aspiration. J Rheumatol. 1997;24(5):912–5.
82. Levy AR, et al. Estimating the occurrence of renal complications among persons with ankylosing spondylitis. Arthritis Care Res (Hoboken). 2014;66(3):440–5.
83. Jakobsen AK, et al. Is nephrolithiasis an unrecognized extra-articular manifestation in ankylosing spondylitis? A prospective population-based Swedish national cohort study with matched general population comparator subjects. PLoS One. 2014;9(11):e113602.
84. Baysal O, et al. Relationship between psychological status and disease activity and quality of life in ankylosing spondylitis. Rheumatol Int. 2011;31(6):795–800.
85. Lim HJ, Moon YI, Lee MS. Effects of home-based daily exercise therapy on joint mobility, daily activity, pain, and depression in patients with ankylosing spondylitis. Rheumatol Int. 2005;25(3):225–9.
86. Karapolat H, et al. Comparison of group-based exercise versus home-based exercise in patients with ankylosing spondylitis: effects on bath ankylosing spondylitis indices, quality of life and depression. Clin Rheumatol. 2008;27(6):695–700.
87. Durmus D, et al. Effects of a home-based exercise program on quality of life, fatigue, and depression in patients with ankylosing spondylitis. Rheumatol Int. 2009;29(6):673–7.
88. Li Y, et al. Sleep disturbances are associated with increased pain, disease activity, depression, and anxiety in ankylosing spondylitis: a case-control study. Arthritis Res Ther. 2012;14(5):R215.

89. Gunaydin R, et al. Fatigue in patients with ankylosing spondylitis: relationships with disease-specific variables, depression, and sleep disturbance. Clin Rheumatol. 2009;28(9):1045–51.
90. Ertenli I, et al. Infliximab, a TNF-alpha antagonist treatment in patients with ankylosing spondylitis: the impact on depression, anxiety and quality of life level. Rheumatol Int. 2012;32(2):323–30.
91. Baillet A, et al. Points to consider for reporting, screening for and preventing selected comorbidities in chronic inflammatory rheumatic diseases in daily practice: a EULAR initiative. Ann Rheum Dis. 2016;75(6):965–73.
92. Peters MJ, Nurmohamed MT. Cardiovascular risk management in rheumatoid arthritis: are we still waiting for the first step? Arthritis Res Ther. 2013;15(2):111.
93. Heslinga SC, et al. Cardiovascular risk management in patients with active ankylosing spondylitis: a detailed evaluation. BMC Musculoskelet Disord. 2015;16:80.
94. Peters MJ, et al. EULAR evidence-based recommendations for cardiovascular risk management in patients with rheumatoid arthritis and other forms of inflammatory arthritis. Ann Rheum Dis. 2010;69(2):325–31.
95. Cantini F, et al. Guidance for the management of patients with latent tuberculosis infection requiring biologic therapy in rheumatology and dermatology clinical practice. Autoimmun Rev. 2015;14(6):503–9.

Chapter 6
Systemic Lupus Erythematosus

Isabel Castrejon, Ailda Nika, Winston Sequeira, and Meenakshi Jolly

Systemic lupus erythematosus (SLE) is a chronic autoimmune disease associated with severe morbidity and increased mortality. The survival of patients with SLE has improved significantly, with a 5-year survival rate increasing from 64–87% in the 1980s to over 95% today [1]. The mortality rates however are three times higher compared to the general population [2]. SLE can potentially affect any organ but the more serious comorbidities and leading causes of death are end-stage renal disease (Standardized mortality ratio (SMR) 7.90), infection (Meta-SMR 4.98), and cardiovascular diseases (CVD) (Meta-SMR 2.72) [2]. In addition, patients with SLE have higher risk of malignancies compared to the general population.

In general, comorbidity imposes an additional burden on SLE patients, reducing their quality of life. The presence of comorbidities is a well-known predictor of greater healthcare utilization and mortality. The larger the number of comorbidities the longer the length of hospital stay and the greater the hospital mortality rates compared to patients with no or fewer number of comorbidities [3]. The Charlson comorbidity index (CCI), an index that assigns a weight for comorbidity, is higher in patients with SLE compared to specific controls matched by age and gender [4]. Furthermore, CCI is an independent and significant predictor of hospital mortality in SLE (hazard ratio 7.8 for high (≥5) vs none, $p < 0.001$) [3]. Besides CCI, infectious diseases are the major independent predictor of hospital mortality. In another study of hospital deaths in SLE, the major acute comorbidity was sepsis (42%) [5].

A comorbid condition can be related to the primary disease by different causal pathways (e.g., end-stage renal disease and SLE) or unrelated to the primary diagnosis but a consequence of the treatment (e.g., osteoporosis and glucocorticoids therapy or infections and immunosuppressive therapy). Sometimes, however, the association and causation is less clear (e.g., cardiovascular or cerebrovascular diseases and SLE).

I. Castrejon, MD, PhD (✉) • A. Nika, MD • W. Sequeira, MD • M. Jolly, MD, MS
Division of Rheumatology, Rush University Medical Center, Chicago, IL, USA
e-mail: isabelcastrejonf@gmail.com; isabel_castrejon@rush.edu

Y. El Miedany (ed.), *Comorbidity in Rheumatic Diseases*,
DOI 10.1007/978-3-319-59963-2_6

In a recent study on the prevalence of self-reported comorbidities in different rheumatic conditions including SLE, it was reported that a substantially increased prevalence (% adjusted rate (95% CI)) of hypertension (HTN) (25.2 (20.6, 29.8)), depression (20.8 (16.9, 24.6)), cataract (7.0 (4.2, 9.8)), thyroid problems (9.8 (7.0, 12.7)), CVD (8.4 (6.1, 10.7)), and diabetes mellitus (DM) (6.4 (4.3, 8.4)). This was reported after adjusting for age and sex in a specific US population with estimates for these conditions [6]. A similar study was done in the UK reviewing clinical practice health records for evaluating adjusted incidence rate ratios (IRR) for comorbidities. In this study, end-stage renal disease (ESRD) was the most common comorbidity (IRR 7.83, 95% CI 4.69–13.08), followed by osteoporosis (incidence rate ratio 2.71, 95% CI 2.43–3.03) [4]. In the same study, men with SLE showed higher rates of CVD and cancer, whereas women had higher rates of infection and osteoporosis. In addition, SLE patients younger than 40 years also had a high incidence for ESRD and CVD with an IRR of 63.06 (95% CI 8.29–479.56) and 40.31 (95% CI 5.11–318.14), respectively, when compared to controls [4].

Among pediatric SLE patients, in a nationwide population-based study in Taiwan, infection was the most common comorbidity [7]. Other comorbidities were musculoskeletal (17%), CVD (16%), ocular disease (11%), and renal disease (11%). Children had a higher risk of heart failure, HTA, osteoporosis, cataracts, glaucoma, dyslipidemia, seizures, encephalopathy, and malignancy compared to non-SLE population [7]. Some of these comorbidities (cataract, DM, malignancy) are also included in irreversible damage assessment in SLE.

In summary, comorbid diseases are prevalent in SLE in comparison with the general population (Table 6.1) and have significant impact on patient's quality of life, healthcare utilization, overall outcomes, and mortality. Here we review some of the most common comorbidities in SLE.

Cardiovascular Diseases

Although SLE can potentially affect any organ system, some of the most serious complications are related to the CVD. A 2.66-fold increased risk of CVD was found in SLE among the Hopkins lupus cohort [13] the risk being fivefold higher in the 35–44-year-old group of patients [14]. SLE patients not only commonly develop coronary artery disease (CAD), but they also frequently develop cerebrovascular (CVA) and peripheral arterial disease (PAD). Overall the prevalence of CAD ranges from 6–12% in SLE patients [15].

Over time, CVD mortality has decreased in the general population; however, a similar level of improvement has not been seen in SLE [2]. It has been estimated that patients with SLE have a threefold increased risk of premature cardiovascular mortality [2]. Rates of hospitalization for acute myocardial infarction and ischemic stroke have increased over time for SLE, while these rates decreased in general population [16].

Table 6.1 Risk of different comorbidities in SLE patients versus the general population in different publications presented in chronological order

Study and population	Comorbidity	Standardized incidence ratios (95%)[a]
Rees et al. [4] Retrospective cohort including 7732 prevalent cases of SLE	Cardiovascular disease[b] Stroke[b] End-stage renal failure[b] Cancer[b] Osteoporosis[b] Infection[b]	1.65 (1.40–1.95) 1.47 (1.20–1.80) 3.41 (1.93–6.05) 1.15 (1.05–1.27) 1.92 (1.70–2.16) 1.10 (1.03–1.18)
Attar et al. [8] Retrospective cohort including 95 SLE patients	Vitamin D deficiency	1.45 (0.53–3.27)
Magder et al. [9] Hopkins lupus cohort of 1874 SLE patients	Cardiovascular events[c]	2.66 (2.16–3.16)
Mok et al. [10] Scandinavian cohort of 490 SLE patients	Cerebrovascular events	2.02 (1.30–3.81)
Bernatsky et al. [11] Multisite international SLE cohort including 16,409 patients linked with regional tumor registries	Cancer: All types	1.14 (1.05–1.23)
	Non-Hodgkin lymphoma	4.39 (3.46–5.49)
	Vulva	3.78 (1.52–7.78)
	Thyroid	1.76 (1.13–2.61)
	Leukemia	1.75 (1.04–2.76)
	Lung	1.30 (1.04–1.60)
	Breast	0.73 (0.61–0.88)
	Endometrial	0.44 (0.23–0.77)
Ramsey-Goldman et al. [12] Self-reported fractures in a large population-based cohort of 792 women with SLE	Osteoporosis Self-reported fractures	4.7 (3.80–5.80)

[a]In comparison with the general population; [b]Adjusted for age and sex, plus alcohol, smoking, hypertension, hyperlipidemia, body mass index, prednisolone use, and baseline Charlson index score; $p < 0.001$ for all. [c]Defined as the occurrence of myocardial infarction, thrombotic stroke, clinically definite angina, percutaneous coronary intervention, a coronary bypass procedure, or claudication

It is unclear why patients with SLE are at a greater risk of accelerated atherosclerosis, but both traditional "Framingham" and nontraditional risk factors certainly play a role. Understanding of pathogenesis and treatment of atherosclerosis in SLE remains challenging and is evolving [17].

Traditional risk factors such as smoking, hyperlipidemia, HTN, DM, and obesity seem to be enhanced by a series of different pathways including ongoing inflammation, disease activity, autoantibodies, or deleterious effect of prolonged corticosteroid exposure in SLE patients. This is manifest with higher rates of complications, such as premature cardiovascular events, including even structural damages, for example, myocardial infarction (MI) and strokes (CVA) in younger ages. It is well known that traditional Framingham risk factor score (FRS) for CVD risk assessment underestimates the CVD risk for patients with SLE. Efforts in finding a better predictor model for SLE patients (e.g., modified FRS in which each item is multiplied by 2 [18]) and biomarkers for CVD risk prediction are ongoing [19].

Common risk factors such as smoking can increase the level of disease activity in general and atherosclerosis complications in particular. Smokers in SLE have a threefold increase in CVD events compared to smokers in general population [20]. In addition, smoking can be an environmental trigger for SLE, and it has been associated with higher disease activity in SLE patients [21]. It is not clear if the greater disease activity and damage (cutaneous) reported among smokers is due to greater immunogenicity (as evident with the presence of DsDNA autoantibodies) or interference with mechanism of action of hydroxychloroquine.

Obesity, an additional cardiovascular risk factor, is more prevalent in SLE and may be associated with prolonged prednisone use, especially central obesity, which is a relative risk for CVD. Using dual x-ray absorptiometry (DXA), 50% of SLE patients reported to be obese, but only 29% were obese when body mass index definition was used [22]. Weight gain in SLE patients is multifactorial. Musculoskeletal manifestations (acute and chronic) may impose physical function limitations contributing to weight gain. Pain, fatigue, sleep, or emotional health issues, fibromyalgia, and medication for fibromyalgia and depression may also contribute. However, the most common reason for SLE patients to gain weight is attributed to corticosteroids used to treat their disease. Petri et al. reported obesity rates in SLE to be mostly associated to corticosteroid use. A 10 mg increase in prednisone dose led to an average 5.50 pounds gain within 3 months [23]. Being overweight is a major contributor to atherosclerosis in SLE patients otherwise at low risk for CVD [24].

Hyperlipidemia is a known risk factor for CVD in SLE, and prednisone use can result in an increase of total cholesterol. Prevalence of dyslipidemia in SLE ranges from 36% at diagnosis to 60% or even higher after 3 years of diagnosis, depending on the definition in the SLICC cohort [25]. Decreased level of high-density lipoprotein (HDL) is the most common abnormality [20]. In SLE, elevated VLDL and triglycerides and lower HDL have been associated with disease activity. In the course of the disease, HDL particles lose their anti-inflammatory and antioxidant properties and become dysfunctional [26]. Paraoxonase-3 (PON3), a potent antioxidant protein, is depleted from the HDL of SLE patients with subclinical atherosclerosis, and PON3 expression in HDL was positively correlated with HDL antioxidant function [26]. The effect of steroids on hyperlipidemia has been well established, but the use of antimalarial drugs on the other hand has been shown to have some protective effect [27]. Dyslipidemia needs to be recognized in SLE and addressed through patient education and lifestyle modifications and if required with medications. Although several randomized clinical trials with statins have failed to prove a clear benefit in halting progression of atherosclerosis [25], yearly monitoring of SLE patients with lipid profile is recommended. In addition, education with lifestyle modifications, use of hydroxychloroquine, or steroid sparing, interventions when possible, along with primary and secondary CVD prevention strategies, is encouraged.

HTN besides being a comorbid condition in itself can cause progression of carotid intima-media thickness leading to strokes and poor renal outcome. Magder and Petri have described a higher risk of cardiovascular events (CVEs) in SLE patients, 2.66 times higher compared with the general population based on Framingham risk scores (95% CI: 2.16–3.16) [9]. In addition, CVE rates were positively associated with blood pressure with a 1.26 for every 10 mmHg increase in systolic blood pressure above 120 mmHg ($p = 0.0054$). In an observational longitudinal study, HTN was an independent risk factor (OR = 5.01, 95% CI 1.38–18.23), besides age, smoking, and dyslipidemia, for MI even before the diagnosis of SLE or shortly thereafter [28].

Considering the crude and adjusted rates for lifetime comorbid conditions, HTN was the most prevalent (55.7%) in SLE followed by other CV events (29.9%) and DM (13.8%) [6]. These rates are higher than in other rheumatic conditions, including rheumatoid arthritis (RA). While for RA and other rheumatic conditions the rates of CVD incidence increase with age, the rates are generally higher in SLE and constant among 35–84-year-old age group [6]. SLE patients with HTN may develop posterior reversible encephalopathy syndrome in the course of the disease [29]. In patients with SLE and HTN, careful workup for renal involvement is suggested along with education and management. In patients with proteinuria and HTN, use of angiotensin-converting enzyme inhibitors may be considered if possible.

End-stage renal disease (ESRD) is seen in SLE and may be related either to greater prevalence of HTN in SLE or directly as result of lupus nephritis.

SLE patients with renal involvement, serositis, Raynaud's phenomenon, and antiphospholipid syndrome have a higher frequency of CV events. The presence of APL antibodies, anti-dsDNA, or low serum complement is associated with CV events as well. APL antibodies might play a role in the development of atherosclerosis via different mechanisms, such as the pro-inflammatory activity or by enhancing the lipid peroxidation of lipoproteins or reducing paraoxonase activity [30]. SLE patients who were positive for APL antibodies had a 57% greater risk of suffering a CV event [31].

Low vitamin D levels are commonly seen among SLE patients. Besides bone health, low vitamin D may have implications for disease activity and CVD in SLE. In a large observational longitudinal study of 890 SLE patients, lower baseline 25(OH)D levels were found to be associated with higher risk for CV risk factors and more active SLE at baseline [32]. There was a trend toward a lower likelihood of CVD events in those with higher baseline 25(OH) D levels in the same study. In another study with 75 women with SLE, higher BMI ($p = 0.014$) and insulin resistance ($p = 0.023$) were noted among those with vitamin D deficiency than those with 25(OH) D > 20 ng/ml [33]. Also, patients with SLEDAI-2 K $\geq$ 4 had lower 25(OH) D than those with SLEDAI-2 K <4 (median 12.9 vs. 20.3 ng/ml, $p = 0.031$). Aortic stiffness was significantly and directly associated with serum 25(OH) D and independently of CVD risk factors and insulin. Furthermore, vitamin D deficiency is associated with hampered vascular repair and reduced endothelial function and may modulate type I IFN responses [34]. Low vitamin D levels are easily modifiable through vigilance, screening, education, and intervention.

Individuals with SLE have a 2.5 times higher risk of cerebrovascular disease (CVA or stroke) than the general population, regardless of the type of stroke [35], which accounts for 10–15% of deaths in SLE [36]. SLE patients have a twofold higher risk of ischemic stroke, a threefold higher risk of intracerebral hemorrhage, and an almost fourfold higher risk of subarachnoid hemorrhage compared to the general population. Relative risk of stroke was highest among individuals younger than 50 years of age [35]. The fact that highest relative risk of stroke was observed at younger ages may be partially explained by the accelerated and premature atherosclerosis seen in SLE. Elevated homocysteine levels in SLE patients have been implicated in higher rates of stroke and arterial thrombosis as well [9]. In addition a more prominent role of thrombotic events in general is becoming evident, affecting late morbidity and mortality in SLE. Thrombosis is becoming the most common cause of death during the late disease course according to [36]. Platelets bearing complement protein C4d (P-C4d) is associated with ischemic stroke (odds ratio 4.54, 95% CI 1.63–12.69, $p = 0.004$) after adjusting for age, ethnicity, and APL antibodies among SLE patients [37]. Furthermore, P-C4d is associated with all-cause mortality and stroke in SLE patients.

PAD is noted to be common among SLE patients [38]. In a Chinese study with 10,144 patients with SLE and 10,144 control patients, incidence of peripheral arterial occlusive disease (PAOD) was 9.39-fold higher (95% confidence interval [CI] = 7.70–11.15) in the SLE cohort than in the non-SLE cohort [39]. Moreover, SLE was an independent risk factor for PAOD. The adjusted risk of PAOD was highest in patients with SLE who were aged ≤34 years (hazard ratio = 47.6, 95% CI = 26.8–84.4). The risk of PAOD was highest during the first year of follow-up and decreased over time.

Pulmonary arterial hypertension (PAH) is commonly associated with connective tissue diseases including systemic sclerosis and SLE. The prevalence of PAH in SLE is estimated to be 0.5–17.5%. Leading predictors of PAH in SLE are Raynaud's phenomenon, anti-U1RNP antibody [40], and anticardiolipin antibody positivity. Among Chinese patients with SLE, pericarditis (odds ratio (OR) = 4.248), pleuritis (OR = 3.061), and anti-RNP (OR = 2.559) were independent risk factors for PAH [41].Although not entirely understood, various elements of SLE, such as vasculitis, APL syndrome causing in situ thrombosis, interstitial pulmonary fibrosis, and hypoxia due to lung disease, can lead to endothelial and smooth muscle proliferation causing damage of the pulmonary vasculature and PAH. Addition of immunosuppressive agent to vasodilators treatment was found to be useful at 6 months in SLE patients with PAH [42].

Some CV events in SLE, particularly heart failure and rhythm disorders, can be the result of several causes, such as lupus activity, fluid overload, anemia, PAH, etc. Over time, cardiovascular mortality has decreased in the general population, but a similar level of improvement was not seen in SLE patients, contributing still to 10–15% of demise rates in SLE [36]. General survival in SLE and that related to CV disease has not improved since 1980 (Centers for Disease Control and Prevention, 2002) [43]. Rates of hospitalizations for CVD events have not decreased. Results from the National Heart, Lung, and Blood Institute Dynamic Registry across 23 clinical centers from 28 consecutive SLE patients undergoing percutaneous coronary intervention (PCI) and compared with non-SLE patients ($n = 3385$) may shed some light to a few potential reasons [44]. As expected, SLE patients were younger and more often female in comparison with non-SLE patients undergoing PCI in this study. SLE patients were less likely than non-SLE patients to have hyperlipidemia but had a similar prevalence of HTA, DM, and tobacco use. The prevalence of multivessel disease was similar between groups. Initial intervention success (by angiographic definition) was not significantly different between groups. However, at 1 year, SLE patients were more likely to experience a myocardial infarction (15.6% versus 4.8%, $p = 0.01$) and more often required repeat PCI (31.3% versus 11.8%, $p = 0.009$) than non-SLE patients, even after adjustment for important covariates [44].

Some of the other potential hurdles may include decreased physician awareness of CVD risks in SLE, lack of a quick CVD assessment risk tool for SLE patients that physicians can employ, need for SLE-specific treatment guidelines for CVD risk management, and limited physician time. Further research into dominant mechanisms underlying CVD in SLE, specific interventions targeting physicians, and patients to lower the risk, their efficiency, and effectiveness are required.

Bone Health and Osteoporosis

Patients with SLE tend more commonly to develop vitamin D deficiency. Because of the photosensitivity and sun exposure avoidance, hypovitaminosis D has been estimated to be more prevalent in lupus patients. The vitamin D deficiency prevalence in SLE patients was reported to be as high as 62.81% in a Chinese population study by Gao et al. and severe vitamin D deficiency in up to 34.71% of patients. This can affect not only the immune system but also bone metabolism and bone health in particular.

SLE patients confront a higher risk of developing bone loss, osteoporosis, and subsequent fragility fractures because of the disease itself and glucocorticoids exposure. Osteoporotic fractures may result in significant additional morbidity, including severe pain, disability, and decreased mobility, and in certain cases increased mortality. Approximately 25–75% of patients with SLE have been found to have osteopenia [45, 46], while osteoporosis rate varies significantly in different studies ranging from 1.4% to 68% [47].

The risk of fracture is nearly fivefold among women with SLE, compared to women from the general US population [48]. The duration of corticosteroid use was furthermore associated with a shorter time from SLE diagnoses to fracture [12]. SLE itself is associated with deterioration in bone structure, cortical microstructure, and bone strength [49]. Besides the traditional risk factors including age, low body weight, low body mass index, and postmenopausal status, SLE-related risk factors including chronic inflammation, increased levels of TNF-alpha and RANKL, can affect osteoclast maturation and activity. Sun avoidance and premature gonadal failure, which cause vitamin D deficiency, are some additional risk factors that can be seen as SLE related [50]. Low C4 has been associated with low spine bone mineral density in the Hopkins lupus cohort [51]. Renal failure, lupus anticoagulant, and Raynaud's phenomenon are other potential risk factors [51]. Daily use of glucocorticoids, not the cumulative dose, was associated with an increased risk of vertebral fractures [52]. Studies with SLE patients have demonstrated that for every 36.5 mg of glucocorticoids, the risk of osteoporosis increased 1.9-fold [53]. In addition to glucocorticoids, other therapeutic agents used in SLE management may promote bone loss, such as cyclophosphamide, leading to premature ovarian failure, placing young women with SLE at a higher risk for bone loss, heparin used in SLE patients which may cause bone loss, via binding to serum calcium, and causing secondary hyperparathyroidism.

Avascular necrosis of the bone is another complication that according to "Euro-lupus project" by Cervera et al. [36] has been noted to be among early complications of SLE patients, therefore not strictly related to long-term exposure to corticosteroid therapy but the current steroid dose exposure as well.

Management of bone health in SLE is particularly difficult, lacking extensive data, and given potential side effects of traditional osteoporosis medications during reproductive age. Hormone therapy can improve BMD in postmenopausal women; however, there has been long-standing concern exposing SLE patients to such therapies knowing that estrogen exposure may enhance SLE itself. How to best treat early osteoporosis in younger SLE patients, who have not yet started or completed their plans for family, beyond traditional calcium and vitamin D supplements remains a clinical dilemma for most treating physicians. Surveillance for bone health, dietary intake of calcium and vitamin D, patient education on bone health – especially for those who are or have been on glucocorticoids or are at risk for poor boner health – are pivotal, as are control of disease activity, use of steroid-lowering/ steroid-sparing treatment strategies, and treatment of vitamin D deficiency.

Malignancy

The combination of intrinsic immune system defect and the exposure to cytotoxic medications are associated with a higher incidence of malignancies in SLE patients. Multiple studies have investigated this association. A recent meta-analysis including 15 studies involving 58,077 patients with SLE summarize the risks of overall and site-specific malignancies in patients with SLE [54]. The overall risk of malignancy in SLE is elevated, compared with the general population, slightly higher in the hospital-based cohorts (pooled RR, 1.33; 95% CI 1.14–1.55) compared with the population-based ones (pooled RR, 1.29; 95% CI 1.09–1.53). Males are at a higher risk to develop a cancer than females (pooled RR 2.41; 95% CI, 1.46–3.98 versus 1.62; 95% CI, 1.36–1.94). The most frequently observed malignancies were non-Hodgkin's lymphoma, Hodgkin's lymphoma, leukemia, and laryngeal, lung, liver, vagina/vulvar, and thyroid malignancies (Table 6.1). The risk was higher for hospital-based cohorts probably because patients with a more severe disease were included.

Diffuse large B-cell lymphoma is the most frequent hematologic cancer seen in SLE. Lymphocytes are the cell line responsible for most of the inflammation in this autoimmune disorder suggesting that the chronic inflammatory state may play a role in the development of cancer. In addition, the Epstein-Barr virus (EBV), which is suggested to have a role in the pathophysiology of SLE [55], has been associated with hematologic malignancies as Burkitt lymphoma and Hodgkin diseases [56].

The increase in human papilloma virus (HPV)-associated cancers reported in women with SLE [57] may be explained by the impaired eradication of this virus and the use of immunosuppressive drugs [58]. Although conflicting data have been published regarding the risk of cervical lesions among women with SLE, a recent meta-analysis has shown a pooled odds ratio for the risk of high-grade squamous intraepithelial lesions of 8.66 (95% CI: 3.75–20.00) in SLE patients, compared to healthy women [59]. Interestingly, when this meta-analysis was performed according to the year of the publication of the study, there was a slight increase in the risk in the periods 2001–2011, with stabilization later. Despite no specific screening tests are recommended for SLE patients [60], these results suggest that women with SLE may benefit from HPV vaccines and specific cervical cancer screening.

Lung cancer also has an increased incidence in SLE patients with an overall histologic distribution comparable to the general population [61]. Possible explanations for this increased risk may be genetically shared susceptibility, pulmonary involvement in SLE with alveolitis or fibrosis playing a role in the development of cancer, or a higher tobacco exposure. Currently there is no robust data showing a clear association with either of these.

A reduced risk for breast cancer and endometrial cancer in women [62, 63] and prostate in men [64] has also been noted. Though reason for this association is uncertain, it suggests a complex interaction between the immune and endocrine system and their role in cancer among SLE patients.

Two studies reported mortality from malignancy in SLE patients. The pooled estimates showed no increase in the risk of death (meta-SMR 1.16, 95% CI 0.57–2.35) [2] from malignancy. Another study evaluated the risk of mortality due to malignancy by gender, in an inception cohort of SLE patients, in Southern Sweden, and compared it with the observed frequencies and spectrum of malignancies in the general population [65]. They reported a twofold increase in the risk of death in men (SMR 2.24, 95% CI 0.6–5.7) and a comparable risk to general population in woman (SMR 1.02, 95% CI 0.4–2.1) from malignancy among SLE patients. Despite conflicting results, age, and gender, appropriate cancer screening is encouraged for all SLE patients.

Infections

Regardless of a dramatic change in survival of patients with SLE, from 50% at 4 years in early studies [66] to 80% at 15 years in more recent studies [67, 68], infections remain a common cause of mortality and morbidity. In a recent meta-analysis of published observational studies, SLE patients exhibited a nearly fivefold increase in the risk of death as a result of infection compared to the general population [2].

Although the etiology of SLE is not completely known, infections can induce the onset and exacerbations of the disease in genetically predisposed individuals [69]. In addition, SLE patients are at an increased risk of developing infections as a result of immunosuppression, the disease activity [70], and some of the medications used to treat SLE (e.g., pneumonia in patients with high doses of steroids) [71].

A wide spectrum of infections has been reported in SLE patients, mostly bacterial infections. The incidence of infections may vary from study to study depending on the type of patients studied (outpatients or hospitalized), presence of renal disease, or the treatments they received (high doses of steroids, cytotoxic, or immunosuppressive drugs). The most common types of infections are pneumonia, urinary tract infection, cellulitis, and bacteremia without focus as in the general population and include similar pathogens (Table 6.2). The most frequent bacterial infections are those caused by *Staphylococcus aureus, E. coli, Salmonella*, and *Streptococcal pneumoniae* (Table 6.2). Although most infections reported in SLE patients are minor in general, it has been also reported opportunistic infections.

Infections with *Salmonella* are more common in SLE patients than in the normal population, probably due to splenic dysfunction [78]. There is an increased risk of mortality if salmonella infection is diagnosed concurrently with the onset of lupus or if a SLE patient is reinfected with *Salmonella* [79]. Patients with active disease (especially nephritis) on intensified immunosuppression appear to be most at risk [71].

Tuberculosis (TB) infection in SLE patients occurs especially in endemic areas, where its prevalence ranges from 5% to 30% [80]. In SLE, TB infections are frequently extrapulmonary and have a higher relapse rate [81]. Mycobacterial infection may affect the skin and mimic vasculitis posing a diagnostic challenge in some lupus patients. In a poor response to more aggressive immunosuppressive therapy, an opportunistic infection must be considered, as a skin biopsy may provide the appropriate diagnosis [82].

SLE patients are also at an increased risk for viral infections [73, 75]. In addition, some viruses such as cytomegalovirus (CMV), Epstein-Barr virus (EBV), and parvovirus B19 play a role as environmental agents that trigger the development of the disease [55]. In contrast, SLE has a decreased incidence in HIV-infected population compared to the general population [83].

A number of factors can increase the risk of infection in SLE patients. The risk factors most frequently associated with infections are prolonged therapy with immunosuppressives, use of high doses of corticosteroids and cyclophosphamide, renal and pulmonary involvement, low complement, and high disease activity.

The first study carefully examining risk factors for infection in SLE patients found an overall infection rate ten times greater in SLE compared to RA patients and patients with nephrotic syndrome. The number of infections was higher in patients with a prednisone dose exceeding 20 mg/day and an impaired renal function [84]. Studies by Urowitz [85] and Lee [86] similarly noted the association of infections with corticosteroid therapy and active renal disease. Although the association of azathioprine with an increased incidence of infections was reported in earlier studies [86], this has not been confirmed in more recent ones [80].

Table 6.2 Characteristics, risk factors, and rates of infections in SLE patients according to recent studies

Study	Population	Infection rate	Infection site	Microorganisms	Risk factors
Ruiz-Irastorza et al. [72] Nested case-control study Follow-up (mean) 8.3 years	83 SLE 166 controls	29%	Pneumonia, bacteremia, cellulitis and skin abscess, TBC	*E. coli*, *S. aureus*, *M. tuberculosis*, *S. pneumoniae*	Lung involvement and prednisone dose
Bosch et al. [73] Prospective controlled study Follow-up (mean) 21 months	110 SLE 220 controls	36% versus 22% (RR = 1.63, $p < 0.05$)	Skin and mucous membranes, urinary tract, pulmonary, bacteremia	*E. coli*, *S. aureus*, *Candida*, h. zoster, *Salmonella*	CH50 < 300, prednisone > 20 mg, and cyclophosphamide
Gladman et al. [74] Nested case-control study Follow-up	93 SLE	25.6%	Pulmonary, skin, genitourinary, soft tissue	*Staphylococcus*, h. zoster, *E. coli*, *streptococcus*, HPV	Steroid use ever and immunosuppressives at time of infection
Noel et al. [75] Cohort study Follow-up	87 SLE	40%	Respiratory tract, bacteremia,	*Staphylococcus*, *S. pneumoniae*, *Salmonella*, h. zoster	Cumulative dose of corticosteroids, cyclophosphamide, flares, and glomerulonephritis
Zonana-Nacach et al. [76] Prospective study Follow-up (mean) 22 months	200 SLE (outpatients)	32%	Urinary, skin, systemic, vaginal	*Bacillus* gram negative, fungi, and coccus gram positive	SLEDAI score ≥ 4, renal activity, prednisone dose, and cyclophosphamide
Suh et al. [77] Retrospective case-control Follow-up	173 SLE	69% 16.9% patient-years of follow-up	Urinary tract, bacteremia, and pneumonia	*E. coli*, *S. aureus*, *Salmonella*, and h. zoster	Cumulative prednisone dose, higher SLEDAI, renal involvement, CRP

Infection rate = (# infection/population at risk) × 100
Abbreviations: *RR* relative risk, *HPV* human papillomavirus

Some studies have found an association between disease activity and increased incidence of infections [70, 76], which may have important clinical considerations. Infections are difficult to assess in SLE patients because some manifestations of infections may be similar to SLE itself. In addition, infections not only may mimic a flare but also may precipitate one causing diagnostic and management challenges. While treatment of disease flare may require escalation of immunosuppressives, the presence of infections may necessitate discontinuation, albeit temporarily, of immunosuppression and use of antibiotics. Some authors have described how high CRP (>50 mg/l) may be of help to differentiate infection from disease activity in SLE patients with fever [77, 87, 88].

With the use of immunosuppressive medications, SLE patients may develop progressive multifocal leukoencephalopathy associated with JC virus, a papovavirus [89]. In addition, SLE patients receiving B-cell-targeted therapy may also experience herpes zoster (HZ) infection. Medications associated with greater HZ risk in patients with SLE include corticosteroids, hydroxychloroquine, cyclophosphamide, azathioprine, methotrexate, and mycophenolate mofetil [90]. Combination immunosuppressive therapy was commonly seen in patients with SLE and was associated with greatly increased HZ risk. For oral corticosteroids and hydroxychloroquine, the risk of HZ was strongly dependent on the medication dose. HZ may also be seen with biologic use such as rituximab.

HPV infection may occur in patients on immunosuppressive medications, as in SLE. This has been well reported from organ transplant literature. Odds ratio for genital HPV infection in women with SLE was 7.2 (95% CI, 2.9–17.8; $p = 0.0001$) [91]. In this study, no association between HPV prevalence and use of immunosuppressive medications was found. In another study, HPV+ viral types were identified using PCR: HPV+ was observed in 14.7% of SLE and 30.8% of controls (87). High-risk HPV types were observed in 11.7% of women with SLE and in 26% of the controls. High-risk viral types 58, 35, and 18 were the most frequently identified in SLE. Herein an association was observed between methotrexate utilization, longer duration of therapy with prednisone, and HPV+ in SLE [92]. In yet another study, SLE patients were found to have a threefold increase in HPV infection, mostly genotypes 53, 58, 45, 66, 6, 84, 83, and 61, as compared with controls, who presented types 6, 18, and 61 more frequently [93]. The higher rate of HPV infection was associated with immunosuppressive therapy. This study provides evidence that SLE patients have a high prevalence of HPV infection, which is even higher with the use of immunosuppressive, a condition that might necessitate a more frequent cervical cancer screening program for these women. The HPV vaccine is well tolerated and reasonably effective in patients with stable SLE and does not induce an increase in lupus activity or flares [94]; however, effectiveness of vaccination in primary prevention of HPV or cervical dysplasia in SLE is not yet established.

In summary, most of the studies have clearly shown that infection is an independent risk factor for death in SLE patients. Because of the independent role of immunosuppressive agents, particularly higher doses of corticosteroids and cyclophosphamide, in the occurrence of infection during SLE and their independent effect on the long-term outcomes, it is important to identify patients who should be targeted for this treatment. To avoid unacceptably high morbidity and mortality, careful follow-up of patients with SLE is recommended, as infection, mainly of bacterial origin, can occur at any time during evolution of the disease and can be related to SLE disease activity.

Fibromyalgia

Fibromyalgia (FM) is a chronic pain syndrome more common in women that often accompanies SLE posing a diagnostic dilemma [95]. The prevalence of FM in SLE patients varies from 22% to 25% in different studies [96, 97] compared to 1–4% in the general population [98]. When no formal criteria are applied and the diagnosis of FM is made by the treating physician, the prevalence can be even higher, around 32% [99]. Caucasian SLE patients have been found to be at higher risk for developing FM compared to African-American and Hispanic ethnic groups in addition to the presence of anxiety or affective disorders [100].

Although the presence of FM is not related to disease activity according to the SLE Disease Activity Index (SLEDAI), it affects the quality of life of these patients as a result of the widespread musculoskeletal pain and pain hypersensitivity [101]. In addition, the clinical features of FM may contribute to a misinterpretation of SLE activity. Both diseases share many symptoms as musculoskeletal pain, fatigue, stiffness, sleep, and cognitive dysfunction. Distinguishing both entities can be especially difficult when a patient with FM have a positive antinuclear antibody (ANA). This test although sensitive is not specific for SLE. A review of 422 positive ANA test at high titers showed that a significant proportion of patients had no connective tissue disorder at the time of testing [102].

In terms of additional comorbidity factors, depression has been highly associated in patients with SLE and FM, but others also presented are autoimmune thyroiditis, arterial hypertension, and dyslipidemia [103].

SLE with FM leads to poorer self-reported health assessments [99] even in early stages of the disease [104], probably related to the mentally, socially, and physically impairing condition a result of FM. Because SLE remains a challenging disease and the prevalence of FM might arise, physicians need to be alert in recognizing the onset of FM when depression and widespread pain coexist. Multidisciplinary approach involving patient education, psychologist, primary care physician, physical therapist, and a pain specialist may be beneficial.

Conclusion

Patients with SLE have experienced a better survival over the last few decades. However, they still present an increased risk of premature mortality compared with the general population, which highlight the importance of a better management of associated comorbidity. Although cardiovascular mortality has decreased in the general population, this improvement has not been seen in SLE patients. For this reason, it has been proposed that SLE should be treated as a "CVD equivalent" such as DM is, with lower lipid goals, more intense aspiring use and potentially more aggressive monitoring. For example, although guidelines recommend a target blood pressure of less than 130/80 mmHg for patients with comorbidities as DM or chronic kidney disease, SLE experts recommend a lower target in SLE patients (120/80 mmHg).

Promotion of preventive measures such as smoking cessation, a low-calorie diet, and aerobic exercise to lose weight should be part of the management of patients with SLE. In addition, they should be encouraged to follow regular screening programs for cervical and breast cancer. The higher prevalence of uterine cervix carcinoma and human papillomavirus infection in lupus patients in comparison with the general population supports an early immunization in teenage patients with lupus. Meticulous exclusion of infections is mandatory, because the potential of infections to masquerade an exacerbation of underlying disease or the catastrophic results if immunosuppression is used when concomitant infection. All patients should be immunized against *Streptococcus pneumoniae* given the incidence and severity of the infections caused by this pathogen. Many patients with SLE suffer from GC-induced osteoporosis, which should prevented by calcium and vitamin D3 supplements and, if necessary, by bisphosphonates. Symptoms affecting quality of life, such as fatigue and fibromyalgia, also need to be addressed with new approaches or therapeutic options.

References

1. Hersh AO, Trupin L, Yazdany J, et al. Childhood-onset disease as a predictor of mortality in an adult cohort of patients with systemic lupus erythematosus. Arthritis Care Res (Hoboken). 2010;62(8):1152–9.
2. Yurkovich M, Vostretsova K, Chen W, Avina-Zubieta JA. Overall and cause-specific mortality in patients with systemic lupus erythematosus: a meta-analysis of observational studies. Arthritis Care Res (Hoboken). 2014;66(4):608–16.
3. Yang Y, Thumboo J, Earnest A, Yong SL, Fong KY. The effect of comorbidity on hospital mortality in patients with SLE from an Asian tertiary hospital. Lupus. 2014;23(7):714–20.
4. Rees F, Doherty M, Grainge M, Lanyon P, Davenport G, Zhang W. Burden of comorbidity in systemic lupus erythematosus in the UK, 1999-2012. Arthritis Care Res (Hoboken). 2016;68(6):819–27.
5. Kang SC, Hwang SJ, Chang YS, Chou CT, Tsai CY. Characteristics of comorbidities and costs among patients who died from systemic lupus erythematosus in Taiwan. Arch Med Sci. 2012;8(4):690–6.
6. Wolfe F, Michaud K, Li T, Katz RS. Chronic conditions and health problems in rheumatic diseases: comparisons with rheumatoid arthritis, noninflammatory rheumatic disorders, systemic lupus erythematosus, and fibromyalgia. J Rheumatol. 2010;37(2):305–15.
7. Chan PC, Yu CH, Yeh KW, Horng JT, Huang JL. Comorbidities of pediatric systemic lupus erythematosus: a 6-year nationwide population-based study. J Microbiol Immunol Infect. 2016;49(2):257–63.

8. Attar SM, Siddiqui AM. Vitamin d deficiency in patients with systemic lupus erythematosus. Oman Med J. 2013;28(1):42–7.
9. Magder LS, Petri M. Incidence of and risk factors for adverse cardiovascular events among patients with systemic lupus erythematosus. Am J Epidemiol. 2012;176(8):708–19.
10. Mok CC, Ho LY, To CH. Annual incidence and standardized incidence ratio of cerebrovascular accidents in patients with systemic lupus erythematosus. Scand J Rheumatol. 2009;38(5):362–8.
11. Bernatsky S, Ramsey-Goldman R, Labrecque J, et al. Cancer risk in systemic lupus an updated international multi-centre cohort study. J Autoimmun. 2013;42:130–5.
12. Ramsey-Goldman R, Dunn JE, Huang CF, et al. Frequency of fractures in women with systemic lupus erythematosus: comparison with United States population data. Arthritis Rheum. 1999;42(5):882–90.
13. Petri M, Orbai AM, Alarcon GS, et al. Derivation and validation of the systemic lupus international collaborating clinics classification criteria for systemic lupus erythematosus. Arthritis Rheum. 2012;64(8):2677–86.
14. Manzi S, Meilahn EN, Rairie JE, et al. Age-specific incidence rates of myocardial infarction and angina in women with systemic lupus erythematosus: comparison with the Framingham study. Am J Epidemiol. 1997;145(5):408–15.
15. Petri M, Spence D, Bone LR, Hochberg MC. Coronary artery disease risk factors in the Johns Hopkins lupus cohort: prevalence, recognition by patients, and preventive practices. Medicine. 1992;71(5):291–302.
16. Tektonidou MG, Wang Z, Ward MM. Trends in hospitalizations due to acute coronary syndromes and stroke in patients with systemic lupus erythematosus, 1996 to 2012. Arthritis & rheumatology. 2016;68(11):2680–5.
17. McMahon M, Skaggs B. Pathogenesis and treatment of atherosclerosis in lupus. Rheum Dis Clin N Am. 2014;40(3):475–95, viii.
18. Urowitz MB, Ibanez D, Su J, Gladman DD. Modified Framingham risk factor score for systemic lupus erythematosus. J Rheumatol. 2016;43(5):875–9.
19. Rho YH, Chung CP, Oeser A, et al. Novel cardiovascular risk factors in premature coronary atherosclerosis associated with systemic lupus erythematosus. J Rheumatol. 2008;35(9):1789–94.
20. Toloza SM, Uribe AG, McGwin G Jr, et al. Systemic lupus erythematosus in a multiethnic US cohort (LUMINA). XXIII. Baseline predictors of vascular events. Arthritis Rheum. 2004;50(12):3947–57.
21. Ghaussy NO, Sibbitt W Jr, Bankhurst AD, Qualls CR. Cigarette smoking and disease activity in systemic lupus erythematosus. J Rheumatol. 2003;30(6):1215–21.
22. Katz P, Gregorich S, Yazdany J, et al. Obesity and its measurement in a community-based sample of women with systemic lupus erythematosus. Arthritis Care Res (Hoboken). 2011;63(2):261–8.
23. Petri M, Lakatta C, Magder L, Goldman D. Effect of prednisone and hydroxychloroquine on coronary artery disease risk factors in systemic lupus erythematosus: a longitudinal data analysis. Am J Med. 1994;96(3):254–9.
24. Sacre K, Escoubet B, Zennaro MC, Chauveheid MP, Gayat E, Papo T. Overweight is a major contributor to atherosclerosis in systemic lupus erythematosus patients at apparent low risk for cardiovascular disease: a cross-sectional controlled study. Medicine. 2015;94(48):e2177.
25. Tselios K, Koumaras C, Gladman DD, Urowitz MB. Dyslipidemia in systemic lupus erythematosus: just another comorbidity? Semin Arthritis Rheum. 2016;45(5):604–10.
26. Marsillach J, Becker JO, Vaisar T, et al. Paraoxonase-3 is depleted from the high-density lipoproteins of autoimmune disease patients with subclinical atherosclerosis. J Proteome Res. 2015;14(5):2046–54.
27. Rahman P, Gladman DD, Urowitz MB, Yuen K, Hallett D, Bruce IN. The cholesterol lowering effect of antimalarial drugs is enhanced in patients with lupus taking corticosteroid drugs. J Rheumatol. 1999;26(2):325–30.

28. Urowitz MB, Gladman DD, Anderson NM, et al. Cardiovascular events prior to or early after diagnosis of systemic lupus erythematosus in the systemic lupus international collaborating clinics cohort. Lupus Sci Med. 2016;3(1):e000143.
29. Gatla N, Annapureddy N, Sequeira W, Jolly M. Posterior reversible encephalopathy syndrome in systemic lupus erythematosus. J Clin Rheumatol Pract Rep Rheum Musculoskelet Dis. 2013;19(6):334–40.
30. Lopez LR, Salazar-Paramo M, Palafox-Sanchez C, Hurley BL, Matsuura E. Garcia-De La Torre I. Oxidized low-density lipoprotein and beta2-glycoprotein I in patients with systemic lupus erythematosus and increased carotid intima-media thickness: implications in autoimmune-mediated atherosclerosis. Lupus. 2006;15(2):80–6.
31. Fernandez-Nebro A, Rua-Figueroa I, Lopez-Longo FJ, et al. Cardiovascular events in systemic lupus erythematosus: a Nationwide study in Spain from the RELESSER registry. Medicine. 2015;94(29):e1183.
32. Lertratanakul A, Wu P, Dyer A, et al. 25-hydroxyvitamin D and cardiovascular disease in patients with systemic lupus erythematosus: data from a large international inception cohort. Arthritis Care Res (Hoboken). 2014;66(8):1167–76.
33. Reynolds JA, Haque S, Berry JL, et al. 25-Hydroxyvitamin D deficiency is associated with increased aortic stiffness in patients with systemic lupus erythematosus. Rheumatology (Oxford). 2012;51(3):544–51.
34. Reynolds JA, Rosenberg AZ, Smith CK, et al. Vitamin D deficiency is associated with endothelial dysfunction and increases type-1 interferon Gene expression in a murine model of SLE. Arthritis & rheumatology. 2016;68(12):2929–35.
35. Holmqvist M, Simard JF, Asplund K, Arkema EV. Stroke in systemic lupus erythematosus: a meta-analysis of population-based cohort studies. RMD Open. 2015;1(1):e000168.
36. Cervera R, Khamashta MA, Font J, et al. Morbidity and mortality in systemic lupus erythematosus during a 10-year period: a comparison of early and late manifestations in a cohort of 1,000 patients. Medicine. 2003;82(5):299–308.
37. Kao AH, McBurney CA, Sattar A, et al. Relation of platelet C4d with all-cause mortality and ischemic stroke in patients with systemic lupus erythematosus. Transl Stroke Res. 2014;5(4):510–8.
38. June RR, Scalzi LV. Peripheral vascular disease in systemic lupus patients. J Clin Rheumatol Pract Rep Rheum Musculoskelet Dis. 2013;19(7):367–72.
39. Chuang YW, Yu MC, Lin CL, Yu TM, Shu KH, Kao CH. Risk of peripheral arterial occlusive disease in patients with systemic lupus erythematosus: a Nationwide population-based cohort study. Medicine. 2015;94(46):e2121.
40. Huang C, Li M, Liu Y, et al. Baseline characteristics and risk factors of pulmonary arterial hypertension in systemic lupus erythematosus patients. Medicine. 2016;95(10):e2761.
41. Li M, Wang Q, Zhao J, et al. Chinese SLE treatment and research group (CSTAR) registry: II. Prevalence and risk factors of pulmonary arterial hypertension in Chinese patients with systemic lupus erythematosus. Lupus. 2014;23(10):1085–91.
42. Kommireddy S, Bhyravavajhala S, Kurimeti K, et al. Pulmonary arterial hypertension in systemic lupus erythematosus may benefit by addition of immunosuppression to vasodilator therapy: an observational study. Rheumatology (Oxford). 2015;54(9):1673–9.
43. Trends in deaths from systemic lupus erythematosus – United States, 1979–1998. 2002. http://www.cdc.gov/mmwr/PDF/wk/mm5117.pdf.
44. Maksimowicz-McKinnon K, Selzer F, Manzi S, et al. Poor 1-year outcomes after percutaneous coronary interventions in systemic lupus erythematosus: report from the National Heart, Lung, and Blood Institute dynamic registry. Circ Cardiovasc Interv. 2008;1(3):201–8.
45. Kalla AA, Fataar AB, Jessop SJ, Bewerunge L. Loss of trabecular bone mineral density in systemic lupus erythematosus. Arthritis Rheum. 1993;36(12):1726–34.
46. Mok CC, Mak A, Ma KM. Bone mineral density in postmenopausal Chinese patients with systemic lupus erythematosus. Lupus. 2005;14(2):106–12.

47. Boyanov M, Robeva R, Popivanov P. Bone mineral density changes in women with systemic lupus erythematosus. Clin Rheumatol. 2003;22(4–5):318–23.
48. Panopalis P, Yazdany J. Bone health in systemic lupus erythematosus. Curr Rheumatol Rep. 2009;11(3):177–84.
49. Bichile T, Petri M. Prevention and management of co-morbidities in SLE. Presse Med. 2014;43(6 Pt 2):e187–95.
50. Lee C, Almagor O, Dunlop DD, Manzi S, Spies S, Ramsey-Goldman R. Self-reported fractures and associated factors in women with systemic lupus erythematosus. J Rheumatol. 2007;34(10):2018–23.
51. Fangtham M, Petri M. 2013 update: Hopkins lupus cohort. Curr Rheumatol Rep. 2013;15(9):360.
52. Van Staa TP, Laan RF, Barton IP, Cohen S, Reid DM, Cooper C. Bone density threshold and other predictors of vertebral fracture in patients receiving oral glucocorticoid therapy. Arthritis Rheum. 2003;48(11):3224–9.
53. Zonana-Nacach A, Barr SG, Magder LS, Petri M. Damage in systemic lupus erythematosus and its association with corticosteroids. Arthritis Rheum. 2000;43(8):1801–8.
54. Cao L, Tong H, Xu G, et al. Systemic lupus erythematous and malignancy risk: a meta-analysis. PLoS One. 2015;10(4):e0122964.
55. Rigante D, Esposito S. Infections and systemic lupus erythematosus: binding or sparring partners? Int J Mol Sci. 2015;16(8):17331–43.
56. Pattle SB, Farrell PJ. The role of Epstein-Barr virus in cancer. Expert Opin Biol Ther. 2006;6(11):1193–205.
57. Dreyer L, Faurschou M, Mogensen M, Jacobsen S. High incidence of potentially virus-induced malignancies in systemic lupus erythematosus: a long-term followup study in a Danish cohort. Arthritis Rheum. 2011;63(10):3032–7.
58. Bernatsky S, Joseph L, Boivin JF, et al. The relationship between cancer and medication exposures in systemic lupus erythaematosus: a case-cohort study. Ann Rheum Dis. 2008;67(1):74–9.
59. Zard E, Arnaud L, Mathian A, et al. Increased risk of high grade cervical squamous intraepithelial lesions in systemic lupus erythematosus: a meta-analysis of the literature. Autoimmun Rev. 2014;13(7):730–5.
60. Tessier-Cloutier B, Clarke AE, Ramsey-Goldman R, Gordon C, Hansen JE, Bernatsky S. Systemic lupus erythematosus and malignancies: a review article. Rheum Dis Clin N Am. 2014;40(3):497–506, viii.
61. Bin J, Bernatsky S, Gordon C, et al. Lung cancer in systemic lupus erythematosus. Lung Cancer. 2007;56(3):303–6.
62. Bernatsky S, Boivin JF, Joseph L, et al. Mortality in systemic lupus erythematosus. Arthritis Rheum. 2006;54(8):2550–7.
63. Bernatsky S, Ramsey-Goldman R, Foulkes WD, Gordon C, Clarke AE. Breast, ovarian and endometrial malignancies in systemic lupus erythematosus: a meta-analysis. Br J Cancer. 2011;104(9):1478–81.
64. Bernatsky S, Ramsey-Goldman R, Gordon C, Clarke AE. Prostate cancer in systemic lupus erythematosus. International journal of cancer. Journal international du cancer. 2011;129(12):2966–9.
65. Nived O, Bengtsson A, Jonsen A, Sturfelt G, Olsson H. Malignancies during follow-up in an epidemiologically defined systemic lupus erythematosus inception cohort in southern Sweden. Lupus. 2001;10(7):500–4.
66. Merrell M, Shulman LE. Determination of prognosis in chronic disease, illustrated by systemic lupus erythematosus. J Chronic Dis. 1955;1(1):12–32.
67. Reveille JD, Bartolucci A, Alarcon GS. Prognosis in systemic lupus erythematosus. Negative impact of increasing age at onset, black race, and thrombocytopenia, as well as causes of death. Arthritis Rheum. 1990;33(1):37–48.

68. Doria A, Iaccarino L, Ghirardello A, et al. Long-term prognosis and causes of death in systemic lupus erythematosus. Am J Med. 2006;119(8):700–6.
69. Rigante D, Mazzoni MB, Esposito S. The cryptic interplay between systemic lupus erythematosus and infections. Autoimmun Rev. 2014;13(2):96–102.
70. Duffy KN, Duffy CM, Gladman DD. Infection and disease activity in systemic lupus erythematosus: a review of hospitalized patients. J Rheumatol. 1991;18(8):1180–4.
71. Kang I, Park SH. Infectious complications in SLE after immunosuppressive therapies. Curr Opin Rheumatol. 2003;15(5):528–34.
72. Ruiz-Irastorza G, Olivares N, Ruiz-Arruza I, Martinez-Berriotxoa A, Egurbide MV, Aguirre C. Predictors of major infections in systemic lupus erythematosus. Arthritis Res Ther. 2009;11(4):R109.
73. Bosch X, Guilabert A, Pallares L, et al. Infections in systemic lupus erythematosus: a prospective and controlled study of 110 patients. Lupus. 2006;15(9):584–9.
74. Gladman DD, Hussain F, Ibanez D, Urowitz MB. The nature and outcome of infection in systemic lupus erythematosus. Lupus. 2002;11(4):234–9.
75. Noel V, Lortholary O, Casassus P, et al. Risk factors and prognostic influence of infection in a single cohort of 87 adults with systemic lupus erythematosus. Ann Rheum Dis. 2001;60(12):1141–4.
76. Zonana-Nacach A, Camargo-Coronel A, Yanez P, Sanchez L, Jimenez-Balderas FJ, Fraga A. Infections in outpatients with systemic lupus erythematosus: a prospective study. Lupus. 2001;10(7):505–10.
77. Suh CH, Jeong YS, Park HC, et al. Risk factors for infection and role of C-reactive protein in Korean patients with systemic lupus erythematosus. Clin Exp Rheumatol. 2001;19(2):191–4.
78. Petri M. Infection in systemic lupus erythematosus. Rheum Dis Clin N Am. 1998;24(2):423–56.
79. Tsao CH, Chen CY, Ou LS, Huang JL. Risk factors of mortality for salmonella infection in systemic lupus erythematosus. J Rheumatol. 2002;29(6):1214–8.
80. Fessler BJ. Infectious diseases in systemic lupus erythematosus: risk factors, management and prophylaxis. Best Pract Res Clin Rheumatol. 2002;16(2):281–91.
81. Yun JE, Lee SW, Kim TH, et al. The incidence and clinical characteristics of mycobacterium tuberculosis infection among systemic lupus erythematosus and rheumatoid arthritis patients in Korea. Clin Exp Rheumatol. 2002;20(2):127–32.
82. Gordon MM, Wilson HE, Duthie FR, Jones B, Field M. When typical is atypical: mycobacterial infection mimicking cutaneous vasculitis. Rheumatology (Oxford). 2002;41(6):685–90.
83. Barthel HR, Wallace DJ. False-positive human immunodeficiency virus testing in patients with lupus erythematosus. Semin Arthritis Rheum. 1993;23(1):1–7.
84. Staples PJ, Gerding DN, Decker JL, Gordon RS Jr. Incidence of infection in systemic lupus erythematosus. Arthritis Rheum. 1974;17(1):1–10.
85. Urowitz MB, Bookman AA, Koehler BE, Gordon DA, Smythe HA, Ogryzlo MA. The bimodal mortality pattern of systemic lupus erythematosus. Am J Med. 1976;60(2):221–5.
86. Lee P, Urowitz MB, Bookman AA, et al. Systemic lupus erythematosus. A review of 110 cases with reference to nephritis, the nervous system, infections, aseptic necrosis and prognosis. Q J Med. 1977;46(181):1–32.
87. Lim E, Koh WH, Loh SF, Lam MS, Howe HS. Non-thyphoidal salmonellosis in patients with systemic lupus erythematosus. A study of fifty patients and a review of the literature. Lupus. 2001;10(2):87–92.
88. Becker GJ, Waldburger M, Hughes GR, Pepys MB. Value of serum C-reactive protein measurement in the investigation of fever in systemic lupus erythematosus. Ann Rheum Dis. 1980;39(1):50–2.
89. Govindappa V, Hicks S, Wichter M, Jolly M. Progressive multifocal leukoencephalopathy in systemic lupus erythematosus. Arthritis Rheum. 2007;57(2):352–4.
90. Hu SC, Yen FL, Wang TN, Lin YC, Lin CL, Chen GS. Immunosuppressive medication use and risk of herpes zoster (HZ) in patients with systemic lupus erythematosus (SLE): a nationwide case-control study. J Am Acad Dermatol. 2016;75(1):49–58.

91. Lyrio LD, Grassi MF, Santana IU, et al. Prevalence of cervical human papillomavirus infection in women with systemic lupus erythematosus. Rheumatol Int. 2013;33(2):335–40.
92. Rojo-Contreras W, Olivas-Flores EM, Gamez-Nava JI, et al. Cervical human papillomavirus infection in Mexican women with systemic lupus erythematosus or rheumatoid arthritis. Lupus. 2012;21(4):365–72.
93. Klumb EM, Pinto AC, Jesus GR, et al. Are women with lupus at higher risk of HPV infection? Lupus. 2010;19(13):1485–91.
94. Mok CC, Ho LY, Fong LS, To CH. Immunogenicity and safety of a quadrivalent human papillomavirus vaccine in patients with systemic lupus erythematosus: a case-control study. Ann Rheum Dis. 2013;72(5):659–64.
95. Bennett R. The concurrence of lupus and fibromyalgia: implications for diagnosis and management. Lupus. 1997;6(6):494–9.
96. Morand EF, Miller MH, Whittingham S, Littlejohn GO. Fibromyalgia syndrome and disease activity in systemic lupus erythematosus. Lupus. 1994;3(3):187–91.
97. Wallace DJ, Schwartz E, Chi-Lin H, Peter JB. The 'rule out lupus' rheumatology consultation: clinical outcomes and perspectives. J Clin Rheumatol Pract Rep Rheum Musculoskelet Dis. 1995;1(3):158–64.
98. Wolfe F, Ross K, Anderson J, Russell IJ, Hebert L. The prevalence and characteristics of fibromyalgia in the general population. Arthritis Rheum. 1995;38(1):19–28.
99. Askanase AD, Castrejon I, Pincus T. Quantitative data for care of patients with systemic lupus erythematosus in usual clinical settings: a patient multidimensional health assessment questionnaire and physician estimate of noninflammatory symptoms. J Rheumatol. 2011;38(7):1309–16.
100. Friedman AW, Tewi MB, Ahn C, et al. Systemic lupus erythematosus in three ethnic groups: XV. Prevalence and correlates of fibromyalgia. Lupus. 2003;12(4):274–9.
101. Gladman DD, Urowitz MB, Gough J, MacKinnon A. Fibromyalgia is a major contributor to quality of life in lupus. J Rheumatol. 1997;24(11):2145–8.
102. Vaile JH, Dyke L, Kherani R, Johnston C, Higgins T, Russell AS. Is high titre ANA specific for connective tissue disease? Clin Exp Rheumatol. 2000;18(4):433–8.
103. Torrente-Segarra V, Salman-Monte TC, Rua-Figueroa I, et al. Fibromyalgia prevalence and related factors in a large registry of patients with systemic lupus erythematosus. Clin Exp Rheumatol. 2016;34(2 Suppl 96):S40–7.
104. Alarcon GS, McGwin G Jr, Uribe A, et al. Systemic lupus erythematosus in a multiethnic lupus cohort (LUMINA). XVII. Predictors of self-reported health-related quality of life early in the disease course. Arthritis Rheum. 2004;51(3):465–74.

Chapter 7
Systemic Sclerosis

Frank A. Wollheim

Let me start with a case history. In 1935 a boy aged 3 attended a marionette theatre for children. Eleven days later he developed high fever and this soon developed into typical measles. Ten days after recovering, the boy developed a sore throat, new fever, and a rash, easily diagnosed as scarlet fever. Since the parents were physicians, the boy was isolated not in an institution, but at home. Three weeks later the young patient developed bilateral otitis media, a condition which carried a serious risk for permanent hearing loss but also could spread to meninges and brain. The boy was saved these complications by a mastoidectomy which drained the pus to the outside and allowed healing with no sequel.

The reader will agree that this patient suffered from three distinct diseases and that one was causing the second which was leading to the third. But clearly one should not call it comorbidity, although an epidemiologic study would have suggested it. A systemic disease like systemic sclerosis (SSc) typically involves pathology in almost all organs of the body resulting in highly heterogeneous disease patterns. When classifying pathology, there is a tremendous semantic problem to distinguish between true *comorbidity, disease manifestation, complication of the disease, and just chance co-occurrence.*

The problem in SSc is well illustrated by a mortality study from our institution (Table 7.1) [1]. A series of 249 patients were followed for at least 10 years. Of the 49 deaths, only 15 could definitely be classified as caused by SSc and 10 definitely as having non-SSc cause. The remaining 24 could only be classified as "possibly" or "probably" disease related. These authors are in good company: in 1991 Alan Silman wrote "Mortality from any disease reflects the summated risk of death as a direct consequence of that disease plus the risks (excess or not) of death from an apparently unrelated cause. The problem of defining a 'related' cause is a real one and the distinction is not always clear" [2]. In other words, comorbidity should be distinguished both from disease manifestation and coincidence which is a special

F.A. Wollheim (✉)
Institute of Clinical Sciences Lund, Rheumatology, Lund University, Lund, Sweden

Y. El Miedany (ed.), *Comorbidity in Rheumatic Diseases*,
DOI 10.1007/978-3-319-59963-2_7

Table 7.1 Causes of death in relation to SSc in 49 patients

Cause of death		Relation with SSc			lSSc/dSSc
		Definite	Probable	Possible	None
Pulmonary disease	10				7/3
Renal disease	1				0/1
Cardiovascular	1	1	4	4	1/9
Gastrointestinal	3	1			4/0
Cancer			7	5	9/3
Infection		7	1	1	2/7
Suicide			2		1/1
Other		1			1/0
lSSc/dSSc	10/5	4/6	8/6	3/7	25/24

From Hesselstrand et al. [1] with permission

challenge in the rare multisystem condition named SSc, where a general vascular dysfunction is a central feature of pathogenesis [3].

Access of comorbidity and its consequence requires ideally prospective studies of population-based well-characterised patient cohorts or population-based material. This is expensive and involves laborious hospital chart work as well as availability of reliable registers. A questionnaire-based instrument was developed [4]. Unfortunately this instrument has been shown to be unreliable [5].

Neither the recent 10th edition of Kelley and Firestein 2000+ page Textbook of Rheumatology nor the multi-authored book "Scleroderma" [6, 7] has separate chapters on comorbidity. Nevertheless, this topic is of interest since associations could contribute to understanding of the pathogenesis of the conditions and also give a warning signal to the clinician to scrutinise some patients for potential malignancy.

Malignancy

The first report of malignancy in SSc may be that of three cases with pulmonary involvement, which at autopsy in addition to fibrosis had alveolar cell carcinoma [8]. The literature since then abounds with papers on cancer risk in various organs, most often the lung and breast (Table 7.2). Many are case reports or cohort studies with or without defined background populations. A Japanese literature search identified almost 2000 publications on the topic. However, the authors could only find six population-based studies published between 1995 and 2012 from Sweden, Scotland, Australia, the USA, Denmark, and Taiwan. 4/6 found a significantly increased standardised incidence ratio, SIR [9]. An exception was a Detroit-based study [10]. The authors commented that their negative result could be explained by a high background incidence of malignancy in the city. The most recent and largest studies from Denmark and Taiwan, respectively [11, 12], based on over 2000 patients each, found an SIR of 1.4 and 1.6, respectively. The pooled SIRs were higher among male patients in both studies. Five of the studies reported SIR of 3.18

Table 7.2 SIRs from six population-based studies of malignancy in SSc

	Total		Men		Women	
Organ	No. of studies	Pooled SIR (95% CI)	No. of studies	Pooled SIR (95% CI)	No. of studies	Pooled SIR (95% CI)
All cancers	6	1.41 (1.18–1.68)*	6	1.85 (1.49–2.31)*	6	1.33 (1.18–1.49)*
Lung	6	3.18 (2.09–4.85)*	5	4.40 (2.73–7.09)*	5	2.73 (1.70–4.39)*
Breast	5	1.10 (0.85–1.42)	–	–	5	1.10 (0.85–1.42)
Prostate	3	1.62 (0.75–3.47)	3	1.62 (0.75–3.47)	–	–
Bladder	2	2.00 (1.06–3.77)*	2	2.51 (0.19–32.5)	2	2.80 (1.36–5.76)*
Hematologic	4	2.57 (1.79–3.68)*	3	3.76 (1.72–8.21)*	4	2.55 (1.24–5.23)*
Non-Hodgkin's lymphoma	2	2.26 (1.21–4.23)*	–	–	2	2.07 (1.00–4.32)
Leukaemia	2	2.75 (1.32–5.73)*	2	7.37 (3.13–17.34)*	–	–
Gastrointestinal	2	0.61 (0.35–1.08)	–	–	2	0.74 (0.31–1.76)
Liver	2	4.36 (2.00–9.51)*	–	–	2	5.81 (0.68–49.75)
Cervix	3	1.33 (0.78–2.24)	–	–	3	1.33 (0.78–2.24)
Nonmelanoma skin cancer	3	2.14 (0.69–6.65)	2	2.34 (1.25–4.59)*	2	2.45 (0.45–13.45)
Corpus uteri	2	0.88 (0.36–2.12)	–	–	2	0.88 (0.36–2.12)

From Onishi et al. [9] with permission
SIR Standardised incidence ratio, *95% CI* 95% confidence interval
*$P < 0.05$

for lung cancer, three found 1.6 for prostate cancer, two 2.0 for bladder cancer, four 2.57 for hematologic, and two 4.36 for liver cancer. The SIR for breast cancer was not significant:1.1 (CI 0.85–1.42). In general, even in these relatively large studies, the correlations were modest and confidence intervals wide.

Another meta-analysis published on the same year, 2013, analysed 16 reports covering 7000 patients and arrived at similar results with an overall RR of 1.75 and most definite correlation between pulmonary and hematologic malignancy [13].

It should come at no surprise that these large population-based inception cohort studies yielded somewhat different results. The Swedish study [14] although covering 85% of the country's 8.5 million population identified only a total of 29 patients with cancer among men and 40 among women. The strongest correlation was with lung cancer, based on a total of 15 patients, and yet this represented a fivefold increase compared to the general population. To summarise the population-based studies confirmed a modest correlation with lung, prostate, liver, bladder, and hematologic cancers. They also confirm higher risks in male patients.

A large prospective cohort study was performed from an SSc centre in Philadelphia [15]. 769 patients were followed between 1987 and 2002 or at total of 3775 patient years. Half of these well-characterised patients were classified as diffuse and half as limited SSc, indicating the influence of referral bias. 90 malignancies were diagnosed. The overall SIR was calculated to 1.55 by using a national cancer registry. The unexpected findings in this study were 12 cases of tongue cancer and pharyngeal cancers (SIR = 15.9). They also had seven cases of oesophageal cancer (SIR 9.63). This could be consequence of the occurrence of Barrett's oesophagus metaplasia. This association was actually confirmed in a large EUSTAR-based study [16]. Similar findings were made in a population-based Australian study [17]. A recent large single centre paper lists 154 malignancies among 2177 patients, 657 of which were diffuse [18]. Breast cancer was most frequent with 65 cases followed by lung (n = 16), gastrointestinal (n = 17), genitourinary (n = 6), gynaecological (n = 17), skin (n = 6), and haematological (n = 19).

Thus it is safe to conclude that SSc is associated with a significant albeit modest increase of cancer. This could be related to increased susceptibility due to environmental or genetic actors or following tissue damage induced by SSc, or to adverse influences from therapeutic agents used in treatment. The last would only favour malignancy occurring well after onset of SSc. Harmful effects of the malignant condition or therapies used to treat them on the other hand would favour SSc onset after malignancy. Coinciding clustering would indicate some common pathogenic mechanism, e.g. genetic susceptibility. These questions have been the subject of some recent work; the temporal clustering of malignancy around the debut of and the immunology of SSc patients was analysed [19–22]. The initial observation based on six patients with anti-RNA polymerase III (RNAP) was that these patients had a short interval between cancer and onset of SSc in contrast to patients with anti-TOPO1 or anticentromere antibodies [19]. A strong link between anti-RNAP and malignancy in SSc was confirmed in the large British study already cited [18]. Multivariable Cox, logistic, and regression analysis all showed RNAP positivity and age reacted to malignancy ($p < 0.001$). Fourteen percent of anti-RNAP positive patients developed malignancy vs only 6% of anti-TOPO-1 and ACA antibody positive patients. The time to cancer onset was significantly shorter among the anti-RNAP positive patients [21]. These findings prompted closer look at the interval between malignancy onsets in relation to SSc onset. The new study showed that anti-RNAP III positive patients had the shortest interval in time of onset between SSc and cancer and also that SSc often occurred in the months preceding the cancer (Fig. 7.1) [19]. The gap was shorter among the anti-RNAP positive patents [19]. This observation was soon confirmed in an Italian survey [19]. Anecdotal reports that cancer treatment resulted in improvement of SSc has added further support to links between the conditions.

An interesting approach was to analyse the gene coding for RNAP in tumours from SSc patients with or without anti-RNAP. Mutations in the *POLR3A* gene were found in 6/8 positive but in none of eight negative patients' tumours [22]. Mutations of this gene in cancer are rare, and the authors speculate that tumour caused by anti-RNAP III antibodies could be instrumental in the triggering of some cases of SSc. In other words, SSc could be a paraneoplastic condition. A practical implication is that some patients with early SSc should be screened for malignancy [23]. A recent case-control study from Italy showed a higher incidence of papillary thyroid cancer. The six cancer patients in this study all had autoantibodies to thyroid antigens compared to 40% in controls. The authors do not disclose interval between onset of the conditions, and the study needs confirmation [24]. In conclusion, SSc like RA and SLE shows several associations to malignant disease although the links do differ in detail.

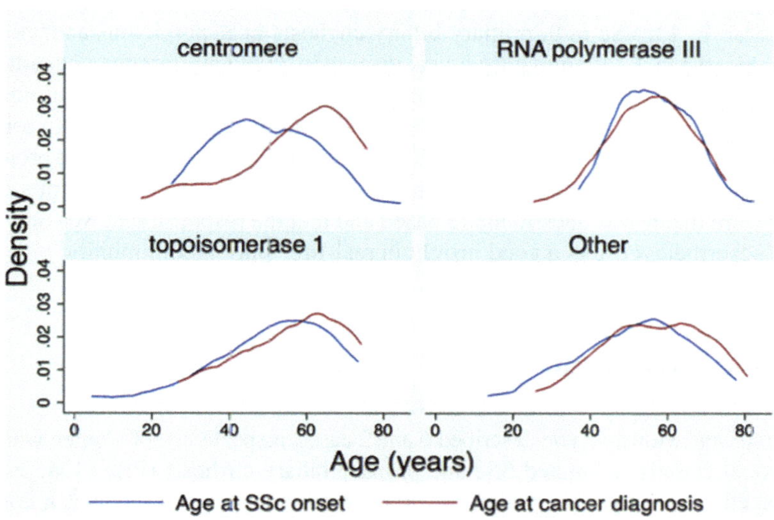

Fig. 7.1 A kernel density function illustrating the distribution of age at cancer n relation to auto-antibody presence (From Shah et al. [21] with permission)

Scleroderma Overlap Syndromes

An extensive literature documents co-occurrence of different systemic autoimmune diseases in SSc patients. A recent representative, single referral centre, found 332 such patients among a total of 1700 SSc patients [25].

The term "SSc overlap syndromes" was used. Myositis was most common (42.8%), followed by RA (32%), Sjögren's syndrome (16.8%), and SLE (8.4%). Anticentromere antibodies were present in 40% of the Sjögren's overlap patients. U1RNP was more common in the SLE overlaps. A prospective French cohort study of 133 patients identified 85 patients (64%) with subjective dry mouth and/or dry eyes, "subjective sicca syndrome". Sixty-one (46%) had abnormal Shirmer test. In all 91 (68%) were considered to have "sicca syndrome" and underwent labial salivary gland biopsy. 50/91 biopsies showed fibrosis, graded as mild, moderate, or severe, and 18/91 had a focus score of at least 1. Therefore, the true incidence of Sjögren's syndrome was 14%. The study explains why several other study reports of up to 80% of Sjögren's are misleading, but they confirm an overrepresentation of true Sjögren's syndrome [26].

Many family studies over decades have shown an overrepresentation of autoimmune diseases among relatives of patients with such diseases. Shared genetic factors in MHC and other susceptibility loci are part of the explanation. A French study looked at this issue among 400 index cases and 313 controls. Data from their 373 and 250 families were collected representing 823 and 318 first-degree relatives [27]. 164 of 373 index cases reported at least one, 35 at least two, and 9 at least 3 first degree relatives with an autoimmune disease. The most common were Sjögren's (72 cases), autoimmune thyroid disease ($n = 49$), and RA ($n = 41$). Vitiligo was found in18, SLE in 13, SSc in 9, primary biliary cirrhosis in 8, pernicious anaemia in 5, celiac disease in 4, inflammatory bowel disease in 3, and autoimmune hepatitis in 3 cases. In all 192 index family and 64 control family members had an autoimmune disease. Significant positive correlations were found for autoimmune thyroid disease and "connective tissue disease" (RA, SLE, and SSc) and in apparent protection for inflammatory bowel disease, when adjusted for family size. The limits of this study were that it was questionnaire based and that the response rate was only 40%, but it nevertheless offers a good insight in real-life "poly-autoimmunity".

Hepatic Involvement

Reynolds and Murray-Lyon described 6 and 2 cases, respectively, of women with what we would classify as limited SSc and primary biliary cirrhosis (PBC) [28, 29]. The combination is sometimes called Reynolds syndrome. They postulated a common immunologic aetiology. We know now that they were on the right track. In a review Kumagi lists a number of comorbidities of PBC [30]. These include other autoimmune conditions like SLE and Sjögren's, but the most common comorbidity was that with "CREST", the limited form of SSc. This was seen in 8% of PBC cases in a population-based study [31]. Among 160 patients with PBC, 12 (8%) has SSc, of which 8 were classified as CREST. Not less than 38/160 had Raynaud's, but it is uncertain how many were related to SSc. Also 40/160 had Sjögren's, but again, the majority may not have been biopsy-confirmed primary Sjögren's [26]. A surprising observation was that patients positive for anti-microsomal antibodies were less likely to express other ANAs. In a more recent study of 80 PBS patients, 5 had "definite" SSc with organ damage, 10 had "early SSc", and another 11 had "isolated SSc features" [32]. This study was done before the new sensitive EULAR/ACR criteria were established. In this study 42/80 patients were ANA positive, 17 had anticentromere antibodies and 15 had anti-CENP-B. Also 15 had scleroderma pattern, Nailfold capillary pattern [32].

An earlier study of T-lymphocytes in patients with the combination of "CREST" SSc and PBS found an overrepresentation of clonally expanded one T-cell receptor beta chain variable region, TCRBV3. The mRNA concentration showed modest increases with PBS alone and SSc without PBS, in sharp contrast to those with both conditions. This clonal expansion was stable over years and may indicate common trigger or pathogenetic pathway [33]. T-cell phenotypic characterisation revealed a defect in the generation and prevalence of regulatory CD8+ cells and also an expansion of the TH17 population [34]. A number of papers have addressed TH17 cell changes in SSc [35–41]. While several studies show increased production of inflammatory cytokines, one also notes a suppression of collagen production, interpreted as a defence against the fibrotic process [39]. A general conclusion is that common immune mechanisms are deranged in SSc and PBC and that both regulatory and effector T cells are involved. However, the detailed pathogenic mechanisms are still not elucidated.

In contrast to PBC, other autoimmune liver diseases, nodular regenerative hyperplasia, chronic active hepatitis, and sclerosing cholangitis have only been reported in case reports or small series, and all these cases most likely represent chance co-occurrence [42–45].

Telocyte loss has been documented in both SSc and liver disease [46–49]. This fascinating newly characterised cell is normally present in the stroma of all organs and interacts with other cells in the tissue. Their long telopods can reach a length of 100 micrometres, but they are only 20–200 nanometres wide. Thus they are only visible by electron microscopy (Fig. 7.2). The podomes form extensive networks and make contact with capillary endothelial cells, fibroblasts, myocytes, macrophages, and stem cells [49]. The aetiology of the telocyte loss in systemic sclerosis and liver fibrosis is unknown, but it is evident that telocytes carry important physiologic functions and that their deficiency could contribute to the comorbidity of scleroderma.

Cardiovascular Disease

Vascular in SSc is manifested by Raynaud's and pathologic nailfold capillaries. Endothelial dysfunction in early SSc was restricted to microcirculation [50]. Digital ulcers are a common complication. The key vascular abnormalities are listed in Table 7.3 [51]. Dysregulation of coagulation and fibrinolysis, platelet activation, and formation of neointima with thickening of vascular walls are some contributors.

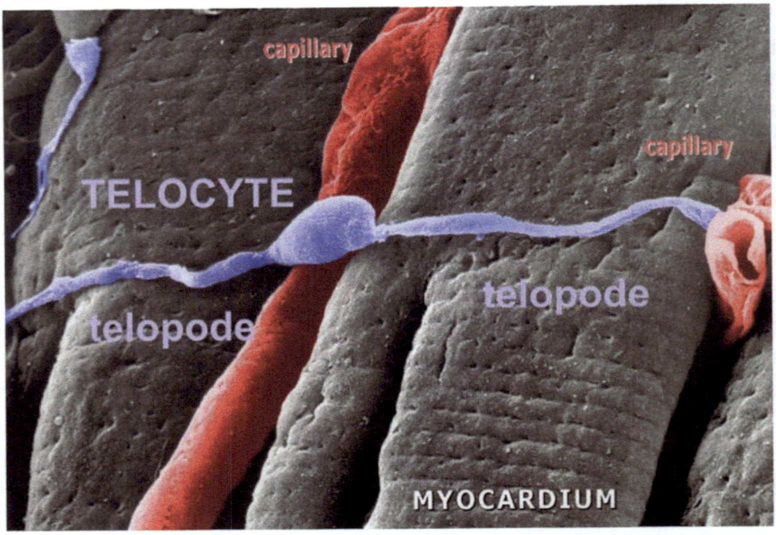

Fig. 7.2 Scanning electron microscopy (SEM) of monkey left ventricular myocardium, showing a typical telocyte with a telopode spanning from a blood vessel (*right*) over myocytes. Another capillary passes under the cell body in the middle (From Wollheim [49] with permission)

Table 7.3 Key vascular abnormalities of SSc

Presence of proliferative vasculopathy with intimal proliferation in peripheral, pulmonary, coronary, and renal arteries in the absence of inflammation is a hallmark feature of scleroderma
Endothelial cell damage is a key and early process. It precedes fibrosis and particularly involves the arterioles
Early detectable changes in the endothelial cells include disappearance of membrane-bound vesicles, vacuolisation of endothelial cell cytoplasm, and gaps between endothelial cells
Defective angiogenesis is an early event in the form of drop out of capillaries and abnormal capillary architecture without a compensatory process
There are conflicting reports regarding the presence and role of circulating endothelial progenitor cells in SSc
There is dysregulation of coagulation and fibrinolysis process
Platelets show enhanced aggregability to various triggers such as type I collagen and adenosine, etc. and are activated throughout the clinical course of SSc
LPA and S1P could potentially contribute to the vasculopathy via endothelial cell activation, neointimal formation, vascular leakiness, increased vasoconstriction, cardiac fibrosis, and hypertension

From Pattanaik et al. [51] with permission

A consequence is hypo-perfusion and tissue anoxia. Morbidity caused by small vessel dysfunction should be regarded as disease manifestations of SSc. Only complications of large vessel abnormality need to be addressed as possible comorbidities. Considering current evidence that atherosclerotic plaque pathophysiology is immune related, it is reasonable to expect an increased prevalence of myocardial infarction, MI, and stroke in patients with chronic autoimmune diseases. Increased risk has been well documented in RA and SLE. An epidemiologic study based on UK primary care data including patients from 1986 to 2011 identified 865 cases of SSc without previous MI or stroke. During a mean follow-up time of 5 years, 20 cases of MI and 22 of stroke occurred. This was significantly more than in the controls with a hazard rate of 1.97 (95% CI 1.21–3.22) for MI and 2.56 (95% CI 1.58–4.41) for stroke. Adjusting for BMI, smoking, hypertension, diabetes, hyperlipidaemia, atrial fibrillation, and aspirin use did not attenuate the correlation [52]. The prevalence of peripheral vascular disease was 4 times higher than in the control's. However, as the authors point out, misdiagnosis may affect the estimate of true peripheral vascular disease.

A Canadian population-based study identified 1239 SSc patients in a cohort of incident cases generated from 1996 to 2010. Each case was matched by 10 non-SSc individuals. After a follow-up time of 2 years, MI occurred with a frequency of 13.0/1000 patient years compared to 4.1 /1000 patient years in the controls. Corresponding figures for stroke were 8.0 vs. 4.1. Adjusted hazard rates were 3.49 (95% CI 2.52–4.83) and 2.35 (95% CI 1.59–348), respectively. In this study the risks were significantly higher in the first year of SSc [53]. Together with numerous less stringent evidence, it is safe to conclude that there is an increased risk of suffering MI and stroke in patients with SSc. This is obviously in part a consequence of the general vascular changes of SSc, but could also have other contributing aetiologies.

Postmortem examination performed in the days when this procedure still was in use clearly showed widespread changes in large vessels more characteristic of vasculopathy than vasculitis [54]. A connection with SSc and large vessel disease was suggested by case histories in the 1980s and 1990s [55–57]. The hypothesis was supported by a case-control study of patients with limited SSc [58]. A study of 33 with limited SSc confirmed increasing loss of elasticity in the carotid arteries [59]. An Australian retrospective study reported ulnar artery occlusion identified by positive Allen tests in patients with digital ulcers [60]. A large French study comparing patients with and without active digital ulcers identified small- and medium-sized arterial pathology but aortic pulse wave velocity abnormality with the ulcers [61]. A recent clinical paper illustrates the mix of causes of ischemic digital ulcers in SSc [62]. Macro vascular comorbidity is particularly prevalent in patients with limited SSc.

Data from hospitalised patients with SSc and atherosclerotic cardiovascular disease (ASCVD) in a sample of 20% of US hospitals analysed data from 1993 to 2007 involving 61,734 patients with SSc compared to 331,235 patients with SLE, 842,787 with RA, and 468,913 with controls. The modified Charlson comorbidity index did not differ among the disease groups. The in-hospital deaths per 1000 hospitalisations were 64.5 for SSc, 26.5 for SLE, 26.1 for RA, and 25.0 for the controls. The mean age of the SLE patients was lower and that of the RA patients higher, but these differences did not explain the higher mortality among the SSc patients. 5.4% of all hospitalisations among SSc patients were related to ASCVD. The study illustrates the high prevalence and severity of ASCVD and points to the need for further analysis of the causes of more efficient management [63].

Myasthenia Gravis

Myasthenia gravis was recognised albeit unusual as a complication of therapy with D-penicillamine in patients with SSc, a drug commonly used to treat SSc over decades until an RTC failed to show efficacy [64]. But co-occurrence has also been observed in patients who were never exposed to this drug. Two such patients were reported in 2007 together with a critical review of the literature [65]. The authors identified a total of 14 patients including their own. All but one were women aged between 24 and 76 years. Eleven were tested for antibodies to the acetylcholine receptor and they were all positive. The authors speculate that this co-occurrence may be more common than reported due to overlapping symptoms. In the absence of recent reports of co-occurrence, it can be concluded that there is no support for comorbidity with myasthenia gravis.

Depression

Anxiety and depression are overrepresented in patients with SSc and not always managed adequately. The question is whether the connection is a disease manifestation, a complication, or a comorbidity or a combination. Mild and transient depression can be observed in nearly 50% of patients in referral centres [66]. Applying stringent criteria and double observation 1 month apart, a recent Canadian study diagnosed major depressive disorder in 5% of all patients, whereas only one quarter of their patients fulfilled criteria at both examinations, and the conclusion was that the majority of depressions were mild and transient [67]. Considering the major impact on quality of life in SSc, this may come as a surprise, but the study illustrates the diagnostic problem. Several studies find correlations with depression and dysfunctional sexual function [68, 69], sleep disturbance [70], and pain [71]. These and several other publications emphasise the reality of increased prevalence of depression but also to its nature as consequence or complications of the disease rather than independent comorbidity. Suicide is probably more prevalent in the general population [72].

Osteoporosis

Osteoporosis is common in SSc and often considered a comorbidity [73–75]. A number of plausible explanations can be considered including reduced physical activity, early menopause, treatment with glucocorticoids and other drugs, malabsorption due to GI involvement, and reduced lean body mass. But they all indicate osteoporosis as an important disease complication rather than comorbidity.

Concluding Remarks

As mentioned in the introduction, comorbidity may often be complication or consequence of SSc. And SSc maybe induced by therapies to other conditions, in particular cancer. In the end the distinction may be less important than the clinician's awareness of unusual or unexpected features of SSc. Vigilance for malignancy, depression, thyroid disease, liver disease, osteoporosis, and Sjögren's are all relevant in the assessment of patients with SSc.

References

1. Hesselstrand R, Scheja A, Åkesson A. Mortality and causes of death in a Swedish series of systemic sclerosis patients. Ann Rheum Dis. 1998;57:682–6.
2. Silman AJ. Scleroderma and survival. Ann Rheum Dis. 1991;50:267–9.
3. Cabral-Marques O, Riemekasten G. Vascular hypothesis revisited: role of stimulating antibodies against angiotensin and endothelin receptors in the pathogenesis of systemic sclerosis. Autoimmun Rev. 2016;15(7):690–4.
4. Sagha O, Stucki G, Liang MH, Fossel AH, Katz JN. The self-administered questionnaire: a new method to assess comorbidity for clinical and health services research. Arthritis Rheum. 2003;49:156–63.
5. Hudson M, Sharma A, Bernstein J, Canadian Scleroderma Research Group, Baron M. Validity of self-reported comorbidities in systemic sclerosis. J Rheumatol. 2009;36(7):1477–80.
6. Kelley, Firestein. Rheumatology. 10th ed. St. Louis: Elsevier; 2016.
7. Varga J, Denton C, editors. Scleroderma: from pathogenesis to comprehensive management. 2nd ed. New York: Springer Science + Business Media; 2017.
8. Zatuchni J, Campbell WN, Zarafonetis CJD. Pulmonary fibrosis and terminal bronchiolar carcinoma in scleroderma. Cancer. 1953;6:1147–58.
9. Onishi A, Sugiyama D, Kumagai S, Morinobu A. Cancer incidence in systemic sclerosis: meta-analysis of population-based cohort studies. Arthritis Rheum. 2013;65(7):1913–21.
10. Chatterjee S, Dombi GW, Severson RK, Mayes MD. Risk of malignancy in scleroderma: a population-based cohort study. Arthritis Rheum. 2005;52:2415–24.
11. Olesen AB, Svaerke C, Farkas DK, Sørensen HT. Systemic sclerosis and the risk of cancer: a nationwide population-based cohort study. Br J Dermatol. 2010;163(4):800–6.
12. Kuo CF, Luo SF, Yu KH, Chou IJ, Tseng WY, Chang HC, et al. Cancer risk among patients with systemic sclerosis: a nationwide population study in Taiwan. Scand J Rheumatol. 2012;41:44–9.
13. Bonifazi M, Tramacere I, Pomponio G, Gabrielli B, Avvedimento EV, La Vecchia C, Negri E, Gabrielli A. Systemic sclerosis (scleroderma) and cancer risk: systematic review and meta-analysis of observational studies. Rheumatology (Oxford). 2013;52(1):143–54.
14. Rosenthal AK, McLaughlin JK, Gridley G, Nyren O. Incidence of cancer among patients with systemic sclerosis. Cancer. 1995;76:910–4.
15. Derk CT, Rasheed M, Artlett CM, Jimenez SA. A cohort study of cancer incidence in systemic sclerosis. J Rheumatol. 2006;33(6):1113–6.
16. Wipff J, Coriat R, Masciocchi M, Caramaschi P, Derk CT, Hachulla E, Riccieri V, Mouthon L, Krasowska D, Ananyeva LP, Kahan A, Matucci-Cerinic M, Chaussade S, Allanore Y. Outcomes of Barrett's oesophagus related to systemic sclerosis: a 3-year EULAR scleroderma trials and research prospective follow-up study. Rheumatology (Oxford). 2011;50(8):1440–4.
17. Hill CL, Nguyen AM, Roder D, Roberts-Thomson P. Risk of cancer in patients with scleroderma: a population based cohort study. Ann Rheum Dis. 2003;62:728–31.

18. Moinzadeh P, Fonseca C, Hellmich M, Shah AA, Chighizola C, Denton CP, Ong VH. Association of anti-RNA polymerase III autoantibodies and cancer in scleroderma. Arthritis Res Ther. 2014;16(1):R53. doi:10.1186/ar448.
19. Shah AA, Rosen A, Hummers L, Wigley F, Casciola-Rosen L. Close temporal relationship between onset of cancer and scleroderma in patients with RNA polymerase I/III antibodies. Arthritis Rheum. 2010;62:2787–95.
20. Airo' P, Ceribelli A, Cavazzana I, Taraborelli M, Zingarelli S, Franceschini F. Malignancies in Italian patients with systemic sclerosis positive for anti-RNA polymerase III antibodies. J Rheumatol. 2011;38(7):1329–34.
21. Shah AA, Hummers LK, Casciola-Rosen L, Visvanathan K, Rosen A, Wigley FM. Examination of autoantibody status and clinical features associated with cancer risk and cancer-associated scleroderma. Arthritis Rheumatol. 2015;67(4):1053–61.
22. Joseph CG, Darrah E, Shah AA, Skora AD, Casciola-Rosen LA, Wigley FM, Boin F, Fava A, Thoburn C, Kinde I, Jiao Y, Papadopoulos N, Kinzler KW, Vogelstein B, Rosen A. Association of the autoimmune disease scleroderma with an immunologic response to cancer. Science. 2014;343(6167):152–7.
23. Shah AA, Casciola-Rosen L. Cancer and scleroderma: a paraneoplastic disease with implications for malignancy screening. Curr Opin Rheumatol. 2015;27(6):563–70.
24. Antonelli A, Ferri C, Ferrari SM, Di Domenicantonio A, Giuggioli D, Galleri D, Miccoli P, Fallahi P. Increased risk of papillary thyroid cancer in systemic sclerosis associated with autoimmune thyroiditis. Rheumatology (Oxford). 2016;55(3):480–4.
25. Pakozdi A, Nihtyanova S, Moinzadeh P, Ong VH, Black CM, Denton CP. Clinical and serological hallmarks of systemic sclerosis overlap syndromes. J Rheumatol. 2011;38(11):2406–9.
26. Avouac J, Sordet C, Depinay C, Ardizonne M, Vacher-Lavenu MC, Sibilia J, Kahan A, Allanore Y. Systemic sclerosis-associated Sjögren's syndrome and relationship to the limited cutaneous subtype: results of a prospective study of sicca syndrome in 133 consecutive patients. Arthritis Rheum. 2006;54(7):2243–9.
27. Koumakis E, Dieudé P, Avouac J, Kahan A, Allanore Y, Association des Sclérodermiques de France. Familial autoimmunity in systemic sclerosis -- results of a French-based case-control family study. J Rheumatol. 2012;39(3):532–8.
28. Murray-Lyon IM, Thompson RP, Ansell ID, Williams R. Scleroderma and primary biliary cirrhosis. Br Med J. 1970;3(5717):258–9.
29. Reynolds TB, Denison EK, Frankl HD, Lieberman FL, Peters RL. Primary biliary cirrhosis with scleroderma, Raynaud's phenomenon and telangiectasia. New syndrome Am J Med. 1971;50(3):302–12.
30. Kumagi T, Heathcote EJ. Primary biliary cirrhosis. Orphanet J Rare Dis. 2008;3:1. doi:10.1186/1750-1172-3-1. Review
31. Watt FE, James OF, Jones DE. Patterns of autoimmunity in primary biliary cirrhosis patients and their families: a population-based cohort study. QJM. 2004;97(7):397–406.
32. Tovoli F, Granito A, Giampaolo L, Frisoni M, Volta U, Fusconi M, Masi C, Lenzi M. Nailfold capillaroscopy in primary biliary cirrhosis: a useful tool for the early diagnosis of scleroderma. J Gastrointestin Liver Dis. 2014;23(1):39–4.
33. Mayo MJ, Jenkins RN, Combes B, Lipsky PE. Association of clonally expanded T cells with the syndrome of primary biliary cirrhosis and limited scleroderma. Hepatology. 1999;29(6):1635–42.
34. Bernuzzi F, Fenoglio D, Battaglia F, Fravega M, Gershwin ME, Indiveri F, Ansari AA, Podda M, Invernizzi P, Filaci G. Phenotypical and functional alterations of CD8 regulatory T cells in primary biliary cirrhosis. J Autoimmun. 2010;35(3):176–80.
35. Deleuran B, Abraham DJ. Possible implication of the effector CD4+ T-cell subpopulation TH17 in the pathogenesis of systemic scleroderma. Nat Clin Pract Rheumatol. 2007;3(12):682–3.
36. Fenoglio D, Battaglia F, Parodi A, Stringara S, Negrini S, Panico N, Rizzi M, Kalli F, Conteduca G, Ghio M, De Palma R, Indiveri F, Filaci G. Alteration of Th17 and Treg cell subpopulations co-exist in patients affected with systemic sclerosis. Clin Immunol. 2011;139(3):249–57.
37. Reilly S, Hügle T, van Laar JM. T cells in systemic sclerosis: a reappraisal. Rheumatology (Oxford). 2012;51(9):1540–9.

38. Brembilla NC, Chizzolini C. T cell abnormalities in systemic sclerosis with a focus on Th17 cells. Eur Cytokine Netw. 2012;23(4):128–39.
39. Brembilla NC, Montanari E, Truchetet ME, Raschi E, Meroni P, Chizzolini C. Th17 cells favor inflammatory responses while inhibiting type I collagen deposition by dermal fibroblasts: differential effects in healthy and systemic sclerosis fibroblasts. Arthritis Res Ther. 2013;15(5):R151. doi:10.1186/ar4334.
40. Yang X, Yang J, Xing X, Wan L, Li M. Increased frequency of Th17 cells in systemic sclerosis is related to disease activity and collagen overproduction. Arthritis Res Ther. 2014;16(1):R4. doi:10.1186/ar4430.
41. Zhou Y, Hou W, Xu K, Han D, Jiang C, Mou K, Li Y, Meng L, Lu S. The elevated expression of Th17-related cytokines and receptors is associated with skin lesion severity in early systemic sclerosis. Hum Immunol. 2015;76(1):22–9.
42. Abraham S, Begum S, Isenberg D. Hepatic manifestations of autoimmune rheumatic diseases. Ann Rheum Dis. 2004;63(2):123–9.
43. Marie I, Levesque H, Tranvouez JL, François A, Riachi G, Cailleux N, Courtois H. Autoimmune hepatitis and systemic sclerosis: a new overlap syndrome? Rheumatology (Oxford). 2001;40(1):102–6.
44. Rodrigues CE, Borges CL, de Carvalho JF. Diffuse systemic sclerosis and autoimmune hepatitis: a unique association. Clin Rheumatol. 2010;29(7):799–801.
45. Assandri R, Monari M, Montanelli A. Development of systemic sclerosis in patients with autoimmune hepatitis: an emerging overlap syndrome. Gastroenterol Hepatol Bed Bench. 2016;9(3):211–9.
46. Manetti M, Guiducci S, Ruffo M, Rosa I, Faussone-Pellegrini MS, Matucci-Cerinic M, Ibba-Manneschi L. Evidence for progressive reduction and loss of telocytes in the dermal cellular network of systemic sclerosis. J Cell Mol Med. 2013;17(4):482–96.
47. Fu S, Wang F, Cao Y, Huang Q, Xiao J, Yang C, Popescu LM. Telocytes in human liver fibrosis. J Cell Mol Med. 2015;19(3):676–83.
48. Liu J, Cao Y, Song Y, Huang Q, Wang F, Yang W, Yang C. Telocytes in liver. Curr Stem Cell Res Ther. 2016;11(5):415–9.
49. Wollheim FA. Telocytes, communicators in healthy stroma and relation to inflammation and fibrosis. Joint Bone Spine. 2016. pii: S1297-319X(16)30109-9. doi: 10.1016/j.jbspin.2016.06.002
50. Domsic RT, Dezfulian C, Shoushtari A, Ivanco D, Kenny E, Kwoh CK, Medsger TA Jr, Champion HC. Endothelial dysfunction is present only in the microvasculature and microcirculation of early diffuse systemic sclerosis patients. Clin Exp Rheumatol. 2014;32(6 Suppl 86):S-154–60.
51. Pattanaik D, Brown M, Postlethwaite BC, Postlethwaite AE. Pathogenesis of systemic sclerosis. Front Immunol. 2015;6:272. doi:10.3389/fimmu.2015.00272.
52. Man A, Zhu Y, Zhang Y, Dubreuil M, Rho YH, Peloquin C, Simms RW, Choi HK. The risk of cardiovascular disease in systemic sclerosis: a population-based cohort study. Ann Rheum Dis. 2013;72(7):1188–93.
53. Aviña-Zubieta JA, Man A, Yurkovich M, Huang K, Sayre EC, Choi HK. Early cardiovascular disease after the diagnosis of systemic sclerosis. Am J Med. 2016;129(3):324–31.
54. D'Angelo WA, Fries JF, Masi AT, Shulman LE. Pathologic observations in systemic sclerosis (scleroderma). A study of fifty-eight autopsy cases and fifty-eight matched controls. Am J Med. 1969;46:428–40.
55. Dorevitch MI, Clemens LE, Webb JB. Lower limb amputation secondary to large vessel involvement in scleroderma. Br J Rheumatol. 1988;27(5):403–6.
56. Alusík S, Kcvác J, Peregrin J. Large arteries involvement in scleroderma--a case report. Angiology. 1990;41(11):973–6.
57. Youssef P, Englert H, Bertouch J. Large vessel occlusive disease associated with CREST syndrome and scleroderma. Ann Rheum Dis. 1993;52(6):464–6.
58. Youssef P, Brama T, Englert H, Bertouch J. Limited scleroderma is associated with increased prevalence of macrovascular disease. J Rheumatol. 1995;22(3):469–72.

59. Cheng KS, Tiwari A, Boutin A, Denton CP, Black CM, Morris R, Hamilton G, Seifalian AM. Carotid and femoral arterial wall mechanics in scleroderma. Rheumatology (Oxford). 2003;42(11):1299–305.
60. Taylor MH, McFadden JA, Bolster MB, Silver RM. Ulnar artery involvement in systemic sclerosis (scleroderma). J Rheumatol. 2002;29(1):102–6.
61. Aïssou L, Meune C, Avouac J, Meunier M, Elhaï M, Sorbets E, Kahan A, Allanore Y. Small, medium but not large arteries are involved in digital ulcers associated with systemic sclerosis. Joint Bone Spine. 2016;83(4):444–7.
62. Sharp CA, Akram Q, Hughes M, Muir L, Herrick AL. Differential diagnosis of critical digital ischemia in systemic sclerosis: report of five cases and review of the literature. Semin Arthritis Rheum. 2016;46(2):209–16.
63. Dave AJ, Fiorentino D, Lingala B, Krishnan E, Chung L. Atherosclerotic cardiovascular disease in hospitalized patients with systemic sclerosis: higher mortality than patients with lupus and rheumatoid arthritis. Arthritis Care Res (Hoboken). 2014;66(2):323–7.
64. Clements PJ, Furst DE, Wong WK, Mayes M, White B, Wigley F, Weisman MH, Barr W, Moreland LW, Medsger TA Jr, Steen V, Martin RW, Collier D, Weinstein A, Lally E, Varga J, Weiner S, Andrews B, Abeles M, Seibold JR. High-dose versus low-dose D-penicillamine in early diffuse systemic sclerosis: analysis of a two-year, double-blind, randomized, controlled clinical trial. Arthritis Rheum. 1999;42(6):1194–203.
65. Zivković SA, Medsger TA Jr. Myasthenia gravis and scleroderma: two cases and a review of the literature. Clin Neurol Neurosurg. 2007;109(4):388–91.
66. Roca RP, Wigley FM, White B. Depressive symptoms associated with scleroderma. Arthritis Rheum. 1996;39(6):1035–40.
67. Thombs BD, Jewett LR, Kwakkenbos L, Hudson M, Baron M, Canadian Scleroderma Research Group. Major depression diagnoses among patients with systemic sclerosis: baseline and one-month followup. Arthritis Care Res (Hoboken). 2015;67(3):411–6.
68. Maddali Bongi S, Del Rosso A, Mikhaylova S, Baccini M, Matucci CM. Sexual function in Italian women with systemic sclerosis is affected by disease-related and psychological concerns. J Rheumatol. 2013;40(10):1697–705.
69. Knafo R, Haythornthwaite JA, Heinberg L, Wigley FM, Thombs BD. The association of body image dissatisfaction and pain with reduced sexual function in women with systemic sclerosis. Rheumatology (Oxford). 2011;50(6):1125–30.
70. Frech T, Hays RD, Maranian P, Clements PJ, Furst DE, Khanna D. Prevalence and correlates of sleep disturbance in systemic sclerosis--results from the UCLA scleroderma quality of life study. Rheumatology (Oxford). 2011;50(7):1280.
71. Milette K, Razykov I, Pope J, Hudson M, Motivala SJ, Baron M, Thombs BD. Clinical correlates of sleep problems in systemic sclerosis: the prominent role of pain. Rheumatology (Oxford). 2011;50(5):921–5.
72. Razykov I, Hudson M, Baron M, Thombs BD, Canadian Scleroderma Research Group. Utility of the patient health questionnaire-9 to assess suicide risk in patients with systemic sclerosis. Arthritis Care Res (Hoboken). 2013;65(5):753–8.
73. Di Munno O, Mazzantini M, Massei P, Ferdeghini M, Pitaro N, Latorraca A, Ferri C. Reduced bone mass and normal calcium metabolism in systemic sclerosis with and without calcinosis. Clin Rheumatol. 1995;14(4):407–12.
74. Frediani B, Baldi F, Falsetti P, Acciai C, Filippou G, Spreafico A, Siagri C, Chellini F, Capperucci C, Filipponi P, Galeazzi M, Marcolongo R. Clinical determinants of bone mass and bone ultrasonometry in patients with systemic sclerosis. Clin Exp Rheumatol. 2004;22(3):313–8.
75. Souza RB, Borges CT, Takayama L, Aldrighi JM, Pereira RM. Systemic sclerosis and bone loss: the role of the disease and body composition. Scand J Rheumatol. 2006;35(5):384–7.

Chapter 8
Gout

Lisa K. Stamp and Peter T. Chapman

Comorbidities are common in patients with gout. Data from NHANES 2007–2008 revealed that of the individuals with gout, 74% had hypertension, 71% had ≥ stage 2 chronic kidney disease, 53% were obese, 26% had diabetes, 14% had a history of myocardial infarction and 10% had a history of stroke [1]. Many people with gout have more than one comorbidity. The metabolic syndrome, which comprises hypertension, cardiovascular disease, chronic kidney disease, type II diabetes, obesity and hyperlipidaemia, is common with a reported prevalence 62.8% (95% CI 51.9–73.6) in people gout compared to 25.4% (95% CI 23.5–27.3) in people without gout in the NHANES 1988–1994 data [2]. Five different combinations of the components of the metabolic syndrome have recently been reported with the authors suggesting these different clinical phenotypes may reflect different pathophysiological processes linked to gout [3].

The presence of comorbidities has important implications, particularly with respect to the choice of therapy for both management of acute gout and long-term urate lowering. The cause-effect relationship between gout/hyperuricaemia and these comorbidities is the subject of ongoing investigation. This chapter will review the evidence for the relationships between gout and these comorbidities and briefly discuss the implications for therapy.

L.K. Stamp (✉)
Department of Medicine, University of Otago, Christchurch, New Zealand
e-mail: Lisa.stamp@cdhb.health.nz

P.T. Chapman
Department of Rheumatology, Immunology and Allergy, Christchurch Hospital, Christchurch, New Zealand

Y. El Miedany (ed.), *Comorbidity in Rheumatic Diseases*,
DOI 10.1007/978-3-319-59963-2_8

Chronic Kidney Disease

Chronic kidney disease is one of the most common comorbidities in gout. A recent systematic review and meta-analysis from six studies reported the pooled prevalence estimate of stage 3 chronic kidney disease in people with gout was 24% (95% CI 19% – 28%); compared to individuals without gout, the odds ratio (OR) for chronic kidney disease stage ≥3 was 2.41 (95% CI 1.86–3.11) after adjustment for age, gender, obesity, diabetes and hypertension [4]. Similarly in a study of 5028 individuals with eGFR 30 – ≤ 60 ml/min/1.73 m^2 or eGFR >60 ml/min/1.73 m^2 with overt proteinuria, the overall prevalence of gout was 24.3% [5]. Chronic kidney disease is a risk factor for gout with a hazard ratio (HR) of 1.88 (95% CI 1.13–3.13) in men and in women HR 2.31 (95% CI 1.25–4.24) [6].

Hyperuricaemia, a critical factor in the development of gout, has been reported to be associated with the development of kidney impairment. In a meta-analysis of 13 observational studies, hyperuricaemia was associated with development of new onset chronic kidney disease in individuals with normal renal function (summary OR 2.35; 95% CI 1.59–3.46) [7]. However, it remains unclear whether urate is causal of impaired kidney function with a recent Mendelian randomisation study failing to show a causal relationship [8].

Impaired kidney function has a significant impact on choice of therapy in gout. Non-steroidal anti-inflammatories (NSAIDs) and colchicine, which are considered first-line treatments for acute gout [9], are both relatively contraindicated in patients with impaired kidney function. Inhibition of prostacyclin and prostaglandin E_2 by NSAIDs in individuals with pre-existing kidney impairment may lead to renal vasoconstriction, reduced renal blood flow and hypertension resulting in acute or worsening kidney impairment. Kidney impairment (creatinine clearance ≤50 ml/min) is an important risk factor for colchicine-induced myotoxicity [10], and the gastrointestinal adverse effects associated with colchicine may be poorly tolerated in those with impaired kidney function.

The use of urate-lowering therapy in individuals with chronic kidney disease remains a challenging clinical issue. The xanthine oxidase inhibitors allopurinol and febuxostat prevent uric acid production and are considered first-line therapy in gout [11]. Allopurinol remains the most commonly used urate-lowering therapy. It is rapidly converted to its active metabolite oxypurinol, which is excreted via the kidneys. Allopurinol can be associated with a rare but potentially life-threatening hypersensitivity syndrome. The association between impaired kidney function and allopurinol hypersensitivity is well recognised [12, 13]. Furthermore, in patients who develop severe adverse reactions with allopurinol, chronic kidney disease is associated with poor clinical outcomes and mortality [14]. The risk of allopurinol hypersensitivity may be minimised by limiting the starting dose of allopurinol to a maximum of 100 mg daily, and lower in those with impaired kidney function, and by avoiding allopurinol in individuals positive for HLA-B*5801 [15]. In patients who tolerate allopurinol, the use of more than 300 mg daily is uncommon despite failure to achieve target urate because of concerns about the risk of allopurinol hypersensitivity. There is increasing evidence that gradual dose escalation is an option even in those with kidney impairment [16]. Whilst larger clinical trials are awaited, current guidelines support the "start low, go slow" dose escalation of allopurinol to achieve target urate even in those with kidney impairment [11].

In comparison to allopurinol, febuxostat is predominantly metabolised in the liver and is not dependent on kidney function for excretion. Therefore dose reduction in individuals with mild-moderate kidney impairment is not required. Data are more limited in individuals with severe kidney impairment (eGFR < 30 ml/min/1.73 m^2). A recent study of 96 patients with gout and moderate-to-severe kidney impairment (eGFR ≥ 15 to ≤ 50 ml/min/1.73 m^2) reported that febuxostat up to 80 mg daily was safe and effective [17].

For those who fail to reach target urate or have adverse effects with a xanthine oxidase inhibitor, the uricosuric agents probenecid or benzbromarone are considered second-line options, whilst pegloticase, a recombinant uricase, is reserved for those individuals with severe gout who have failed or cannot tolerate other urate-lowering therapies [11]. Because of a more acceptable safety profile, probenecid is generally considered the first-line uricosuric and can have a moderate urate-lowering effect even in those with eGFR < 50 ml/min/1.72m^2 [18]. Benzbromarone is not widely available as it has been associated with hepatotoxicity but may be an effective urate-lowering therapy in those with impaired kidney function [19], although efficacy reduces once eGFR is <30 ml/min/1.72m^2. There is limited experience in using pegloticase in kidney impairment. In a post-hoc analysis of two phase 3 clinical trials which included patients with chronic kidney disease stage 3 and 4, there was no significant change in renal function, and the efficacy and safety of pegloticase did not appear to be affected by renal function [20].

Urate lowering may also improve kidney function in those with gout. For example, in a post-hoc analysis of the FOCUS study in which 116 patients with gout received febuxostat for up to 5 years, there was an inverse correlation between maintenance or improvement in eGFR and reduction in serum urate [21].

Hypertension

Hypertension is common in patients with hyperuricaemia and gout and vice versa. In a recent large prospective cohort study, this bidirectional association was observed with an 18% increased risk of developing hypertension in those with gout compared to those without gout (HR 1.18; 95% CI 1.02–1.367), and hypertensive patients had an 88% increased risk of developing gout compared to normotensive individuals (HR1.88; 95% CI 1.61–2.21) [22]. Although observational studies have suggested that hyperuricaemia is associated with development of hypertension [23], a causal association was not confirmed in a recent Mendelian randomisation study [24].

Loop and thiazide diuretics which are used in the management of hypertension increase serum urate, whilst other antihypertensives such as losartan and amlodipine reduce serum urate. The relationship between diuretic use and incident gout is well established [25–27]. For example, in the Atherosclerosis Risk in Communities Study (ARIC), incident gout was associated with use of any diuretic (HR 1.48; 95% CI 1.11–1.98), a thiazide diuretic (HR 1.44; 95% CI 1.0–2.01) or a loop diuretic (HR 2.31; 95% CI 1.36–3.91) an effect that was mediated by alterations in serum urate [28]. The use of other antihypertensives has been associated with a reduced risk of gout. In a nested case-control study of 24,768 people with newly diagnosed gout and 50,000 controls, the relative risk of incident gout was 0.87 (95% CI 0.82–0.93) for calcium channel blockers and 0.81 (95% CI 0.70–0.94) for losartan [29].

The use of diuretics may also make urate lowering therapy more challenging. People with gout receiving allopurinol and the loop diuretic furosemide have significantly higher plasma oxypurinol concentration for any given allopurinol dose compared with those not receiving furosemide [30], and those receiving furosemide require higher doses of allopurinol to achieve serum urate <0.36 mmol/l [16]. Although there are no specific studies on the effects stopping diuretics in people with gout, concomitant use may make urate-lowering treatment more difficult, and where possible alternate medications for hypertension which do not increase serum urate should be used.

Urate-lowering therapies may also have beneficial effects on blood pressure. Allopurinol has also been reported to reduce blood pressure in hyperuricaemic adults and adolescents with essential hypertension [31, 32], and in a study of hyperuricaemic patients undergoing cardiac surgery who were treated with up to 60 mg daily of febuxostat for 6 months, a significant reduction in blood pressure was observed [33]. In men with gout, 4 weeks of either allopurinol 300 mg daily or febuxostat 40 mg, 80 mg or 120 mg daily was associated with a significant decrease in diastolic blood pressure compared to placebo [34].

Cardiovascular Disease

Gout has been associated with an increased risk of coronary artery disease [1, 35–37], death due to cardiovascular causes [38, 39], stroke [40], peripheral artery disease [41] and heart failure [42]. The association between gout and cardiovascular disease is stronger in women than men [37, 43].

Observational studies have reported associations between hyperuricaemia and increased risk of coronary heart disease [44], stroke [45] and cardiovascular and all-cause mortality [46]. However, Mendelian randomisation studies are conflicting with one reporting no evidence of causal association between uric acid and cardiovascular disease [24] and another reporting evidence of causal association between uric acid and adverse cardiovascular outcomes, particularly sudden cardiac death [47]. Notwithstanding uncertainty around the causal relationship, a recent study reported a statistically significant association between the presence of asymptomatic monosodium urate crystal deposition in joints and moderate-severe coronary artery calcification [48]. Subclinical inflammation associated with monosodium urate crystals is one potential mechanism for this observation.

NSAIDs, which may be used for management of acute gout, have been associated with an increased risk of major cardiovascular events such as myocardial infarction, stroke and death. In a recent meta-analysis of >300,000 participants from >600 trials after 1 year, there was a significantly increased risk of major cardiovascular events with diclofenac and the coxibs but not with naproxen [49]. The effect of colchicine on risk of cardiovascular events is of considerable interest. In the general population, a recent meta-analysis of five studies reported a reduction in composite cardiovascular outcomes in patients with established cardiovascular disease [50]. In an observational study of people with gout, the use of colchicine was associated with a reduced risk of myocardial infarction, stroke or transient ischaemic attack (HR 0.51; 95% CI 0.30–0.88) [51]. Although large-scale randomised controlled trials are required, colchicine may be an appropriate therapy for acute gout and prophylaxis when starting urate-lowering therapy in patients with cardiovascular disease where NSAIDS may be contraindicated. However, clinicians must be cognisant of the interactions between colchicine and cytochrome P45 3A4 (CYP3A4) and P-glycoprotein (Gp) inhibitors such as verapamil and diltiazem which can result in raised plasma colchicine concentrations [52].

Whether urate-lowering therapy reduces cardiovascular events is the subject of ongoing clinical trials in people with and without gout. Data in people with gout are conflicting. In a retrospective cohort study in Taiwan of people with gout and no prior history of cardiovascular disease, allopurinol appeared to increase the risk and uricosuric therapy reduce the risk of cardiovascular events [53]. However, whilst cases and controls were matched on age, gender, diabetes, hypertension and hyperlipidaemia, they were not matched on the presence of chronic kidney disease; there were significantly more patients in the allopurinol group with chronic kidney disease. Details on important cardiovascular risk factors including blood pressure and smoking were lacking. In addition, the majority of patients in this study were receiving ≤100 mg daily of allopurinol with only 15% receiving ≥300 mg daily, and those patients receiving higher doses of allopurinol had a lower risk of cardiovascular events compared to those on low dose suggesting that the dose of allopurinol and the degree of serum urate reduction may be important [53]. In a large cohort study using US insurance claims data, initiation of a xanthine oxidase inhibitor in people with gout was not associated with an increase or a decrease in composite nonfatal cardiovascular outcome (including myocardial infarction, coronary revascularization, stroke and heart failure) compared to those with gout not starting urate-lowering therapy [54]. However, as the authors comment, adherence with urate-lowering therapy was low. In comparison, in a prospective case-matched cohort study, people with gout who received urate-lowering therapy had a lower risk of cardiovascular disease (HR0.29; 95% CI 0.11–0.80) and all-cause mortality (HR 0.47; 95% CI 0.29–0.79) compared to those who did not receive urate-lowering therapy [55].

Hyperlipidaemia

Gout is associated with increased very-low-density lipoproteins (VLDL) triglycerides [56, 57]. An association between the apolipoprotein A1-C3-A4 gene cluster and gout has also been observed [58, 59]. Fenofibrate, which is used in the management of hypertriglyceridaemia, increases urinary urate excretion thereby reducing serum urate [60–62]. In people with gout receiving urate-lowering therapy with allopurinol or benzbromarone, fenofibrate further lowers serum urate [63–65].

Obesity

Over 50% of people with gout are obese. A recent meta-analysis reported that the risk of gout increases as BMI increases with relative risk of 1.78, 2.67, 3.62 and 4.64 for people with BMI of 25 kg/m^2, 30 kg/m^2, 35 kg/m^2 and 40 kg/m^2, respectively, compared with persons with a BMI of 20 kg/m^2 [66]. The distribution of fat may also be important. Visceral fat obesity, defined as visceral fat area >100 cm^2, has been reported to be an independent risk factor for gout (OR 2.488, 95% CI 1.04–4.44) [67]. Furthermore, whilst both subcutaneous fat obesity and abdominal fat obesity are associated with hyperuricaemia, the mechanisms appear different with reduced urinary urate excretion dominant in those with subcutaneous fat obesity and urate overproduction dominant in those with visceral fat obesity [68].

Obesity is one of the few modifiable risk factors for gout. However, weight loss is challenging and difficult to sustain for many people. In obese individuals with gout, an average weight loss of 7.7 kg has been associated with a significant reduction in serum urate (baseline serum urate, 9.6 ± 1.7 mg/dl, falling to 7.9 ± 1.5 mg/dl; $p = 0.001$) and a decrease in frequency of gouty attacks (2.1 ± 0.8 attacks/month to 0.6 ± 0.7 attacks/month ($p = 0.002$)) [69]. More substantial weight loss, such as is achieved through bariatric surgery, has also been associated with a significant reduction in serum urate and gout attacks [70, 71].

Diabetes

Whilst both insulin resistance and type 2 diabetes have been associated with gout, the relationship is complex, and risk appears different for men and women. Using data from a US insurance plan, people with gout had an increased risk of developing diabetes even after adjustment for co-founders including age and comorbidities (HR 1.45; 95% CI 1.37–1.54). Furthermore, risk is greater in women (HR 1.78; 95% CI 1.51–2.09) compared to men (HR 1.41; 95% CI 1.33–1.50) [72]. Similar findings for increased risk of diabetes in people with gout and a stronger association in women than men has been reported in the UK [73]. The observation that gout and type 2 diabetes share common genetic risk alleles adds support to the association between these conditions [74]. Whether effective urate lowering in people with gout can reduce the risk of developing diabetes is unknown. However, there has been the suggestion that colchicine use in people with gout might reduce the risk of diabetes [75].

Management of acute gout in people with concomitant diabetes can be challenging. There is a frequent reluctance to use corticosteroids, although many individuals with gout and diabetes also have kidney impairment which precludes the use of NSAIDS and colchicine. Intra-articular steroids are a useful option in this group of patients, particularly if only one or two larger joints are involved. Oral prednisone is an alternative, and in general the associated increase in blood sugars can be managed given the short-term duration of therapy for acute gout.

Solid Organ Transplantation

Gout can occur in approximately one-quarter of people with renal and cardiac transplants [76]. Cyclosporine which is used for immunosuppression post-transplant is associated with an increase in serum urate and an increased risk of gout [77].

The goals of gout management in transplant recipients are the same as the general population. However, special care must be given to drug interactions (Table 8.1). Concomitant use of NSAIDs and calcineurin inhibitors (e.g. cyclosporine, tacrolimus) increases the risk of acute calcineurin nephrotoxicity [79]. Colchicine neuromyotoxicity may be more common in renal and cardiac transplant recipients [80]. The combination of cyclosporine and colchicine may predispose to myotoxicity [81]. Whilst allopurinol and febuxostat remain first-line urate-lowering therapies, there is a clinically important interaction between these agents and azathioprine. 6-Mercaptopurine, the active metabolite of azathioprine, is partly inactivated by xanthine oxidase; thus inhibition of xanthine oxidase by allopurinol or febuxostat may increase 6-mercaptopurine levels resulting in myelosuppression. This combination of a xanthine oxidase inhibitor and azathioprine should be used with great caution. Changing to an immunosuppressive agent that does not interact with a xanthine oxidase inhibitor (e.g. mycophenolate mofetil) may be clinically appropriate.

Other Comorbidities

A number of other comorbidities are increasingly recognised in association with gout. The Charlson index, a general health status measure which has been a predictor of mortality, includes information on different health categories (myocardial infarction, congestive heart failure, peripheral vascular disease, cerebrovascular disease, dementia, chronic pulmonary disease, rheumatological disease, peptic ulcer disease, liver disease, diabetes mellitus, renal diseases, malignancy and HIV infection). A recent case-controlled study using the UK Clinical Practice Research Datalink examined the burden of a wide range comorbidities in people with and without gout. At gout diagnosis, 38.25% of those with gout had a Charlson index ≥ 1 compared to 27.97% of controls ($p < 0.001$) [82]. The risk of developing incident comorbidities was significantly higher in those with gout compared to controls. Interestingly there was a higher risk of developing hemiplegia, depression, anaemia, hypothyroidism and psoriasis in addition to those comorbidities more traditionally associated with gout such as renal and cardiovascular disease [82].

Table 8.1 Summary of important comorbidities in gout and implications for therapy

Comorbidity	Association in gout	Effect of urate-lowering therapy on comorbidity in people with gout	Implications for acute gout management	Implications for urate-lowering therapy
Impaired kidney function	Chronic kidney disease associated with gout – HR 1.88 (95% CI 1.13–3.13) among men and 2.31 (95% CI 1.25–4.24) among women [6]	In people with gout, urate lowering may improve kidney function	NSAIDs and colchicine relatively contraindicated	Associated with increased risk of allopurinol-related serious adverse events especially in those with HLA-B*5801 Start low, go slow allopurinol dosing strategy advised Reduced efficacy of uricosuric agents
Hypertension		Allopurinol, febuxostat and probenecid shown to reduce blood pressure in small studies	NSAIDs may contribute to hypertension, consideration of interactions with diuretics and ACEI	
Cardiovascular disease	Gout associated with an increased risk of coronary artery disease [1, 35–37], death due to cardiovascular causes [38, 39], stroke [40], peripheral artery disease [41] and heart failure [42]	Data on urate-lowering therapy conflicting Currently there are ongoing clinical trials on the effects of urate-lowering therapy on cardiovascular in those with and without gout	NSAIDs may be associated with increased risk CVD events Colchicine may be associated with decreased risk of events	Febuxostat caution in CHF
Diabetes	Increased risk of incident diabetes in patients with gout [72, 73]	No evidence	Colchicine may reduce risk of incident diabetes Corticosteroids may increase blood sugars, but this can usually be managed for the short duration of therapy for acute gout	
Obesity	BMI associated with increased risk of gout [67, 78]	No evidence urate lowering decreases weight	Prednisone may contribute to increased weight	

Comorbidity	Association in gout	Effect of urate-lowering therapy on comorbidity in people with gout	Implications for acute gout management	Implications for urate-lowering therapy
Solid organ transplantation	Gout occurs in ~25% of renal and cardiac transplant recipients		NSAIDs may increase risk of calcineurin nephrotoxicity	Clinically significant interaction between xanthine oxidase inhibitors (allopurinol, febuxostat) and azathioprine use combination with caution and monitor FBC
			Increased risk colchicine neuro-myotoxicity	

A number of other comorbidities have been reported to be associated with gout including erectile dysfunction [83, 84], atrial fibrillation [85], increased risk of depression [86] and increased risk of deep vein thrombosis and pulmonary embolism [87]. Gout has also been associated with a reduced risk of vascular and non-vascular dementia [88] and Alzheimer's disease [89]. A recent meta-analysis reported no decrease in the risk of Parkinson's disease in people with gout [90] although a reduced risk of gout in people with Parkinson's disease has been reported [91].

Screening

Screening for comorbidities including obesity, diabetes, hypertension, hyperlipidaemia and modifiable risk factors for cardiovascular disease is recommended in gout management guidelines [11, 92]. Primary care is an ideal setting for comorbidity screening given the majority of people with gout are managed in primary care. However, appropriate systems need to be developed in both primary and secondary care settings to ensure screening is undertaken at appropriate intervals. If comorbidities are identified, then appropriate management should be instituted with consideration of how therapy may influence gout and its management as discussed in this chapter.

Emerging Therapies

Pegloticase, a recombinant urate oxidase (uricase), was developed for the treatment of refractory chronic gout. Uricases convert uric acid to the more water-soluble and hence readily excretable allantoin and the potent oxidant H_2O_2. In the absence of glucose-6-phosphate dehydrogenase (G6PD), red blood cells are unable to generate sufficient NAPDH to counteract the oxidative stress caused by H_2O_2, resulting in cell lysis and haemolytic anaemia [93]. The use of uricases is therefore contraindicated in G6PD deficiency [94]. H_2O_2 also oxidises haemoglobulin to cause methaemoglobineamia which leads to cyanosis and can result in seizures and death. G6DP deficiency is the most common enzyme deficiency in the world, affecting over 400 million people, and both the FDA and EMA recommend individuals at high risk of G6PD deficiency are screened prior to therapy with pegloticase and the drug avoided in the presence of deficiency [93] (http://www.accessdata.fda.gov/) (http://www.ema.europa.eu/). Pegloticase and rasburicase (another available uricase) should be reserved for patients with resistant gout flares and/or a high urate burden refractory to standard therapies. Identifying the ideal patient group, optimal treatment regimens and prevention of neutralising antibody formation remain challenges in uricase therapy.

A number of novel hypouricaemic drugs are in development and/or have recently been approved for clinical use. Lesinurad, a proximal tubule urate transport inhibitor (of URAT1 and OAT4) prescribed in combination with allopurinol, has been shown to be efficacious, but there is limited data in patients with renal impairment. This applies to other selective urate reabsorption inhibitors (SURIs) currently being investigated (e.g. arhoalfenate, levotofisospam). As with all clinical studies, inclusion of patients with comorbidities will be important in determining their safety and efficacy for the diverse group of patients with gout.

Summary

Screening and management of common comorbidities is strongly recommended in the overall treatment strategy of patients with gout. This is particularly relevant in gout patients with the metabolic syndrome. Attention to changing wherever possible pharmacological therapies which may worsen hyperuricaemia and gout (e.g. diuretics) and avoiding gout medications which may adversely impact on comorbidities (e.g. NSAIDs in chronic kidney disease) or enhance drug interactions is important for optimal management (summarised in Tables 8.1 and 8.2). Treating to target (sustained urate <0.36 mmol/L, <0.30 mmol/L in tophaceous gout) underpins successful gout therapy and may infer additional beneficial outcomes for several comorbidities, particularly those associated with the metabolic syndrome.

Table 8.2 Medications used to treat comorbidities associated with gout and their effect on gout management

Medications	Effect	Interactions with medication used in gout	Dosing adjustment/ monitoring
Furosemide	Increase in serum urate	Allopurinol – increase plasma oxypurinol concentration – may increase risk of AHS in those with kidney impairment	Start allopurinol at no more than 100 mg daily and less in those with ≥CKD stage 4
	Increase risk of gout		May require higher doses of allopurinol to achieve target SU
		NSAIDs – may increase risk of deterioration in kidney function	
Thiazide diuretics	Increase serum urate	Allopurinol – may increase risk of AHS in those with kidney impairment	Start allopurinol at no more than 100 mg daily and less in those with ≥CKD stage 4
	Increase risk of gout		

(continued)

Table 8.2 (continued)

Medications	Effect	Interactions with medication used in gout	Dosing adjustment/ monitoring
Aspirin	Increase serum urate	High-dose aspirin decreases uricosuric effect of probenecid	–
Warfarin	Increased risk gastrointestinal bleeding	Allopurinol – increase anticoagulant effect	Monitor INR
		NSAID increase risk GI bleeding if get peptic ulceration or gastritis	
ACE inhibitors		NSAID – may increase risk of deterioration in kidney function	
CYP3A4 and P-glycoprotein inhibitors e.g., diltiazem, verapamil, cyclosporine, clarithromycin		Colchicine	Reduce colchicine dose by 33–66%
Azathioprine		Allopurinol and febuxostat – increased risk bone marrow toxicity	Avoid combination, if use combination reduce azathioprine by 50–75% and use lower dose of allopurinol with frequent monitoring of FBC

References

1. Zhu Y, Pandya B, Choi H. Comorbidities of gout and hyperuricemia in the US general population: NHANES 2007-2008. Am J Med. 2012;125:679–87.
2. Choi H, Ford E, Li C, Curhan G. Prevalence of the metabolic syndrome in patients with gout: the Third National Health and Nutrition Examination Survey. Arthritis Care Res. 2007;57(1):109–15.
3. Richette P, Clerson P, Perissin L, Flipo R, Bardin T. Revisiting co-morbidities in gout: a cluster analysis. Ann Rheum Dis. 2015;74:142–7.
4. Roughley M, Belcher J, Mallen C, Roddy E. Gout and risk of chronic kidney disease and nephrolithiasis: meta-analysis of observational studies. Arthritis Res Ther. 2015;17:90.
5. Jing J, Kielstein J, Schultheiss U, Sitter T, Titze S, Schaeffner E, et al. Prevalence and correlates of gout in a large cohort of patients with chronic kidney disease: the German Chronic Kidney Disease (GCKD) study. Nephrol Dial Transplant. 2015;30(4):613–21.
6. Wang W, Bhole V, Krishnan E. Chronic kidney disease as a risk factor for incident gout among men and women: retrospective cohort study using data from the Framingham Heart Study. BMJ Open. 2015;5:e006843.

7. Li L, Yang C, Zhao Y, Zeng X, Liu F, Fu P. Is hyperuricemia an independent risk factor for new-onset chronic kidney disease?: a systematic review and meta-analysis based on observational cohort studies. BMC Nephrol. 2014;15:122. doi:10.1186/471-2369-15-122.
8. Hughes K, Flynn T, de Zoysa J, Dalbeth N, Merriman T. Mendelian randomization analysis associates increased serum urate, due to genetic variation in uric acid transporters, with improved renal function. Kidney Int. 2013;85(2):344–51.
9. Khanna D, Khanna P, Fitzgerald J, Singh M, Sangmee B, Neogi T, et al. 2012 American College of Rheumatology Guidelines for the Management of Gout. Part 2: therapy and antiinflammatory prophylaxis of acute gouty arthritis. Arthritis Care Res. 2012;64(10):1447–61.
10. Wallace S, Singer J, Duncan G, Wigley F, Kuncl R. Renal function predicts colchicine toxicity: guidelines for the prophylactic use of colchicine in gout. J Rheumatol. 1991;18(2):264–9.
11. Khanna D, Fitzgerald J, Khanna P, Sangmee B, Singh M, Neogi T, et al. 2012 American College of Rheumatology Guidelines for the Management of Gout. Part 1: systematic nonpharmacologic and pharmacologic therapeutic approaches to hyperuricaemia. Arthritis Care Res. 2012;64(10):1431–46.
12. Hande K, Noone R, Stone W. Severe allopurinol toxicity. Description and guidelines for prevention in patients with renal insufficiency. Am J Med. 1984;76:47–56.
13. Ramasamy S, Korb-Wells C, Kannangara D, Smith M, Wang N, Roberts D, et al. Allopurinol hypersensitivity: a systematic review of all published cases, 1950-2012. Drug Saf. 2013;36:953–80.
14. Chung W-H, Chang W-C, Stocker S, Juo C-G, Graham G, Lee M-H, et al. Insights into the poor prognosis of allopurinol-induced severe cutaneous adverse reactions: the impact of renal insufficiency, high plasma levels of oxypurinol and granulysin. Ann Rheum Dis. 2015;74(12):2157–64. doi:10.1136/annrheumdis-2014-205577.
15. Stamp L, Day R, Yun J. Allopurinol hypersensitivity: investigating the cause and minimizing the risk. Nat Rev Rheumatol. 2016;12(4):235–42.
16. Stamp L, O'Donnell J, Zhang M, James J, Frampton C, Barclay M, et al. Using allopurinol above the dose based on creatinine clearance is effective and safe in chronic gout, including in those with renal impairment. Arthritis Rheum. 2011;63(2):412–21.
17. Saag K, Whelton A, Becker M, MacDonald P, Hunt B, Gunawardhana L. Impact of febuxostat on renal function in gout subjects with moderate-to-severe renal impairment. Arthritis Rheum. 2016;68(8):2035–43. doi:10.1002/art.39654.
18. Pui K, Gow P, Dalbeth N. Efficacy and tolerability of probenecid as urate-lowering therapy in gout; clinical experience in high-prevalence population. J Rheumatol. 2013;40(6):872–6.
19. Stamp LH, Hslett J, Frampton C, White D, Gardner D, Stebbings S, Taylor G, et al. The safety and efficacy of benzbromarone in gout in Aotearoa New Zealand. Intern Med J. 2016;46(9):1075–80.
20. Yood R, Ottery F, Irish W, Wolfson M. Effect of pegloticase on renal function in patients with chronic kidney disease: a post hoc subgroup analysis of 2 randomized, placebo-controlled, phase 3 clinical trials. BMC Res Notes. 2014;7:51.
21. Whelton A, MacDonald P, Zhao L, Hunt B, Gunawardhana L. Renal function in gout: long-term treatment effects of febuxostat. J Clin Rheumatol. 2011;17(1):7–13.
22. Pan A, Teng G, Yuan J-M, Koh W-P. Bi-directional association between self reported hypertension and gout: the Singapore Chinese health study. PLoS One. 2015;10(10):e0141749.
23. Wang J, Qin T, Chen J, Li Y, Wang L, Huang H, Li J. Hyperuricemia and risk of incident hypertension: a systematic review and meta-analysis of observational studies. PLoS One. 2014;9(12):e114259.
24. Palmer T, Nordestgaard B, Benn M, Tybjærg-Hansen A, Davey Smith G, Lawlor D, et al. Association of plasma uric acid with ischaemic heart disease and blood pressure: mendelian randomisation analysis of two large cohorts. Br Med J. 2013;347:f4262. doi:10.1136/bmj.f4262.
25. McAdams-Demarco M, Maynard J, Baer A, Kao L, Kottgen A, Coresh J. A urate gene-by-diuretic interaction and gout risk in participants with hypertension: results from the ARIC study. Ann Rheum Dis. 2013;72:701–6.

26. Bao Y, Curhan G, Merriman T, Plenge R, Kraft P, Choi H. Lack of gene-diuretic interactions on the risk of incident gout: the Nurses' Health Study and Health Professionals Follow-up Study. Ann Rheum Dis. 2015;74:1394–8.
27. Bruderer S, Bodmer M, Jick S, Meier C. Use of diuretics and risk of incident gout. A population-based case-control study. Arthritis Rheum. 2014;66(1):185–96.
28. McAdams DeMArco M, Maynard J, Baer A, Gelber A, Young J, Alonso A, et al. Diuretic use, increased serum urate levels and risk of incident gout in a population-based study of adults with hypertension. Arthritis Rheum. 2012;64(1):121–9.
29. Choi H, Soriano L, Zhang Y, Rodriguez L. Anti-hypertensive drugs and risk of incident gout among patients with hypertension: population based case-control study. Br Med J. 2012;344:d8190. doi:10.1136/bmj.d8190.
30. Stamp L, O'Donnell J, Zhang M, Frampton C, Chapman P, Barclay M. Relationship between serum urate and plasma oxypurinol – is there a target plasma oxypurinol to achieve serum urate <6mg/dL? Arthritis Rheum. 2009;60(10 Suppl):S561.
31. Kanbay M, Ozkara A, Selcoki Y, Isik B, Turgut F, Bavbek N, et al. Effect of treatment of hyperuricemia with allopurinol on blood pressure, creatinine clearance, and proteinuria in patients with normal renal function. Int Urol Nephrol. 2007;39(4):1227–33.
32. Feig D, Soletsky B, Johnson R. Effect of allopurinol on blood pressure of adolescents with newly diagnosed essential hypertension. JAMA. 2008;300(8):924–32.
33. Sezai A, Soma M, Nakata K, Hata M, Yoshitake I, Wakui SH, Hata H, et al. Comparison of febuxostat and allopurinol for hyperuricemia in cardiac surgery patients (NU-FLASH Trial). Circ J. 2013;77:2043–9.
34. Kim H, Seo Y-I, Song Y. Four-week effects of allopurinol and febuxostat treatments on blood pressure and serum creatinine level in gouty men. J Korean Med Sci. 2014;29:1077–81.
35. Krishnan E, Baker J, Furst D, Schumacher HR. Gout and the risk of acute myocardial infarction. Arthritis Rheum. 2006;54(8):2688–96.
36. Choi H, Curhan G. Independent impact of gout on mortality and risk for coronary heart disease. Circulation. 2007;116:894–900.
37. De Vera M, Raheem K, Bhole V, Kopec J, Choi H. The independent impact of gout on the risk of acute myocardial infarction among elderly women: a population-based study. Ann Rheum Dis. 2010;69(6):1162–4.
38. Teng G, Ang L-W, Saag K, Yu M, Yuan J-M, Koh W-P. Mortality due to coronary heart disease and kidney disease among middle-aged and elderly men and women with gout in the Singapore Chinese Health Study. Ann Rheum Dis. 2012;71:924–8.
39. Stack A, Hanley A, Casserly L, Cronin C, Abdalla A, Kiernan T, et al. Independent and conjoint associations of gout and hyperuricaemia with total and cardiovascular mortality. QJM. 2013;106(4):647–58.
40. Seminog O, Goldacre M. Gout as a risk factor for myocardial infarction and stroke in England: evidence from record linkage studies. Rheumatology. 2013;52:2251–9.
41. Baker J, Schumacher H, Krishnan E. Serum uric acid level and risk for peripheral arterial disease: analysis of data from the multiple risk factor intervention trial. Angiology. 2007;58(4):450–7.
42. Krishnan E. Gout and the risk for incident heart failure and systolic dysfunction. BMJ Open. 2013;15(2):e000282.
43. Clarson L, Hider S, Belch JJF, Heneghan C, Roddy E, Mallen C. Increased risk of vascular disease associated with gout: a retrospective, matched cohort study in the UK Clinical Practice Research Datalink. Ann Rheum Dis. 2015;74:642–7.
44. Kim S, Guevara J, Kim K, Choi H, Heitjan D, Albert D. Hyperuricaemia and coronary heart disease: a systematic review and meta-analysis. Arthritis Care Res. 2010;62(2):170–80.
45. Kim S, Guevara J, Kim K, Choi H, Heitjan D, Albert D. Hyperuricaemia and risk of stroke: a systematic review and meta-analysis. Arthritis Care Res. 2009;61(7):885–92.
46. Zhao G, Huang L, Song M, Song L. Baseline serum uric acid level as a predictor of cardiovascular disease related mortality and all-cause mortality: a meta-analysis of prospective studies. Atherosclerosis. 2013;231(1):61–8.

47. Kleber ME, Delgado G, Grammer TB, Silbernagel G, Huang J, Krämer BK, Ritz E, März W. Uric acid and cardiovascular events: a mendelian randomization study. J Am Soc Nephrol. 2015;26(11):2831–8. doi: 10.1681/ASN.2014070660
48. Andres M, Quintanilla M-A, Sivera F, Sanchez-PAya J, Pascual E, Vela P, et al. Silent monosodium urate crystals deposits associate with severe coronary calcification in asymptomatic hyperuricemia: "an exploratory study". Arthritis Rheum. 2016; doi:10.1002/art.39581.
49. Bhala N, Emberson J, Merhi A, Abramson S, Arber N, Baron J, et al. Vascular and upper gastrointestinal effects of non-steroidal anti-inflammatory drugs: meta-analyses of individual participant data from randomised trials. Lancet. 2013;382(9894):769–79.
50. Verma S, Eikelboom J, Nidorf S, Al-Omran M, Gupta N, Teoh H, et al. Colchicine in cardiac disease: a systematic review and meta-analysis of randomized controlled trials. BMC Cardiovasc Disord. 2015;18:969.
51. Solomon D, Liu CC, Kuo IH, Zak A, Kim S. Effects of colchicine on risk of cardiovascular events and mortality among patients with gout: a cohort study using electronic medical records linked with Medicare claims. Ann Rheum Dis. 2015; doi:10.1136/annrheumdis-2015-207984.
52. Terkeltaub R, Furst D, Kook K, DiGiacinto J, Davis M. New dosing guidelines for colchicine to avoid toxicity when used with Ca2+ channel blockers: the potent P-Gp/CYP3A4 inhibitor verapamil increases maximal concentration of single dose colchicine by 30% and exposure by ~100% in healthy subjects. Arthritis Rheum. 2009;60(10 Suppl):S414.
53. Kok V, Horng J-T, Chang W-S, Hong Y-F, Chang T-H. Allopurinol therapy in gout patients does not associate with beneficial cardiovascular outcomes: a population based matched-cohort study. PLoS One. 2014;9(6):e99102.
54. Kim S, Schneeweiss S, Choudhry N, Liu J, Glynn R, Solomon D. Effects of xanthine oxidase inhibition on cardiovascular disease in patients with gout: a cohort study. Am J Med. 2015;128(6):553. e7.
55. Chen J-H, Lan J-L, Cheng C-F, Liang W-M, Lin H-Y, Tsay G, et al. Effect of urate lowering therapy on the risk of cardiovascular disease and all-cause mortality in patients with gout: a case matched cohort study. J Rheumatol. 2015;42(9):1694–701.
56. Matsubara K, Matsuzawa Y, Jiao S, Takama T, Kubo M, Tarui S. Relationship between hypertriglyceridemia and uric acid production in primary gout. Metabolism. 1999;38(7):698–701.
57. Rasheed H, Hsu A, Dalbeth N, Stamp L, McCormick S, Merriman T. The relationship of apolipoprotein B and very low density lipoprotein triglyceride with hyperuricaemia and gout. Arthritis Res Ther. 2014;16:495.
58. Rasheed H, Phipps-Green A, Topless R, Smith M, Hill C, Lester S, et al. Replication of association of the apolipoprotein A1-C3-A4 gene cluster with the risk of gout. Rheumatology. 2016; doi:10.1093/rheumatology/kew057.
59. Cardona F, Tinahones F, Collantes E, Escudero A, Garcia-Fuentes E, Soriguer F. Contribution of polymorphisms in the apolipoprotein AI-CIII-AIV cluster to hyperlipidaemia in patients with gout. Ann Rheum Dis. 2005;64:85–8.
60. Desager J, Hulhoven R, Harvengt C. Uricosuric effect of fenofibrate in healthy volunteers. J Clin Pharmacol. 1980;20:560–4.
61. Yamamoto T, Moriwaki Y, Takahashi S, Tsutsumi Z, Hada T. Effect of fenofibrate on plasma concentration and urinary excretion of purine bases and oxypurinol. J Rheumatol. 2001;28:2294–7.
62. Bastow M, Durrington P, Ishola M. Hypertriglyceridaemia and hyperuricaemia: effects of two fibric acid derivatives (Bezafibrate and fenofibrate) in a double-blind, placebo-controlled trial. Metabolism. 1988;37(3):217–20.
63. Hepburn A, Kaye S, Feher M. Fenofibrate: a new treatment for hyperuricaemia and gout? Ann Rheum Dis. 2001;60:984–6.
64. Feher M, Hepburn A, Hogarth M, Ball S, Kaye S. Fenofibrate enhances urate reduction in men treated with allopurinol for hyperuricaemia and gout. Rheumatology. 2003;42(2):321–5.
65. Takahashi S, Moriwaki Y, Yamamoto T, Tsutsumi Z, Ka T, Fukuchi M. Effects of combination treatment using anti-hyperuricaemic agents with fenofibrate and/or losartan on uric acid metabolism. Ann Rheum Dis. 2003;62:572–5.

66. Aune D, Norat T, Vatten L. Body mass index and the risk of gout: a systematic review and dose–response meta-analysis of prospective studies. Eur J Nutr. 2014;53:1591–601.
67. Lee J, Lee J, Lee J, Jung S, Suh Y, Koh J, et al. Visceral fat obesity is highly associated with primary gout in a metabolically obese but normal weighted population: a case control study. Arthritis Res Ther. 2015;17(1):79.
68. Matsuura F, Yamashita S, Nakamura T, Nishida M, Nozaki S, Funahashi T, et al. Effects of visceral fat accumulation on uric acid metabolism in male obese subjects: visceral fat obesity is linked more closely to overproduction of uric acid than subcutaneous fat obesity. Metabolism. 1998;47(8):929–33.
69. Dessein P, Shipton E, Stanwix A, Joffe B, Ramokgadi J. Beneficial effects of weight loss associated with moderate calorie/carbohydrate restriction, and increased proportional intake of protein and unsaturated fat on serum urate and lipoprotein levels in gout: a pilot study. Ann Rheum Dis. 2000;59:539–43.
70. Romero-Talamás H, Daigle C, Aminian A, Corcelles R, Brethauer SA, Schauer PR. The effect of bariatric surgery on gout: a comparative study. Surg Obes Relat Dis. 2014;10:1161–5.
71. Dalbeth N, Chen P, White M, Gamble G, Barratt-Boyes C, Gow P, et al. Impact of bariatric surgery on serum urate targets in people with morbid obesity and diabetes: a prospective longitudinal study. Ann Rheum Dis. 2014;73:797–802.
72. Kim S, Liu J, Solomon D. Risk of incident diabetes in patients with gout: a cohort study. Arthritis Rheum. 2015;67(1):273–80.
73. Rho Y, Lu N, Peloquin C, Man A, Zhu Y, Zhang Y, et al. Independent impact of gout on the risk of diabetes among women and men: a population based, BMI-matched cohort study. Ann Rheum Dis. 2016;75(1):91–5.
74. Lai H-M, Chen C-J, Yu-Jih Su B, Chen Y-C, Yu S-F, Yen J-H, et al. Gout and type 2 diabetes have a mutual inter-dependent effect on genetic risk factors and higher incidences. Rheumatology. 2012;51:715–20.
75. Wang L, Sawhney M, Zhao Y, Carpio G, Fonseca V, Shi L. Association between colchicine and risk of diabetes among veterans affairs population with gout. Clin Ther. 2015; doi:10.1016/j.clinthera.2015.03.010.
76. Stamp L, Ha L, Searle M, O'Donnell J, Frampton C, Chapman P. Gout in renal transplant recipients. Nephrology. 2006;11:367–71.
77. Stamp L, Searle M, O'Donnell J, Chapman P. Gout in solid organ transplantation: a challenging clinical problem. Drugs. 2005;65(18):2593–611.
78. Campion E, Glynn R, DeLabry L. Asymptomatic hyperuricaemia: risks and consequence in the normative aging study. Am J Med. 1987;82:421–6.
79. Naesens M, Kuypers D, Sarwal M. Calcineurin Inhibitor Nephrotoxicity. Clin J Am Soc Nephrol. 2009;4(2):481–508.
80. Wluka A, Ryan P, Miller A, Richardson M, Bergin P, Page J, et al. Post-cardiac transplantation gout: incidence and therapeutic complications. J Heart Lung Transplant. 2000;19:951–6.
81. Ducloux D, Schuller V, Bresson-Vautrin C, Chalopin JM. Colchicine myopathy in renal transplant recipients on cyclosporin. Nephrol Dial Transplant. 1997;12:2389–92.
82. Kuo C, Grainge M, Mallen C, Zhang W, Doherty M. Comorbidities in patients with gout prior to and following diagnosis: case-control study. Ann Rheum Dis. 2014; doi:10.1136/annrheumdis-2014-206410.
83. Schlesinger N, Radvanski D, Cheng J, Kostis J. Erectile dysfunction is common among patients with gout. J Rheumatol. 2015;42(10):1893–7.
84. Hsu C-Y, Lin C-L, Kao C-H. Gout is associated with organic and psychogenic erectile dysfunction. Eur J Intern Med. 2015;26:691–5.
85. Kim S, Liu J, Solomon D. Risk of incident atrial fibrillation in gout: a cohort study. Ann Rheum Dis. 2015; doi:10.1136/annrheumdis-2015-208161.
86. Changchien T-C, Yen Y-C, Lin C-L, Lin M-C, Liang J-A, Kao C-H. High risk of depressive disorders in patients with gout: a nationwide population-based cohort study. Medicine. 2015;94(52):e2401.

87. Huang C-C, Huang P-H, Chen J-H, Lan J-L, Tsay G, Lin H-Y, et al. An independent risk of gout on the development of deep vein thrombosis and pulmonary embolism: a nationwide population-based cohort study. Medicine. 2015;94(51):e2143.
88. Hong J-Y, Lan T-Y, Tang G-J, Tang C-H, Chen T-J, Lin H-Y. Gout and the risk of dementia: a nationwide population-based cohort study. Arthritis Res Ther. 2015;17(1):139.
89. Lu N, Dubreuil M, Zhang Y, Neogi T, Rai SK, Ascherio A, et al. Gout and the risk of Alzheimer's disease: a population-based, BMI-matched cohort study. Ann Rheum Dis. 2016;75(3):547–51.
90. Ungprasert P, Srivali N, Thongprayoon C. Gout is not associated with a lower risk of Parkinson's disease: a systematic review and meta-analysis. Parkinsonism Relat Disord. 2015;21(10):1238–42.
91. Pakpoor J, Seminog O, Ramagopalan S, Goldacre M. Clinical associations between gout and multiple sclerosis, Parkinson's disease and motor neuron disease: record-linkage studies. BMC Neurol 2015;15(1):art16, 1–6.
92. Zhang W, Doherty M, Bardin T, Pascual E, Barskova V, Conaghan P, et al. EULAR evidence based recommendations for gout. Part II: management. Report of a task force of the EULAR Standing Committee for International Clinical Studies Including Therapeutics (ESCISIT). Ann Rheum Dis. 2006;65(10):1312–24.
93. Cappellini M, Fiorelli G. Glucose-6-phosphate dehydrogenase deficiency. Lancet. 2008;37:64–74.
94. McDonagh E, Thorn C, Callaghan J, Altman R, Klein T. PharmGKB summary: uric acid-lowering drugs pathway, pharmacodynamics. Pharmacogenet Genomics. 2014;24:464–76.

Chapter 9
Osteoarthritis

Cristina Hernández-Díaz, Natasja van Schoor, and Adham Aboul Fotouh Khalil

Epidemiology

Osteoarthritis (OA) can be considered as a disease defined by characteristic structural alterations of the joint, including focal degradation of articular cartilage and remodeling of subchondral bone with the formation of osteophytes at the joint margins, as well as an illness defined by a person's symptoms, including pain, fatigue, mood alterations, and sleep disturbance [1].

The prevalence of OA depends on several factors such as the definition used and site of interest [2]. In the Hertfordshire Cohort Study, the only modest agreement between radiographic, clinical, and self-reported methods of diagnosis of knee OA (KOA) was observed [3]. The sites most affected by the disease are the knee, hip, and hand [2]. In the European Project on Osteoarthritis (EPOSA), using preharmonized data from population-based cohort studies from Germany, Italy, Sweden, the Netherlands, Spain, and the United Kingdom, 20.2% of the subjects aged 65–80 years had clinical OA of the knee, 6.1% had clinical OA of the hip, and 17.1% had clinical OA of the hand based on the American College of Rheumatology (ACR) criteria [4]. Using data from the National Health and Nutrition Examination Survey I (NHANES I), it was estimated that nearly 27 million adults from the United States aged 25 years or over had clinical OA of any joint [5].

C. Hernández-Díaz (✉)
Laboratorio de Ultrasonido Musculoesqueletico y Articular, Instituto Nacional de Rehabilitación, Calzada México-Xochimilco, Ciudad de México, Mexico
e-mail: cristy_hernandez@hotmail.com

N. van Schoor
Department of Epidemiology and Biostatistics, VU University Medical Center, EMGO Institute for Health and Care Research, Amsterdam, The Netherlands

A.A.F. Khalil
New Kasr El Aini Teaching Hospital, Cairo University, Cairo, Egypt

Y. El Miedany (ed.), *Comorbidity in Rheumatic Diseases*,
DOI 10.1007/978-3-319-59963-2_9

Pain, stiffness, and loss of movement and function are important reasons for patients to visit their family doctor [2]. According to the Global Burden of Disease 2010 study, hip and knee OA is one of the leading causes of disability. Out of 291 conditions, hip and knee OA was ranked as the 11th highest contributor to global disability and 38th highest in disability-adjusted life years (DALYs) [6]. Because of the aging of the population and consequent increase in the absolute number of older persons and as a consequence to the global epidemic of overweight and obesity, the number of persons with OA is expected to rise in the coming years [2, 6].

Obesity

Overweight and obesity are highly prevalent. Worldwide, the proportion of adults with a body mass index (BMI) of 25 kg/m^2 or greater increased between 1980 and 2013 from 28.8% to 36.9% in men and from 29.8% to 38.0% in women [7]. Overweight and obesity are important risk factors for OA because of the higher stress on weight-bearing joints. In a large population-based cohort using primary care records, 1,764,061 persons were followed for a median follow-up duration of 4.45 years [8]. In persons with normal weight (BMI < 25 kg/m^2), incidence rates (per 1000 person-years at risk) were 3.7, 1.7, and 2.6 for the knee, hip, and hand OA, respectively. In persons with obesity grade II (BMI ≥ 35 kg/m^2), the incidence rates were 19.5, 3.8, and 4.0, respectively [8]. For the knee, this is a more than five-fold increased risk. Interestingly, also an increased risk for hand OA was observed, indicating that the higher mechanical load on the joints is not the only explanation for the increased OA risk in case of overweight/obesity.

As weight is a modifiable risk factor, it is interesting to study the relationship between weight change and OA. The Framingham study showed that a weight reduction of 5 kg over a period of 10 years decreases the risk for developing KOA by more than 50% [9]. A systematic review suggests that weight loss following bariatric surgery may improve hip and knee pain in OA [10]. However, as the authors indicate, there is a paucity of evidence and large variability between studies.

Cardiovascular Disease

Cardiovascular disease (CVD) is the leading cause of death worldwide with stroke and myocardial infarction being among the main mortality factors. By 2030, mortality is expected to increase up to 23.3 million people with CVD. Several reports discussed the association of musculoskeletal symptoms with CVD, especially rheumatoid arthritis, fibromyalgia, and low back pain, as well as the association between CVD and obesity, diabetes, and smoking, which are related to OA [11].

Very little is known about the association between CVD and OA; its association has been described in elderly patients, but no prevalence has been described. Association has been attributed to several factors such as the arthritis-associated pain, muscle weakness, and NSAID prescription. [12]. By itself, OA pain can lead to immobility and consequently considered as an inherent risk for CVD. In concordance, muscle weakness can contribute to stopping physical activities, whereas medications to treat pain like nonsteroidal anti-inflammatory drugs (NSAIDs) are frequently associated with increased CVD risk. Chronic systemic-related inflammation due to inflammatory arthritis has been linked to both OA and CVD [11].

Patients known to have hypertension were assessed for a possible pathologic link to OA. It has been proposed that persistent hypertension promotes episodically reduced blood flow causing subchondral ischemia, especially at the end of long bones, as well as reduced interstitial blood flow in the small bones. These mechanisms can compromise nutrient and gas exchange into the cartilage surface, initiating degradative changes, apoptosis of osteocytes, and osteoclastic resorption [13–15].

Dyslipidemia and cholesterol levels can induce OA by an excessive amount of fatty acid in the bone. Similarly, the excessive intake of polyunsaturated fatty acids can cause bone marrow lesions. Both scenarios can lead to/influence hand and knee OA risk without a clear link with BMI. Earlier studies revealed that in women with hypercholesterolemia and hypertriglyceridemia, subchondral bone lesions can be detected as early as 2 years of the onset of these metabolic conditions [13, 16].

Impact of Comorbidity Outcomes in OA

Depending on the comorbidity, OA symptoms are linked to the underlying pathology whether inflammatory or mechanical (such as cartilage damage). For example, in metabolic syndrome patients, OA is mainly linked to chronic inflammation or an insulin-resistance state. Insulin resistance was found able to initiate cartilage damage; this state was also reported in patients with hyperglycemia and hyperinsulinemia [17].

Other studies revealed that overweight increases the risk of developing osteophytes and radiographic progression. In women, a 35% higher risk of KOA was observed when BMI increased 5 units. This relation was not clear for hip OA [17].

Also, dietary intake can influence developing of the cartilage as well as OA susceptibility. Nutrients such as vitamin D are linked to cartilage and bone metabolism. Results of earlier research studies showed that low levels of vitamin D increase the risk of hip OA, was associated with rapid progression of KOA, and predicted loss of joint space as well as increase osteophyte formation in KOA. Low levels of vitamin K were also associated with joint space narrowing and osteophyte formation, while low levels of vitamin C are related to increasing KOA progression and high levels prevent radiographic progression [17].

As mechanical stress is expected to impact mainly on the lower limb joints, living longer promotes cumulative joint loads; consequently, chondrocytes release inflammatory and degradation-promoting mediators that lead to cartilage matrix breakdown. However, this explanation is not fully adequate for OA joints of the hands. On the other hand, some theories suggest that osteoblasts release soluble mediators with deleterious effects which lead to cartilage breakdown. Another study suggested that adipose tissue may act as a specialized endocrine tissue which releases cytokines such as adiponectin, leptin, and visfatin that regulates glucose and adipocyte metabolism as well as inflammatory and immune responses, hence able to modulate the chondrocyte and osteoblast responses to cartilage breakdown. In hands' OA, this adipose tissue response might lead to the inflammatory reaction and radiographic progression; in the knee, Hoffa's fat pad would do the same job [16]. This association suggests a systemic link mediated by adipokines. This notion is supported by the results of studies carried out on patients with metabolic syndrome or any of its components. When having more than one component of the metabolic syndrome, there are much higher possibilities to develop hand or knee OA. In women, there is a higher risk for KOA when several components of the metabolic syndrome are present as compared with obesity alone; the similar additive effect was reported in OA of the hand joints, particularly in the combined presence of obesity and hypertension [16].

Diabetes was suggested as a possible mechanism to develop OA since 1961. Considering the several studies carried out to probe this association, glucose intolerance and the insulin-resistance state can increase the risk for KOA progression. The difference in the gender, joint affection distribution, and severity were attributed to hormonal and anatomical factors as well as the severity of the associated comorbidity. It has also been hypothesized that the association has been linked also to the decline in cell function with aging, pancreatic beta-cell decrease function, and senescent chondrocytes [13, 18].

Glucose is necessary for chondrocyte homeostasis. Elevation of the serum glucose level can disrupt chondrocyte metabolism mainly by losing the regulation of the expression of the main membrane glucose transporter (GLUT-1) and intracellular chondrocyte glucose uptake. As a result, larger amounts of reactive oxygen species (ROSs) start to form and generate glucose and pro-inflammatory cytokines, such as TNFα, which, in association with fibroblast-like synoviocyte (FLS) response, play a major role in promoting matrix cartilage breakdown and chondrocyte death. This is achieved by inducing metalloprotease 1 and 13 release which will initiate a catabolic program [releasing metalloprotease with thrombospondin motifs 4 and 5 (ADAMTS 4–5)] in an acute response reaction enhanced by TNFα and fibroblast-like synoviocyte (FLS) cellular exposure. Chronic hyperglycemia may increase nonenzymatic glycation reactions associated with oxidative stress that generates advanced glycation end products (AGEs) which eventually add to ROSs producing numerous inflammatory events (inflammation, tissue remodeling, apoptosis). Meanwhile, FLS secretes proteases into synovial fluid which contribute to the degradation of joint cartilage matrix. All the events get enhanced in advanced age patients known to have chronic diabetes. Insulin was reported not able to inhibit TNFα and IL1B.

Another theory suggests that glycation of cartilage leads to changing physical properties of the cartilage proteins and increase of the cartilage collagen stiffness network reducing its resistance to mechanical stress [14].

Clinical Manifestations Between OA and Comorbidities

Although OA is the disease that most commonly causes pain and physical disability, the real extension of the impact of its combination with other chronic diseases on the patient may lead to a greater impairment of the patients' physical functions and quality of life, in addition to worsening the prognosis of arthroplasties. Therefore, it is important to identify whether the patient's symptoms reflect the true severity of the osteoarthritic process or has been accentuated by the associated comorbidity(ies).

In OA, pain, stiffness, limited range of motion, and decreasing quality of life are the general signs and symptoms of the disease, not different for primary or secondary OA [19]. Usually, pain is the first and predominant symptom. Buckling of the knee joints and sometimes the feeling of instability could influence the fear of falling, poor balance confidence, and activity limitation. Similarly, varus-valgus motion and increasing pain while bending, as well as muscle weakness, are frequently associated with poor knee function [20, 21].

Hip OA pain is associated with limited function especially abduction strength; the symptom is not always present, but still the limited range of motion can be present. In the hand, the poor function and fist limitation with the loss of strength may be the reason for consulting [20, 21]. Foot OA presents in early stages associated with mechanical factors such as hallux valgus, first interphalangeal hyperextension, and decreased metatarsophalangeal dorsiflexion, all accompanied with loss of foot arch, which are the main signs; pain is usually the last symptom and consultation and is related to worse function or knee pain [20, 21].

Sedentary habits can impact the blood pressure by increasing it and limiting exercise habits. Multi-joint or single pain is related to OA severity, especially knee OA with no influence of BMI and obesity-associated factors; pain is often characterized by its quality, timing, antecedents, and consequences; and these characteristics are also associated with sleep quality and fatigue [15]. There has not been demonstrated that self-limited physical function is present when OA is related to obesity, CVD or osteoporosis; instead, obesity and CVD may affect musculoskeletal system limiting physical activity especially in the knee or hip for the elderly population [22, 23]. Another clinical aspect is the soft tissue rheumatism related initially to limited joint activity and therefore OA; in spite of this relation not well studied, it has been observed that a higher glucose level is related to a 5.5% risk of developing OA, but no clear association between soft tissue lesions and OA [24, 25] has been established.

Focusing attention on pain, chronic diabetes associated with neuropathy can increase pain perception and thus increase sensitivity and joint damage [16, 18].

The clinical and functional evaluation is the same as in primary OA; there are not any study that has described a different or specific clinical OA pattern that we are aware of; published data related to the influence of diabetes, hypertension, or dyslipidemia on OA progression or establishment have not proved clearly a different core set of symptoms; as we pointed before, these data center on the impact of the progression of OA (hand, knee, or hip mainly) related to pain and/or radiographic evolution with the associated disease [26, 27].

Imaging Between OA and Comorbidities

Despite the many studies on imaging in OA, there is relatively few relating OA with obesity and/or CVD. Imaging may help to identify whether the patient's symptoms reflect true joint damage or have been aggravated by the disease-associated comorbidities. Imaging can help identify the chronicity of the disease and the status of the underlying bones and rule out the presence of other local joint disorders. Furthermore, it is important to look for early signs in people without any symptom.

Imaging techniques such as conventional radiology (Rx) and ultrasound (US) are widely used to evaluate the disease, either in early or late stages, as well as magnetic resonance image (MRI) with relaxation time and T2 map generation. Each technique has set the benefits to using, and each has an advantage over the other. However, the whole scenario differs in the presence of comorbidities. For example, early in the disease course, and whatever diagnostic technique used, imaging signs of cartilage damage may not be related to the presence of pain in patients with metabolic diseases. However, later in the disease course, whether US or MRI was used to assess for the risk for developing OA or subclinical lesions, synovitis seen on US grayscale with power Doppler enhancement, or MRI with T2 relaxation time, had a clear association with the progression or development of knee OA, when compared to radiographic progression according to Kellgren-Lawrence (KL) score [27–29].

An MRI study on the hip in obese people without pain has demonstrated that bone marrow lesions can be present without any symptom, as well as the increasing of 6 mm in the acetabular weight for each year, that causes an increase in the body mass index, which lead to reduce cartilage volume and cartilage defects and bone marrow lesions located in the central region of the femoral head. This may be explained with the axial load and contact stress that obesity causes on the hip that can influence early cartilage defects and damage [30].

There is no data related to hand OA and comorbidity.

Medical Management Between OA and Comorbidity

Current treatment focuses on pain relief and/or control and cartilage damage reduction; with several guidelines and strategies handling both, no recommendations have been published in relation to managing OA patients who have an associated comorbidity(ies). Chronic disease management (CDM) or chronic disease care is the wide term used to refer to the treatment of people with chronic diseases.

CDM includes a variety of actions that involve a systematic approach to care planning, utilization of multiple treatment modalities tailored to the patient's needs, and use of multidisciplinary teams and if available health-care providers [31]. Such strategy in managing patients living with OA and comorbidities such as obesity, metabolic syndrome, diabetes, and CVD should be considered to help in overcoming the different challenges.

A meta-analysis performed by Brand et al. in 2014 [31] identified 13 randomized controlled trials that mainly focus on generalized or lower limb OA treatment sources or primary outcomes with or without surgical intervention; the interesting issues in this paper were the focus on knee and hip OA, physiotherapy outcomes, strength-training program outcomes, and the many ways a patient with OA can be treated. Unfortunately, none of these interventions may influence the outcome measures in the comorbidities when related to OA.

A smart approach can help to reduce cartilage damage; the individual approach is mandatory, and probably even in the lack of meta-analysis or controlled studies that associated OA with comorbidity treatment, the recommendations to reduce risk in each disease can help relieve OA pain.

Independent of the individualized medication related to OA and each of the comorbidities associated, physical activity or aerobic or resistance training is recommended [32]. As OA joint pain tends to migrate to adjacent joints, a positive impact of the physical training can be observed in the affected as well as the nearby non-affected joints [32]. In acute inflammation, local management of the affected joint might be the best approach. Patients with OA and comorbidities can exercise if adequate adaptations in the exercise program are made. In a randomized controlled trial carried out by de Rooij et al. [33] on knee OA and exercise therapy, the authors studied the impact of a supervised exercise program, of no more than 60 min a week, adapted to the state of the associated comorbid disease in each patient. Results reported significant improvement of the patients' physical as well as clinical status and revealed how educational and coaching strategies were important in maintaining patients' adherence to the exercise program and improving physical functioning.

While weight loss through physical training, combined with dietary counseling and restricted diet, was effective in reducing the mechanical load on the joints, amending such programs might be advised in the presence of associated comorbidities. Walking alone as an exercise for 40–60 min a day, at least 3–5 times a week, was recommended to maintain a healthy joint and muscle status as well as reduce the risk for CVD. Two studies carried out on OA patients revealed that the patients who kept on doing the exercise program for 2–5 years not only maintained their weight loss but also had a positive impact on other comorbidities such as cardiovascular disease, diabetes, and depression [33, 34].

On another front, if dyslipidemia was the main disease, training must be up to 120 min a week to reduce cholesterol levels. Intense exercise is better compared to moderate physical activities, and both aerobic and resistance training showed the best outcomes with significant positive impact on serum lipids level [34]. Recently, it has been reported that hip OA progression was reduced through time if patients are using statins to treat hypercholesterolemia, which is supported by the hypothesis that statins reduce subchondral bone ischemia thus causing cartilage degeneration [35]; however, further clinical controlled trials are needed to fully support this hypothesis.

Metabolic syndrome can be treated with physical activities with training programs that include walking, running, and cycling in different intensities; diet is another factor to add to the exercise program [34]. In diabetes the physical training increases insulin sensitivity and muscle glucose uptake, whereas leptin control in diet can contribute to reducing inflammatory parameters. This is attributed to the finding that skeletal muscles produce IL6 while exercising. Earlier studies revealed that this cytokine can regulate energy expenditure and lipolysis, appetite, as well as body composition. This also could be the reason why omega-3 and six unsaturated fatty acids are now being used as adjuvant treatment in OA. Furthermore, exercise induces smooth muscle relaxation and vasodilatation. In patients with associated neuropathy, attention should be paid to avoid foot ulcers or signs of ischemia [32–34].

Medication either for OA or the comorbid disease is mandatory to treat existent symptoms, and it requires individualized approach and follow-up, as needed; associations and secondary effects should be observed and a multidisciplinary approach established is required. The interaction between medications and the associated comorbidities will be discussed in a separate chapter later in this book.

Conclusions

Osteoarthritis is a multifactorial, multi-joint progressive disease. It requires individualized and multidisciplinary approach tailored to the patients' health status, considering the associated comorbidities before advising the management plan. Patients should be aware that it is not only a matter of pain but also a matter of function, quality of life, and long-term actions to keep a good joint health. Knowing how comorbid diseases influence cartilage damage is mandatory to improve strategies to keep cartilage healthy.

References

1. Hochberg MC. Osteoarthritis year 2012 in review: clinical. Osteoarthr Cartil. 2012;20:1465–9.
2. Bijlsma JW, Berenbaum F, Lafeber FP. Osteoarthritis: an update with relevance for clinical practice. Lancet. 2011;377:2115–26.
3. Parsons C, Clynes M, Syddall H, Jagannath D, Litwit A, van der Pas S, et al. How well do radiographic, clinical and self-reported diagnoses of knee osteoarthritis agree? Findings from the Hertfordshire cohort study. Spring. 2015;4:177.

4. van der Pas S, Castell MV, Cooper C, Denkinger M, Dennison EM, Edwards MH, et al. European project on osteoarthritis: design of a six-cohort study on the personal and societal burden of osteoarthritis in an older European population. BMC Musculoskelet Disord. 2013;14:138.
5. Lawrence RC, Felson DT, Helmick CG, Arnaold LM, Choi H, Deyo RA, et al. Estimates of the prevalence of arthritis and other rheumatic conditions in the United States. Part II. Arthritis Rheum. 2008;58:26–35.
6. Cross M, Smith E, Hoy D, Nolte S, Ackerman I, Fransen M, et al. The global burden of hip and knee osteoarthritis: estimates from the global burden of disease 2010 study. Ann Rheum Dis. 2014;73:1323–30.
7. Ng M, Fleming T, Robinson M, Thompson B, Graetz N, Margono C, et al. Global, regional, and national prevalence of overweight and obesity in children and adults during 1980–2013: a systematic analysis for the global burden of disease study 2013. Lancet. 2014;384:766–81.
8. Reyes C, Leyland KM, Peat G, Cooper C, Arden NK, Prieto-Alhambra D. Association between overweight and obesity and risk of clinically diagnosed knee, hip, and hand osteoarthritis: a population-based cohort study. Arthritis Rheumatol. 2016;68:1869–75.
9. Felson DT, Zhang Y, Anthony JM, Naimark A, Anderson JJ. Weight loss reduces the risk for symptomatic knee osteoarthritis in women. The Framingham study. Ann Intern Med. 1992;116:535–9.
10. Gill RS, Al-Adra DP, Shi X, Sharma AM, Birch DW, Karmali S. The benefits of bariatric surgery in obese patients with hip and knee osteoarthritis: a systematic review. Obes Rev. 2011;12:1083–9.
11. Hall JA, Stubbs B, Mamas AM, Myint PK, Smith TO. Association between osteoarthritis and cardiovascular disease: systematic review and meta-analysis. Eur J Prev Cardiol. 2016;23(3):938–46.
12. Rahman MM, Kopec JA, Cibere J, Goldsmith CH, Anis AH. The relationship between osteoarthritis and cardiovascular disease in a population health survey: a cross-sectional study. BMJ Open. 2013;3(5):pii:e002624
13. Piva SR, Susko AM, Samannaaz SK, Josbeno DA, Fitzgerald KG, FGS T. Links between osteoarthritis and diabetes: implications for management from physical activity perspective. Clin Geriatr Med. 2015;31(1):67–87.
14. Eymard F, Oarsons C, Edwards MH, Petit-Dop F, Reginster JY, Bruyére O, et al. Diabetes is a risk factor for knee osteoarthritis progression. Osteoarthr Cartil. 2015;23:851–9.
15. Chadha R. Revealed aspect of metabolic osteoarthritis. J Orthop. 2016;13:347–51.
16. Sellam J, Berenbaum F. Is osteoarthritis a metabolic disease? Joint Bone Spine. 2013;80:568–73.
17. Hamada D, Maynard R, Schott E, Drinkwater CJ, Ketz JP, Kates SL, et al. Insulin suppresses TNF-dependent early osteoarthritic changes associated with obesity and type 2 diabetes. Arthritis Rheumatol. 2016;68(6):1392–402.
18. Anton SD, Karabetian C, Naugle K, Buford TW. Obesity and diabetes as accelerators of functional decline; can lifestyle interventions maintain functional status in high risk older adults? Exp Gerontol. 2013;48(9):888–97. doi:10.1016/j.exger.2013.06.007.
19. Calvet J, Orellana C, Larrosa M, Navarro N, Chillaron JJ, Pedro-Botet J, et al. High prevalence of cardiovascular co-morbidities in patients with symptomatic knee or hand osteoarthritis. Scand J Rheumatol. 2015;27:1–4.
20. Hooper MH, Moskowitz R. Chapter 7. Osteoarthritis: clinical presentations. In: Kluwer W, editor. Osteoarthritis, diagnosis, and medical/surgical management. 4th ed. Philadelphia: Lippincott Williams & Wilkins. p. 139–45.
21. Sharma L. Osteoarthritis year in review 2015: clinical. Osteoarthr Cartil. 2016;24:36–48.
22. Zambon S, Siviero P, Denkinger M, Limongi F, Castell MV, van der Pas S, et al. Role of osteoarthritis, comorbidity, and pain in determining functional limitations in older populations: European project on osteoarthritis. Arthritis Care Res. 2016;6:801–10.
23. Duclos M. Osteoarthritis, obesity and type 2 diabetes: the weight of waist circumference. Ann Phys Rehabil Med. 2016;29:157–60.

24. Arkkila PE, Gautier JF. Musculoskeletal disorders in diabetes mellitus: an update. Best Prac Res Clin Rheumatol. 2004;17(6):945–70.
25. Kirkman MS. Osteoarthritis progression: is diabetes a culprit? Osteoarthr Cartil. 2015;23:839–40.
26. Adriaanse MC, Hanneke WD, van der Heide I, Struijs JN, Baan CA. The impact of comorbid chronic conditions on quality of life in type 2 diabetes patients. Qual Life Res. 2016;25:175–82.
27. Frey N, Hügle T, Jick SS, Meier CR, Spoendlin J. Type II diabetes and incident osteoarthritis of the hand: a population-base case-control analysis. Osteoarthr Cartil. 2016;24:1535–40.
28. Mathiesen A, Slatkowsky-Christensen B, Kvien TK, Berner-Hammer H, Haugen IK. Ultrasound-detected inflammation predicts radiographic progression in hand osteoarthritis after 5 years. Ann Rheum Dis. 2016; 75:825–30.
29. Jungmann PM, Kraus MS, Alizai H, Nardo L, Baum T, Nevitt MC, et al. Metabolic risk factors are associated with cartilage degradation assessed by T_2 relaxation time at the knee: data from the osteoarthritis initiative. Arthritis Care Res. 2013;62(12):1942–50.
30. Teichtahl AJ, Wang Y, Smith S, Wluka AE, Zhu M, Urquhart D, et al. Bone geometry of the hip is associated with obesity and early structural damage – a 3.0 T magnetic resonance imaging study of community-based adults. Arthritis Res Ther. 2015;17:112.
31. Brand CA, Ackerman IN, Tropea J. Chronic disease management: improving care for people with osteoarthritis. Best Prac Res Clin Rheumatol. 2014;28:119–42.
32. Pedersen BK, Saltin B. Exercise as medicine-evidence for prescribing exercise as therapy in 26 different chronic diseases. Scand J Med Sci Sports. 2015;25(Suppl 3):1–72.
33. de Rooij M, van der Leeden M, Cheung J, van der Esch M, Häkkinen A, Hverkamp D, et al. Efficacy of tailored exercise therapy on physical function in patients with knee osteoarthritis and comorbidity: a randomized controlled trial. Arthritis Care Res. 2016; doi:10.1002/acr.23013.
34. Sartori-Cintra AR, Aikawa P, Cintra DE. Obesity versus osteoarthritis: beyond the mechanical overload. Einstein (Sao Paulo). 2014;12(3):374–9.
35. Baker JF, Walsh P, Mulhall KJ. Statins: a potential role in the management of osteoarthritis? Joint Bone Spine. 2011;78:31–4.

Chapter 10
Sjögren's Syndrome

Sadik A. Khuder, Ibtisam Al-Hashimi, and Anand B. Mutgi

Sjögren's syndrome (SS) is an inflammatory systemic disease characterized by lymphocytic infiltration of the exocrine glands leading to a widespread exocrinopathy, often manifested as dry mouth and dry eyes [1, 2]. The prevalence of SS ranges from 0.05% to 4.8% worldwide with female to male prevalence of 9:1 [3, 4]. However, the majority of patients remain undiagnosed [1].

The pathophysiology and/or the triggering factor(s) of SS are not well known. A combination of genetic predisposition and viral infections has been proposed as potential triggering factor for the abnormal activation of the inflammatory response both locally and systemically in the exocrine glands [5]. It has been suggested that the pathogenesis of SS follows a typical multistep model of human autoimmune diseases, which is characterized by the loss of immunologic tolerance to self-antigens leading to the production of autoantibodies with subsequent emergence of autoimmune disease [6, 7]. Although the manifestations of SS can be mild and subclinical, it often compromises the overall health and well-being of the affected individuals [8]. SS can also be associated with serious and potentially life-threatening complications [9].

Clinical Manifestations

The clinical manifestation of SS varies widely, ranging from subclinical or mild sicca symptoms to a life-threatening disease. SS is primarily a disease of the exocrine glands that result in reduction in their secretory capacity and secretory

S.A. Khuder (✉) • A.B. Mutgi
Department of Medicine, The University of Toledo, Toledo, Ohio, USA
e-mail: sadik.khuder@utoledo.edu

I. Al-Hashimi
Deparment of Surgery, The University of Texas Southwestern Medical Center, Dallas, Texas

Y. El Miedany (ed.), *Comorbidity in Rheumatic Diseases*,
DOI 10.1007/978-3-319-59963-2_10

products. The exocrine system includes not only the salivary and lacrimal glands but also all the mucus secreting glands in the respiratory and gastrointestinal systems, the vagina, sweat glands, gallbladder, and digestive enzymes in the liver and pancreas [1]. The reduction of the secretory fluids of the exocrine glands compromises the homeostasis, functions, and the physiology of the entire body.

There are two types of SS, primary SS (pSS) and secondary SS (sSS). pSS affects primarily the exocrine glands, while sSS affects the exocrine system in conjunction with connective tissue and/or autoimmune disease [10]. Both pSS and sSS might also be associated with fibromyalgia, thyroid disease, Raynaud's syndrome, vasculitis, peripheral neuropathy, or glomerulonephritis [11]. Severe extraglandular manifestations are observed in 15% of SS patients [12] and might occur early or late in the course of the disease [13]. Due to the broad distribution of the exocrine system, the initial manifestations of SS may appear unrelated, which often delays the diagnosis, especially when the classic clinical findings of xerostomia and xerophthalmia are not the presenting manifestation of the disease [14].

Sjögren's syndrome is an under-recognized condition, and its classical sicca symptoms (dry mouth and dry eyes) are often dismissed as medications side effect. Consequently, SS remains underdiagnosed, and its associated comorbidities are overlooked leading to poor quality of life and serious complications. Improving our understanding of SS and its associated comorbidities might increase awareness of healthcare providers and facilitate timely diagnosis of the disease. Appropriate timely diagnosis of SS would allow for a more efficient treatment and minimize the potential of life-threatening complications.

Sjögren's Syndrome-Associated Comorbidities

A part from the comorbidity associated with dry eyes and dry mouth, approximately 20–40% of SS patients experience other comorbidities that extend beyond the exocrine glands. At least one third of SS patients has additional extraglandular manifestations such as neurological, vascular, or fatigue [4]. SS-associated comorbidities might be manifested as lymphocytic infiltration of the lung, liver, or kidneys or as vasculitis, peripheral neuropathy, and/ or by immune complex-mediated glomerulonephritis [11]. Sjögren's syndrome-associated comorbidities can be sufficiently serious to cause increase in mortality rate. A recent meta-analysis attributed the increased mortality among SS patients to three main causes: cardiovascular events, infections, and malignant lymphoproliferative disorders [15]. The following sections summarize the prevalence and clinical manifestation of comorbid conditions in SS, and their impact on patients' overall health and well-being.

Gastrointestinal (GI), Liver, Gallbladder, and Pancreas

The entire gastrointestinal tract may be involved in SS. SS has been associated with a broad spectrum of organic GI diseases, including gastroesophageal reflux, esophagitis, chronic atrophic gastritis, and celiac disease [16]. GI symptoms have been reported to affect a large number of SS patients and are frequently debilitating [17, 18]. Various gastrointestinal symptoms occur including epigastric pain, nausea, and dyspepsia; due to chronic atrophic gastritis; and cramps and constipation from the involvement of the small and large intestines [19, 20].

Patients with SS are at an increased risk for gastroesophageal reflux disease [21]. The reduction in the production of the exocrine secretory fluids, including saliva, mucus, bile, digestive enzymes (liver and pancreas), and hypochlorhydria, results in delayed digestion and stomach emptying, which might contribute to the occurrence of esophageal and dyspeptic diseases. Gastroesophageal acid reflux provokes symptoms that may include difficulty swallowing, persistent heartburn, delayed digestion, regurgitation of acid, with extra-esophageal complications including cough, laryngitis, asthma, and dental erosion [22]. The pathogenesis of gastroesophageal reflux disease is multifactorial and includes motor abnormalities, such as impaired lower esophageal sphincter resting tone and delayed gastric emptying; anatomical factors, such as hiatal hernia; impaired mucosal resistance; and visceral hypersensitivity [23]. Signs of gastroparesis and functional dyspepsia are higher among SS patients than the general population [24, 25].

Esophageal hypomotility and delayed gastric emptying have also been reported in SS [26]. Due to the combination of difficulty in swallowing and impaired esophageal motility, dysphagia occurs in approximately 75% of SS patients [27]. The low lubrication and prolonged pharyngeal transit time could also lessen the acid clearance capacity of the esophagus. Defective peristalsis is found in one third or more of SS patients, resulting in decreased or absent of contractility in the upper third of the esophagus [28]. Gastroesophageal reflux disease in patients with Sjögren's syndrome may not always be manifested as heartburn and acid regurgitation when it is caused by hypochlorhydria [29].

SS patients may also develop dysmotility in the small and large intestines; a significant number of the patients suffer from irritable bowel syndrome (IBS) [30]. Other SS-associated gastrointestinal symptoms include colitis, pancreatitis, gastritis, and celiac disease [31]. Celiac disease appears more frequently among SS patients than the general population. Studies have shown that the incidence of celiac disease is ten-fold higher among SS patients than non-SS population [32]. Gastrointestinal manifestations, and in particular gastroesophageal reflux, may be the initial presentation of SS, but they may also be related to medication treatment [21].

Pulmonary

Pulmonary manifestations are among the most prevalent complications in SS. The reported prevalence rate of pulmonary involvement varies usually between 9% and 75%, depending on the methods of detection and patient selection [33]. Moreover, SS patients have 3.2 fold increases in respiratory failure compared to the general population [34]. Pulmonary lesions, such as diffuse interstitial fibrosis, recurrent pneumonitis, pleural effusions, and suspected lymphoma or pseudolymphoma were observed in patients with SS [35]. Progressive pulmonary inflammation leads to airway obstruction [36, 37], alveolitis [38], interstitial fibrosis [35], and pulmonary arterial hypertension [39, 40] and lymphoma. The positive association of SS with ailments in airways, alveoli, interstitia, and vessels of the lung may explain the high incidence of respiratory failure and lung impairment in SS patients [41, 42]. Routine chest CT scans of SS patients revealed varying abnormalities in 34–50% of patients [43, 44]. The common patterns of lung involvement identified with high-resolution CT scan included honeycomb formation, ground-glass attenuation, centrilobular nodules, reticular pattern, and bronchiectasis [45]. Although patients with SS may present with the entire spectrum of interstitial lung disease (nonspecific interstitial pneumonia, usual interstitial pneumonia, and cryptogenic organizing pneumonia), the most frequent disorder is lymphocytic interstitial pneumonia [46]. Airway abnormalities include follicular bronchitis, bronchiectasis, and bronchiolitis. Pulmonary inflammation, mainly alveolar lymphocytosis, was detected in 55% of the patients using bronchoalveolar lavage as a screening test in patients without any respiratory symptoms [47].

Pulmonary involvement in SS may be manifested as chest pain (pleuritis), interstitial pneumonia, and lung fibrosis (cough and shortness of breath). Among the variety of histologic patterns observed in SS are interstitial pneumonia, nonspecific interstitial pneumonia, bronchiolitis, and amyloidosis [48]. The lesions may involve the trachea, bronchi, and bronchioles [49]. Small airways disease, such as follicular bronchiolitis, is a common histologic finding in patients with pulmonary involvement in SS. Impairment and destruction of the pulmonary exocrine glands could be due to the lymphocytic infiltration of the respiratory tract. Despite being the most frequent complication, pulmonary manifestations in SS generally develop late in the course of disease and are rarely the presenting feature [46]. Patients who have related lung diseases have reduced quality of life and compromised physical functionality; they are also at four-fold higher risk for mortality within10 years following of the diagnosis [50].

Neurological

Varieties of neuropathies have been reported with SS including sensory, peripheral, and cranial and myelopathic neuropathies. In addition to central nervous system (CNS) involvement, other neuropathic patterns may include polyradiculopathies, mononeuritis multiplex, autonomic neuropathies, and cranial neuropathies [51]. Neurological involvement could be due to the direct lymphocytic infiltration of the central nervous tissue, vascular injury caused by anti-neuronal and anti-SSA antibodies, and/or as a result of ischemia secondary to small vessel vasculitis [52]. The neurological manifestations may precede the onset of SS in 40–80% of patients [51].

The prevalence of neurological manifestations in SS ranges between 10% and 60%, with pure or predominantly sensory polyneuropathies as the most common neurological manifestations [53]. Mononeuropathy multiplex, polyradiculopathy, symptomatic dysautonomia, cranial neuropathy, myopathy, and central nervous system involvement are less common [54].

Several neuropathy subtypes have been described in SS patients. Sensory, sensorimotor, and small fiber neuropathy (SFN) are the most common types seen in SS [51]. Sensory disturbances due to small fiber dysfunction or loss include negative symptoms (such as thermal cutaneous hypoesthesia) and positive symptoms (such as spontaneous burning pain or thermal allodynia or hyperalgesia) [55].

The reported frequency of peripheral nervous system symptoms (PNS) in literature varies based on the patients' population and the objectives of the studies. PNS symptoms were reported to occur as frequently as 87% in patients exhibiting any type of neuropathy [56]. In patients with peripheral neuropathies, symptoms may include numbness, paresthesia, and/or pain in the extremities.

A pure sensory trigeminal neuropathy has been described in patients with SS [57, 58]. SS patients with pure sensory neuropathy display an abnormal blink reflex and a normal jaw jerk possibly due to damage involving the neurons of the Gasser ganglion where the trigeminal sensory neurons conducing cutaneous stimuli are located [59].

SS patients may suffer from changes in visual acuity or disturbances in visual quality as a result of optic neuropathy, which may occur before or at the same time as the diagnosis of SS [60]. It has been reported that anti-Ro and anti-La autoantibodies might play a role in mediating or potentiating vascular injury in the central nervous system of SS patients [61].

Cardiovascular

Asymptomatic cardiac involvement is common in patients with SS, sclerosis of the aortic valve cusps and a slight aortic regurgitation are reported [62]. Although heart diseases are rarely reported in SS [63], clinical evidence suggests that SS patients have higher frequency of cardiovascular and metabolic abnormalities, such as altered lipid profiles, hypertriglyceridemia, increased LDL and uric acid, hypertension, atherosclerosis and increased risk for myocardial infarction; they also appear to have higher frequency of diabetes mellitus [33, 64–70].

Enhanced atherogenesis has also been reported in SS [65, 71, 72]. Several factors have been suggested as possible contributing factors for atherosclerosis in SS patients including the duration of the disease, joint involvement, Raynaud's phenomenon, leucopenia, anti-SSA/Ro and anti-SSB/La autoantibodies, and swelling of the salivary glands [65, 66, 73, 74]. The mechanism for atherosclerosis in SS is not clear. The dysregulation of T and B cell have been suggested to enhance the production of interferon α (IFNα), a central cytokine in SS, which could contribute to cardiovascular risk in SS patients [66]. The impairment of endothelial repair through accelerated apoptosis of endothelial progenitor cells, along with the enhancement of foam cell formation in the atherosclerotic plaque, could be due to the atherogenic potential of IFNα [75].

A great majority of SS patients have a restricted variability in both heart rate and blood pressure, both of which could be a symptom of cardiovascular autonomic nervous system dysfunction [76]. A few studies (and case reports) have reported pericarditis, systolic, and diastolic dysfunction of the left ventricle, valve disorders, and autoimmune myocarditis [62, 77–80]. Studies have also suggested that the incidence of valvular regurgitation, pericardial effusion, pulmonary hypertension, and increased left ventricular mass index are disproportionately higher in SS patients with and without clinical manifestations of heart disease.

It has been estimated that cardiovascular events occur in approximately 5–7.7% of SS patients including stroke, myocardial infarction, deep venous thrombosis, and, most frequently, arrhythmias [81–85]. Tricuspid regurgitation, injured mitral and/ or aortic valves, pulmonary hypertension, and increased left ventricular mass have also been reported [86].

SS patients are also at higher risk for stroke than the general population [64, 65]. Zoller and coworkers reported that hospitalization for SS was associated with an increased risk of ischemic or hemorrhagic stroke in Sweden [87]. Another study reported a significantly higher incidence of cerebrovascular (ischemic stroke) and cardiovascular events (heart attacks) compared to healthy controls, which could be also related to the fact that SS patients have higher prevalence of hypertension and hypercholesterolemia [67]. Only one study by Chiang and coworkers reported that SS is not associated with an increased risk of ischemic stroke [88].

Cutaneous

Nearly half of the patients with SS develop cutaneous manifestations, which may include dry skin, purpura, and/or urticaria-like lesions [89]. Dry skin (xerosis) is the most frequent and characteristic cutaneous manifestation of SS. Angular cheilitis is a common finding and is associated with xerosis and xerostomia [90].

Cutaneous vasculitis is common, specifically on lower extremities, and is often associated with serologic abnormalities [91]. Vasculitis is more common in patients with early onset of SS, and the prevalence increases in patients with a long duration of disease [92]. Adults with SS are also at a higher risk for shingles; it has been suggested that the use of medications could increase the risk for shingles in SS patients [93].

Autoimmune

Sjögren's syndrome is often associated with other autoimmune disorders such as autoimmune thyroid disease, multiple sclerosis, lupus erythematosus, scleroderma, spondyloarthropathy, myositis, or inflammatory rheumatoid arthritis [33, 62–65]. The prevalence of autoimmune diseases is also higher among individuals who have first-degree relative with SS or other autoimmune disease [67]. In general, individuals who suffer from one autoimmune disease have a higher probability of being affected by other autoimmune disorders [68]. The increased susceptibility to another autoimmune disease could be an indication of a possible common pathogenic mechanism(s) among various autoimmune diseases. SS shares several clinical and laboratory findings with lupus erythematosus and rheumatoid arthritis, such as polyclonal hypergammaglobulinemia, circulating autoantibodies, chronic inflammation, and frequent joint involvement during the course of disease [69].

Thyroid Disorders

One in two SS patients has clinical or subclinical thyroid disease with greater incidence in primary than secondary SS [1]. Autoimmune thyroid disease (AITD), thyroid dysfunction, and the presence of thyroid antibodies are well documented in patients with SS [94]. The most common cause of thyroiditis is Hashimoto's disease [95, 96]. There is literature evidence for the coexistence of thyroiditis with SS [97, 98]. A 24% increase in the risk of hypothyroidism was reported among hospitalized SS patients [33].

The risk for SS is significantly increased in female patients with thyroid diseases, particularly those in their mid-40s to mid-60s [99].

Though an endocrine organ, the thyroid gland is histologically and functionally similar to the lacrimal and salivary glands [100], and the histopathologic changes in SS and autoimmune thyroiditis display similar lymphocytic infiltration [101, 102].

Chronic Fatigue

Fatigue is one of the most common systemic manifestations of SS [94]. The reported prevalence ranges between 38% and 88% of the patients [103–106]. Fatigue is therefore a major contributor to the impaired quality of life seen in SS patients [107]. Younger age, xerostomia, and pain are significantly correlated with fatigue [108].

Results of studies using multidimensional assessment tools suggest that physical/somatic fatigue is more severe and more prevalent than mental fatigue. One study reported that 96% of SS patients suffer from significant physical fatigue while only 48% of patients report significant mental fatigue [105]. Another study examined fatigue in SS, using the Multidimensional Fatigue Inventory (MFI), found that SS patients were more fatigued than healthy controls in three dimensions (the "general fatigue," "physical fatigue," and the "reduced activity" dimension), but there were no differences between patients and controls in the "reduced motivation" and "mental fatigue" dimensions [109].

Several studies have shown correlations between the levels of fatigue and various surrogate "disease activity" markers such as serum levels of immunoglobulins, lymphocyte counts, and ANA and anti-Ro (SSA) antibodies [105, 110, 111]. It has been suggested that IL-6 might play an important role in the pathogenesis of fatigue in SS. Serum IL-6 correlates inversely with general fatigue domain of MFI in patients with detectable levels of serum IL-6 [112]. Associations between fatigue and arthralgia/myalgia, fibromyalgia, both state and trait anxiety scores, depression, and neuroticism, as well as impaired sleep patterns were also suggested as potential contributors to the fatigue symptoms [113]. Studies have shown that pSS patients have a significantly higher level of sleep deficit [114, 115].

Muscle involvement may occur in the course of SS. A study by Colafrancesco et al. reported that 1.3% of SS patients showed muscle weakness [116]. However, only small number of patients with myalgia exhibited changes in (CPK) serum level and electromyography.

Psychological

Approximately 20% of SS patients develop cognitive impairments such as dementia, lack of concentration, memory loss, and various psychiatric disorders [117–119]. Approximately 12% of hospitalized SS patients suffer from depression, and there is an 18% increase in the risk of depression in these patients [33]. About 33% of the patients suffer from clinical anxiety [120], although anxiety is more common than depression [121]. Both anxiety and/or depression generally show a negative effect on quality of life [122].

Headaches

The prevalence of headaches in SS remains controversial. A large cohort study reported no significant difference in the frequency of headaches among SS patients compared to healthy controls [123]. However, other studies have reported significant differences in prevalence of headaches in SS patients than healthy controls [123, 124]. Both the magnitude and severity of the impact were considerably higher among SS patients than non- Sjögren's headache sufferers [123].

Gynecological

Gynecologic symptoms are common in SS and can be a significant source of morbidity [125]. The prevalence of vaginal dryness, dyspareunia, and reduced sexual drive are high in women with SS, especially among women with vulvar and vaginal dryness. Studies have shown that women with SS have impaired sexual function and more sexual distress compared with healthy controls; approximately 68% of SS patients report changes in their sexual ability because of the dryness. Sexual dysfunction and distress are influenced by vaginal dryness as well as psychosocial factors [126], some of which might be worsened by menopausal status.

Renal Involvement

A significant number of SS patients report frequent urinary tract infections. The prevalence of renal involvement varies greatly from 4.2% [127] to 67% [127, 128]. Tubulointerstitial nephritis (TIN) is the most common presentation of renal involvement in SS. TIN is the result of epithelial disease with a predominantly mononuclear lymphocytic infiltration with CD4/CD8 T cell [128, 129] and is often characterized by distal renal tubular acidosis (dRTA) [130]. Several case series reports have suggested a decreased bone mineral density in SS patients with dRTA [131, 132]. The incidence of osteomalacia in SS patients with renal tubular acidosis ranges between 25% and 45% [133].

Glomerular involvement is less commonly observed in SS. The most common glomerular disease is mesangioproliferative glomerulonephritis, which is caused by the deposition of immune complexes, most frequently cryoglobulins. Previous studies suggested that 64% of all patients with glomerulonephritis were due to cryoglobulinemia [134]. Glomerulonephritis tends to occur at a later stage of the disease course than TIN and may be associated with the development of lymphoma [134, 135].

Osteoporosis and Changes in Bone Mineral Composition

Patients with primary SS share a number of clinical and serological features which theoretically could predispose to decrease in bone mineralization; these include low vitamin D levels, hypercalciuria related to underlying interstitial nephritis, steroid use for systemic involvement, and coexistence with other organ-specific autoimmune disorders known to increase osteoporosis risk, such as primary biliary cirrhosis and celiac disease [127, 136].

Almost two thirds of patients with SS have evidence of impaired bone density, which may be attributed in part to the presence of traditional risk factors as well as disease-related features [66]. Several case series reported low bone mineral density (BMD) in patients with SS [131, 132].

Lymphoma and Other Malignancies

Among autoimmune diseases, SS has the highest incidence of malignant lymphoproliferative transformation, and these malignancies are the most serious complication of the disease. SS is often considered an intermediate between autoimmune disease and lymphoproliferative disorder [137]. The prevalence of lymphoma in SS ranges from 4% to 9% [138–140]. Lymphoma in SS might be localized in extranodal areas such as salivary glands, the gastrointestinal tract, the thyroid gland, lungs, kidneys, or orbit [9]. There is also an increased incidence of lymphoma with extensive mediastinal adenopathy [139].

Studies have suggested that SS patients show a 2.6-fold greater risk for developing a malignancy and a 37.5-fold greater risk for developing non-Hodgkin's lymphoma (NHL) compared to healthy individuals [141]. NHL affects 5–10% of pSS patients [137, 142–144]; patients with sSS are at a higher risk for lymphoma than patients with pSS. Age and sex-adjusted standardized mortality ratio of SS with and without NHL is 3.25 and 1.08, respectively, which suggest that patients with SS have a shorter life expectancy [138].

SS patients are also at nine-fold higher risk for developing diffuse large B-cell lymphoma in the lymph nodes or extranodal sites [145–149]. Indolent extranodal marginal zone B-cell lymphoma of the mucosa-associated lymphoid tissue (MALT) has been identified as the most common SS-associated lymphoma subtype, whereas MALT lymphoma (MALTL) in the salivary gland is consistently associated with underlying SS [137, 140, 146, 150]. Marginal zone lymphoma was reported to associate with SS [151] and to lesser extent diffuse large B-cell lymphoma (DLBCL). Malignant lymphoma is thought to be a consequence of the inflammation, which promotes the release of cytokines that cause B-lymphocyte proliferation [152]. Over the years, B-cell hyperplasia could subsequently progress to MALT lymphoma [153]. Low C4 levels and palpable purpura were found to be associated with increased risk for malignancy [142]. Other risk factors for lymphoma include persistent parotid glands enlargement, splenomegaly, lymphadenopathy, leg ulcers, peripheral nerve involvement, anemia, neutropenia, low-grade fever, low levels of C3, and mixed cryoglobulinemia [147]. B-cell-activating factor (BAFF), a member of the tumor necrosis factor family, enhances the survival of B cells and was found to be overexpressed in SS and lymphomas [154]. Human herpesvirus-6 and herpesvirus-8, and *Helicobacter pylori* have been proposed as potential contributing factors in the development of lymphoproliferative lesions [155, 156].

In addition to lymphoma, other organ malignancies can also occur in patients with SS such as lung, breast, gastrointestinal, gynecological, renal, and skin cancers [147, 157–160]. However, an increase in the incidence of these cancers has not been demonstrated.

Conclusions

In conclusion our review confirms that SS is associated with several comorbidities and that patients with SS have higher rate of hospitalization and mortality. Among the prevalent comorbidities in SS patients are pulmonary and cardiovascular diseases, neurological and thyroid disorders, cutaneous diseases, vasculitis, fatigue, psychological disorders, and lymphoma. The broad distribution of the comorbidities necessitates multidisciplinary approach for the treatment of SS patients. Optimal management of SS patients requires timely identification of risk factors for comorbidities, effective treatment of concurrent illness, and psychological distress in order to achieve a long-term control of the disease and improve patients' quality of life.

References

1. Al-Hashimi I. Sjögren's syndrome: diagnosis and management: review. Womens Health. 2007;3:107–22.
2. Khuder SA, Al-Hashimi I, Mutgi AB, Altorok N. Identification of potential genomic biomarkers for Sjögren's syndrome using data pooling of gene expression microarrays. Rheumatol Int. 2015;35:829–36.
3. Bowman SJ, Ibrahim GH, Holmes G, Hamburger J, Ainsworth JR. Estimating the prevalence among Caucasian women of primary Sjögren's syndrome in two general practices in Birmingham, UK. Scand J Rheumatol. 2004;33:39–43.
4. Vitali C, Bombardieri S, Jonsson R, Moutsopoulos HM, Alexander EL, Carsons SE, et al. Classification criteria for Sjögren's syndrome: a revised version of the European criteria proposed by the American-European consensus group. Ann Rheum Dis. 2002;61:554–8.
5. Nikolov NP, Illei GG. Pathogenesis of Sjögren's syndrome. Curr Opin Rheumatol. 2009;21:465–70.
6. Brennan MT, Sankar V, Leakan RA, Grisius MM, Collins MT, Fox PC, et al. Sex steroid hormones in primary Sjögren's syndrome. J Rheumatol. 2003;30:1267–71.
7. Kivity S, Arango MT, Ehrenfeld M, Tehori O, Shoenfeld Y, Anaya JM, et al. Infection and autoimmunity in Sjögren's syndrome: a clinical study and comprehensive review. J Autoimmun. 2014;51:17–22.
8. Thomas E, Hay EM, Hajeer A, Silman AJ. Sjögren's syndrome: a community-based study of prevalence and impact. Br J Rheumatol. 1998;37:1069–76.
9. Kassan SS, Moutsopoulos HM. Clinical manifestations and early diagnosis of Sjogren syndrome. Arch Intern Med. 2004;164:1275–84.
10. Al-Hashimi I, Khuder S, Haghighat N. Frequency and predictive value of the clinical manifestations in Sjögren's syndrome. J Oral Pathol Med. 2001;30:1–6.
11. Skopouli FN, Dafni U, Ioannidis JP, Moutsopoulos HM. Clinical evolution, and morbidity and mortality of primary Sjogren's syndrome. Semin Arthritis Rheum. 2000;29:296–304.
12. Baldini C, Pepe P, Quartuccio L, Priori R, Bartoloni E, Alunno A, et al. Primary Sjogren's syndrome as a multi-organ disease: impact of the serological profile on the clinical presentation of the disease in a large cohort of Italian patients. Rheumatology (Oxford). 2014;53:839–44.
13. Baldini C, Pepe P, Luciano N, Ferro F, Talarico R, Gossi S, et al. A clinical prediction rule for lymphoma development in primary Sjögren's syndrome. J Rheumatol. 2012;39:804–8.
14. Pavlakis PP, Alexopoulos H, Kosmidis ML, Mamali I, Moutsopoulos HM, Tzioufas AG, et al. Peripheral neuropathies in Sjögren's syndrome: a critical update on clinical features and pathogenetic mechanisms. J Autoimmun. 2012;39:27–33.
15. Singh AG, Singh S, Matteson EL. Rate, risk factors and causes of mortality in patients with Sjögren's syndrome: a systematic review and meta-analysis of cohort studies. Rheumatology (Oxford). 2016;55:450–60.
16. Palm Ø, Moum B, Gran JT. Estimation of Sjögren's syndrome among IBD patients: a six year post-diagnostic prevalence study. Scand J Rheumatol. 2002;31(3):140–5.
17. Tsianos EB, Vasakos S, Drosos AA, Malamou-Mitsi VD, Moutsopoulos HM. The gastrointestinal involvement in primary Sjögren's syndrome. Scand J Rheumatol. 1986;61:151–5.
18. Ostuni PA, Germana B, Di Mario F, Rugge M, Plebani M, De Zambiasi P, et al. Gastric involvement in primary Sjögren's syndrome. Clin Exp Rheumatol. 1993;11:21–5.

19. Sheikh SH, Shaw-Stiffel TA. The gastrointestinal manifestations of Sjögren's syndrome. Am J Gastroenterol. 1995;90:9–14.
20. Constantopoulos SH, Tsianos EV, Moutsopoulos HM. Pulmonary and gastrointestinal manifestations of Sjögren's syndrome. Rheum Dis Clin N Am. 1992;18:617–35.
21. Chang CS, Liao CH, Muo CH, Kao CH. Increased risk of concurrent gastroesophageal reflux disease among patients with Sjögren's syndrome: a nationwide population-based study. Eur J Intern Med. 2016;31:73–8.
22. Vakil N, van Zanten SV, Kahrilas P, Dent J, Jones R, Global Consensus Group. The Montreal definition and classification of gastroesophageal reflux disease: a global evidence-based consensus. Am J Gastroenterol. 2006;101:1900–20.
23. De Giorgi F, Palmiero M, Esposito I, Mosca F, Cuomo R. Pathophysiology of gastro-oesophageal reflux disease. Acta Otorhinolaryngol Ital. 2006;26:241–6.
24. Saito YA, Schoenfeld P, Locke GR III. The epidemiology of irritable bowel syndrome in North America: a systemic review. Am J Gastroenterol. 2002;97:1910–5. 35.
25. Hungin AP, Whorwell PJ, Tack J, Mearin F. The prevalence, patterns and impact of irritable bowel syndrome: an international survey of 40 000 subjects. Aliment Pharmacol Ther. 2003;17:643–50.
26. Park K, Haberberger RV, Gordon TP, Jackson MW. Antibodies interfering with the type 3 muscarinic receptor pathway inhibit gastrointestinal motility and cholinergic neurotransmission in Sjögren's syndrome. Arthritis Rheum. 2011;63:1426–34.
27. Anselmino M, Zaninotto G, Costantini M, Ostuni P, Ianniello A, Boccú C, et al. Esophageal motor function in primary Sjögren's syndrome: correlation with dysphagia and xerostomia. Dig Dis Sci. 1997;42:113–8.
28. Tsianos EB, Chiras CD, Drosos AA, Moutsopoulos HM. Oesophageal dysfunction in patients with primary Sjögren's syndrome. Ann Rheum Dis. 1985;44:610–3.
29. Ebert EC. Gastrointestinal and hepatic manifestations of Sjogren syndrome. J Clin Gastroenterol. 2012;46:25–30.
30. Ohlsson B, Scheja A, Janciauskiene S, Mandl T. Functional bowel symptoms and GnRH antibodies: common findings in patients with primary Sjögren's syndrome but not in systemic sclerosis. Scand J Rheumatol. 2009;38:391–3.
31. Teppo AM, Maury CP. Antibodies to gliadin, gluten and reticulin glycoprotein in rheumatic diseases: elevated levels in Sjögren's syndrome. Clin Exp Immunol. 1984;57:73–8.
32. Szodoray P, Barta Z, Lakos G, Szakall S, Zeher M. Coeliac disease in Sjögren's syndrome—a study of 111 Hungarian patients. Rheumatol Int. 2004;24:278–82.
33. Koch T, Al-Hashimi I, Koffman BM, Deshpande A, Khuder SA. Comorbidities associated with Sjögren's syndrome: results from the Nationwide Inpatient Sample. Univ Toledo J Med Sci. 2014;1:4–7.
34. Yeh JJ, Chen HJ, Li TC, Wong YS, Tang HC, Yeh TC, et al. Association between Sjogren's syndrome and respiratory failure: put airway, interstitia, and vessels close together: a national cohort study. PLoS One. 2014;9:e110783.
35. Strimlan CV, Rosenow EC 3rd, Divertie MB, Harrison EG Jr. Pulmonary manifestations of Sjögren's syndrome. Chest. 1976;70:354–61.
36. Segal I, Fink G, Machtey I, Gura V, Spitzer SA. Pulmonary function abnormalities in Sjögren's syndrome and the sicca complex. Thorax. 1981;36:286–9.
37. Ismael S, Wermert D, Dang-Tran KD, Venot M, Fagon JY, Diehl JL. Severe excessive dynamic airway collapse in a patient with primary Sjögren's syndrome. Respir Care. 2014;59:e156–9.
38. Dalavanga YA, Constantopoulos SH, Galanopoulou V, Zerva L, Moutsopoulos HM. Alveolitis correlates with clinical pulmonary involvement in primary Sjögren's syndrome. Chest. 1991;99:1394–7.
39. Asherson RA, Cervera R. Pulmonary hypertension, antiphospholipid antibodies, and syndromes. Clin Rev Allergy Immunol. 2007;32:153–8.
40. Launay D, Hachulla E, Hatron PY, Jais X, Simonneau G, Humbert M. Pulmonary arterial hypertension: a rare complication of primary Sjogren syndrome: report of 9 new cases and review of the literature. Medicine (Baltimore). 2007;86:299–315.

41. Chung WS, Lin CL, Ho FM, Li RY, Sung FC, Kao CH, et al. Asthma increases pulmonary thromboembolism risk: a nationwide population cohort study. Eur Respir J. 2014;43:801–7.
42. Konstantinides SV. Asthma and pulmonary embolism: bringing airways and vessels closer together. Eur Respir J. 2014;43:694–6.
43. Franquet T, Giménez A, Monill JM, Díaz C, Geli C. Primary Sjögren's syndrome and associated lung disease: CT findings in 50 patients. Am J Roentgenol. 1997;169:655–8.
44. Matsuyama N, Ashizawa K, Okimoto T, Kadota J, Amano H, Hayashi K. Pulmonary lesions associated with Sjögren's syndrome: radiographic and CT findings. Br J Radiol. 2003;76:880–4.
45. Ito I, Nagai S, Kitaichi M, Nicholson AG, Johkoh T, Noma S, et al. Pulmonary manifestations of primary Sjogren's syndrome: a clinical, radiologic, and pathologic study. Am J Respir Crit Care Med. 2005;171:632–8.
46. Cain HC, Noble PW, Matthay RA. Pulmonary manifestations of Sjögren's syndrome. Clin Chest Med. 1998;19:687–99.
47. Hatron PY, Wallaert B, Gosset D, Tonnel AB, Gosselin B, Voisin C, et al. Subclinical lung inflammation in primary Sjögren's syndrome. Relationship between bronchoalveolar lavage cellular analysis findings and characteristics of the disease. Arthritis Rheum. 1987;30:1226–31.
48. Yamadori I, Fujita J, Bandoh S, Tokuda M, Tanimoto Y, Kataoka M, et al. Nonspecific interstitial pneumonia as pulmonary involvement of primary Sjögren's syndrome. Rheumatol Int. 2002;22:89–92.
49. Papadimitraki ED, Kyrmizakis DE, Kritikos I, Boumpas DT. Ear-nose-throat manifestations of autoimmune rheumatic diseases. Clin Exp Rheumatol. 2004;22:485–94.
50. Palm O, Garen T, Bergen Enger T, Jensen JL, Lund MB, Aaløkken TM, et al. Clinical pulmonary involvement in primary Sjögren's syndrome: prevalence, quality of life and mortality-a retrospective study based on registry data. Rheumatology. 2013;52:173–9.
51. Chai J, Logigian EL. Neurological manifestations of primary Sjögren's syndrome. Curr Opin Neurol. 2010;23:509–13.
52. Tobón GJ, Pers JO, Devauchelle-Pensec V, Youinou P. Neurological disorders in primary Sjögren's syndrome. Autoimmune Dis. 2012;2012:645967.
53. Paşcalău NA, Cioară FL, Roşca E, MuŢiu G, Pobirci LO, Jinca CM, et al. Atypical case of Sjögren's syndrome with psychiatric and peripheral neurological disorder. Romanian J Morphol Embryol. 2016;57:307–11.
54. Santosa A, Lim AY, Vasoo S, Lau TC, Teng GG. Neurosjögren: early therapy is associated with successful outcomes. J Clin Rheumatol. 2012;18:389–92.
55. Lefaucheur JP, Wahab A, Plante-Bordeneuve V, Sene D, Měnard-Lefaucheur I, Rouie D, et al. Diagnosis of small fiber neuropathy: a comparative study of five neurophysiological tests. Neurophysiol Clin. 2015;45:445–55.
56. Tajima Y, Mito Y, Owada Y, Tsukishima E, Moriwaka F, Tashiro K. Neurological manifestations of primary Sjögren's Japanese patients. Intern Med. 1997;36:690–3.
57. Kaltreider HB, Talal N. The neuropathy of Sjögren's syndrome: trigeminal nerve involvement. Ann Intern Med. 1969;70:751–62.
58. Dumas M, Perusse R. Trigeminal sensory neuropathy. Oral Surg Oral Med Oral Pathol Oral Radiol Endod. 1999;87:577–82.
59. Valls-Sole J, Graus F, Font J, Pou A, Tolosa ES. Normal proprioceptive trigeminal afferents in patients with Sjögren's syndrome and sensory neuronopathy. Ann Neurol. 1990;28:786–90.
60. Wise CM, Agudelo CA. Optic neuropathy as an initial manifestation of Sjögren's syndrome. J Rheumatol. 1998;15:799–802.
61. Alexander EL, Ranzenbach MR, Kumar AJ, Kozachuk WE, Rosenbaum AE, Patronas N, et al. Anti-Ro(SS-A) autoantibodies in central nervous system disease associated with Sjögren's syndrome (CNS-SS): clinical, neuroimaging, and angiographic correlates. Neurology. 1994;44:899–908.
62. Rantapää-Dahlqvist S, Backman C, Sandgren H, Östberg Y. Echocardiographic findings in patients with primary Sjögren's syndrome. Clin Rheumatol. 1993;12:214–8.

63. Lee LA, Pickrell MB, Reichlin M. Development of complete heart block in an adult patient with Sjögren's syndrome and anti-Ro/SS-A autoantibodies. Arthritis Rheum. 1996;39:1427–9.
64. Lodde BM, Sankar V, Kok MR, Leakan AR, Tak PP, Pillemer SR. Serum lipid levels in Sjögren's syndrome. Rheumatology (Oxford). 2006;45:481–4.
65. Vaudo G, Bocci EB, Shoenfeld Y, Schillaci G, Wu R, Del Papa N, et al. Precocious intima-media thickening in patients with primary Sjögren's syndrome. Arthritis Rheum. 2005;52:3890–7.
66. Gravani F, Papadaki I, Antypa E, Nezos A, Masselou K, Ioakeimidis D, et al. Subclinical atherosclerosis and impaired bone health in patients with primary Sjogren's syndrome: prevalence, clinical and laboratory associations. Arthritis Res Ther. 2015;17:99.
67. Bartoloni E, Baldini C, Schillaci G, Quartuccio L, Priori R, Carubbi F, et al. Cardiovascular disease risk burden in primary Sjogren's syndrome: results of a population-based multicentre cohort study. J Intern Med. 2015;278:185–92.
68. Perez-De-Lis M, Akasbi M, Siso A, Diez-Cascon P, Brito-Zeron P, Diaz-Lagares C, et al. Cardiovascular risk factors in primary Sjögren's syndrome: a case–control study in 624 patients. Lupus. 2010;19:941–8.
69. Juarez M, Toms TE, de Pablo P, Mitchell S, Bowman S, Nightingale P, et al. Cardiovascular risk factors in women with primary Sjogren's syndrome: United Kingdom primary Sjögren's syndrome registry results. Arthritis Care Res. 2014;66:757–64.
70. Cruz W, Fialho S, Morato E, Castro G, Zimmermann A, Ribeiro G, et al. Is there a link between inflammation and abnormal lipoprotein profile in Sjögren's syndrome? Joint Bone Spine. 2010;77:229–31.
71. van Leuven SI, Franssen R, Kastelein JJ, Levi M, Stroes ES, Tak PP. Systemic inflammation as a risk factor for atherothrombosis. Rheumatology(Oxford). 2008;47:3–7.
72. Shoenfeld Y, Gerli R, Doria A, Matsuura E, Cerinic MM, Ronda N, et al. Accelerated atherosclerosis in autoimmune rheumatic diseases. Circulation. 2005;112:3337–47.
73. Gerli R, Vaudo G, Bocci EB, Schillaci G, Alunno A, Luccioli F, et al. Functional impairment of the arterial wall in primary Sjögren's syndrome: combined action of immunologic and inflammatory factors. Arthritis Care Res (Hoboken). 2010;62:712–8.
74. Atzeni F, Sarzi-Puttini P, Signorello MC, Gianturco L, Stella D, Boccassini L, et al. New parameters for identifying subclinical atherosclerosis in patients with primary Sjögren's syndrome: a pilot study. Clin Exp Rheumatol. 2014;32:361–8.
75. Kaplan MJ, Salmon JE. How does interferon-alpha insult the vasculature? Let me count the ways. Arthritis Rheum. 2011;63:334–6.
76. Kovács L, Papós M, Takács R, Róka R, Csenke Z, Kovács A, et al. Autonomic nervous system dysfunction involving the gastrointestinal and the urinary tracts in primary Sjögren's syndrome. Clin Exp Rheumatol. 2003;21:697–703.
77. Gyongyosi N, Pokorny G, Jambrik Z, Kovacs L, Makula E, Csanady M. Cardiac manifestations in primary Sjögren's syndrome. Ann Rheum Dis. 1996;55:450–4.
78. Levin MD, Zoet-Nugteren SK, Markusse HM. Myocarditis and primary Sjögren's syndrome. Lancet. 1999;354:128–9.
79. Yoshioka K, Tegoshi H, Yoshida T, Uoshima N, Kasamatsu Y. Myocarditis and primary Sjögren's syndrome. Lancet. 1999;354:1996.
80. Golan TD, Keren D, Elias N, Naschitz JE, Toubi E, Misselevich I, et al. Severe reversible cardiomyopathy associated with systemic vasculitis in primary Sjögren's syndrome. Lupus. 1997;6:505–8.
81. Haga HJ, Jacobsen EM, Peen E. Incidence of thromboembolic events in patients with primary Sjögren's syndrome. Scand J Rheumatol. 2008;37(2):127–9.
82. Pasoto SG, Chakkour HP, Natalino RR, Viana VS, Bueno C, Lianza AC, et al. Lupus anticoagulant: a marker for stroke and venous thrombosis in primary Sjögren's syndrome. Clin Rheumatol. 2012;31:1331–8.
83. Lodde BM, Sankar V, Kok MR, Leakan RA, Tak PP, Pillemer SR. Adult heart block is associated with disease activity in primary Sjögren's syndrome. Scand J Rheumatol. 2005;34:383–6.

84. Kang J, Lin H. Comorbidities in patients with primary Sjögren's syndrome: a registry-based case-control study. J Rheumatol. 2010;37:1188–94.
85. Ungprasert P, Srivali N, Kittanamongkolchai W. Risk of venous thromboembolism in patients with Sjögren's syndrome: a systematic review and meta-analysis. Clin Exp Rheumatol. 2015;33:746–50.
86. Vassiliou VA, Moyssakis I, Boki KA, Moutsopoulos HM. Is the heart affected in primary Sjögren's syndrome? An echocardiographic study. Clin Exp Rheumatol. 2008;26:109–12.
87. Zöller B, Li X, Sundquist J, Sundquist K. Risk of subsequent ischemic and hemorrhagic stroke in patients hospitalized for immune-mediated diseases: a nationwide follow-up study from Sweden. BMC Neurol. 2012;12:41.
88. Chiang CH, Liu CJ, Chen PJ, Huang CC, Hsu CY, Chan WL, et al. Primary Sjögren's syndrome and risk of ischemic stroke: a nationwide study. Clin Rheumatol. 2014;33:931–7.
89. Kittridge A, Routhouska SB, Korman NJ. Dermatologic manifestations of Sjögren syndrome. J Cutan Med Surg. 2011;15:8–14.
90. Bernacchi E, Amato L, Parodi A, Cottoni F, Rubegni P, De Pità O, et al. Sjögren's syndrome: a retrospective review of the cutaneous features of 93 patients by the Italian Group of Immunodermatology. Clin Exp Rheumatol. 2004;22:55–62.
91. Ramos-Casals M, Anaya JM, Garcia-Carrasco M, Rosas J, Bove A, Claver G, et al. Cutaneous vasculitis in primary Sjögren syndrome: classification and clinical significance of 52 patients. Medicine. 2004;83:96–106.
92. Ramos-Casals M, Solans R, Rosas J, Camps MT, Gil A, Del Pino-Montes J, et al. Primary Sjögren syndrome in Spain—clinical and immunologic expression in 1010 patients. Medicine. 2008;87:210–9.
93. Chen JY, Wang LK, Feng PH, Chu CC, Cheng TJ, Weng SF, et al. Risk of shingles in adults with primary Sjögren's syndrome and treatments: a nationwide population-based cohort study. PLoS One. 2015;10:e0134930.
94. Mavragani CP, Moutsopoulos HM. The geoepidemiology of Sjögren's syndrome. Autoimmun Rev. 2010;9:A305–10.
95. Biró E, Szekanecz Z, Czirják L, Dankó K, Kiss E, et al. Association of systemic and thyroid autoimmune diseases. Clin Rheumatol. 2006;25:240–5.
96. Chen WS, Lin HD, Su KY, Lin DC, Wang HP. A cohort study of autoimmune thyroid diseases in primary Sjögren's syndrome in northern Taiwan. Formosan J Rheumatology. 2007;21:20–5.
97. Coll J, Anglada J, Tomas S, Reth P, Goday A, Millan M, et al. High prevalence of subclinical Sjögren's syndrome features in patients with autoimmune thyroid disease. J Rheumatol. 1997;24:1719–24.
98. Robazzi TC, Adan LF. Autoimmune thyroid disease in patients with rheumatic diseases. Rev Bras Reumatol. 2012;52:417–30.
99. Lu MC, Yin WY, Tsai TY, Koo M, Lai NS. Increased risk of primary Sjögren's syndrome in female patients with thyroid disorders: a longitudinal population-based study in Taiwan. PLoS One. 2013;8:e77210.
100. Jara LJ, Navarro C, Brito-Zerón Mdel P, García-Carrasco M, Escárcega RO, Ramos-Casals M, et al. Thyroid disease in Sjögren's syndrome. Clin Rheumatol. 2007;26:1601–6.
101. Adamson TC 3rd, Fox RI, Frisman DM, Howell FV. Immunohistologic analysis of lymphoid infiltrates in primary Sjogren's syndrome using monoclonal antibodies. J Immunol. 1983;130:203–8.
102. Kromer G, Sundick RS, Schauenstein K, Hála K, Wick G. Analysis of lymphocytes infiltrating the thyroid gland of obese strain chickens. J Immunol. 1985;135:2452–7.
103. Haldorsen K, Bjelland I, Bolstad AI, Jonsson R, Brun JG. A five-year prospective study of fatigue in primary Sjögren's syndrome. Arthritis Res Ther. 2011;13:R167.
104. Theander L, Strombeck B, Mandl T, Theander E. Sleepiness or fatigue? Can we detect treatable causes of tiredness in primary Sjögren's syndrome? Rheumatology (Oxford). 2010;49:1177–83.

105. Segal B, Thomas W, Rogers T, Leon JM, Hughes P, Patel D, et al. Prevalence, severity, and predictors of fatigue in subjects with primary Sjögren's syndrome. Arthritis Rheum. 2008;59:1780–7.
106. Iannuccelli C, Spinelli FR, Guzzo MP, Priori R, Conti F, Ceccarelli F, et al. Fatigue and widespread pain in systemic lupus erythematosus and Sjögren's syndrome: symptoms of the inflammatory disease or associated fibromyalgia? Clin Exp Rheumatol. 2012;30(Suppl 74):117–21.
107. Champey J, Corruble E, Gottenberg JE, Buhl C, Meyer T, Caudmont C, et al. Quality of life and psychological status in patients with primary Sjögren's syndrome and sicca symptoms without autoimmune features. Arthritis Rheum. 2006;55:451–7.
108. Koh JH, Kwok SK, Lee J, Son CN, Kim JM, Kim HO, et al. Pain, xerostomia, and younger age are major determinants of fatigue in Korean patients with primary Sjögren's syndrome: a cohort study. Scand J Rheumatol. 2016;21:1–7.
109. Godaert GL, Hartkamp A, Geenen R, Garssen A, Kruize AA, Bijlsma JW, et al. Fatigue in daily life in patients with primary Sjögren's syndrome and systemic lupus erythematosus. Ann N Y Acad Sci. 2002;966:320–6.
110. Hansen B, Manthorpe R. Antibodies against SS-B/La and SS-A/Ro antigens in patients with primary Sjögren's syndrome. Scand J Rheumatol. 1986;61:93–7.
111. Bax HI, Vriesendorp TM, Kallenberg CG, Kalk WW. Fatigue and immune activity in Sjögren's syndrome. Ann Rheum Dis. 2002;61:284.
112. d'Elia HF, Bjurman C, Rehnberg E, Kvist G, Konttinen YT. Interleukin 6 and its soluble receptor in a central role at the neuroimmunoendocrine interface in Sjogren's syndrome: an explanatory interventional study. Ann Rheum Dis. 2009;68:285–6.
113. Karageorgas T, Fragioudaki S, Nezos A, Karaiskos D, Moutsopoulos HM, Mavragani CP. Fatigue in primary Sjögren's syndrome: clinical, laboratory, psychometric, and biologic associations. Arthritis Care Res (Hoboken). 2016;68:123–31.
114. Gudbjörnsson B, Karlsson-Parra A, Karlsson E, Hällgren R, Kämpe O. Clinical and laboratory features of Sjögren's syndrome in young women with previous postpartum thyroiditis. J Rheumatol. 1994;21:215–9.
115. Tishler M, Barak Y, Paran D, Yaron M. Sleep disturbances, fibromyalgia and primary Sjögren's syndrome. Clin Exp Rheumatol. 1997;15:71–4.
116. Colafrancesco S, Priori R, Gattamelata A, Picarelli G, Minniti A, Brancatisano F, et al. Myositis in primary Sjögren's syndrome: data from a multicentre cohort. Clin Exp Rheumatol. 2015;33:457–64.
117. Malinow KL, Molina R, Gordon B, Selnes OA, Provost TT, Alexander EL, et al. Neuropsychiatric dysfunction in primary Sjögren's syndrome. Ann Intern Med. 1985;103:344–50.
118. Bowman SJ, Pillemer S, Jonsson R, Asmussen K, Vitali C, Manthorpe R, et al. Revisiting Sjögren's syndrome in the new millennium: perspectives on assessment and outcome measures. Report of a workshop held on 23 March 2000 at Oxford, UK. Rheumatology (Oxford). 2001;40:1180–8.
119. Delalande S, de Seze J, Fauchais A-L, Hachulla E, Stojkovic T, Ferriby D, et al. Neurologic manifestations in primary Sjögren's syndrome: a study of 82 patients. Medicine (Baltimore). 2004;83:280–29.
120. Strombeck B, Ekdahl C, Manthorpe R, Jacobsson LT. Physical capacity in women with primary Sjögren's syndrome: a controlled study. Arthritis Rheum. 2003;49:681–8.
121. Milin M, Cornec D, Chastaing M, Griner V, Berrouiguet S, Nowak E, et al. Sicca symptoms are associated with similar fatigue, anxiety, depression, and quality-of-life impairments in patients with and without primary Sjögren's syndrome. Joint Bone Spine. 2016;83(6):681–5. pii:S1297-319X(15)00312-7.
122. Inal V, Kitapcioglu G, Karabulut G, Keser G, Kabasakal Y. Evaluation of quality of life in relation to anxiety and depression in primary Sjögren's syndrome. Mod Rheumatol. 2010;20:588–97.

123. Tjensvoll AB, Gøransson LG, Harboe E, Kvaløy JT, Omdal R. High headache-related disability in patients with systemic lupus erythematosus and primary Sjögren's syndrome. Eur J Neurol. 2014;21:1124–30.
124. Harboe E, Tjensvoll AB, Maroni S, Gøransson LG, Greve OJ, Beyer MK, et al. Neuropsychiatric syndromes in patients with systemic lupus erythematosus and primary Sjögren syndrome: a comparative population-based study. Ann Rheum Dis. 2009;68:1541–6.
125. Lehrer S, Bogursky E, Yemini M, Kase NG, Birkenfeld A. Gynecologic manifestations of Sjögren's syndrome. Am J Obstet Gynecol. 1994;170:835–7.
126. van Nimwegen JF, Arends S, van Zuiden GS, Vissink A, Kroese FG, Bootsma H. The impact of primary Sjögren's syndrome on female sexual function. Rheumatology (Oxford). 2015;54:1286–93.
127. Goules A, Masouridi S, Tzioufas AG, Ioannidis JP, Skopouli FN, Moutsopoulos HM. Clinically significant and biopsy-documented renal involvement in primary Sjögren syndrome. Medicine (Baltimore). 2000;79:241–9.
128. Bossini N, Savoldi S, Franceschini F, Mombelloni S, Baronio M, Cavazzana I, et al. Clinical and morphological features of kidney involvement in primary Sjögren's syndrome. Nephrol Dial Transplant. 2001;16:2328–36.
129. Matsumura R, Kondo Y, Sugiyama T, Sueishi M, Koike T, Takabayashi K, et al. Immunohistochemical identification of infiltrating mononuclear cells in tubulointerstitial nephritis associated with Sjögren's syndrome. Clin Nephrol. 1988;30:335–40.
130. Kobayashi T, Muto S, Nemoto J, Miyata Y, Ishiharajima S, Hironaka M, et al. Fanconi's syndrome and distal (type 1) renal tubular acidosis in a patient with primary Sjögren's syndrome with monoclonal gammopathy of undetermined significance. Clin Nephrol. 2006;65:427–32.
131. Aerts J, Vigouroux C, Fournier P, Cariou D, Pasquier P. Osteomalacia of renal origin disclosing Gougerot-Sjögren syndrome. Rev Med Intern. 1994;15:43–7.
132. Cherif E, Ben Hassine L, Kaoueche Z, Khalfallah N. Osteomalacia as inaugural manifestation of Sjögren syndrome. BMJ Case Rep. 2013;2013:pii:bcr2013201345.
133. Richards P, Chamberlain MJ, Wrong OM. Treatment of osteomalacia of renal tubular acidosis by sodium bicarbonate alone. Lancet. 1972;2:994–7.
134. Goules AV, Tatouli IP, Moutsopoulos HM, Tzioufas AG. Clinically significant renal involvement in primary Sjögren's syndrome: clinical presentation and outcome. Arthritis Rheum. 2013;65:2945–53.
135. Voulgarelis M, Skopouli FN. Clinical, immunologic, and molecular factors predicting lymphoma development in Sjögren's syndrome patients. Clin Rev Allergy Immunol. 2007;32:265–74.
136. Selmi C, Meroni PL, Gershwin ME. Primary biliary cirrhosis and Sjögren's syndrome: autoimmune epithelitis. J Autoimmun. 2012;39:34–42.
137. Zintzaras E, Voulgarelis M, Moutsopoulos HM. The risk of lymphoma development in autoimmune diseases: a meta-analysis. Arch Intern Med. 2005;165:2337–44.
138. Martel C, Gondran G, Launay D, Lalloué F, Palat S, Lambert M, et al. Active immunological profile is associated with systemic Sjögren's syndrome. J Clin Immunol. 2011;31:840–7.
139. Solans-Laque R, Lopez-Hernandez A, Bosch-Gil JA, Palacios A, Campillo M, Vilardell-Tarres M. Risk, predictors, and clinical characteristics of lymphoma development in primary Sjögren's syndrome. Semin Arthritis Rheum. 2011;41:415–23.
140. Voulgarelis M, Ziakas PD, Papageorgiou A, Baimpa E, Tzioufas AG, Moutsopoulos HM. Prognosis and outcome of non-Hodgkin lymphoma in primary Sjögren syndrome. Medicine. 2012;91:1–9.
141. Lazarus MN, Robinson D, Mak V, Møller H, Isenberg DA. Incidence of cancer in a cohort of patients with primary Sjogren's syndrome. Rheumatology. 2006;45:1012–5.
142. Ioannidis JPA, Vassiliou VA, Moutsopoulos HM. Long-term risk of mortality and lymphoproliferative disease and predictive classifi cation of primary Sjögren's syndrome. Arthritis Rheum. 2002;46:741–7.

143. Theander E, Manthorpe R, Jacobsson LT. Mortality and causes of death in primary Sjögren's syndrome: a prospective cohort study. Arthritis Rheum. 2004;50:1262–9.
144. Brito-Zeron P, Ramos-Casals M, Bove A, Sentis J, Font J. Predicting adverse outcomes in primary Sjögren's syndrome: identification of prognostic factors. Rheumatology (Oxford). 2007;46:1359–62.
145. Smedby KE, Vajdic CM, Falster M, Engels EA, Martinez-Maza O, Turner J, et al. Autoimmune disorders and risk of non-Hodgkin lymphoma subtypes: a pooled analysis within the InterLymph consortium. Blood. 2008;111:4029–38.
146. Royer B, Cazals-Hatem D, Sibilia J, Agbalika F, Cayuela JM, Soussi T, et al. Lymphomas in patients with Sjogren's syndrome are marginal zone B-cell neoplasms, arise in diverse extra-nodal and nodal sites, and are not associated with viruses. Blood. 1997;90:766–75.
147. Theander E, Henriksson G, Ljungberg O, Mandl T, Manthorpe R, Jacobsson LT. Lymphoma and other malignancies in primary Sjögren's syndrome: a cohort study on cancer incidence and lymphoma predictors. Ann Rheum Dis. 2006;65:796–803.
148. Kojima M, Tsukamoto N, Yokohama A, Suzuki Y, Shimizu K, Nishikawa M, et al. B-cell lymphoma associated with Sjögren's syndrome among Japanese patients: a clinicopathologic and immunohistochemical study of 15 cases. J Clin Exp Hematop. 2009;49:89–95.
149. Patel S, Kramer N, Cohen AJ, Rosenstein ED. Renal lymphoma: unusual lymphoproliferative manifestation of Sjogren's syndrome. J Rheumatol. 2013;40:102–3.
150. Baimpa E, Dahabreh IJ, Voulgarelis M, Moutsopoulos HM. Hematologic manifestations and predictors of lymphoma development in primary Sjögren syndrome: clinical and pathophysiologic aspects. Medicine (Baltimore). 2009;88:284–93.
151. Anderson LA, Gadalla S, Morton LM, Landgren O, Pfeiffer R, Warren JL, et al. Population-based study of autoimmune conditions and the risk of specific lymphoid malignancies. Int J Cancer. 2009;125:398–405.
152. Sun Y, Zhang W, Li B, Zou Z, Selmi C, Gershwin ME. The coexistence of Sjogren's syndrome and primary biliary cirrhosis: a comprehensive review. Clin Rev Allergy Immunol. 2015;48:301–15.
153. Schmid U, Helbron D, Lennert K. Development of malignant lymphoma in myoepithelial sialadenitis. Vrichows Arch A Pathol Anat Histol. 1982;395:11–43.
154. Hansen A, Lipsky PE, Dorner T. B-cell lymphoproliferation in chronic inflammatory rheumatic diseases. Nat Clin Pract Rheumatol. 2007;3:561–9.
155. Engels AE. Infectious agents as causes of non-Hodgkin lymphoma. Cancer Epidemiol Biomark Prev. 2007;16:401–4.
156. Martin DN, Mikhail IS, Landgren O. Autoimmunity and hematologic malignancies: associations and mechanisms. Leuk Lymphoma. 2009;50:541–50.
157. Adzic TN, Pesut DP, Nagorni-Obradovic LM, Stojsic JM, Vasiljevic MD, Bouros D. Clinical features of lung cancer in patients with connective tissue diseases: a 10-year hospital based study. Respir Med. 2008;102:620–4.
158. Xu Y, Fei Y, Zhong W, Zhang L, Zhao J, Li L, Wang M. The prevalence and clinical characteristics of primary Sjogren's syndrome patients with lung cancer: an analysis of ten cases in China and literature review. Thorac Cancer. 2015;6:475–9.
159. Zhang W, Feng S, Yan S, Zhao Y, Li M, Sun J, et al. Incidence of malignancy in primary Sjogren's syndrome in a Chinese cohort. Rheumatology (Oxford). 2010;49:571–7.
160. Gadalla SM, Amr S, Langenberg P, Baumgarten M, Davidson WF, Schairer C, et al. Breast cancer risk in elderly women with systemic autoimmune rheumatic diseases: a population-based case–control study. Br J Cancer. 2009;100:817–21.

Chapter 11
Fibromyalgia

Mohamed Osama Hegazi and Mihaela Comina Micu

The term fibromyalgia (FM) is derived from the New Latin term "fibro" (fibrous tissues) and the Greek terms "myo" (muscle) and "algos" (pain). FM represents one of a group of soft tissue pain disorders that affect muscles and soft tissues, such as tendons and ligaments. It is a medical diagnosis used to describe the diminished quality of life related to generalized body pains and physical and psychological symptoms that occur in the absence of a clear pathologic cause [1]. Not infrequently, the disorder is termed FM syndrome because the widespread chronic pain seldom occurs alone [2]. FM is often accompanied with fatigue, headache, cognitive disturbances, and sleep disorders (Table 11.1). The disorder is one of the most common causes of chronic widespread pain. The widespread musculoskeletal pain that constitutes the hallmark of FM is usually associated with increased pain perception characterized by allodynia (a heightened sensitivity to stimuli that is not normally painful) and hyperalgesia (an accentuated response to painful stimuli) [3]. The amplified pain perception in FM is typically manifested as sensitivity to blunt pressure and is clinically detected as multiple tender points.

History of Fibromyalgia

FM remained to be a matter of skepticism throughout its history. People with FM suffer not only from constant widespread pain, but they also sometimes face judgment and distrust from medical professionals who doubt if their condition is real.

M.O. Hegazi
Al Adan Hospital, Hadiya, Kuwait

M.C. Micu (✉)
Rheumatology Division, Rehabilitation Department, Rehabilitation Clinical Hospital, Cluj-Napoca, Romania
e-mail: mcmicu@yahoo.com

Y. El Miedany (ed.), *Comorbidity in Rheumatic Diseases*,
DOI 10.1007/978-3-319-59963-2_11

Table 11.1 Comorbidities with fibromyalgia

Intimate FM symptoms or comorbidities that may constitute part of the syndrome:	
Main	
Fatigue (may overlap with chronic fatigue syndrome)	
Psychiatric disorder (anxiety, depression, and post-traumatic stress disorder)	
Headaches (tension-type headache and migraine)	
Cognitive dysfunctions “fibrofog”(decline in memory, attention, and executive functions)	
Sleep disturbances (nonrestorative sleep and sleep interruption)	
Paresthesias (limb paresthesias with normal neurologic testing)	
Irritable bowel syndrome (may be considered as one of the central pain syndromes)	
Other	
Costochondritis, TMJ disease	
Dysmenorrhea, interstitial cystitis	
Restless leg syndrome	
Autonomic dysfunction	
FM comorbidities that are considered as separate associated disease entities:	
Rheumatologic:	Rheumatoid arthritis, systemic lupus erythematosus, Sjögren’s syndrome, psoriatic arthritis, and ankylosing spondylitis
Musculoskeletal:	Low back pain and cervical spondylosis
Cardiovascular:	Hypertension and atherosclerotic cardiovascular disease
Inflammatory bowel disease:	Crohn’s disease and ulcerative colitis
Endocrinologic:	Autoimmune thyroid disease
Obesity	
Obstructive sleep apnea	
Chronic rhinitis	
Chronic urticaria	
Gluten hypersensitivity	

In the early 1820s, a disorder with multiple tender points was first identified. Gowers coined the term “fibrositis” in 1904. Later on, it was shown that FM is associated with non-inflammatory pain and tenderness in muscles, ligaments, and joints, and the term was changed to “fibromyalgia” [4]. In the mid-1940s, researchers discovered FM syndrome was associated with depression and stress. This correlation led to the common thought that FM was purely a psychological disorder. However recently, FM is thought to be one of the centralized pain states in which there are central nervous system (CNS) origins of or amplification of pain [5]. The first controlled clinical study with validation of known symptoms and tender points was published in 1981 [4]. In 1990, The American College of Rheumatology wrote the first set of guidelines to help diagnose FM [6].

Epidemiology

At least 10% of the general population has chronic widespread pain, and the majority of these individuals do not have any specific disease or structural abnormality to account for the pain; many of these patients have symptoms and findings compatible with FM [7]. More than 40% of patients referred to a tertiary pain clinic meet the diagnostic criteria for FM [8]. FM is now considered the most common cause of generalized musculoskeletal pain in women between the ages of 20 and 55 years [9]. The worldwide prevalence of FM in the general population is approximately 2–3% and increases with age [10]. It is much more common in women than men [9, 10]. In spite of the fact that FM is mainly a disease of adults, recognition of the juvenile fibromyalgia syndrome is now increasing [11].

Pathogenesis

The root cause of FM is poorly understood, which may partly explain why its legitimacy might have been questioned by some healthcare professionals. The disorder has been categorized as either primary or secondary. In primary FM, there is no underlying diagnosis or precipitating cause, while with secondary FM, a probable cause exists. There is no evidence that a single event "causes" secondary FM. Rather, many physical and/or emotional stressors may trigger or aggravate symptoms. These have included certain infections, such as a viral illness or Lyme disease, as well as emotional or physical trauma [12]. The disorder may present after several years of living with hypothyroidism, lupus, or rheumatoid arthritis. The exact pathogenesis of FM is unclear. FM is considered a disorder of pain regulation, classified often under the term central sensitization [5, 12]. Experimental pain testing has identified attenuated descending analgesic activity as at least one potential reason for the widespread pain sensitivity [12]. Evidence from functional MRI has shown that individuals with FM have increased neuronal activation in pain processing regions of the brain following the application of otherwise innocuous stimuli [12]. Furthermore, brain imaging studies have reported a hypoperfusion of the striatum and thalamus at rest, decreased dopamine binding in the striatum in response to experimental pain, as well as changes in brain structure in the cingulate cortex, insular cortex, striatum, and thalamus in patients with FM [12]. These findings suggest that functional and morphological changes occur in the forebrain of individuals with FM, especially in structures known to be involved in pain systems [12]. The risk of developing FM is eightfold higher for first-degree relatives of patients with FM than for an unrelated individual [12]. Genetic factors may explain the strong familial predisposition to FM [5]. Genes modulate neurotransmitters and other inflammatory pathways involved in pain sensation [5]. Specific genetic polymorphisms (occurrence of two or more alleles in one locus) associated with an increased risk of developing FM pertain to genes that involved in serotonin and catecholamine metabolism [12]. Twin studies suggest that approximately 50% of the risk of developing fibromyalgia and related conditions such as irritable bowel syndrome (IBS) and headache is genetic and 50% is environmental [13]. An individual's "set point" or "volume control" for pain is set by a variety of factors, including the levels of neurotransmitters that facilitate pain transmission and those that reduce pain transmission [5]. Many of the neurotransmitters known to facilitate the transmission of pain in the CNS, such as substance P, glutamate, and nerve growth factor, were found to be increased in the cerebrospinal fluid of individuals with FM, whereas levels of metabolites of neurotransmitters that typically inhibit pain transmission, such as serotonin, norepinephrine, and dopamine, are reduced [12]. Neurotransmitters mediating pain transmission may also affect mood, memory, fatigue, and sleep [5]. Potentially modifiable risk factors for developing fibromyalgia include poor sleep, obesity, physical inactivity, and poor job or life satisfaction.

Diagnosis

FM is a chronic functional illness that presents with widespread musculoskeletal pain as well as a constellation of symptoms including fatigue, cognitive dysfunction, sleep difficulties, stiffness, anxiety, and depressed mood [14]. People with FM typically see many doctors before receiving the diagnosis. One reason for this may be that pain and fatigue, the main symptoms of FM, overlap with those of many other conditions. Doctors often have to rule out other potential causes of the symptoms before making a diagnosis of FM. The cardinal manifestation of FM is widespread musculoskeletal pain involving both sides of the body and present above and below the waist. However, the pain may initially be localized, often in the neck and shoulders. Common patient descriptions include "I feel as if I hurt all over," or "it feels as if I always have the flu." Patients typically describe pain predominantly throughout the muscles, but often state that their joints hurt, and sometimes describe joint swelling, although synovitis is not present on examination. In patients with FM, the one finding that is usually present on physical examination is tenderness in soft tissue anatomic locations [6]. FM characteristically shows no abnormal laboratory results. Laboratory or imaging workup is not needed unless it is required to rule out other conditions with a similar clinical presentation.

The diagnosis of FM may be under-recognized in clinical practice; prevalence estimates in one US county using surveys with standardized criteria were higher than estimates based upon medical record documentation of the diagnosis (6.4 versus 1.1%) [15]. The 1990 American College of Rheumatology criteria for FM were research classification criteria and were never intended to be used as strict diagnostic criteria for use in clinical practice [5]. These criteria require that individuals have widespread pain as well as tenderness in 11 or more of 18 possible "tender points" [6]. Many individuals who clearly have FM do not have pain throughout their entire body or may not have at least 11 tender points [5]. The alternative 2011 FM survey criteria were intended for use in epidemiological studies and represent an alternative method to assess FM [16]. These criteria include a patient self-report survey that is administered on a single piece of paper. Patients fill out a symptom survey asking about the locations of pain as well as the presence and severity of fatigue, sleep disturbances, memory difficulties, headaches, irritable bowel, and mood problems. Practitioners may prefer this approach of assessment for FM because it does not require performing a tender point examination [5]. These criteria identify most of the same individuals who meet the 1990 criteria but identify many more male patients (who rarely meet the 1990 criteria because of inadequate numbers of tender points) [5]. In clinical practice, FM should be suspected in patients having multifocal pain not fully explained by injury or inflammation [5].

Therapy

Patients should be educated regarding the diagnosis and treatment, the uncertainty regarding pathogenesis of FM, and the patient's role in their own treatment. Treatment of FM includes both non-pharmacologic and drug therapies. Drug treatment is reserved to patients who do not respond to non-pharmacologic therapy alone (usually the majority). Exercise may produce an appreciable benefit regarding pain and fatigue. Aerobic exercise has been best studied, but strengthening and stretching have also been shown to be of value [5]. Other non-pharmacologic forms of therapy include cognitive behavioral therapy and complementary and alternative medicine therapies [5]. The approved drugs for the treatment of FM include pregabalin, milnacipran, duloxetine, and amitriptyline [5, 12]. One of these drugs could be introduced in patients not responding to non-pharmacologic alone. In general, drugs should be started at low doses and should be built up slowly. Drug therapy is effective in controlling pain as well as other symptoms including fatigue, mood changes, and sleep disturbances. Individual variations between drugs concerning efficacy and side effects should be considered while selecting a drug for a specific patient. In patients unresponsive to a program including education, exercise, and drug monotherapy, additional interventions, such as drug combinations, psychological interventions, and supervised physical therapy, may be considered. After a review of a very large number of studies, reviews, and meta-analyses, the European League Against Rheumatism (EULAR) revised recommendations for the management of FM were published in 2016 [17]. The recommendations include a multidisciplinary approach that starts with patient education followed by physical and other non-pharmacological therapies "e.g. acupuncture biofeedback and cognitive behavioral therapy." If the response is inadequate, patient is reassessed, and further treatment is individualized according to patient needs. Further steps include psychological therapy, pharmacological therapy, and multimodal rehabilitation programs [17]. With the better understanding of the nature of the disorder, the increased recognition of the syndrome and the introduction of new effective drugs, the outcome of FM is expected to further improve [12].

Fibromyalgia Comorbidities

As mentioned above, FM is characterized by chronic widespread pain and is generally accompanied by one or more concomitant symptoms including fatigue, sleep disturbances, cognitive dysfunction, anxiety, and/or depressive episodes. These symptoms or comorbidities are intimately related to FM and may be considered as elements of the syndrome rather than comorbid conditions (Table 11.1). Fatigue is one of the most common symptoms associated with the pain in FM patients. Overlap exists between the FM-related fatigue and that of the chronic fatigue syndrome (also known as systemic exertion intolerance disease). Psychiatric disorders, including depressive disorders, anxiety disorders, and post-traumatic stress disorder, are more prominent in FM than in other rheumatic diseases, such as rheumatoid arthritis. Approximately 25% of patients with FM have concurrent major depression, and 50% have a lifetime history of depression. Headache in the form of migraine and/or tension-type headache affects 50% or more of FM sufferers [18]. Patients also often report paresthesias, including numbness, tingling, burning, or creeping or crawling sensations, especially in both arms and both legs. However, unless a concurrent neurologic disorder, such as carpal tunnel syndrome or a cervical radiculopathy, is present, a detailed neurologic evaluation or formal testing is usually unremarkable. Symptoms suggestive of IBS occur also frequently in patients with FM. Other visceral types of pain such as pelvic pain, dysmenorrhea, and bladder symptoms (suggestive of interstitial cystitis) are also common in patients with FM. Patients also may have a variety of poorly understood symptoms such as costochondritis-related chest pain, temporomandibular joint (TMJ) disease, dysgeusia (distortion of the sense of taste), vulvodynia, palpitations, dyspnea, and orthostatic intolerance. Autonomic dysfunction has been reported at rest and after a physiological stressor such as exercise in FM patients especially women [3].

There is an array of separate disease entities that are reported with high frequency in FM patients and are considered as comorbid conditions (Table 11.1). In a study of 11,704 patients with selected conditions, FM was the highest in its association with comorbidities compared to SLE, RA, and non-inflammatory rheumatic diseases [19]. The EPIFFAC study, in Spain, reported that 84% of patients with FM have one or more comorbid diseases: 67% have other musculoskeletal conditions, 35% psychological disorders, 27% gastrointestinal disorders, 23.5% cardiovascular disorders, and 19% endocrinological disorders [20]. In hospitalized patients in the USA, the most common comorbidities when FM was the primary diagnosis were nonspecific chest pain, mood disorders, and spondylosis/intervertebral disk disorders/other back problems; with FM as a secondary diagnosis, the most common primary diagnoses were essential hypertension, disorders of lipid metabolism, coronary atherosclerosis/other heart diseases, and mental disorders [21]. In the study conducted by Wolfe et al., in the USA, there was a significant association of FM with hypertension, other cardiovascular conditions, depression, diabetes, lung diseases, asthma, liver diseases, neurological diseases, thyroid diseases, gastrointestinal disorders, mental illnesses, renal diseases, severe allergies, and genitourinary disorders [19]. FM patients have stronger comorbidity with these disorders than patients with rheumatoid arthritis [19]. In a large health insurance database review, in the USA, Weir et al. described that patients with FM were two to seven times more likely to have one or more of the following comorbid conditions: depression, anxiety, headache, IBS, chronic fatigue syndrome, systemic lupus erythematosus, and rheumatoid arthritis [22].

On the other hand, FM can exist along with a number of diseases in a higher frequency than that observed in the general population. FM is observed to coexist with other rheumatologic diseases, such as, SLE (30%), RA (25%), psoriatic arthritis (24%), and ankylosing spondylitis (15%) [23].

FM is significantly associated also with primary Sjögren's syndrome (pSS) with a prevalence that approaches 30% in pSS patients [24].

FM was documented in 30 of 113 patients with inflammatory bowel disease, specifically in 49% of patients with Crohn's disease and 19% with ulcerative colitis ($p = 0.001$) [25]. Being overweight or obese was associated with an increased risk of FM, especially among women who also reported low levels of physical exercise [26].

The relation of FM to a number of allergic or hypersensitivity conditions has been well observed. FM is associated with chronic urticarial [27], chronic allergic rhinitis [28], and non-celiac gluten hypersensitivity [29].

Diagnostic Challenges

The multiple symptoms of fibromyalgia often simulate those of related disorders and may further complicate the diagnosis. There is an overlap in the symptomatology and also disease comorbidity among some "functional" conditions, including FM, chronic headache, chronic fatigue syndrome, IBS, TMJ disorders, major depression, anxiety, panic attack, and post-traumatic stress disorder.

Differentiation from Other Pain Disorders

A variety of chronic or recurrent pain disorders such as tension type headache, migraine, TMJ disease, IBS, and painful bladder syndrome may occur as isolated pain disorders or may constitute a part of the spectrum of the FM syndrome. The presence of concomitant fatigue, and/or sleep, cognitive, and psychiatric disorders is suggestive of FM. Laboratory testing may be unnecessary as it yields normal results in the majority of cases. Paresthesias likewise show normal neurologic testing results in FM unless they are related to cervical spondylosis or carpal tunnel syndrome. Laboratory and imaging modalities are required only to rule out organic or structural causes for the patients' symptoms whenever the physician suspects these causes. Osteoarthritis causes stiffness, tenderness, pain, and potential deformity of affected joints, and it most commonly occurs in older individuals. It is differentiated from FM based upon a patient's history, clinical examination, and degenerative joint changes seen on x-ray in people with osteoarthritis. However, it is important to note that FM can co-occur in people with osteoarthritis.

Differentiation from Rheumatologic Disorders

Differentiation of FM from autoimmune or rheumatologic diseases is a challenge. That is mainly due to symptom overlap. Given also that FM coexists specifically in a higher than usual frequency with some of these disorders, the situation becomes more complex. The physician is here facing one of three possibilities: FM alone, the autoimmune condition alone, or FM and its comorbid rheumatic disease. Polymyalgia rheumatica is a chronic, inflammatory condition that causes stiffness and pain in the shoulders, hips, or other regions. The disorder, which primarily affects individuals over age 50, is frequently associated with inflammation of certain large arteries. PMR is differentiated from fibromyalgia based upon a person's medical history, physical examination, and blood tests notably erythrocyte sedimentation rate and C-reactive protein. RA is a chronic disease that causes inflammation of joints, resulting in pain, swelling, and potential deformity of the affected joints. SLE is also a chronic, inflammatory disorder of connective tissue. Patients may be affected by abnormalities involving multiple organ systems. Although both disorders (RA and SLE) share many symptoms with FM, they have other features that are not usually seen in people with FM, including inflammation of the synovial membranes and high titers of autoantibodies. A detailed discussion about the mutual impact of SLE or RA and FM will come later in this chapter. Ankylosing spondylitis is a chronic, progressive, inflammatory disease involving joints of the spine. This condition leads to stiffness, pain, and decreased movement of the spine. Ankylosing spondylitis also causes characteristic findings that can be seen on x-ray, which are absent in people with FM. By contrast, spinal motion and x-rays are usually normal in people with FM.

Additional Diagnostic Possibilities

Some other conditions that could lead to symptoms similar to those of FM may be investigated according to the physicians' suspicion and preference. These include vitamin D deficiency, hypothyroidism, metabolic and inflammatory myopathies, and systemic viral illnesses.

Impact of Fibromyalgia Comorbidities

Fibromyalgia and Autoimmune Rheumatic Diseases

FM and chronic inflammatory or autoimmune rheumatic diseases show several overlapping features such as joint pain, fatigue, morning stiffness, depression, and sleep disturbances that make their differentiation very problematic in clinical practice as well as in epidemiological surveys.

The baseline assessment together with the monitoring of disease activity, functional status, and quality of life provides the physician with the necessary information to manage the autoimmune rheumatic condition. The presence of FM as an associated condition may artificially modify these parameters. On the other hand, comorbid inflammatory or autoimmune diseases may have a negative impact on FM symptoms leading to unjustified medication escalation, potential toxicity, and higher management costs.

Mutual Impact of Rheumatoid Arthritis and Fibromyalgia

FM is present in a variable percentage (10–25%) of RA patients defining a RA subset so-called fibromyalgic RA [30–34]. The high pain and disability scores seen in these patients suggest that they will have high RA activity scores at baseline (especially in early disease) and during follow-up, discordant to the inflammatory parameters [30, 35]. Indeed, remission status quantification may be controversial. Disease activity measures such as Disease Activity Score (DAS) and Simplified Disease Activity Index (SDAI) are popular disease activity indexes, very important in the treatment decision for disease-modifying antirheumatic drugs (DMARDs) as well as for biologic therapies. In "fibromyalgic RA," an overestimated disease activity may be taken into consideration especially when inflammatory parameters are weak or negative [33, 36]. This subset of patients may have greater benefit by using other than disease-modifying antirheumatic drug (DMARD) escalation strategies (painkillers, physiotherapy, and psychological treatment) to control symptoms [33].

DAS 28 is a composite activity index which combines four components: 28 swollen joint count (SJC), 28 tender-joint count (TJC), acute-phase response (erythrocyte sedimentation rate (ESR) or C- reactive protein (CRP)), and a general health assessment using a visual analogue score (VAS-GH). SJC are evaluated by the assessor, in contrast to TJC and VAS which are patient reported. Tenderness may be associated with augmented pain processing in FM and RA, and DAS28 scores may overestimate inflammatory disease activity in people with a high TJC [33, 37]. Similar magnification may be applied to other disease activity indices such as SDAI, clinical disease activity index (CDAI), and other composite disease activity indexes.

Although anti-citrullinated protein antibody (ACPA) positivity is usually inversely associated with the clinical diagnosis of FM, one should not omit the fact that early and very early RA may present with oligoarthritis and negative ACPA [35, 38, 39].

In this regard, some authors suggest different tools helpful for identifying fibromyalgic RA patients such as "the Fibromyalgia Rapid Screening Tool" (FiRST), the number of painful joints minus swollen joints or musculoskeletal ultrasound, as a high-resolution imaging method for clinical and subclinical synovitis detection [37, 40, 41]. The FiRST is a self-administered questionnaire consisting of six questions covering several domains of FM: widespread pain, fatigue, pain characteristics, non-painful abnormal sensations, functional somatic symptoms, sleep, and cognitive problems. The options to answer are yes (1 point) and no (zero points); with the maximum score of 6 and a cutoff value of ≥5 associated with the highest sensitivity and specificity for FM (it detects ACR 90-defined FM patients with a sensitivity of 74.5% and a specificity of 80.4%, with a negative predictive value of 97% and a positive predictive value of 26.6%) [40].

Similar results were obtained in the study by Pollard et al. [33]. The authors demonstrate that a score of ≥7 (tender minus swollen joints) can reach a sensitivity of 83% and specificity of 80% for identifying "fibromyalgic RA" patients [33]. Furthermore, Ghib et al. compared US evaluation "grayscale (GS) and power Doppler (PD)" and DAS 28 scores in patients with RA, FM-RA, and FM alone concluding that DAS 28 is not a reliable measure of disease activity in patients with RA and associated FM, due to the higher TJC and patient global health assessment. In this study, SJC and ESR were similar in the RA and FM-RA groups and lower in the FM group. Median PD-US scores proved to be significantly different between the FM and RA groups and between FM-RA and FM groups. No significant differences were noted between US scores in the RA and FM-RA groups. Indeed, US scores correlated moderately only with DAS28 and CDAI in patients with RA, and not in patients with FM-RA. These scores were inversely correlated with DAS28 and CDAI in FM patients, the authors concluding that US evaluation may be more accurate (in comparison to clinical evaluation) for disease activity evaluation in FM-RA patients [41].

Patients' self-evaluation regarding pain level, physical functioning, mental well-being, and social functioning was subject to dispute in the last years due to its low credibility. A recent study conducted by Kool et al. concluded that spouses and patients (group with RA and group with FM) appraise patients' health status in a similar way, but with worse outcome for all parameters in the FM group in comparison to the RA group, results supported also by other authors when comparing FM patients with patients with other painful conditions [42, 43].

FM associated with chronic inflammatory rheumatologic or autoimmune diseases tends to have a profound impact on health-related quality of life (HRQL) and has been found to be associated with high treatment costs [44, 45]. In this regard, the "OMERACT fibromyalgia syndrome workshop" tried to highlight those domains that should be consistently measured in clinical trials such as pain, physical and emotional functioning, patient global satisfaction ratings, negative health states, and adverse events [46].

The patients' perception of HRQL is quantified by using generic instruments and questionnaires that provide a general picture or specific instruments or questionnaires that focus on several aspects relevant for a disease or patient group. The Short Form 36-item Health Survey Questionnaire (SF-36) is a validated, generic instrument covering eight domains of HRQL – physical functioning, physical role, social functioning, bodily pain, general health, vitality, emotional role, and mental health scores [47]. Several studies performed by now, comparing HRQL of patients with RA and FM, suggest that all domains had lower scores in FM-RA patients and that FM patients have lower mental health scores in comparison to those with RA [30, 48–50]. Salaffi et al. concluded in a recent study that the domains typically affected by FM were mental health, social functioning, vitality, pain, and general health. Somatization rates were higher in this category of patients. Indeed, FM patients considered widespread pain, fatigue, and unrefreshing sleep as the most significant factors with negative impact on working performance. In contrast, physical functioning and role limitations due to physical function were more impaired in RA [30, 48, 50, 51].

Sleep disturbance has a major influence on the quality of life and is prevalent in patients with FM and RA [52]. Still, comparative studies focused on sleep quality are scarce. Ulus et al. focused in his study on sleep quality evaluation using a questionnaire (the Pittsburgh Sleep Quality Index (PSQI)) consisting of 19 items (4-point scale) defining seven subcategories – sleep duration, sleep disturbances, sleep latency, daytime dysfunction, sleep efficiency, sleep quality, and medication use [53]. Apart from this, the impact of pain, fatigue, depression, and disease activity on sleep quality was evaluated. Patients with FM-RA showed higher fatigue scores than controls, and FM patients demonstrated higher scores, which correlated to PSQI, compared to RA patients [54]. Indeed, patients with FM-RA and high depression scores may have more sleep problems (quality and duration) when compared to subjects without rheumatologic disorders. The negative impact is even higher when pain, fatigue, and disease activity are added [54].

Mutual Impact of Spondyloarthritis Group (Spa) and Fibromyalgia

The SpA includes several related pathologic entities such as ankylosing spondylitis, psoriatic arthritis, reactive arthritis, juvenile SpA, and inflammatory bowel disease-related and undifferentiated SpA. The presence of FM clinical features in this group has been evaluated in several papers that confirm a prevalence of 4–25% in comparison to only 2–4% in the general population [9, 55, 56]. FM patients express continuously a higher level of fatigue and intensity of pain in comparison to SpA patients. Activity and functional indexes such as Bath Ankylosing Spondylitis Disease Activity Index (BASDAI) and Bath Ankylosing Spondylitis Functional Index (BASFI) are strongly influenced by the presence of FM. The BASDAI score comprises six items based on the subjective assessment of pain, stiffness, and fatigue, all overlapping FM symptoms. Therefore, activity assessment, patient selection, and treatment evaluation may become very challenging in FM-SpA patients. BASFI score determines the degree of functional limitation in patients with SpA and comprises of ten questions – the first eight questions evaluating activities related to functional anatomical limitations determined by the inflammatory lesions associated to the disease and the last two questions evaluating the patients' ability to cope with everyday life. Almodovar et al. performed a recent study focused on the analysis of those factors that best characterize FM-AS patients; in addition they studied the extent in which FM affects the activity and functional disease parameters. Finally, a correlation with a radiologic score was made. The authors concluded that associated FM would modify (increase) the measures of activity and functional damage and that an increased ratio BASDAI/Bath Ankylosing Spondylitis Radiology Index (BASRI) ≥1.5 or BASFI/BASRI ≥1.08 would identify with high probability the FM-SpA subset. Indeed, higher activity index would lead to some extent to overtreatment with lesser efficacy and higher medical costs [56]. Another study conducted by Roussou et al. attempted to assess the concomitant presence of clinical symptoms in patients with SpAs and FM and investigated the potential overlap between the defined tender points characteristic for FM and enthesitis in SpA patients [55]. The authors used for enthesitis assessment the Mander scoring system and pointed out an interesting finding regarding the low discriminatory capacity of the examiner in differentiating the specific FM tender points from the enthesitis sites, raising the problem of mislabeling patients with SpA as FM when concomitant fatigue, sleep disturbance, and improvement of pain with exercises occurs. This fact would lead to inappropriate treatment recommendations [55, 57]. The tender point examination reliability has been questioned, and concerns were raised about it as a clinical outcome measure. Of note, the new preliminary FM diagnostic criteria do not include the tender point evaluation anymore, but validation in prospective studies is still missing. Moreover, one of the critics regarding these new diagnostic criteria is that establishing a diagnosis without physical examination would omit other comorbidities and potential causes for the present patients' symptoms [58, 59].

Fatigue and sleep disturbances are important symptoms interfering with all aspects of life in patients with SpA, similar to other chronic rheumatologic diseases [54, 60, 61]. Several quality-of-life assessment questionnaires such as the Stanford Health Assessment Questionnaire (HAQ) and arthritis impact measurement scales (AIMS) contain questions about this item but showing limits in fully reflecting the complete spectrum of FM-related symptoms [54, 62–64]. In this sense, the Fibromyalgia Impact Questionnaire (FIQ) was developed, consisting of ten questions that capture the overall effect of FM symptoms. By now, it is a validated tool, showing a very good responsiveness to change and good correlation with similar questionnaires such as HAQ, AIMS, and SF-36 [65]. Overall, in SpA patients, fatigue appears to be a common symptom associated with pain, female gender, physical functional disability, medication status, and physiological distress [54].

Mutual Impact of Systemic Lupus Erythematosus and Fibromyalgia

Some studies reported antinuclear antibody (ANA) positivity, photosensitivity, Raynaud phenomenon, oral ulcers, or sicca symptoms in FM patients. In spite of the fact that these manifestations are characteristic of SLE, Sjögren's syndrome, or systemic sclerosis, they were found in a quite consistent percentage of patients with the FM syndrome [66, 67]. They were ambiguously considered as part of the FM clinical spectrum, or otherwise they could represent a partial, early, or mild form of the autoimmune disease. These manifestations may indeed cause problems in establishing the differential diagnosis, especially in patients with milder clinical presentation of the autoimmune disease. Inadequate treatment recommendations may also occur in misdiagnosed patients [68].

Neuropsychiatric symptoms present in SLE and in FM patients represent another important challenge for the practitioner. Neuropsychiatric symptoms can be among the earliest manifestations of SLE, with a prevalence reaching up to 40%, some of them showing a very high mortality rate [69]. The overlapping clinical spectrum comprises headaches, psychiatric disorders (depression and anxiety), cognitive impairment, ischemic transient attacks, and demyelination, the first three being the most frequent manifestations. In addition, sleep disorders, fatigue, and musculoskeletal symptoms are found in both entities [70, 71].

Surveys of the medical literature show a high prevalence of FM (8–45%) in SLE patients. This prevalence is correlated with SLE duration of >5 years. FM-SLE patients have similar sociodemographic, characteristics, treatment strategies, severity, and activity index [72–76]. In a recent study conducted by Torrente-Segarra et al., the authors found a significantly higher prevalence of psychiatric symptoms in patients with SLE and FM compared to the non-FM-SLE patients. They suggested that FM in SLE patients strongly predisposes to psychiatric disorders. However, the authors concluded that the psychiatric manifestations were not linked to a higher SLE activity in the study group and therefore should benefit from a different treatment approach [75]. The presence of FM has been recognized as having a significant negative impact on the physical and mental status in SLE – active and inactive patients – reducing their self-reported quality of life. In fact, depression is the major factor associated with the presence of FM in SLE patients [75–77]. Other findings like photosensitivity, oral ulcers, secondary sicca syndrome, and a higher daily dosage of corticosteroids correlated with the presence of FM in SLE patients. Several comorbidities like autoimmune thyroiditis, arterial hypertension, and dyslipidemia were found to occur more frequently in the subset of FM/SLE patients [76].

Mutual Impact of Primary Sjögren's Syndrome (Pss) and Fibromyalgia

Most individuals with Sjögren's syndrome present with sicca symptoms, parotid gland enlargement, and variable extra-glandular features among which arthralgia, myalgia, and chronic fatigue are frequent and disabling symptoms [78]. The aforementioned symptoms may overlap with FM features. Recent data show that FM prevalence in pSS patients is around 30% vs 20% when using ACR 2010 FM classification criteria vs ACR 1990 criteria [24]. FM-pSS patients tend to have significantly higher tender point counts and widespread pain index compared to pSS patients without FM. Tender point counts correlate significantly with the pain and depression level as well as with the EULAR Sjögren's Syndrome Patient Reported Index (ESSPRI) but not with disease activity according to Choi et al. [24, 79]. Indeed, insomnia and cognitive dysfunction were more often encountered in FM-pSS in comparison to only pSS patients [79]. In contrast to all these remarks, FM was not associated with the presence of autoantibodies, extra-glandular features, and disease activity [79].

Fatigue is a common shared feature in both FM and Sjögren's syndrome. Fatigue is reported in a very high percentage "in some studies up to 85%" in pSS patients, and 50% of them consider it the most disabling symptom. Some authors consider fatigue a clear feature of active disease; however, no statistically significant correlation between fatigue and p SS activity was demonstrated by now [80–83]. Furthermore, fatigue was found to correlate with the depression and anxiety scales, disease duration, and FIQ score [84].

Other Comorbidities and Fibromyalgia

Clinical manifestations such as fatigue, widespread musculoskeletal pain, depression, anxiety disorders, memory loss, abdominal pain, diarrhea alternating with constipation, and bloating are common in celiac disease (CD), IBD, and FM. CD typically presents in childhood with gastrointestinal symptoms but, often in adulthood several other non-gastrointestinal manifestations, tend to dominate the clinical picture. In fact, the similarities in symptomatology between FM and CD triggered the hypothesis that FM has a higher prevalence in CD patients in comparison to general population and secondly that a percentage of FM patients could have subclinical CD [84–86]. Another hypothesis would be the fact that vitamin D deficiency, a common finding in CD patients, could mimic FM features [84, 87, 88].

FM occurs in 20–30% of IBS patients, and more than 30% (up to 70%) of the FM patients meet the criteria for IBS [89, 90]. Indeed, the incidence of CD in IBS patients is four to seven times higher than in controls without IBS [21, 87, 91].

As mentioned above, in a study of hospitalized patients in the USA, essential hypertension, disorders of lipid metabolism, and coronary atherosclerosis/other heart diseases were among the most common primary diagnoses when FM was the secondary diagnosis [21]. This and other similar findings led researchers to explore this issue. In a health insurance database cohort study from Taiwan, FM patients showed a significantly higher subsequent risk of a coronary heart disease event than the patients without FM [92]. Researchers from Turkey evaluated mean platelet volume, which is a determinant of platelet activation and is a newly emerging independent risk factor for cardiovascular disease. Results showed that the levels of mean platelet volume were significantly higher in the FM group than in the control group, suggesting an early atherosclerotic marker in patients with FM [93]. Mortality does not appear to be increased due to FM itself; however, death due to suicide and accidents is increased [94]. Confirming the relation between FM and cardiovascular disease, although still a matter of research, may change this concept. The association of obesity and FM may also have morbidity and mortality implications. Quality of life and FM symptomatology were found to be worse in obese FM patients [95].

Impact on Healthcare and Community

Patients with FM have comparatively high levels of comorbidities and high levels of healthcare utilization and cost [96]. In "real life," FM impact on primary healthcare resources is expressed mainly due to higher visit rates for at least 10 years prior to FM diagnosis. Depression, fatigue, chest pain, sleep disturbance, dizziness, and IBS are the main causes for these visits. In fact, FM patients are more prone to develop depression and vice versa [97].

Indeed, more medical prescriptions were recorded in FM patients in comparison to controls prior to diagnosis and after, and overall rates of diagnosis-related procedures and tests referrals were higher especially prior to FM diagnosis [98]. In addition to the increased healthcare utilization, a significant individual and social burden of FM will reflect also in a negative impact on work participation and productivity [96–99].

Implications for Science/Research

Now, suggestions for several research priorities should be taken into consideration and may be synthetized as follows:

- A better definition of the OMERACT core domains that should be consistently measured in clinical trials.
- The development of validated tools for patients' evaluation in clinical practice in cases of FM comorbidities.
- The increased utilization of musculoskeletal ultrasound evaluation in clinical practice as a more accurate and noninvasive method for clinical and subclinical inflammatory and/or structural musculoskeletal lesion detection [41, 100]. This will help solve diagnostic dilemmas whenever FM is suspected to accompany another autoimmune or rheumatic condition.
- Research priorities regarding FM management were formulated in the EULAR revised recommendations for the management of FM (2016) [17]. Some of these research areas look to be attractive to rheumatologists who deal with FM and its associated comorbid conditions. These recommendations include:
  - Are there characteristics of patients with fibromyalgia that predict response to specific therapies?
  - How should fibromyalgia be managed when it occurs as a comorbidity with inflammatory arthritis?

  - What aspects of a healthcare system optimize outcome for the patients (who is best for the management of FM patients)?

- We believe also that the association of FM with cardiovascular disease, FM with obesity, and FM with autonomic dysfunction constitutes rich areas of future research.

References

1. Walitt B, Nahin RL, Katz RS, et al. The prevalence and characteristics of fibromyalgia in the 2012 national health interview survey. PLoS One. 2015;10:e0138024.
2. Mease P, Arnold LM, Choy EH, OMERACT Fibromyalgia Working Group, et al. Fibromyalgia syndrome module at OMERACT 9: domain construct. J Rheumatol. 2009;36:2318–29.
3. Clauw DJ, Arnold LM, BH MC, Fibro Collaborative. The science of fibromyalgia. Mayo Clin Proc. 2011;86:907–11.
4. Inanici F, Yunus MB. History of fibromyalgia: past to present. Curr Pain Headache Rep. 2004;8:369–78.
5. Clauw DJ. Fibromyalgia: a clinical review. JAMA. 2014;311:1547–55.
6. Wolfe F, Smythe HA, Yunus MB, et al. The American College of Rheumatology 1990 criteria for the classification of fibromyalgia. Report of the Multicenter Criteria Committee. Arthritis Rheum. 1990;33(2):160–72.
7. Croft P, Rigby AS, Boswell R, et al. The prevalence of chronic widespread pain in the general population. J Rheumatol. 1993;20:710–3.
8. Brill S, Ablin JN, Goor-Aryeh I, et al. Prevalence of fibromyalgia syndrome in patients referred to a tertiary pain clinic. J Investig Med. 2012;60:685–8.
9. Aloush V, Ablin JN, Reitblat T, et al. Fibromyalgia in women with ankylosing spondylitis. Rheumatol Int. 2007;27:865–8.
10. Queiroz LP. Worldwide epidemiology of fibromyalgia. Curr Pain Headache Rep. 2013;17:356.
11. McLeod JD. Juvenile fibromyalgia syndrome and improved recognition by pediatric primary care providers. J Pediatr Health Care. 2014;28:e9–18.
12. Schmidt-Wilcke T, Clauw DJ. Fibromyalgia: from pathophysiology to therapy. Nat Rev Rheumatol. 2011;7:518–27.
13. Kato K, Sullivan PF, Evengård B, et al. A population-based twin study of functional somatic syndromes. Psychol Med. 2009;39:497–505.
14. Goldenberg DL. Diagnosis and differential diagnosis of fibromyalgia. Am J Med. 2009;122:S14–21.
15. Vincent A, Lahr BD, Wolfe F, et al. Prevalence of fibromyalgia: a population-based study in Olmsted County, Minnesota, utilizing the Rochester Epidemiology Project. Arthritis Care Res (Hoboken). 2013;65:786–92.
16. Wolfe F, Clauw DJ, Fitz Charles MA, et al. Fibromyalgia criteria and severity scales for clinical and epidemiological studies: a modification of the ACR preliminary diagnostic criteria for fibromyalgia. J Rheumatol. 2011;38:1113–22.
17. Macfarlane GJ, Kronisch C, Dean LE, et al. EULAR revised recommendations for the management of fibromyalgia. Ann Rheum Dis. 2016;76(2):318–28. pii: annrheumdis-2016-209724.
18. Marcus DA, Bernstein C, Rudy TE. Fibromyalgia and headache: an epidemiological study supporting migraine as part of the fibromyalgia syndrome. Clin Rheumatol. 2005;24:595–601.
19. Wolfe F, Michaud K, Li T, et al. Chronic conditions and health problems in rheumatic diseases: comparisons with rheumatoid arthritis, noninflammatory rheumatic disorders, systemic lupus erythematosus, and fibromyalgia. J Rheumatol. 2010;37:305–15.

20. Collado A, Gomez E, Coscolla R, et al. Work, family and social environment in patients with Fibromyalgia in Spain: an epidemiological study: EPIFFAC study. BMC Health Serv Res. 2014;14:513.
21. Haviland MG, Banta JE, Przekop P. Fibromyalgia: prevalence, course, and co-morbidities in hospitalized patients in the United States, 1999–2007. Clin Exp Rheumatol. 2011;29:S79–87.
22. Weir PT, Harlan GA, Nkoy FL, et al. The incidence of fibromyalgia and its associated comorbidities: a population-based retrospective cohort study based on International Classification of Diseases, 9th Revision codes. J Clin Rheumatol. 2006;12:124–8.
23. Azevedo VF, PaivaEdos S, Felippe LR, et al. Occurrence of fibromyalgia in patients with ankylosing spondylitis. Rev Bras Reumatol. 2010;50:646–50.
24. Choi BY, Oh HJ, Lee YJ, Song YW. Prevalence and clinical impact of fibromyalgia in patients with primary Sjögren's syndrome. Clin Exp Rheumatol. 2016;34:S9–13.
25. Buskila D, Odes LR, Neumann L, et al. Fibromyalgia in inflammatory bowel disease. J Rheumatol. 1999;26:1167–71.
26. Mork PJ, Vasseljen O, Nilsen TI. Association between physical exercise, body mass index, and risk of fibromyalgia: longitudinal data from the Norwegian Nord-Trøndelag Health Study. Arthritis Care Res (Hoboken). 2010;62:611–7.
27. Torresani C, Bellafiore S, De Panfilis G. Chronic urticaria is usually associated with fibromyalgia syndrome. Acta Derm Venereol. 2009;89:389–92.
28. Frieri M, Argyriou A. Is there a relationship between fibromyalgia and rhinitis? Allergy Asthma Proc. 2012;33:443–9.
29. Isasi C, Colmenero I, Casco F. Fibromyalgia and non-celiac gluten sensitivity: a description with remission of fibromyalgia. Rheumatol Int. 2014;34:1607–12.
30. Ranzolin A, Brenol JC, Bredemeier M, et al. Association of concomitant fibromyalgia with worse disease activity score in 28 joints, health assessment questionnaire, and short form 36 scores in patients with rheumatoid arthritis. Arthritis Rheum. 2009;61:794–800.
31. Atzeni F, Cazzola M, Benucci M, Franco MD, Salaffi F, Sarzi-Puttini P. Chronic widespread pain in the spectrum of rheumatological diseases. Best Pract Res Clin Rheumatol. 2011;25:165–71.
32. Wolfe F, Michaud K. Severe rheumatoid arthritis (RA), worse outcomes, comorbid illness, and sociodemographic disadvantage characterize RA patients with fibromyalgia. J Rheumatol. 2004;31:695–700.
33. Pollard LC, Kingsley GH, Choy EHS, et al. Fibromyalgic rheumatoid arthritis and disease assessment. Rheumatology (Oxford). 2010;49:924–8.
34. Branco JC, Bannwarth B, Failde I, et al. Prevalence of fibromyalgia: a survey in five European countries. Semin Arthritis Rheum. 2010;39:448–53.
35. Lee YC, Lu B, Boire G, Haraoui BP, Hitchon CA, Pope JE, et al. Incidence and predictors of secondary fibromyalgia in an early arthritis cohort. Ann Rheum Dis. 2013;72:949–54.
36. Coury F, Rossat A, Tebib A, et al. Rheumatoid arthritis and fibromyalgia: a frequent unrelated association complicating disease management. J Rheumatol. 2009;36:58–62.
37. Leeb BF, Andel I, Sautner J, Nothnagl T, Rintelen B. The DAS28 in rheumatoid arthritis and fibromyalgia patients. Rheumatology. 2004;43:1504–7.
38. Felson DT, Smolen JS, Wells G, et al. American College of Rheumatology/European League against Rheumatism provisional definition of remission in rheumatoid arthritis for clinical trials. Ann Rheum Dis. 2011;70:404–13.
39. Cader MZ, Filer A, Hazlehurst J, de Pablo P, Buckley CD, Raza K. Performance of the 2010 ACR/EULAR criteria for rheumatoid arthritis: comparison with 1987 ACR criteria in a very early synovitis cohort. Ann Rheum Dis. 2011;70:949–55.
40. Fan A, Tournadre A, Pereira B, et al. Performance of Fibromyalgia Rapid Screening Tool (FiRST) to detect fibromyalgia syndrome in rheumatic diseases. Rheumatology (Oxford). 2016;55(10):1746–50. pii: kew244.

41. Ghib LJ, Tămaş MM, Damian LO, et al. The role of ultrasonography in assessing disease activity in patients with rheumatoid arthritis and associated fibromyalgia. Med Ultrason. 2015;17(3):339–44.
42. Kool MB, Van Middendorp H, Bijlsma JWJ, Geenen R. Patient and spouse appraisals of health status in rheumatoid arthritis and fibromyalgia: discrepancies and associations with invalidation. Clin Exp Rheumatol. 2011;29(Suppl 69):S63–9.
43. Levy O, Segal R, Maslakov I, Markov A, Tishler M, Amit-Vazina M. The impact of concomitant fibromyalgia on visual analogue scales of pain, fatigue and function in patients with various rheumatic disorders. Clin Exp Rheumatol. 2016;34(Suppl 96):S120–4.
44. Mas AJ, Carmona LM, Valverde M, Ribas B, the EPISER study group. Prevalence and impact of fibromyalgia on function and quality of life in individuals from the general population: results from a nationwide study in Spain. Clin Exp Rheumatol. 2008;26:519–26.
45. Hughes G, Martinez C, Myon E, et al. The impact of a diagnosis of fibromyalgia on health care resource use by primary care patients in the UK: an observational study based on clinical practice. Arthtitis Rheum. 2006;54:177–83.
46. Mease PJ, Arnold LM, Bennet R, et al. Identifying the clinical domains of fibromyalgia: contributions from clinician and patient Delphi exercises. Arthritis Rheum. 2008;15:952–60.
47. Ware J, Sherbourne CD. The MOS 36-item short form health survey (SF-36). 1. Conceptual frame-work and item selection. Med Care. 1992;30:473–81.
48. Birtane M, Kaan Uzunca K, Tastekin N, et al. The evaluation of quality of life in fibromyalgia syndrome: a comparison with rheumatoid arthritis by using SF-36 Health Survey. Clin Rheumatol. 2007;26:679–84.
49. Strombeck B, Ekdahl C, Manthorpe R, et al. Health-related quality of life in primary Sjögren's syndrome, rheumatoid arthritis and fibromyalgia compared to normal population data using SF-36. Scand J Rheumatol. 2000;29:20–8.
50. Salaffi F, Sarzi Puttini P, Girolimetti R, Atzeni F, GaspariniS GW. Health-related quality of life in fibromyalgia patients: a comparison with rheumatoid arthritis patients and the general population using the SF-36 health survey. Clin Exp Rheumatol. 2009;27(Suppl 56):S67–74.
51. Verbunt JA, Pernot DHFM, Smeets RJEM. Disability and quality of life in patients with fibromyalgia. Health Qual Life Outcomes. 2008;6:8.
52. Belt NK, Kronholm E, Kauppi MJ. Sleep problems in fibromyalgia and rheumatoid arthritis compared with the general population. Clin Exp Rheumatol. 2009;27:35–41.
53. Ulus Y, Akyol Y, Tander B, Durmus D, Bilgici A, Kuru O. Sleep quality in fibromyalgia and rheumatoid arthritis: associations with pain, fatigue, depression, and disease activity. Clin Exp Rheumatol. 2011;29(Suppl 61):S92–6.
54. Husted JA, Tom BD, Schentag CT, Farewell VT, Gladmann DD. Occurrence and correlates of fatigue in PsA. Ann Rheum Dis. 2009;68:1553–8.
55. Roussou E, Ciurtin C. Clinical overlap between fibromyalgia tender points and enthesitis sites in patients with spondyloarthritis who present with inflammatory back pain. Clin Exp Rheumatol. 2012;30(Suppl 74):S24–30.
56. Almodóvar R, Carmona L, Zarco P, et al. Fibromyalgia in patients with ankylosing spondylitis: prevalence and utility of the measures of activity, function and radiological damage. Clin Exp Rheumatol. 2010;28(Suppl 63):S33–9.
57. Mander M, Simpson JM, McLellan A, Walker D, Goodcare JA, Dick WC. Studies with enthesitis index as a method of clinical assessment in ankylosing spondylitis. Ann Rheum Dis. 1987;46:197–202.
58. Wolfe F, Clauw DJ, Fitzcharles MA, et al. The American College of Rheumatology preliminary diagnostic criteria for fibromyalgia and measurement of symptom severity. Arthritis Care Res (Hoboken). 2010;62(5):600–10.
59. Mease PJ, Clauw JD, Arnold LM, et al. Fibromyalgia syndrome-OMERACT 7 workshop. J Rheumatol. 2005;32:2270–7.
60. Sokoll KB, Helliwell PS. Comparison of disability and quality of life in rheumatoid and psoriatic arthritis. J Rheumatol. 2001;28:1842–6.

61. Chandran V, Bhella S, Schentag C, et al. Functional assessment of chronic illness therapy-fatigue scale is valid in patients with psoriatic arthritis. Ann Rheum Dis. 2007;66:936–9.
62. Blackmore M, Gladman DD, Husted J, et al. Measuring health status in psoriatic arthritis: the Health Assessment Questionnaire and its modification. J Rheumatol. 1995;22:886–93.
63. Duffy CM, Watanabe Duffy KN, Gladman DD, et al. Utilization of the Arthritis Impact Measurement Scales (AIMS) for patients with psoriatic arthritis. J Rheumatol. 1992;19:1727–32.
64. Husted J, Gladman DD, Long JA, et al. Validating the SF-36 health questionnaire in patients with psoriatic arthritis. J Rheumatol. 1997;24:511–7.
65. Bennet R. The Fibromyalgia Impact Questionnaire (FIQ): a review of its development, current version, operating characteristics and uses. Clin Exp Rheumatol. 2005;23(Suppl 39):S154–62.
66. Al-AllF AW, Ottewell L, Pullar T. The prevalence and significance of positive antinuclear antibodies in patients with fibromyalgia syndrome: 2–4 years' follow-up. Clin Rheumatol. 2002;21:472–7.
67. Dinerman H, Goldenberg DL, Felson DT. A prospective evaluation of 118 patients with the fibromyalgia syndrome: prevalence of Raynaud's phenomenon, sicca symptoms, ANA, low complement, and Ig deposition at the dermal-epidermal junction. J Rheumatol. 1986;13:368–73.
68. Dönmez S, Pamuk ON, Ümit EG, Top MS. Autoimmune rheumatic disease associated symptoms in fibromyalgia patients and their influence on anxiety, depression and somatisation: a comparative study. Clin Exp Rheumatol. 2012;30(Suppl 74):S65–9.
69. Unterman A, Nolte JE, Boaz M, Abady M, Shoenfeld Y, Zandman-Goddard G. Neuropsychiatric syndromes in systemic lupus erythematosus: a meta-analysis. Semin Arthritis Rheum. 2011;41:1–11.
70. Bachen E, Chesney M, Criswell A. Prevalence of mood and anxiety disorders in women with systemic lupus erythematosus. Arthritis Rheum. 2009;61:822–9.
71. Palagini L, Carmassi C, Conversano C, et al. Transdiagnostic factors across fibromyalgia and mental disorders: sleep disturbances may play a key role. A clinical review. Clin Exp Rheumatol. 2016;34(Suppl 96):S140–4.
72. Friedman AW, Tew MB, Ahn C, et al. For the LUMINA Study Group. Lupus. 2003;12:274–9.
73. Middleton G, Mc Farlin J, Lipsky P. The prevalence and clinical impact of fibromyalgia in systemic lupus erythematosus. Arthritis Rheum. 1994;37:1181–8.
74. Handra R, Aggrawal P, Wali JP, Wig N, Dwivedi SN. Fibromyalgia in Indian patients with systemic lupus erythematosus. Lupus. 1998;7:475–8.
75. Torrente-Segarra V, Carbonell Abelló J, Castro Oreiro S, Manresa Domínguez JM. Association between fibromyalgia and psychiatric disorders in systemic lupus erythematosus. Clin Exp Rheumatol. 2010;28(Suppl 63):S22–6.
76. Torrente-Segarra V, Salman-Monte TC, Rúa-Figueroa I, RELESSER study Group of the Spanish Society of Rheumatology (SER) and the study Group of Systemic Autoimmune Diseases of the SER (EAS-SER), et al. Fibromyalgia prevalence and related factors in a large registry of patients with systemic lupus erythematosus. Clin Exp Rheumatol. 2016;34(Suppl 96):S40–7.
77. Waldheim E, Elkan AC, Pettersoson S, et al. Health-related quality of life, fatigue and mood in patients with SLE and high levels of pain compared to controls and patients with low levels of pain. Lupus. 2013;22:1118–27.
78. Ng WF, Bowman SJ. Primary Sjögren's syndrome: too dry and too tired. Rheumatology (Oxford). 2010;49:844–53.
79. Seror R, Ravaud P, Mariette X, et al. EULAR Sjögren's Syndrome Patient Reported Index (ESSPRI): development of a consensus patient index for primary Sjögren's syndrome. Ann Rheum Dis. 2011;70:968–72.
80. Priori R, Iannucelli C, Alessandri C, et al. Fatigue in Sjögren's syndrome: relationship with fibromyalgia, clinical and biologic features. Clin Exp Rheumatol. 2010;28(Suppl 63):S82–6.

81. Barendregt PJ, Arendregt PJ, Visser M, Smets E, et al. Fatigue in primary Sjögren's syndrome. Ann Rheum Dis. 1998;57:291–5.
82. Giles I, Isenberg D. Fatigue in primary Sjögren's syndrome: is there a link with the fibromyalgia syndrome? Ann Rheum Dis. 2000;59:875–8.
83. Iannuccelli C, Spinelli FR, Guzzo MP, et al. Fatigue and widespread pain in systemic lupus erythematosus and Sjögren's syndrome: symptoms of inflammatory disease or associated fibromyalgia? Clin Exp Rheumatol. 2012;30(Suppl 74):S117–21.
84. Tovoli F, Giampaolo L, Caio G, et al. Fibromyalgia and coeliac disease: a media hype or an emerging clinical problem? Clin Exp Rheumatol. 2013;31(Suppl 79):S50–2.
85. García-Leiva JM, Carrasco JL, Slim M, Calandre EP. Celiac symptoms in patients with fibromyalgia: a cross-sectional study. Rheumatol Int. 2015;35(3):561–7.
86. Zipser RD, Patel S, Yahaya KZ, Baisch DW, Monarch E. Presentations of adult celiac disease in a nationwide patient support group. Dig Dis Sci. 2003;48:761–4.
87. Straube S, Andrew MR, Derry S, McQuay HJ. Vitamin D and chronic pain. Pain. 2009;141:10–3.
88. Daniel D, Pirotta MV. Fibromyalgia- should we be testing and treating for vitamin D deficiency? Aust Fam Physician. 2011;40:712–6.
89. Rodrigo L, Blanco I, Bobes J, de Serres FJ. Remarkable prevalence of coeliac disease in patients with irritable bowel syndrome plus fibromyalgia in comparison with those with isolated irritable bowel syndrome: a case-finding study. Arthritis Res Ther. 2013;15:R201.
90. Sperber AD, Atzmon Y, Neumann L, et al. Fibromyalgia in the irritable bowel syndrome: studies of prevalence and clinical implications. Am J Gastroenterol. 1999;94:3541–6.
91. Ford AC, Chey WD, Talley NJ, Malhotra A, Spiegel BM, Moayyedi P. Yield of diagnostic tests for celiac disease in individuals with symptoms suggestive of irritable bowel syndrome: systematic review and meta-analysis. Arch Intern Med. 2009;169:651–8.
92. Tsai PS, Fan YC, Huang CJ. Fibromyalgia is associated with coronary heart disease: a population-based cohort study. Reg Anesth Pain Med. 2015;40:37–42.
93. Haliloğlu S, Carlioglu A, Sahiner E, Karaaslan Y, Kosar A. Mean platelet volume in patients with fibromyalgia. Z Rheumatol. 2014;73:742–5.
94. Wolfe F, Hassett AL, Walitt B, Michaud K. Mortality in fibromyalgia: a study of 8,186 patients over thirty-five years. Arthritis Care Res (Hoboken). 2011;63:94–101.
95. Aparicio VA, Segura-Jiménez V, Alvarez-Gallardo IC, et al. Are there differences in quality of life, symptomatology and functional capacity among different obesity classes in women with fibromyalgia? The al-Ándalus project. Rheumatol Int. 2014;34:811–21.
96. Berger A, Dukes E, Martin S, Edelsberg J, et al. Characteristics and healthcare costs of patients with fibromyalgia syndrome. Int J Clin Pract. 2007;61:1498–508.
97. Fuller-Thomson E, Nimigon-Young J, Brennenstuhl S. Individuals with fibromyalgia and depression: findings from a nationally representative Canadian survey. Rheumatol Int. 2012;32:853–62.
98. Spaeth M. Epidemiology, costs, and the economic burden of fibromyalgia. Arthritis Res Ther. 2009;11:117.
99. Perrot S, Schaefer C, Knight T, Hufstader M, Chandran AB, Zlateva G. Societal and individual burden of illness among fibromyalgia patients in France: association between disease severity and OMERACT core domains. BMC Musculoskelet Disord. 2012;13:22.
100. Meenagh G, Sakellariou G, Iagnocco A, et al. Ultrasound imaging for the rheumatologist XXXIX. Sonographic assessment of the hip in fibromyalgia. Clin Exp Rheumatol. 2012;30:319–21.

Chapter 12
Vasculitis

Yair Molad

Vasculitis is a heterogeneous group of disorders characterized by inflammation of the blood vessel walls. It can results in vessel wall destruction leading to aneurysm or rupture or in stenosis with tissue damage from ischemia and subsequent activation of the inflammatory cascade [1]. The different vasculitides may be categorized by the size of the involved vessel: large – aorta and its main branches; medium – visceral arteries; small – capillaries and intraparenchymal arteries, arterioles, and venules [1]. They may occur as a primary disorder or secondary to infection (particularly hepatitis B and C); malignancy; autoimmune disease such as rheumatoid arthritis, systemic lupus erythematosus, and Sjogren's syndrome; intake of certain drugs, and exposure to allergens.

Comorbidities may be an intrinsic component of systemic vasculitis, or they may present as adverse events following treatment with corticosteroids, immunosuppressive drugs, biological drugs, or other agents. This chapter describes the main comorbidities attributed to the inflammatory pathological process that underlies the vasculitides and to the immunoregulatory drugs used to treat them. The associations of vasculitis in adults with cardiovascular diseases, metabolic syndrome, arterial hypertension, infectious complications, malignancy, and thrombosis are highlighted.

Y. Molad (✉)
Rheumatology Unit, Rabin Medical Center – Beilinson Hospital, Petach Tikva and Sackler Faculty of Medicine, Tel Aviv, Israel
e-mail: ymolad@post.tau.ac.il

Y. El Miedany (ed.), *Comorbidity in Rheumatic Diseases*,
DOI 10.1007/978-3-319-59963-2_12

Large-Vessel Vasculitis

In large-vessel vasculitis, the vasculitic process is predominantly confined to the aorta and its major branches. The most common form, particularly in the white, over-50-year-old population, is giant cell arteritis (GCA). GCA is characterized histopathologically by invasion of the entire vessel wall with macrophages, lymphocytes, and plasma cells, with focal accumulation of giant cells, and clinically by headache, tenderness of the scalp, claudication of the jaw and/or tongue, loss of vision, and polymyalgia rheumatica. Systemic symptoms, such as fatigue, malaise, and fever, and a highly elevated erythrocyte sedimentation rate are almost invariably present. Corticosteroids are the mainstay of treatment. Patients are usually started on prednisone 40–60 mg/day followed by gradual dose tapering sometimes over several years [2].

Another major form of large-vessel vasculitis is Takayasu arteritis (TA), which usually affects the aorta and its brachiocephalic branches but may sometimes affect the pulmonary arteries, other visceral arteries, and arteries of the lower extremities. TA is characterized histopathologically by granulomatous inflammation with infiltrates of lymphocytes, plasma cells, eosinophils, histiocytes, and Langerhans cells. The active inflammation results in segmental narrowing of the arteries with aneurysm formation, which presents clinically with a myriad of ischemic symptoms including claudication of the upper and lower extremities, cerebral ischemia, ischemic bowel disease, renal vascular hypertension, aortic insufficiency, and others. TA occurs at a younger age than GCA, between 15 and 45 years, predominantly in women of Oriental, African, and Latin-American descent [3]. Treatment consists of corticosteroids for more than 1 year, often accompanied by other immunosuppressive drugs, such as methotrexate, azathioprine, mycophenolate mofetil, tocilizumab, and/or antitumor necrosis factor (TNF) agents [4, 5].

Comorbidities of Large-Vessel Vasculitis

Cardiovascular Disease

Premature accelerated atherosclerosis is a common finding in many of the inflammatory rheumatic diseases and one of the main causes of premature cardiovascular morbidity and mortality [6, 7]. The high rate of conventional risk factors such as diabetes mellitus, hypertension, dyslipidemia, metabolic syndrome, chronic kidney disease, and persistent proteinuria contributes to the underlying pathologic mechanism. Inflammation-mediated endothelial cell dysfunction and activation and increased production of C-reactive protein are involved as well [7].

Epidemiological studies suggest that the overall mortality of patients with GCA is similar to or only slightly higher than that of the age-matched general population [8, 9], but cardiovascular morbidity and mortality is significantly increased [10]. Patients are at higher-than-normal risk of early and late ischemic stroke, mainly at the time of GCA presentation. Reported rates of stroke associated with biopsy-proven GCA, especially in the vertebrobasilar territory, range from 2.8% in a retrospective review study of 287 consecutive patients followed for a 27-year period in a single center in Spain [11] to 7% in a French population-based study of 57 patients [12]. Most of the affected patients in the latter study were older men with vascular risk factors [12]. Similarly, a Canadian population-based study reported an increased incidence of stroke during the first year after GCA diagnosis [13]. Among three comparative population-based studies of patients with and without GCA, two found no difference in the incidence of ischemic heart disease due to coronary artery atherosclerosis [14, 15], and one found an increase in the GCA group [16].

TA was found to be associated with accelerated atherosclerosis in autopsy [17, 18] and carotid artery ultrasonography [19] studies. Risk factors are older age and high blood lipid levels. Stroke occurs in 10–20% of patients with TA, which is a remarkably high prevalence given that TA affects predominantly young women [20]. Left main coronary artery occlusion can occur as result of active ostial arteritis. Coronary artery involvement is detected in 10–30% of patients with TA [21].

Although aortitis is frequently associated with TA, patients with GCA appear to have an elevated incidence of aortic aneurysm, particularly of the thoracic aorta, compared with the general population [22]. A UK General Practice Research Database parallel cohort study of 6999 patients with GCA and 41,994 controls found a twofold increase in the rate of aortic aneurysm in patients with GCA compared to an age-matched general population [23]. Aortic aneurysm may appear many years after the diagnosis of GCA, even after treatment has been completed. Therefore diagnosis requires a high index of clinical suspicion and imaging workup [24].

Hypertension and Metabolic Syndrome

Renovascular hypertension due to renal artery stenosis or aortic coarctation is a frequent finding in patients with large-vessel vasculitis. In patients with TA, it may be the presenting complaint that leads to diagnosis [25]. In a retrospective analysis of 180 patients with biopsy-proven GCA from Italy, hypertension was found to be significantly associated with an increased risk of the development of severe cranial ischemic events [odds ratio (OR) = 7.77, 95% confidence interval (CI) 0.83, 72.76] [26]. Interestingly, a retrospective study of 286 patients with GCA from the United States found that those with hypertension or diabetes mellitus at diagnosis had more relapses during follow-up than those without these comorbidities [27]. This finding emphasizes the prognostic importance of early and tight control of blood pressure in patients with GCA.

Metabolic syndrome is a cluster of conditions, namely, high body mass index, hypertension, diabetes mellitus, and hypertriglyceridemia, that occur together and increase the risk of cardiovascular disease. A high prevalence of metabolic syndrome has been observed in patients with TA, regardless of disease duration, disease activity, use of glucocorticoids, or level of inflammatory cytokines [28].

Infections

Corticosteroids and immunosuppressive, cytotoxic, and biologic drugs, all used in the treatment of systemic vasculitis, are associated with an increased risk of systemic infections, one of the leading causes of death in patients with GCA. A study of 1664 patients with GCA found that 48% had at least one episode of systemic infection; the risk was highest in the first 6 months of corticosteroid treatment [29]. However, a retrospective population-based study showed that patients with corticosteroid-treated CGA were not at an overall higher-than-normal risk of infections requiring hospitalization or acquired during hospitalization, but they seemed to be at increased risk specifically of gastrointestinal infections [30]. Nevertheless, although the overall mortality rate of patients with GCA is not different from that of the general population, infection is a significantly more common cause of death in the first year after diagnosis [8, 31].

Thrombosis

The relationship between vasculitis and thrombosis has been established in recent years. The underlying mechanism involves endothelial cell adhesiveness, endothelial cell activation, and tissue factor production, as well as the procoagulable state of patients with active vasculitis [32, 33]. In a large population-based study, the risk of venous thromboembolism was significantly high in patients with recent-onset GCA, independent of age and gender [34]. Moreover, deep venous thrombosis was found to be among the mortality risk factors in a cohort of 9311 hospitalized patients with GCA in the United States [35]. There are no available studies describing the risk and prevalence of thromboembolism in patients with TA.

Malignancy

Whether cancer and/or lympho- or myeloproliferative disorders are more frequent in patients with GCA remains unclear. Several population-based, case-control studies performed in countries where GCA is prevalent concluded that affected patients are not at increased risk of cancer either before [36] or after [37, 38] diagnosis. However, a meta-analysis of cohort studies of patients with GCA and/or polymyalgia rheumatic [39] and a retrospective analysis of 271 consecutive patients [40] found a slightly increased risk of malignancy at the time of GCA diagnosis. One South Korean retrospective cohort study failed to demonstrate an increased risk of malignancy in patients with TA compared to the general population [41].

Medium-Vessel Vasculitis

Polyarteritis nodosa (PAN) is a multi-organ necrotizing form of vasculitis that affects medium- and small-sized vessels. It commonly involves the kidneys, gastrointestinal tract, skin, peripheral nerves, and muscles.

Comorbidities

Cardiovascular Disease

Cardiovascular disease associated with PAN usually presents as congestive heart failure (27%), hypertension (37%), and less commonly as myocardial infarction (2%) [42]. Coronary arteritis with multiple coronary aneurysms is very rare [43]. There are no published case studies of the prevalence of hypertension and metabolic syndrome in PAN.

Infections

Classical PAN is usually treated with corticosteroids and cytotoxic drugs which pose an increased risk of infectious complications. However, there are no case studies specifically addressing this adverse effect in patients with PAN.

Thrombosis

The association of PAN with an increased risk of arterial and venous thrombosis has been documented in several studies [44–46]. A retrospective, systematic analysis of 1130 patients with PAN or small-sized vessel vasculitis derived from the French Vasculitis Study Group cohort found a significantly lower frequency of venous thromboembolism in the PAN group, although the risk was relatively higher during active than inactive disease (3.27 events/person-year versus 0.58 events/person-year) [47].

Malignancy

Despite the well-recognized association between hairy-cell leukemia and PAN [48], case studies report a lower risk of the development of cancer after diagnosis of either hepatitis B-associated or nonviral-associated PAN [49–51].

Small-Vessel Vasculitis

Patients with small-vessel vasculitis may be classified according to the presence or absence of immune complexes. The immune-complex-mediated small-vessel vasculitides include IgA vasculitis (Henoch-Schönlein purpura), essential cryoglobulinemic vasculitis, hypocomplementemic urticarial vasculitis, and anti-glomerular basement membrane disease. All these forms are characterized by attacks of purpura, urticaria, arthralgias/arthritis, gastrointestinal symptoms, and/or glomerulonephritis. The pauci-immune small-vessel vasculitides are associated with the presence of proteinase-3 (c-ANCA)- or myeloperoxidase (p-ANCA)-specific anti-neutrophilic cytoplasmic antibodies (ANCA). They include granulomatosis with polyangiitis (GPA or Wegener's granulomatosis), eosinophilic granulomatosis with polyangiitis (EGPA or Churg-Strauss syndrome), and microscopic polyangiitis (MPA). Clinically, ANCA-associated vasculitis (AAV) is characterized by cutaneous, upper and lower respiratory tract, neurological, and renal manifestations that lead to death within weeks to months if left untreated. Currently, treatment consists of corticosteroids; cytotoxic drugs such as cyclophosphamide (until recently, the standard of care for the majority of patients [52]), azathioprine, and methotrexate; and a B-cell-depleting drug (rituximab). The use of these drugs has considerably improved patient outcome, but it has also raised concerns about disease- and treatment-related sequelae. According to the prospective multicenter European Vasculitis Study Group (EUVAS) trials, survival rates in patients with AAV treated according to strictly defined protocols at presentation were 88% at 1 year, 85% at 2 years, and 78% at 5 years. However, the mortality ratio was 2.6 compared with the general population [53].

Comorbidities

Atherosclerosis

Early mortality in AAV is due mostly to disease complications and/or severe treatment-associated infections; late mortality is attributed to cardiovascular disease and/or malignancy. Coronary artery disease has been found to be two to four times more frequent in patients with AAV than the age-matched general population [54–56]. A logistic regression model fitted to data derived from the first four trials of the EUVAS trials revealed that 14% of patients with Wegener's granulomatosis or MPA have an episode of cardiovascular disease within 5 years of diagnosis [57]. Moreover, accelerated subclinical atherosclerosis has emerged as a significant morbidity in AAV. It is apparently associated with the systemic active inflammatory state of the vasculitis itself, as demonstrated by the increase in plasma microparticles [58], and occurs independently of traditional cardiovascular risk factors [54, 57, 59, 60]. Manifestations include endothelial dysfunction [61], increased intima-media thickness of the carotid artery [58], and plaque burden in the carotid arteries, aorta, and femoral arteries [60]. Interestingly, a Danish cohort of patients with GPA did not show an increased prevalence of stroke compared to controls [62].

Metabolic Syndrome

A case-control, cross-sectional study showed that metabolic syndrome is more prevalent in patients with AAV (43%) than in healthy individuals (25%; $P = 0.012$) [63], unrelated to current or cumulative prednisone use.

Thrombosis

The frequency of venous thromboembolism is increased in patients with AAV, especially when it is concurrent with active disease [47, 62–67]. The prospective 2-year Wegener's Granulomatosis Etanercept Trial [64] included 180 patients with GPA, of whom 7.2% had a history of venous thromboembolism before enrolment and 8.9% had an event of venous thromboembolism during follow-up. In a retrospective study of 19 patients with EGPA (Churg-Strauss syndrome), 31.6% were found to have evidence of thrombosis [67]. This finding was supported by a meta-analysis of retrospective case series of EGPA showing that 3.1–30% of patients had arterial and venous thromboembolic events [68]. Other studies of AAV noted arterial thrombosis rates of 18.7% [54, 56], mostly cardiovascular events.

Infections

In patients with AAV treated with high-dose corticosteroids, cytotoxic drugs such as cyclophosphamide, and biologic agents such as rituximab, infections are a major and sometimes life-threatening complication and a leading cause of death [53, 69–71]. The burden of infection is greatest during remission induction, reflecting the intensity of immunosuppression. In observational studies, 20–60% of patients with AAV acquired significant infections [72, 73]. Others reported 53 episodes of major infections during induction and maintenance treatment in 35 French patients with Wegener's granulomatosis followed for 6 years [74], similar to the 33% rate reported in a Norwegian cohort [75]. A 48% rate of severe infection was found in a cohort of patients with GPA diagnosed between 1984 and 1999 and followed for 4.5 years [76]. Multivariate analysis of the causes of early death in the EUVAS trials revealed that infection, leukopenia, and adverse event scores were each independently associated with early mortality [69]. Half of the infections occurred within the first 2 months of diagnosis, in agreement with the findings of an international, prospective, multicenter study showing that 48% of deaths of patients with AAV treated according to strictly defined protocols were due to infections [53]. Accordingly, the cumulative incidence of infection of a prospectively followed inception cohort of patients with biopsy-proven AAV was 51% at 1 year, 58% at 2 years, and 65% at 5 years; corresponding rates of severe infection were 22%, 23%, and 26% [77, 78]. Infection-induced death in AAV cohort studies was significantly predicted by disease activity at diagnosis and severity of organ damage at remission but not by cyclophosphamide treatment for remission induction [72] or remission maintenance therapy [78]. Older age at disease onset not only increases the risk of infection but also the resulting morbidity and mortality [79]. Leukopenia and renal failure were also associated with a higher rate of infections [79, 80].

Drug schedules may also affect the infection rate. In a comparative cohort study, 147 patients with AAV at 6 months after initiation were treated with cyclophosphamide and either 0 mg, 5 mg, or >5 mg prednisone daily. Those who received glucocorticosteroids beyond 6 months had a significantly higher incidence of infections (0.64 infections/person-year versus 0.39 infections/person-year, $P < 0.0001$) [81]. Others found that patients receiving intravenous pulses of cyclophosphamide for induction of AAV remission were at lower risk of infection than patients treated with daily oral cyclophosphamide [80, 82, 83]. However, the incidence was similar when daily oral cyclophosphamide induction was followed by azathioprine maintenance therapy [81].

Rituximab is a chimeric monoclonal CD20 antibody that depletes B cells. In a randomized control trial, rituximab proved effective for induction and maintenance of remission in AAV [84]. There was no difference between rituximab and cyclophosphamide in either effectiveness for remission induction or rate of serious infections [84]. In two retrospective studies, rates of severe infections in patients on rituximab maintenance treatment were 24% [85] and 41% [86]. Putative factors associated with an increased risk included older age, cumulative dose of cyclophosphamide, kidney involvement, low CD4 cell count, and decrease in total immunoglobulins after the first 2 g of rituximab treatment [85]. The rate of hypogammaglobulinemia seemed to be associated with cyclophosphamide use [87–89] and with the type of rituximab maintenance regimen [89], independent of the rituximab cumulative dose [88, 89]. Rituximab treatment, either a single or repeated courses, has also been associated with late-onset neutropenia in patients with GPA and MPA, with a consequent high incidence of infection [90]. These findings emphasize the importance of regular monitoring of absolute neutrophil count along with serum immunoglobulin level during and following rituximab treatment.

Malignancy

Malignancy accounts for 22% of the mortality in the first year of diagnosis of AAV [53]. Studies estimate an increased global risk of both solid and hematologic malignancies, from 1.6 to 18 times higher than that in the general population [91–98]. However, whether this risk is inherent to the disease or related to its treatment is difficult to determine for several reasons: the low prevalence of AAV; the relatively short patient survival time; and the well-documented carcinogenic properties of the alkylating agent cyclophosphamide. A longitudinal study of the risk of malignancy in a Dutch cohort of patients who were diagnosed with histopathologically confirmed AAV between 1991 and 2013 and treated with immunosuppressive agents reported a 2.21-fold higher risk (95% CI 64–2.92) than in the general population [99]. The most frequent type of malignancy was nonmelanoma skin cancer [standardized incidence ratio (SIR) 4.23, 95% CI 2.76–6.19]. The incidence rates of other malignancies were not significantly increased. Malignancy risk was significantly associated with the duration of cyclophosphamide therapy for more than 1 year. (Interestingly, it was not increased in patients who had received cyclophosphamide for less than 1 year.) A Danish study of 293 patients diagnosed with GPA from 1973 to 1999 and followed through 2010 found an increased risk of nonmelanoma skin cancers. There were also

11 cases of cyclophosphamide-associated bladder carcinomas and cases of myeloid leukemia [100]. The incidence of nonmelanoma skin cancers increased from the second year of follow-up onward, with SIR 7.0 (95% CI 2.3–16) for cancers diagnosed at 20 years or more after the diagnosis of GPA. The incidence of bladder cancer increased after 5–9 years (SIR 5.3, 95% CI 1.1–15), 10–14 years (SIR 14.4, 95% CI 5.3–31), and 15–19 years (SIR 10.5, 95% CI 1.2–38). The incidence of myeloid leukemia was significantly increased during years 5–9 (SIR 23.9, 95% CI 2.7–86). Rates of all three malignancies rose in patients exposed to cumulative cyclophosphamide doses of more than 36 g; in those treated with lower doses, the only malignancy type in excess was nonmelanoma skin cancer. The cancer risk among cyclophosphamide-naive patients was not significantly increased. These findings were confirmed by a meta-analysis of 6 studies including a total of 2578 patients which yielded an overall pooled SIR of 1.74 for cancer in patients with AAV (95% CI = 1.37–2.21) [101], with higher risks specifically of nonmelanoma skin cancer (SIR 5.18, 95% CI 3.47–7.73), leukemia (SIR 4.89, 95% CI 2.93–8.16), and bladder cancer (SIR 3.84, 95%CI 2.72–5.42).

Impact of Comorbidity on Disease Outcome and Mortality in AAV

AAV comorbidities impact the overall survival and quality of life of patients. To assess and predict disease outcome and patient survival with respect to comorbidities, researchers have developed various integrated scores for use in daily practice as well as clinical trials. The current gold standard tool in the clinical research setting is the 1987 Charlson Comorbidity Index (CCI) which was designed to predict the 1- or 10-year mortality risks in 16 diseases or conditions, each of which is assigned a weight of 1–6 [102, 103]. The CCI was found to be a valuable measure when used with the International Classification of Diseases, Ninth Revision [104]. An age-adjusted CCI index [CCI(a)] was introduced in 1984 which takes the effect of aging on mortality into account by assigning one extra point for each decade above 50 years [103]. The predictive value of the CCI was assessed in a longitudinal observational study of 30 consecutive patients with AAV attending a university-affiliated medical center in Israel from January 1996 to December 2011 [105]. The main comorbidities that occurred during the study period were hypertension (12 patients, 40%), diabetes mellitus (7 patients, 23.3%), stroke/transient ischemic attack (2 patients, 6.7%), and coronary heart disease (1 patient, 3.3%). Five patients (16.7%) acquired a malignant disease during the study period: four solid tumors (13.3%) and one (3.3%) hematologic malignancy. Five patients (16.67%) died during follow-up: one from malignancy and four from infection. A higher CCI(a) score at diagnosis was significantly correlated with active disease at diagnosis ($P = 0.021$), higher CCI(a) score at the last follow-up visit ($P = 0.001$), and a high value on the Birmingham Vasculitis Activity Score ($P = 0.02$). A CCI(a) score of 5 or more at diagnosis was significantly associated with a greater risk of death (OR 12; 95% CI 1.8–79.68, $P = 0.014$), and an increment of more than 1 in the CCI(a) score from diagnosis of AAV to the last follow-up was significantly associated with reduced patient survival. In accordance, in a study of patients with GPA and preexisting comorbidities [106], the calculated odds ratios for mortality for patients with a CCI score of 1 or more at diagnosis were 13.3 during years 0–2 of follow-up and 1.9 thereafter, compared to 0 and 1.4, respectively, for patients with a CCI score of 0 at diagnosis. These studies [105, 106] emphasize the pivotal effect of preexisting comorbidities, defined as an increased CCI score at AAV diagnosis, on the risk of early and late death during the disease course. The data support the need to assess comorbidities at the time of AAV diagnosis and treatment planning.

Behçet's Disease

Behçet's disease (BD) is a chronic vasculitis affecting vessels of any size, with no predominant type (variable-vessel vasculitis) [1]. It is characterized clinically by oral and genital ulcers, papulopustular and nodular skin lesions, pathergy, vascular involvement, uveitis, and central nervous system and gastrointestinal involvement [107]. The disease is particularly prevalent along the Silk Road, extending from Japan to the Middle Eastern and the Mediterranean countries; reported rates range from 14/100,000 to 20/100,000 population [108]. It is also often more severe in these regions. BD has been associated with the HLA-B*51 antigen [109]. The European League Against Rheumatism recommends immunosuppressive treatment for patients with BD, including corticosteroids, azathioprine, cyclophosphamide, or cyclosporine A [110].

Comorbidities

Cardiovascular Disease

The heart is one of the major organs involved in BD. Common cardiac manifestations include intracardiac thrombus, endocarditis, myocarditis, pericarditis, endomyocardial fibrosis, coronary arteritis, myocardial infarction, and valvular disease [111, 112]. Patients with vascular BD and coronary artery involvement may present with coronary thrombosis, aneurysm, or rupture. Coronary aneurysms may be asymptomatic or manifest with acute coronary syndrome; they are usually detected during angiography procedures [113]. The pulmonary artery is the most common large artery affected in BD [114, 115], and pulmonary artery aneurysm is associated with an increased risk of death [116, 117]. Peripheral arteries in the lower extremities are also commonly involved [113, 118]. Peripheral arterial aneurysms, pseudoaneurysms, stenosis, and occlusion frequently require invasive endovascular and/

or surgical intervention [118]. In a study of 796 Chinese patients with BD, 12.8% had evidence of involvement mainly of the abdominal aorta and lower extremities (28.6% each), followed by the pulmonary artery (23.2%), coronary artery (8.9%), and carotid artery (7.1%) [113].

Despite the relatively increased prevalence of arterial involvement in BD and the prolonged inflammatory course of the disease, atherosclerosis was not found to be more prevalent in patients with BD than in healthy control subjects [119–121]. In a study of 239 Turkish patients with BD [119], the rate of subclinical atherosclerosis was similar to that in matched healthy subjects and significantly lower than in patients with rheumatoid arthritis. Another case-controlled Turkish study [121] found no between-group difference in the risk of angina pectoris, myocardial infarction, and ischemic heart disease. Interestingly, a systematic review and meta-analysis of cardiac disease in BD reported an increase in cardiac diastolic dysfunction [122].

In the Chinese cohort study of BD, 70.6% of the vascular lesions were in veins and 54.9% in arteries [113]. Venous involvement predominately took the form of thrombophlebitis, mainly in the lower extremities, followed by the superior vena cava and inferior vena cava. In a chart review of 5970 Turkish patients with BD, 882 (14.7%) had vascular involvement (14.7%), mostly deep vein thrombosis (67.1%), almost always in the legs [123]. Venous disease was more common in patients from the Middle East [124].

Thrombosis

The prevalence of thrombosis in BD ranges between 10% and 30% [125–128]. Arterial and vascular thrombotic events usually occur early in the disease course and are believed to result from active vasculitis [129]. They may involve multiple arteries as well as deep and superficial veins. Budd-Chiari syndrome and vena cava thrombosis account for a significant proportion of the morbidity in BD [130, 131]. The increased risk of thrombosis as well as the low frequency of venous thromboembolic complications may be explained by the procoagulable and adherent endovascular changes that occur in BD as a result of the inflammatory process in the blood vessel walls [132, 133]. Besides venous thrombosis of the lower extremity veins, dural cerebral venous thrombosis is a common vascular manifestation in BD, more frequently seen in youth and in males [133]. It usually causes increased intracranial pressure and presents with headache, blurred vision with papilledema and sixth nerve palsy, and vomiting [133, 134]. A systematic review of 249 patients with BD reported an overall incidence of cerebral venous thrombosis of 3.1/1000 person-years [134]. The sagittal and transverse sinuses were the most frequent sites affected (almost 60% of cases each), and treatment usually consisted of corticosteroids, immunosuppressive drugs, and, less frequently, anticoagulation. Sequelae were present in 20% of patients. The predominant complication was optic nerve atrophy/blindness/reduced visual acuity [134]. Usually, treatment with anticoagulants alone is not recommended, but in patients with cerebral venous thrombosis, anticoagulation may sometimes be combined with corticosteroids [133, 135]. Pulmonary artery thrombosis is rare in BD, usually found in association with pulmonary artery aneurysm. It accounts for significant morbidity and mortality [114, 136]. Intracardiac wall thrombosis has also been reported in BD, frequently in association with pulmonary artery disease [137].

Infections

There are no studies to suggest an increased risk of serious bacterial or viral infections associated with BD. Nevertheless, serious infections have been reported in 16.3% of patients with BD treated with biologic drugs such as TNF inhibitors [138].

Malignancy

Because BD is a rare disease, only a few studies have addressed the risk of malignancy. A nationwide population-based study of 1314 patients in Taiwan reported an overall higher risk of cancer in patients with BD than in the general population (2.3%, SIR 1.8) but only in females [139]. Specifically, risks were highest for hematological malignancy (SIR 4.21), especially non-Hodgkin's lymphoma, and breast cancer (SIR 2.16). The cancer prevalence in a retrospective cohort of 1769 Korean patients with BD was 1.8% [140]. Thyroid cancer was the most common type of solid cancer, followed by breast, cervix, and stomach cancer; myelodysplastic syndrome was the most common hematological cancer, followed by aplastic anemia and lymphoma [140]. The predominance of hematologic malignancy, especially myelodysplastic syndrome, was supported by a review study of 651 Chinese patients with BD hospitalized in Peking Union Medical College Hospital from 1995 to 2012 [141]. Other studies [142, 143] in addition to a systematic review [144] observed that myelodysplastic syndrome was more common in patients with gastrointestinal involvement of BD, with an increased association with trisomy 8 [144]. The association of trisomy 8 and myelodysplastic syndrome in BD was also reported in a review study of 54 Japanese patients, mostly elderly (70–90 years old), with gastrointestinal involvement [145].

Conclusion

Comorbidities affect the course and outcome of vasculitis. They reflect both the diminished preexisting health status of the patient at the time of initiation of immunosuppressive therapy as well as the accrual of organ damage and treatment-related morbidity during the period of active disease and remission-induction and maintenance therapy. Comorbidities are common in all types of vasculitis. Special emphasis should be placed on the high risk of treatment-induced severe infections and atherosclerotic as well as thrombotic vascular morbidity and mortality. Careful and meticulous assessment of the presence of comorbidities is mandatory at diagnosis of the various vasculitides, during the active phase of disease, and at remission.

References

1. Jennette JC, Falk RJ, Bacon PA, Basu N, Cid MC, Ferrario F, et al. 2012 revised international Chapel Hill consensus conference nomenclature of vasculitides. Arthritis Rheum. 2013;65(1):1–11.
2. Matteson EL, Buttgereit F, Dejaco C, Dasgupta B. Glucocorticoids for management of polymyalgia rheumatica and giant cell arteritis. Rheum Dis Clin N Am. 2016;42(1):75–90.
3. de Souza AW, de Carvalho JF. Diagnostic and classification criteria of Takayasu arteritis. J Autoimmun. 2014;48-49:79–83.
4. Mukhtyar C, Guillevin L, Cid MC, Dasgupta B, de Groot K, Gross W, et al. European Vasculitis Study Group. EULAR recommendations for the management of large vessel vasculitis. Ann Rheum Dis. 2009;68(3):318–23.
5. Ferfar Y, Mirault T, Desbois AC, Comarmond C, Messas E, Savey L, et al. Biotherapies in large vessel vasculitis. Autoimmun Rev. 2016;15(6):544–51.
6. Hollan I, Meroni PL, Ahearn JM, Cohen Tervaert JW, Curran S, Goodyear CS, et al. Cardiovascular disease in autoimmune rheumatic diseases. Autoimmun Rev. 2013;12(10):1004–15.
7. Mason JC, Libby P. Cardiovascular disease in patients with chronic inflammation: mechanisms underlying premature cardiovascular events in rheumatologic conditions. Eur Heart J. 2015;36(8):482–9c.
8. Ninan J, Nguyen AM, Cole A, Rischmueller M, Dodd T, Roberts-Thomson P, et al. Mortality in patients with biopsy-proven giant cell arteritis: a south Australian population-based study. J Rheumatol. 2011;38(10):2215–7.
9. Baslund B, Helleberg M, Faurschou M, Obel N. Mortality in patients with giant cell arteritis. Rheumatology (Oxford). 2015;54(1):139–43.
10. Tomasson G, Peloquin C, Mohammad A, Love TJ, Zhang Y, Choi HK, et al. Risk for cardiovascular disease early and late after a diagnosis of giant-cell arteritis: a cohort study. Ann Intern Med. 2014;160(2):73–80.
11. Gonzalez-Gay MA, Vazquez-Rodriguez TR, Gomez-Acebo I, Pego-Reigosa R, Lopez-Diaz MJ, Vazquez-Triñanes MC, et al. Strokes at time of disease diagnosis in a series of 287 patients with biopsy-proven giant cell arteritis. Medicine (Baltimore). 2009;88(4):227–35.
12. Samson M, Jacquin A, Audia S, Daubail B, Devilliers H, Petrella T, et al. Stroke associated with giant cell arteritis: a population-based study. J Neurol Neurosurg Psychiatry. 2015;86(2):216–21.
13. Amiri N, De Vera M, Choi HK, Sayre EC, Avina-Zubieta JA. Increased risk of cardiovascular disease in giant cell arteritis: a general population-based study. Rheumatology (Oxford). 2016;55(1):33–40.
14. González-Gay MA, Blanco R, Abraira V, García-Porrúa C, Ibáñez D, García-Pais MJ, et al. Giant cell arteritis in Lugo, Spain, is associated with low long-term mortality. J Rheumatol. 1997;24(11):2171–6.
15. Udayakumar PD, Chandran AK, Crowson CS, Warrington KJ, Matteson EL. Cardiovascular risk and acute coronary syndrome in giant cell arteritis: a population-based retrospective cohort study. Arthritis Care Res (Hoboken). 2015;67(3):396–402.
16. Petri H, Nevitt A, Sarsour K, Napalkov P, Collinson N. Incidence of giant cell arteritis and characteristics of patients: data-driven analysis of comorbidities. Arthritis Care Res (Hoboken). 2015;67(3):390–5.
17. Filer A, Nicholls D, Corston R, Carey P, Bacon P. Takayasu arteritis and atherosclerosis: illustrating the consequences of endothelial damage. J Rheumatol. 2001;28(12):2752–3.
18. Numano F, Okawara M, Inomata H, Kobayashi Y. Takayasu's arteritis. Lancet. 2000;356:1023–5.
19. Seyahi E, Ugurlu S, Cumali R, Balci H, Seyahi N, Yurdakul S, et al. Atherosclerosis in Takayasu arteritis. Ann Rheum Dis. 2006;65(9):1202–7.
20. Duarte MM, Geraldes R, Sousa R, Alarcão J, Costa J. Stroke and transient ischemic attack in Takayasu's arteritis: a systematic review and meta-analysis. J Stroke Cerebrovasc Dis. 2016;25(4):781–91.

21. Rav-Acha M, Plot L, Peled N, Amital H. Coronary involvement in Takayasu's arteritis. Autoimmun Rev. 2007;6(8):566–71.
22. Bossert M, Prati C, Balblanc JC, Lohse A, Wendling D. Aortic involvement in giant cell arteritis: current data. Joint Bone Spine. 2011;78(3):246–51.
23. Robson JC, Kiran A, Maskell J, Hutchings A, Arden N, Dasgupta B, et al. The relative risk of aortic aneurysm in patients with giant cell arteritis compared with the general population of the UK. Ann Rheum Dis. 2015;74(1):129–35.
24. Mackie SL, Hensor EM, Morgan AW, Pease CT. Should I send my patient with previous giant cell arteritis for imaging of the thoracic aorta? A systematic literature review and meta-analysis. Ann Rheum Dis. 2014;73(1):143–8.
25. Mwipatayi BP, Jeffery PC, Beningfield SJ, Matley PJ, Naidoo NG, Kalla AA, et al. Takayasu arteritis: clinical features and management: report of 272 cases. ANZ J Surg. 2005;75(3):110–7.
26. Salvarani C, Della Bella C, Cimino L, Macchioni P, Formisano D, Bajocchi G, et al. Risk factors for severe cranial ischaemic events in an Italian population-based cohort of patients with giant cell arteritis. Rheumatology (Oxford). 2009;48(3):250–3.
27. Labarca C, Koster MJ, Crowson CS, Makol A, Ytterberg SR, Matteson EL, et al. Predictors of relapse and treatment outcomes in biopsy-proven giant cell arteritis: a retrospective cohort study. Rheumatology (Oxford). 2016;55(2):347–56.
28. da Silva TF, Levy-Neto M, Bonfá E, Pereira RM. High prevalence of metabolic syndrome in Takayasu arteritis: increased cardiovascular risk and lower adiponectin serum levels. J Rheumatol. 2013;40(11):1897–904.
29. Durand M, Thomas SL. Incidence of infections in patients with giant cell arteritis: a cohort study. Arthritis Care Res (Hoboken). 2012;64(4):581–8.
30. Udayakumar PD, Chandran AK, Crowson CS, Warrington KJ, Matteson EL. Hospitalized infections in giant cell arteritis: a population-based retrospective cohort study. J Rheumatol. 2014;41(12):2447–51.
31. Schmidt J, Smail A, Roche B, Gay P, Salle V, Pellet H, et al. Incidence of severe infections and infection-related mortality during the course of Giant cell arteritis: a multicenter, prospective. Double-Cohort Study Arthritis Rheumatol. 2016;68(6):1477–82.
32. Gaffo AL. Thrombosis in vasculitis. Best Pract Res Clin Rheumatol. 2013;27(1):57–67.
33. Emmi G, Silvestri E, Squatrito D, Amedei A, Niccolai E, D'Elios MM, et al. Thrombosis in vasculitis: from pathogenesis to treatment. Thromb J. 2015;13:15.
34. Aviña-Zubieta JA, Bhole VM, Amiri N, Sayre EC, Choi HK. The risk of deep venous thrombosis and pulmonary embolism in giant cell arteritis: a general population-based study. Ann Rheum Dis. 2016;75(1):148–54.
35. Unizony S, Menendez ME, Rastalsky N, Stone JH. Inpatient complications in patients with giant cell arteritis: decreased mortality and increased risk of thromboembolism, delirium and adrenal insufficiency. Rheumatology (Oxford). 2015;54(8):1360–8.
36. Kermani TA, Schäfer VS, Crowson CS, Hunder GG, Ytterberg SR, Matteson EL, et al. Cancer preceding giant cell arteritis: a case-control study. Arthritis Rheum. 2010;62(6):1763–9.
37. Kermani TA, Schäfer VS, Crowson CS, Hunder GG, Gabriel SE, Ytterberg SR, et al. Malignancy risk in patients with giant cell arteritis: a population-based cohort study. Arthritis Care Res (Hoboken). 2010;62(2):149–54.
38. Gonzalez-Gay MA, Lopez-Diaz MJ, Martinez-Lado L, Peña-Sagredo JL, Lopez-Agreda H, Miranda-Filloy JA, et al. Cancer in biopsy-proven giant cell arteritis. A population-based study. Semin Arthritis Rheum. 2007;37(3):156–63.
39. Ungprasert P, Sanguankeo A, Upala S, Knight EL. Risk of malignancy in patients with giant cell arteritis and polymyalgia rheumatica: a systematic review and meta-analysis. Semin Arthritis Rheum. 2014;44(3):366–70.
40. Liozon E, Loustaud V, Fauchais AL, Soria P, Ly K, Ouattara B, et al. Concurrent temporal (giant cell) arteritis and malignancy: report of 20 patients with review of the literature. J Rheumatol. 2006;33(8):1606–14.

41. Park JK, Choi IA, Lee EY, Song YW, Lee EB. Incidence of malignancy in Takayasu arteritis in Korea. Rheumatol Int. 2014;34(4):517–21.
42. Cassling RS, Lortz JB, Olson DR, Hubbard TF, McManus BM. Fatal vasculitis (periarteritis nodosa) of the coronary arteries: angiographic ambiguities and absence of aneurysms at autopsy. J Am Coll Cardiol. 1985;6(3):707–14.
43. Kastner D, Gaffney M, Tak T. Polyarteritis nodosa and myocardial infarction. Can J Cardiol. 2000;16:515–8.
44. Zoller B, Li X, Sundquist J, Sundquist K. Risk of pulmonary embolism in patients with autoimmune disorders: a nationwide follow-up study from Sweden. Lancet 2012;379:244–9.
45. Zöller B, Li X, Sundquist J, Sundquist K. Risk of subsequent ischemic and hemorrhagic stroke in patients hospitalized for immune-mediated diseases: a nationwide follow-up study from Sweden. BMC Neurol. 2012;12:41.
46. Zöller B, Li X, Sundquist J, Sundquist K. Risk of subsequent coronary heart disease in patients hospitalized for immune-mediated diseases: a nationwide follow-up study from Sweden. PLoS One. 2012;7:e33442.
47. Allenbach Y, Seror R, Pagnoux C, Teixeira L, Guilpain P. Guillevin L; French Vasculitis study group. High frequency of venous thromboembolic events in Churg-Strauss syndrome, Wegener's granulomatosis and microscopic polyangiitis but not polyarteritis nodosa: a systematic retrospective study on 1130 patients. Ann Rheum Dis. 2009;68(4):564–7.
48. Hasler P, Kistler H, Gerber H. Vasculitides in hairy cell leukemia. Semin Arthritis Rheum. 1995;25(2):134–42.
49. Pagnoux C, Seror R, Henegar C, Mahr A, Cohen P, Le Guern V, et al. French Vasculitis study group. Clinical features and outcomes in 348 patients with polyarteritis nodosa: a systematic retrospective study of patients diagnosed between 1963 and 2005 and entered into the French Vasculitis study group database. Arthritis Rheum. 2010;62(2):616–26.
50. Guillevin L, Mahr A, Callard P, Godmer P, Pagnoux C, Leray E, et al; French Vasculitis Study Group. Hepatitis B virus-associated polyarteritis nodosa: clinical characteristics, outcome, and impact of treatment in 115 patients. Medicine (Baltimore) 2005;84(5):313–322.
51. Ribi C, Cohen P, Pagnoux C, Mahr A, Arène JP, Puéchal X, et al. French Vasculitis study group. Treatment of polyarteritis nodosa and microscopic polyangiitis without poor-prognosis factors: a prospective randomized study of one hundred twenty-four patients. Arthritis Rheum. 2010;62(4):1186–97.
52. Hoffman GS, Kerr GS, Leavitt RY, Hallahan CW, Lebovics RS, Travis WD, et al. Wegener granulomatosis: an analysis of 158 patients. Ann Intern Med. 1992;116(6):488–98.
53. Flossmann O, Berden A, de Groot K, Hagen C, Harper L, Heijl C, et al. European Vasculitis Study Group. Long-term patient survival in ANCA-associated vasculitis. Ann Rheum Dis. 2011;70(3):488–94.
54. Morgan MD, Turnbull J, Selamet U, Kaur-Hayer M, Nightingale P, Ferro CJ, et al. Increased incidence of cardiovascular events in patients with antineutrophil cytoplasmic antibody-associated vasculitides: a matched-pair cohort study. Arthritis Rheum. 2009;60(11):3493–500.
55. Tervaert JW. Translational mini-review series on immunology of vascular disease: accelerated atherosclerosis in vasculitis. Clin Exp Immunol. 2009;156(3):377–85.
56. Faurschou M, Mellemkjaer L, Sorensen IJ, Svalgaard Thomsen B, Dreyer L, et al. Increased morbidity from ischemic heart disease in patients with Wegener's granulomatosis. Arthritis Rheum. 2009;60(4):1187–92.
57. Suppiah R, Judge A, Batra R, Flossmann O, Harper L, Höglund P, et al. A model to predict ardiovascular events in patients with newly diagnosed Wegener's granulomatosis and microscopic polyangiitis. Arthritis Care Res (Hoboken). 2011;63(4):588–96.
58. de Leeuw K, Sanders JS, Stegeman C, Smit A, Kallenberg CG, Bijl M. Accelerated atherosclerosis in patients with Wegener's granulomatosis. Ann Rheum Dis. 2005;64(5):753–9.
59. Chironi G, Pagnoux C, Simon A, Pasquinelli-Balice M, Del-Pino M, Gariepy J, et al. Increased prevalence of subclinical atherosclerosis in patients with small-vessel vasculitis. Heart. 2007;93(1):96–9.

60. Filer AD, Gardner-Medwin JM, Thambyrajah J, Raza K, Carruthers DM, Stevens RJ, et al. Diffuse endothelial dysfunction is common to ANCA associated systemic vasculitis and polyarteritis nodosa. Ann Rheum Dis. 2003;62(2):162–7.
61. Hajj-Ali RA, Major J, Langford C, Hoffman GS, Clark T, Zhang L, et al. The interface of inflammation and subclinical atherosclerosis in granulomatosis with polyangiitis (Wegener's): a preliminary study. Transl Res. 2015;166(4):366–74.
62. Faurschou M, Obel N, Baslund B. High risk of pulmonary embolism and deep venous thrombosis but not of stroke in granulomatosis with polyangiitis (Wegener's). Arthritis Care Res (Hoboken). 2014;66(12):1910–4.
63. Petermann Smits DR, Wilde B, Kianersi Adegani M, de Jongh H, van Paassen P, Cohen Tervaert JW. Metabolic syndrome in ANCA-associated vasculitis. Rheumatology (Oxford). 2013;52(1):197–203.
64. Merkel PA, Lo GH, Holbrook JT, Tibbs AK, Allen NB, Davis JC Jr, et al. Wegener's Granulomatosis Etanercept Trial Research Group. Brief communication: high incidence of venous thrombotic events among patients with Wegener granulomatosis: the Wegener's Clinical Occurrence of Thrombosis (WeCLOT) Study. Ann Intern Med. 2005;142(8):620–6.
65. Weidner S, Hafezi-Rachti S, Rupprecht HD. Thromboembolic events as a complication of antineutrophil cytoplasmic antibody-associated vasculitis. Arthritis Rheum. 2006;55(1):146–9.
66. Stassen PM, Derks RP, Kallenberg CG, Stegeman CA. Venous thromboembolism in ANCA-associated vasculitis--incidence and risk factors. Rheumatology (Oxford). 2008;47(4):530–4.
67. Whyte AF, Smith WB, Sinkar SN, Kette FE, Hissaria P. Clinical and laboratory characteristics of 19 patients with Churg-Strauss syndrome from a single South Australian centre. Intern Med J. 2013;43(7):784–90.
68. Ames PR, Margaglione M, Mackie S, Alves JD. Eosinophilia and thrombophilia in Churg Strauss syndrome: a clinical and pathogenetic overview. Clin Appl Thromb Hemost. 2010;16(6):628–36.
69. Little MA, Nightingale P, Verburgh CA, Hauser T, De Groot K, Savage C, et al. European Vasculitis Study (EUVAS) Group. Early mortality in systemic vasculitis: relative contribution of adverse events and active vasculitis. Ann Rheum Dis. 2010;69(6):1036–43.
70. Wall N, Harper L. Complications of long-term therapy for ANCA-associated systemic vasculitis. Nat Rev Nephrol. 2012;8(9):523–32.
71. Lai QY, Ma TT, Li ZY, Chang DY, Zhao MH, Chen M. Predictors for mortality in patients with antineutrophil cytoplasmic autoantibody-associated vasculitis: a study of 398 Chinese patients. J Rheumatol. 2014;41(9):1849–55.
72. Holle JU, Gross WL, Latza U, Nölle B, Ambrosch P, Heller M, et al. Improved outcome in 445 patients with Wegener's granulomatosis in a German vasculitis center over four decades. Arthritis Rheum. 2011;63(1):257–66.
73. Cartin-Ceba R, Golbin JM, Keogh KA, Peikert T, Sánchez-Menéndez M, Ytterberg SR, et al. Rituximab for remission induction and maintenance in refractory granulomatosis with polyangiitis (Wegener's): ten-year experience at a single center. Arthritis Rheum. 2012;64(11):3770–8.
74. Charlier C, Henegar C, Launay O, Pagnoux C, Berezné A, Bienvenu B, et al. Risk factors for major infections in Wegener granulomatosis: analysis of 113 patients. Ann Rheum Dis. 2009;68(5):658–63.
75. Aasarød K, Iversen BM, Hammerstrøm J, Bostad L, Vatten L, Jørstad S. Wegener's granulomatosis: clinical course in 108 patients with renal involvement. Nephrol Dial Transplant. 2000;15(5):611–8.
76. Bligny D, Mahr A, Toumelin PL, Mouthon L, Guillevin L. Predicting mortality in systemic Wegener's granulomatosis: a survival analysis based on 93 patients. Arthritis Rheum. 2004;51(1):83–91.
77. McGregor JG, Negrete-Lopez R, Poulton CJ, Kidd JM, Katsanos SL, Goetz L, et al. Adverse events and infectious burden, microbes and temporal outline from immunosuppressive therapy in antineutrophil cytoplasmic antibody-associated vasculitis with native renal function. Nephrol Dial Transplant. 2015;30 Suppl 1:Si171–81.

78. Kitagawa K, Furuichi K, Sagara A, Shinozaki Y, Kitajima S, Toyama T, et al. Kanazawa Study Group for Renal Diseases and Hypertension. Risk factors associated with relapse or infectious complications in Japanese patients with microscopic polyangiitis. Clin Exp Nephrol. 2016;20(5):703–11.
79. Harper L, Savage CO. ANCA-associated renal vasculitis at the end of the twentieth century-a disease of older patients. Rheumatology. 2005;44:495–501.
80. Booth AD, Almond MK, Burns A, Ellis P, Gaskin G, Neild GH, et al. Pan-Thames Renal Research Group. Outcome of ANCA-associated renal vasculitis: a 5-year retrospective study. Am J Kidney Dis. 2003;41(4):776–84.
81. McGregor JG, Hogan SL, Hu Y, Jennette CE, Falk RJ, Nachman PH. Glucocorticoids and relapse and infection rates in anti-neutrophil cytoplasmic antibody disease. Clin J Am Soc Nephrol. 2012;7(2):240–7.
82. Turnbull J, Harper L. Adverse effects of therapy for ANCA-associated vasculitis. Best Pract Res Clin Rheumatol. 2009;23(3):391–401.
83. Guillevin L, Cordier JF, Lhote F, Cohen P, Jarrousse B, Royer I, et al. A prospective, multicenter, randomized trial comparing steroids and pulse cyclophosphamide versus steroids and oral cyclophosphamide in the treatment of generalized Wegener's granulomatosis. Arthritis Rheum. 1997;40(12):2187–98.
84. Nossent JC. Rituximab or cyclophosphamide in ANCA-associated renal vasculitis. N Engl J Med. 2010;363(21):2072–4. author reply 2073-4
85. Besada E, Koldingsnes W, Nossent JC. Long-term efficacy and safety of pre-emptive maintenance therapy with rituximab in granulomatosis with polyangiitis: results from a single centre. Rheumatology. 2013;52(11):2041–7.
86. Alberici F, Smith RM, Jones RB, Roberts DM, Willcocks LC, Chaudhry A, et al. Long-term follow-up of patients who received repeat-dose rituximab as maintenance therapy for ANCA-associated vasculitis. Rheumatology (Oxford). 2015;54(7):1153–60.
87. Marco H, Smith RM, Jones RB, Guerry MJ, Catapano F, Burns S, et al. The effect of rituximab therapy on immunoglobulin levels in patients with multisystem autoimmune disease. BMC Musculoskelet Disord. 2014;15:178.
88. Venhoff N, Effelsberg NM, Salzer U, Warnatz K, Peter HH, Lebrecht D, et al. Impact of rituximab on immunoglobulin concentrations and B cell numbers after cyclophosphamide treatment in patients with ANCA-associated vasculitides. PLoS One. 2012;7(5):e37626.
89. Besada E, Koldingsnes W, Nossent JC. Serum immunoglobulin levels and risk factors for hypogammaglobulinemia during long-term maintenance therapy with rituximab in patients with granulomatosis with polyangiitis. Rheumatology. 2014;53(10):1818–24.
90. Knight A, Sundström Y, Börjesson O, Bruchfeld A, Malmström V, Gunnarsson I. Late-onset neutropenia after rituximab in ANCA-associated vasculitis. Scand J Rheumatol. 2016;7:1–4.
91. Gayraud M, Guillevin L, Cohen P, Lhote F, Cacoub P, Deblois P, et al. Treatment of good-prognosis polyarteritis nodosa and Churg-Strauss syndrome: comparison of steroids and oral or pulse cyclophosphamide in 25 patients. French Cooperative Study Group for Vasculitides. Br J Rheumatol. 1997;36(12):1290–7.
92. Haubitz M, Schellong S, Göbel U, Schurek HJ, Schaumann D, Koch KM, et al. Intravenous pulse administration of cyclophosphamide versus daily oral treatment in patients with anti-neutrophil cytoplasmic antibody-associated vasculitis and renal involvement: a prospective, randomized study. Arthritis Rheum. 1998;41(10):1835–44.
93. Adu D, Pall A, Luqmani RA, Richards NT, Howie AJ, Emery P, et al. Controlled trial of pulse versus continuous prednisolone and cyclophosphamide in the treatment of systemic vasculitis. QJM. 1997;90(6):401–9.
94. Edgar JD, Rooney DP, McNamee P, McNeill TA. An association between ANCA positive renal disease and malignancy. Clin Nephrol. 1993;40(1):22–5.
95. Westman KW, Bygren PG, Olsson H, Ranstam J, Wieslander J. Relapse rate, renal survival, and cancer morbidity in patients with Wegener's granulomatosis or microscopic polyangiitis with renal involvement. J Am Soc Nephrol. 1998;9(5):842–52.

96. Knight A, Askling J, Ekbom A. Cancer incidence in a population-based cohort of patients with Wegener's granulomatosis. Int J Cancer. 2002;100(1):82–5.
97. Pankhurst T, Savage CO, Gordon C, Harper L. Malignancy is increased in ANCA-associated vasculitis. Rheumatology (Oxford). 2004;43(12):1532–5.
98. Tatsis E, Reinhold-Keller E, Steindorf K, Feller AC, Gross WL. Wegener's granulomatosis associated with renal cell carcinoma. Arthritis Rheum. 1999;42(4):751–6.
99. Rahmattulla C, Berden AE, Wakker SC, Reinders ME, Hagen EC, Wolterbeek R, et al. Incidence of malignancies in patients with antineutrophil cytoplasmic antibody-associated vasculitis diagnosed between 1991 and 2013. Arthritis Rheumatol. 2015;67(12):3270–8.
100. Faurschou M, Mellemkjaer L, Voss A, Keller KK, Hansen IT, Baslund B. Prolonged risk of specific malignancies following cyclophosphamide therapy among patients with granulomatosis with polyangiitis. Rheumatology (Oxford). 2015;54(8):1345–50.
101. Shang W, Ning Y, Xu X, Li M, Guo S, Han M, et al. Incidence of cancer in ANCA-associated vasculitis: a meta-analysis of observational studies. PLoS One. 2015;10(5):e0126016.
102. Charlson ME, Pompei P, Ales KL, MacKenzie CR. A new method of classifying prognostic comorbidity in longitudinal studies: development and validation. J Chronic Dis. 1987;40(5):373–83.
103. Charlson M, Szatrowski TP, Peterson J, Gold J. Validation of a combined comorbidity index. J Clin Epidemiol. 1994;47(11):1245–51.
104. Deyo RA, Cherkin DC, Ciol MA. Adapting a clinical comorbidity index for use with ICD-9-CM administrative databases. J Clin Epidemiol. 1992;45(6):613–9.
105. Ofer-Shiber S, Molad Y. Association of the Charlson comorbidity index with renal outcome and all-cause mortality in antineutrophil cytoplasmatic antibody-associated vasculitis. Medicine (Baltimore). 2014;93(25):e152.
106. Faurschou M, Ahlström MG, Lindhardsen J, Baslund B, Obel N. Impact of pre-existing comorbidities on mortality in granulomatosis with polyangiitis: a cohort study. Rheumatology (Oxford). 2016;55(4):649–53.
107. Hatemi G, Yazici Y, Yazici H. Behçet's syndrome. Rheum Dis Clin N Am. 2013;39(2):245–61.
108. Sazzini M, Garagnani P, Sarno S, De Fanti S, Lazzano T, Yang Yao D, et al. Tracing Behçet's disease origins along the silk road: an anthropological evolutionary genetics perspective. Clin Exp Rheumatol. 2015;33(6 Suppl 94):S60–6.
109. Gul A, Ohno S. HLA-B*51 and Behçet disease. Ocul Immunol Inflamm. 2012;20(1):37–43.
110. Hatemi G, Silman A, Bang D, Bodaghi B, Chamberlain AM, Gul A, et al. EULAR Expert Committee. EULAR recommendations for the management of Behçet disease. Ann Rheum Dis. 2008;67(12):1656–62.
111. Demirelli S, Degirmenci H, Inci S, Arisoy A. Cardiac manifestations in Behcet's disease. Intractable Rare Dis Res. 2015;4(2):70–5.
112. Geri G, Wechsler B, Thi Huon du L, Isnard R, Piette JC, Amoura Z, et al. Spectrum of cardiac lesions in Behçet disease: a series of 52 patients and review of the literature. Medicine (Baltimore) 2012;91(1):25–34.
113. Fei Y, Li X, Lin S, Song X, Wu Q, Zhu Y, et al. Major vascular involvement in Behçet's disease: a retrospective study of 796 patients. Clin Rheumatol. 2013;32(6):845–52.
114. Seyahi E, Yazici H. Behçet's syndrome: pulmonary vascular disease. Curr Opin Rheumatol. 2015;27(1):18–23.
115. Celik S, Yazici Y, Sut N, Yazici H. Pulmonary artery aneurysms in Behçet's syndrome: a review of the literature with emphasis on geographical differences. Clin Exp Rheumatol. 2015;33(6 Suppl 94):S54–9.
116. Yazici H, Esen F. Mortality in Behçet's syndrome. Clin Exp Rheumatol. 2008;26(5 Suppl 51):S138–40.
117. Saadoun D, Wechsler B, Desseaux K, Le Thi HD, Amoura Z, Resche-Rigon M, et al. Mortality in Behçet's disease. Arthritis Rheum. 2010;62(9):2806–12.
118. Yang SS, Park KM, Park YJ, Kim YW, Do YS, Park HS, et al. Peripheral arterial involvement in Behcet's disease: an analysis of the results from a Korean referral center. Rheumatol Int. 2013;33(8):2101–8.

119. Seyahi E, Ugurlu S, Cumali R, Balci H, Ozdemir O, Melikoglu M, et al. Atherosclerosis in Behçet's syndrome. Semin Arthritis Rheum. 2008;38(1):1–12.
120. Marzban M, Mandegar MH, Karimi A, Abbasi K, Movahedi N, Navabi MA, et al. Cardiac and great vessel involvement in "Behcet's disease". J Card Surg. 2008;23(6):765–8.
121. Ugurlu S, Seyahi E, Yazici H. Prevalence of angina, myocardial infarction and intermittent claudication assessed by Rose Questionnaire among patients with Behcet's syndrome. Rheumatology (Oxford). 2008;47(4):472–5.
122. Aslam F, Bandeali SJ, Crowson C, Alam M. Cardiac function and diastolic dysfunction in Behcet's disease: a systematic review and meta-analysis. Int J Rheumatol. 2016;2016:9837184.
123. Tascilar K, Melikoglu M, Ugurlu S, Sut N, Caglar E, Yazici H. Vascular involvement in Behçet's syndrome: a retrospective analysis of associations and the time course. Rheumatology (Oxford). 2014;53(11):2018–22.
124. Davatchi F, Shahram F, Chams-Davatchi C, Shams H, Nadji A, Akhlaghi M, et al. Behcet's disease: from East to West. Clin Rheumatol. 2010;29(8):823–33.
125. Koç Y, Güllü I, Akpek G, Akpolat T, Kansu E, Kiraz S, et al. Vascular involvement in Behçet's disease. J Rheumatol. 1992;19(3):402–10.
126. Gürler A, Boyvat A, Türsen U. Clinical manifestations of Behçet's disease: an analysis of 2147 patients. Yonsei Med J. 1997;38(6):423–7.
127. Ames PR, Steuer A, Pap A, Denman AM. Thrombosis in Behçet's disease: a retrospective survey from a single UK center. Rheumatology (Oxford). 2001;40(6):652–5.
128. Sarica-Kucukoglu R, Akdag-Kose A, KayabalI M, Yazganoglu KD, Disci R, Erzengin D, et al. Vascular involvement in Behçet's disease: a retrospective analysis of 2319 cases. Int J Dermatol. 2006;45(8):919–21.
129. La Regina M, Gasparyan AY, Orlandini F, Prisco D. Behcet's disease as a model of venous thrombosis. Open Cardiovasc Med J. 2010;4:71–7.
130. Seyahi E, Caglar E, Ugurlu S, Kantarci F, Hamuryudan V, Sonsuz A, et al. An outcome survey of 43 patients with Budd-Chiari syndrome due to Behçet's syndrome followed up at a single, dedicated center. Semin Arthritis Rheum. 2015;44(5):602–9.
131. Desbois AC, Rautou PE, Biard L, Belmatoug N, Wechsler B, Resche-Rigon M, et al. Behcet's disease in Budd-Chiari syndrome. Orphanet J Rare Dis. 2014;9:104.
132. Fernández-Bello I, López-Longo FJ, Arias-Salgado EG, Jiménez-Yuste V, Butta NV. Behçet's disease: new insight into the relationship between procoagulant state, endothelial activation/damage and disease activity. Orphanet J Rare Dis. 2013;8:81.
133. Saadoun D, Wechsler B, Resche-Rigon M, Trad S, Le Thi HD, Sbai A, et al. Cerebral venous thrombosis in Behçet's disease. Arthritis Rheum. 2009;61(4):518–26.
134. Aguiar de Sousa D, Mestre T, Ferro JM. Cerebral venous thrombosis in Behçet's disease: a systematic review. J Neurol. 2011;258(5):719–27.
135. Alexoudi I, Kapsimali V, Vaiopoulos A, Kanakis M, Vaiopoulos G. Evaluation of current therapeutic strategies in Behçet's disease. Clin Rheumatol. 2011;30(2):157–63.
136. Seyahi E, Melikoglu M, Akman C, Hamuryudan V, Ozer H, Hatemi G, et al. Pulmonary artery involvement and associated lung disease in Behçet disease: a series of 47 patients. Medicine (Baltimore). 2012;91(1):35–48.
137. Mogulkoc N, Burgess MI, Bishop PW. Intracardiac thrombus in Behçet's disease: a systematic review. Chest. 2000;118(2):479–87.
138. Vallet H, Riviere S, Sanna A, Deroux A, Moulis G, Addimanda O. French Behçet Network. Efficacy of anti-TNF alpha in severe and/or refractory Behçet's disease: multicenter study of 124 patients. J Autoimmun. 2015;62:67–74.
139. Wang LH, Wang WM, Hsu SM, Lin SH, Shieh CC. Risk of overall and site-specific cancers in Behçet disease: a nationwide population-based study in Taiwan. J Rheumatol. 2015;42(5):879–84.
140. Ahn JK, Oh JM, Lee J, Koh EM, Cha HS. Behcet's disease associated with malignancy in Korea: a single center experience. Rheumatol Int. 2010;30(6):831–5.
141. Lin Y, Li G, Zheng W, Tian X, Zhang F. Behcet's disease associated with malignancy: a report of 41 Chinese cases. Int J Rheum Dis. 2014;17(4):459–65.

142. Cheon JH, Celik AF, Kim WH. Behcet's disease: gastrointestinal involvement. In: Yazici Y, Yazici H, editors. Behcet's syndrome. New York: Springer; 2010. p. 165–88.
143. Yurdakul S, Tüzüner N, Yurdakul I, Hamuryudan V, Yazici H. Gastrointestinal involvement in Behçet's syndrome: a controlled study. Ann Rheum Dis. 1996;55(3):208–10.
144. Esatoglu SN, Hatemi G, Salihoglu A, Hatemi I, Soysal T, Celik AF. A reappraisal of the association between Behçet's disease, myelodysplastic syndrome and the presence of trisomy 8: a systematic literature review. Clin Exp Rheumatol. 2015;33(6 Suppl 94):S145–51.
145. Tada Y, Koarada S, Haruta Y, Mitamura M, Ohta A, Nagasawa K. The association of Behçet's disease with myelodysplastic syndrome in Japan: a review of the literature. Clin Exp Rheumatol. 2006;24(5 Suppl 42):S115–9.

Chapter 13
Juvenile Idiopathic Arthritis

Emanuela Del Giudice, Joost F. Swart, and N.M. Wulffraat

In the United States, around 80% of Medicare spending is allocated to patients with four or more chronic conditions, with the costs exponentially increasing per number of chronic conditions [1]. More research into patients' perspectives on the ways in which multiple conditions affect their health, well-being, and clinical care is needed to complement the professional perspective and ensure that care is truly patient-centered [2]. The coexistence of two or more diseases (multimorbidity) in the same individual also raises the question whether there is an underlying common etiological pathway. Comorbidity is mostly defined as any distinct additional entity that has existed or may occur during the clinical course of a patient who has the index disease under study [3]. Comorbidity can be concordant if the diseases are parts of the same pathophysiologic risk profile and more likely to share the same management and are more likely to be the focus of the same disease management plan (e.g., type 2 diabetes mellitus and hypertension) [4]. Discordant comorbidity on the other hand means that the diseases are "not directly related in either pathogenesis or management and do not share an underlying predisposing factor" (e.g., type 2 diabetes mellitus and irritable bowel syndrome) [4]. Comorbidity may represent an active, past, or transient illness [5]. The patient's complexity is the overall impact of the different diseases in an individual taking into account their severity and other health-related attributes (e.g., socioeconomic, cultural, environmental, and patient behavior characteristics) [2].

E. Del Giudice
Department of Pediatric Immunology and Rheumatology, UMC Utrecht, Wilhelmina Children's Hospital, Utrecht, The Netherlands

Department of Paediatrics and Infant Neuropsychiatry, Sapienza University of Rome, Rome, Italy

J.F. Swart (✉) • N.M. Wulffraat
Department of Pediatric Immunology and Rheumatology, UMC Utrecht, Wilhelmina Children's Hospital, Utrecht, The Netherlands
e-mail: jswart@umcutrecht.nl; N.Wulffraat@umcutrecht.nl

Y. El Miedany (ed.), *Comorbidity in Rheumatic Diseases*,
DOI 10.1007/978-3-319-59963-2_13

A chronic disease is a disease lasting 3 months or more, by the definition of the US National Center for Health Statistics. Chronic diseases generally cannot be prevented by vaccines or cured by medication, nor do they just disappear. The US National Health Council summarized the facts on chronic disease in 2014 and stated that about 40 million Americans are limited in their usual activities due to one or more chronic health conditions [6]. Generally incurable and ongoing, chronic diseases affect approximately 133 million Americans, representing more than 40% of the total population of the United States [7]. By 2020, that number is projected to grow to an estimated 157 million, with 81 million having multiple conditions [8]. About half of all adults have a chronic condition, and approximately 8% of children ages 5–17 were reported by their parents to have limited activities due to at least one chronic disease or disability [9]. More and more people are living with not just one chronic illness, such as diabetes, heart disease, arthritis, or depression, but with two or more conditions. Almost a third of the population is now living with multiple chronic conditions [10]. In 2009, 7 out of 10 deaths in the United States are due to chronic diseases. Heart disease, cancer, and stroke account for more than half of all deaths each year [7]. More than 75% of all health-care costs are due to chronic conditions [7]. A 2007 study reported that seven chronic diseases – cancer, diabetes, hypertension, stroke, heart disease, pulmonary conditions, and mental illness – have a total impact on the economy of $1,300,000,000,000 (1.3 trillion) annually. By the year 2023, this number is projected to increase to $4.2 trillion in treatment costs and lost economic output [11].

In rheumatoid arthritis (RA), many studies on comorbidities exist reporting cardiovascular, renal, lung, gastrointestinal diseases, infections, depression, osteoporosis, and malignancies occurring in RA. These studies indicate that these events occur more frequently in RA compared to the general population [12]. This higher prevalence is usually explained by either the activity of the disease itself, or by its treatment, in particular glucocorticoids [12]. Juvenile idiopathic arthritis (JIA) is the most common occurring chronic rheumatic disease in childhood with a population-based estimate indicating a prevalence of approximately 1–2 per 1000 children and an incidence of 11–14 new cases per 100,000 children [13]. JIA is defined as arthritis of unknown origin starting before the age of 16 and persisting for at least 6 weeks with other known conditions excluded [14]. JIA has variable rates in course and activity of disease; it is not a single disorder but consists of a heterogeneous group of autoimmune inflammatory diseases [15]. Only one JIA subtype, rheumatoid factor (RF)-positive polyarticular JIA, is similar to rheumatoid arthritis (RA) in adults, but this subtype only affects 2–7% of the children with JIA [15]. Although biologic therapy can dramatically improve disease outcomes, many children with arthritis will continue to have active disease as adults, some with severe disability. Furthermore potential adverse effects include infections, and its use imposes substantial economic burdens on patients, families, and society. Childhood arthritis is costly to society, in both personal and economic terms. For 2012 it was calculated that the average annual cost for a JIA patient in the United Kingdom was €31,546, with direct health-care costs equaling to €14,509, direct non-health-care costs amounting to €8323, and productivity losses being €8715 [16]. Another study confirmed that

Table 13.1 Prevalences for the main comorbidities in JIA

Comorbidity in JIA	Prevalence
Uveitis	11.6–30% [21]
Diabetes	3.5% [22]
Inflammatory bowel disease	0.131% [23]
Asthma and atopic disease	10.8% [own data]
Malignancy	0.17% after median 6.8 years [24]
Cardiovascular disease	2% after median 29 years of JIA [25]

EU country-specific annual health-care costs for JIA in 2012 ranged from €18,913 to €36,396 [17]. This was a remarkable increase in annual health-care costs for JIA patients compared to previous studies due to the inclusion of nonprofessional caregiver costs, a wider use of biologics, and longer hospital stays. Patients with JIA also show a medium impairment in health status and caregivers have a life burden [17].

Over the last decade, interest in the concept of comorbidity and multimorbidity has increased [18–20]. This is likely due to the fact that clinicians are facing an aging population with multiple morbid conditions occurring in one individual especially for the adult rheumatologists where comorbidity is frequent. Also in children, it is important to understand all potential interactions of co-existing diseases and its impact on the patient's overall well-being, in order to provide safe, efficient, and optimal care of our patients (Table 13.1). In most chronic pediatric disorders, comorbidity prior to or following the index disease comprises rare events, and thus large numbers of children are required for study. For juvenile arthritis, the burden of comorbidity is largely unknown, while one can imagine that with modifiable risk factors (e.g., healthy diet, physical activity, and no tobacco use), a huge impact can be gained in even preventing a chronic disease in these patients.

JIA-Associated Uveitis

Background

JIA-associated uveitis (JIA-U) is the most frequent extra-articular manifestation of JIA. Uveitis is the inflammation of the uvea (comprising the iris, choroid, and retina) according to the Standardization of Uveitis Nomenclature (SUN) criteria to define the anatomical location and time course of uveitis [18, 26, 27]. Anatomically, uveitis can be defined as anterior, intermediate, posterior, or panuveitis, while the time course of uveitis is classified as acute, subacute, chronic, or recurrent. The most common form of uveitis is chronic (silent) anterior uveitis. This form of uveitis is most frequently associated with oligoarticular and rheumatoid factor negative polyarticular categories of JIA. Acute anterior uveitis can also occur in JIA, which is generally directly symptomatic (red and painful eye), unilateral, and episodic and is usually associated with the enthesitis-related arthritis (ERA) category of JIA and HLA-B27 positivity [28].

Epidemiology

In long-term follow-up data, JIA-associated uveitis with onset in early childhood seems to have a biphasic course, with a reduction in anterior chamber activity at around age 9 years, after which it increases again in the early teenage years [29]. The reported prevalence of uveitis among children with JIA varies from 11.6% to 30% [21]. In another study of 1081 patients with JIA, 13.1% of whom developed uveitis, chronic anterior disease was the most frequent type (68.3%), followed by acute anterior disease (16.2%), recurrent anterior disease (12%), and panuveitis (3.5%) [30]. According to the results of a US study that compared two JIA cohorts with onset of joint symptoms before and after 1993, the year when JIA-associated uveitis screening guidelines were published, the frequency of severe uveitis at diagnosis did not decrease over time [31].

Pathogenesis

The pathophysiology of JIA-U is not well understood, likely both genetic and environmental factors are involved. Studies looking at the association between the risk of JIA-U and HLA-subtype are conflicting but have identified several HLA alleles within different specific JIA categories. In oligoarticular JIA, the HLA DR5 haplotype [32] and the HLA DRB1 1104 allele (in particular the combination between HLA DRB1 1104 and HLA DPB1 0201) are linked to a major risk to have chronic anterior uveitis [33], while in ERA patients HLA B27 is involved [34]. Otherwise HLA-DR1 seems to have a protective role against JIA-U [35]. There is an evidence for the involvement of both T and B lymphocytes, from immunohistochemistry of eye biopsies from patients with JIA which show a predominance of CD4+ rather than CD8+ T lymphocytes as well as variable levels of CD20+ B lymphocytes. CD4+ lymphocytes include pro-inflammatory Th1 cells (producing interferon gamma) and Th17 cells (producing interleukin-17), which are regulated by both CD4 + CD25 + FoxP3 + T regulatory cells (Tregs) and inducible Tregs. It is likely that autoimmunity results from imbalance between an immune response against native intraocular antigens after a loss of tolerance to self-antigens. In addition to the adaptive immune response, also the innate immune system has been implicated in the pathogenesis of JIA-U [35].

Prognosis

At 24 years' follow-up, 49% of patients with JIA-U treated at a single center had signs of active uveitis or were receiving topical corticosteroids to treat flares [36]. A similar rate of persistence into adulthood of asymptomatic uveitis (almost 50%) was seen in a cohort of 19 patients with JIA-associated uveitis who were born in 1976–1980 [37].

A systematic literature analysis of outcomes in patients with JIA-associated uveitis in 2006 showed an adverse visual outcome (visual acuity <20/40 in both eyes) in 9.2% of patients as well as cataracts (20.5%), glaucoma (18.9%), and band keratopathy (15.7%) [38]. The outcome of uveitis in patients with newly diagnosed juvenile idiopathic arthritis in two 4-year cohorts from 1990–1993 and 2000–2003 showed complications rates of 35% and 21%, respectively [39]. The frequency of complications decreasing with time could be related to earlier use of systemic immunosuppressive agents, such as methotrexate, to treat joint disease. In the retrospective study of Bolt et al., 34% of 35 JIA uveitis patients recruited during 1997–2005 developed complications during follow-up (mean 5.62 years) [40]. Although 91% of eyes had normal best corrected visual acuity, 5.6% were legally blind, and the remainder had some reduction in visual acuity [40]. The recent multicenter study of Haasnoot et al. showed that about one third of the adult patients with JIA-uveitis developed one visually impaired or blind eye [41].

Skarin et al. described long-term complications in a cohort of 55 patients with JIA-associated uveitis treated at a single center between 1973 and 1982: at 7 years after uveitis onset, 42% had cataracts and 5% had glaucoma. At 24 years' follow-up, 51% had cataracts and 22% had glaucoma [36]. A retrospective study of 327 patients with JIA-associated uveitis examined long-term outcome risk factors for visual loss [42]. Several factors are involved in a severe course of uveitis and the development of complications: male sex, a young age at onset of uveitis; a short duration between onset of arthritis and development of uveitis; and the presence of synechiae at first diagnosis of uveitis. These adverse prognostic factors overlap to some extent with the risk factors for initial development of uveitis [21, 31, 43, 44]. The main predictor of uveitis severity might be the time interval between arthritis and uveitis onset; a short interval is associated with an increase in ocular complications, mainly found in oligoarticular juvenile arthritis [45].

Early identification and treatment of JIA-U is important to avoid the risk of ocular sight-threatening complications including cataracts, glaucoma, band keratopathy, and persistent cystoid macular edema and can ultimately result in visual impairment and blindness [38]. Despite this, a fair amount of the patients suffered from ongoing uveitis activity and needed ongoing treatment as well as surgical interventions [41].

Therapy

Initial treatment is with topical corticosteroids, but evidence supports the early introduction of systemic immunosuppressive drugs, such as methotrexate (MTX), as steroid-sparing agents. An indication for systemic immunosuppression with a DMARD is failure to achieve adequate control of inflammation after 3 months of topical treatment (corticosteroids eye drops cannot be reduced $\leq$3 drops/day) or systemic corticosteroids cannot be reduced <0.15 mg/kg body weight or in case of a new inflammation-related complication [46].

Moreover, cumulative long-term use of systemic steroids is associated with well-known adverse effects, and these agents should be tapered to zero as early as possible. A systematic review and meta-analysis identified nine eligible studies of methotrexate use in noninfectious uveitis, including a total of 135 patients of whom 121 had JIA [47]. Improvements in intraocular inflammation were seen in 73% (the most commonly used MTX dose was 15 mg/m^2/week, although doses of up to 30 mg/m^2/week have been used given as subcutaneous injections) [47].

Also other nonbiologic DMARDs are used in the treatment of JIA-associated uveitis, including azathioprine, mycophenolate mofetil, ciclosporin, and tacrolimus, but methotrexate remains the preferred second-line therapy after topical corticosteroids [48, 49]. In the last decade, biologic therapy has started to play a central role in the management of JIA-associated uveitis [50]. The strongest evidence supports the use of adalimumab in the treatment of JIA-associated uveitis. Otherwise numerous studies have reported new-onset uveitis or flares of uveitis in patients receiving etanercept [51–54], and data from national registries show that etanercept treatment is associated with a greater incidence of uveitis than is seen with either adalimumab or infliximab therapy [55]. Therefore, etanercept is not recommended in patients with JIA-associated uveitis. A 2014 meta-analysis including 229 children with JIA-associated uveitis showed that the efficacy of infliximab and adalimumab was similar and that both are superior to etanercept [56]. During the follow-up, uveitis more commonly remained in remission in those treated with adalimumab rather than infliximab (60% versus 18.8%) [57]. Management of JIA-U includes the use of both topical and systemic anti-inflammatory agents and is an active area of research, and prospective controlled studies of biologic therapies, including adalimumab, tocilizumab, and abatacept, are underway or planned. Future research into the pathogenesis of JIA-associated uveitis and the identification of novel biomarkers could enable earlier diagnosis and more personalized treatment.

Diabetes and Other Autoimmune Diseases

Background

Type 1 diabetes mellitus (DM1) is known to be associated with juvenile idiopathic arthritis (JIA), celiac disease (CD), and autoimmune thyroiditis (AIT) [58–61]. Children with JIA have an increased prevalence of type 1 diabetes and autoimmune thyroiditis, but studies describing the comorbidity of DM1 and JIA in larger cohorts are rare [60, 62–64]. The first pediatric patient was a 7-year-old girl with arthritis and diabetes who was reported in 1968 [65]. Afterwards several case reports were described [66, 67] on patients having both JIA and DM1. The coexistence of celiac disease (CD) with autoimmune diseases including JIA is largely documented [68]. Several case reports have described a concomitant association between CD and JIA even a case of systemic JIA [69].

Epidemiology

Rudolf, et al. [22] in 1986 identified seven patients with JIA among 200 diabetic children which would be a prevalence of 3.5%. In a standardized longitudinal data study from 330 German/Austrian centers [64], the data of 54,911 patients with DM1, who were younger than 16 years of age, were prospectively collected from 1995 up to September 2013. The prevalence of JIA in these children and adolescents with DM1 was significantly greater than in patients without diabetes, 106 of 54,911 patients (0.19% versus 0.07%) [70]. In children and adolescents with JIA, 88% had diabetes before the rheumatic disease. Age at diabetes onset (median 7.2 years) was 5 years lower than age at first JIA documentation (12.0 years) for these patients. In children without JIA, diabetes onset was later (8.3 years, $p = 0.04$) [64]. Another study from Finnish national registers enrolled all patients with both JIA and DM1, covering a period of 30 years (1976–2005), within a population of about 5 million [62]. During the 30-year surveillance period, 240 patients were reimbursed for drugs to treat both chronic arthritis and DM. One hundred twelve patients were excluded because they were reimbursed for drugs to treat arthritis at age >21 years and for DM drugs at <30 years of age. After a further check to ascertain the diagnoses and the exact age at the onset of the diseases, they found that the remaining 82 patients had JIA classified according to ILAR criteria and DM1 (55 girls, 27 boys). Forty-nine patients had DM1 prior to JIA (59.8) and 33 had JIA prior to DM1 (41.2%). In this study, they showed a 4.5-fold increase in the number of patients with both JIA and DM1 during the three decades, a high prevalence of RF positivity (15%), and a low proportion of uveitis (7%) [62].

Another study also found significantly more often CD in children with both JIA and DM1 in comparison with patients with DM1 only ($p = 0.002$); for AIT this was not significant ($p = 0.06$) [64]. Previous studies have reported a prevalence of JIA co-occurring with CD in children of approximately 3–7% [60, 71].

Pathogenesis

Children with JIA enrolled in the CARRA Registry between May 2010 and May 2012 were investigated for differences in proportion of subjects who had first-degree relatives (FDR) with autoimmunity. There were 4677 JIA and about 31.8% subjects having FDR with any autoimmune disease [72]. First-degree relatives with DM1 were present in 3.1% for JIA patients [72]. According to literature, autoimmune diseases in general and DM1 with JIA specifically must have common genetic features. A comparative analysis with 15 immune diseases showed that DM1 is more similar genetically to other autoantibody-positive diseases, significantly most similar to juvenile idiopathic arthritis, and significantly least similar to ulcerative colitis and provided support for three additional new DM1 risk loci [73]. Before that a number of different single genes have shown susceptibility for both JIA and DM1

[68, 74, 75]. In the study of Alpigiani et al. [76], 66 Italian patients with JIA were screened, and antithyroid autoantibody frequency was with 14% higher in JIA than in the general population, while DM1 markers (islet autoantibodies and genetic markers) were with only 3% not frequent at all, and furthermore no clinical evidence for DM1 could be found.

In the 1272 first-degree relatives of 205 CD cases, a total of 62 autoimmune diseases were reported in 58 individuals [77]. A significant increase in IDDM was found at less than 20 years of age (SR 4.0, CI 2.0–7.0), and also the prevalence of JIA at any age was significantly higher than expected (SR 5.7; CI 1.5–12.7) [77]. There is increasing evidence that CD shares many predisposing susceptibility loci with JIA [68].

Prognosis

Growth is influenced negatively by JIA, in fact patients with DM1 and JIA were smaller and slimmer than their peers without JIA [64]. A third AI disease was found in 22% of the patients with both DM1 and JIA, being hypothyroidism in 67% and celiac disease in 33% [62]. Serious psychiatric problems were found in 20% of patients with depression as the most frequent diagnosis [62]. Patients with multiple AI diseases need well-coordinated multi-professional approach, and care support is necessary not only for patients but also for parents.

Inflammatory Bowel Disease

Background

Inflammatory bowel disease (IBD) as diagnosed with endoscopy and/or pathology is a growing field of interest in patients with JIA because new-onset IBD cases have been described under treatment with etanercept (ETN) [78–80]. However, arthritis is the most frequent extraintestinal manifestation in children with IBD, occurring in 7–25% of patients, and it may precede the onset of gastrointestinal symptoms by years [81–84]. It appears to be more prevalent in patients with large bowel than those with small bowel involvement and in those with complications such as abscesses, pseudomembranous polyposis, perianal disease, etc. [85]. One could argue that the diagnosis of JIA immediately expires, when IBD occurs in a "JIA" patient. The ILAR classification for JIA clearly demands that the arthritis is of unknown etiology with other conditions excluded, and since the arthritis could now be considered as a preceding extra-articular manifestation of the IBD, this is no longer the case [14]. Whether the JIA was wrongly diagnosed or the IBD was provoked by ETN remains uncertain.

Epidemiology

In the data from the German biologics registry collected from 2001 to 2013, 3071 JIA patients with 8389 patient-years (PY) of observation were followed, and IBD was diagnosed in 11 patients, 8 with Crohn disease, and 3 with ulcerative colitis [23]. IBD incidence in patients with JIA was therefore 1.31/1000 PY and is much higher than published IBD incidence of 0.083/1000 in pediatric populations [86]. IBD more commonly had ERA, extended oligoarthritis, psoriatic arthritis, and also rheumatoid factor (RF)-negative polyarthritis. No IBD occurred in patients with systemic JIA or RF-positive polyarthritis. In patients treated with methotrexate (MTX), the IBD incidence was significantly lower, while etanercept (ETN) monotherapy was associated with an increased incidence of IBD. In this study, IBD occurred only during treatment with ETN but not with other TNF inhibitors or biologics [23].

Pathogenesis

Tumor necrosis factor α (TNF- α) and a dysfunction of regulatory T cells seem to have a key role in the linkage between gut and joint inflammation [87, 88]. Alterations in key molecules that regulate the immune response in the gut of patients with enthesitis-related JIA arthritis are similar to those with CD. The interaction between antigen-presenting cells (APCs) and intestinal bacterial flora contributes to the development of uncontrolled CD4+ cell activation, which leads to the release of pro-inflammatory cytokines such as TNF-α, IL-6, IL-12, IL-23, and IL-17 [89]. Etanercept may induce the production of TNF- α and IFN- γ, favoring inflammation in the bowel mucosa [90], and IFN-γ is thought to contribute to granuloma formation [90, 91].

Many studies showed that alteration of gut microbiota is involved in subclinical gut inflammation and promotion of joint inflammation. Gut microbial “pro-arthritogenic” profiles have been hypothesized, also with differential microbial profiles and intragroup variability among active disease and remission, and in different JIA subgroups, suggesting instability of microbial ecosystem in autoimmune diseases compared to healthy status. Similar to other chronic autoimmune and inflammatory diseases, different microbial profiles could promote inflammation and contribute to the disease pathogenesis [92, 93].

Prognosis

As soon as a JIA patient is diagnosed with IBD while on etanercept, the patient has to stop etanercept and may be switched to adalimumab or infliximab treatment, since these anti-TNF agents are effective against IBD as well.

Asthma and Atopy

Background

Allergic conjunctivitis, allergic rhinitis, atopic dermatitis (AD), and asthma are all considered clinical manifestations of allergy or atopy.

Epidemiology

Over the last two decades, the incidences of autoimmune diseases and allergic diseases have been increasing [94]. AD is among the most prevalent chronic inflammatory diseases, and it was classified as first among common skin diseases in the World Health Organization 2010 Global Burden of Disease survey [95] with a social and economic impact. There have been numerous epidemiological reports on the coexistence of autoimmune diseases and atopic diseases, both being chronic inflammatory diseases, in adults. As for childhood onset diseases, it is known that patients with JIA can develop atopic diseases. A recent study reported that Taiwanese children with allergic diseases even had an increased risk of developing JIA [94]. The children with a single allergic disease had adjusted odds ratios for developing JIA of 1.44 for asthma, and the adjusted odds ratios increased to 1.72 for those with at least two allergic diseases. Unfortunately, for JIA patients, it is not published in what rate atopic diseases coexist.

In our own cohort of 446 JIA patients (36% male and 64% female), we found 29 patients with AD and 23 with asthma [own data]. Therefore 10.8% in our JIA-population did have either eczema or asthma. Compared to the Dutch prevalence of asthma and eczema retrieved from the CBS database, the RR for JIA patients to develop asthma is 1.155 and 1.168 for atopic eczema (both nonsignificant).

Pathogenesis

Until recently JIA and other autoimmune diseases were solely seen as typical T-helper cell type 1 (Th1) mediated diseases [94, 96]. In contrary, asthma and other atopic diseases are typically seen as Th2 mediated diseases [97]. According to this Th1-Th2 paradigm, people with autoimmune diseases have a reduced risk for developing atopic diseases and vice versa [93, 95]. This paradigm has helped in explaining the etiology of these different diseases and has even resulted in the development of new therapies. However, recent discoveries have served to dispute this paradigm and have provided additional insight into the roles of Th17 cells, B lymphocytes, and T regulatory cells as well as the considerable communication and commonalities between the complex signaling pathways. Most likely there are additional explanations and other cell types that play a significant role in the pathogenesis of both diseases [97, 98]. In addition, according to the paradigm, specific sets of cytokines characterize Th1 and Th2 diseases. Th1 diseases are associated with IL-1, IL-6, IL-12, TNF-alpha, and IFN-gamma, whereas Th2 diseases are typically associated with high levels of IL-4 and IL-13 [94, 99, 100]. However, this paradigm fails to explain some contradictory results; animal studies reveal conflictingly that INF-gamma seems to have different roles during the course of arthritis, either an enhancing one or a regulating one; further, the lack of efficacy of anti-IFN-gamma therapy in patients with RA does not support the thought of only Th1 to characterize auto-inflammatory diseases [101]. It is likely that there is more to this than the acknowledged dichotomy of these cytokine groups. Furthermore, IL-18, a cytokine that is associated with both Th1 as Th2 mediated disease, could have an important role in the pathogenesis of both disease types [100]. Moreover, the model of the pathogenic process of rheumatoid arthritis has changed since the identification of Th17 and regulatory T cells [101]. Perhaps there are more cell types associated with these diseases. Conceivably, evaluating these distinctive cytokines could provide better understanding in the future.

Prognosis

A study from China described a prospective cohort of enthesitis-related arthritis (ERA) patients with co-existing atopy [102]. A total of 151 ERA patients were enrolled at diagnosis and were divided into those with atopy ($n = 62$, 41%) and those without ($n = 89$, 59%). A diagnosis of atopy at study entry was made when at least two of the following three criteria were present: a positive serum-specific IgE concentration of >0.70 kU/L, positive skin prick test results, or an individual and family history of atopy However also 91.9% of the atopic group did not have clinical allergy, urticaria, allergic rhinitis, eczema, or asthma [102]. "Atopic" patients had significantly more active joints at disease onset, joint pain, and limitation compared to non-atopic group, and during the 2 years of follow-up, the number of flares was significantly higher in atopic ERA patients [102]. Another study also had emphasized that allergic and autoimmune disease may coexist and even that allergic disorders may exacerbate autoimmune disease [97]. The presence of coexistent atopy could add greater difficulty in successful management of ERA. In the study of Guo et al. [102], significantly more ERA patients with atopy were receiving biologics and there was a significantly lower rate of responses in the atopic group compared with the nonatopic group at 12 and 18 months. This might suggest that coexistent atopy in ERA patients might complicate the response to therapy. Likewise, the 61 systemic onset juvenile idiopathic arthritis (sJIA) patients enrolled in the study of Zhang et al. [103] were divided into an atopic group ($n = 27$) and a nonatopic one ($n = 34$) using the same definition as Guo. The first group of patients with co-existing atopy at diagnosis had significantly more affected joints and significantly higher ferritin levels and IgE serum levels than sJIA patients without atopy, and also the JIA flares of the atopic group were significantly higher than that of the nonatopic group ($p = 0.016$) [103].

Malignancies

Background

In recent years, concern has been raised about JIA and its possible risk for malignancies. It has been discussed if the disease itself might be associated with an increased cancer risk, and there is a limited evidence for an association with increased cancer rates [104]. Concerning JIA there are conflicting data, in fact some studies found an elevated risk of malignancies [105–107] whereas others did not find an increased cancer risk [108, 109]. Also Simard et al. [106] studied the risk of cancer occurrence in a nationwide Swedish population-based cohort of 9020 JIA patients, and they concluded that there was an elevated risk of malignancy among biologic therapy naive JIA patients during the last 20 years. Several studies concluded that JIA group appear to have an increased rate of incident malignancies compared to children without JIA, but this risk did not seem to be significantly associated with the concomitant use of therapy such as MTX or TNF inhibitors [107, 110].

An overview of the literature showed a risk for developing cancer of 0.033–0.046% per year of follow-up for JIA patients using MTX and 0.025% for JIA patients not using MTX, steroids or anti-TNF [111].

This was lower than compared to the general healthy population with an incidence of 0.032% and came even further down when treated with etanercept with 0.015% [111]. In a large study by Horneff et al. 3695 JIA patients were prospectively followed with a total of more than 13,198 observation years [112]. Twelve cases of suspected malignancies, including seven lymphoid neoplasms, have been reported in patients treated with methotrexate (MTX), and /or TNF-α inhibitors. Ten patients were exposed to biologics, nine etanercept, two adalimumab, one infliximab and one case was consecutively treated with adalimumab, etanercept, infliximab and abatacept.

In a retrospective single-center hospital-based cohort study by Barth et al. [113] performed using data on the 3691 JIA patients (3–73 years old, 64% female) treated between 1952 and 2010 at Garmisch-Partenkirchen, the cancer incidence in JIA patients was compared to cancer registry rates in the German population. A history of malignancy was reported by 47 patients without an overall increased cancer risk, although the most common types of cancer were melanoma ($n = 11$), cervical cancer ($n = 8$), and breast cancer ($n = 7$). This could be also due to a large range of age of patients, with a greater risk in the older. Patients with pJIA were prospectively observed in the German national JIA biological register and its follow-up register to investigate the rates of serious adverse events (SAE) and of events of special interest (ESI) under ETA and ADA treatment compared with methotrexate (MTX) [114]. The risk for malignancies was not significantly increased for ETA and ADA compared with MTX. Also in an open-label multicenter study performed in 38 centers in 19 countries, a prospective long-term efficacy and safety of etanercept in patients with JIA categories of extended oligoarthritis (eoJIA), enthesitis-related arthritis

(ERA), or psoriatic arthritis (PsA), without cases of malignancy reported, was showed [115, 116]. Patients were allowed different concomitant therapies as MTX, hydroxychloroquine, chloroquine, or sulfasalazine. Otherwise this study was limited by the open-label design and the lack of a placebo control group as a comparator.

Epidemiology

In the study by Niaki et al. [24], the combined data from six existing North American juvenile-onset arthritis cohorts were collected and linked to regional cancer registries to detect incident cancers after cohort entry, defined as first date seen in the pediatric rheumatology clinic and then followed for an average of 6.8 years. The six juvenile arthritis registries provided a total of 5294 patients (mean age was 8.9 years), and during follow-up nine invasive cancers occurred; three of these were hematological (Hodgkin's, non-Hodgkin's lymphoma, and leukemia). Six of nine (two-thirds) of the malignancies occurred in patients who had been exposed to disease-modifying antirheumatic drugs (DMARDs), and five of these had also been exposed to biological agents. This study provides unique data on a large number of JIA patients clinically confirmed with a cancer registry linkage, but few patients were followed in their past early adulthood for the short follow-up, and further studies should investigate cancer risk in patients with juvenile arthritis in mid to late adulthood.

Pathogenesis

It has already been established for other chronic inflammatory disorders such as rheumatoid arthritis (RA) that the disease itself favors the occurrence of malignant tumors [117] and an increased incidence of cancer (lung cancer, lymphoma, and also melanoma) has been shown compared to the general population, mainly in patients with highly active diseases [118–120]. However additional data are still necessary to quantify differences in malignancy between nonbiologic and biologic DMARD-treated patients with RA to study the rates related to treatment rather than to the underlying disease.

Several potential pathogenic mechanisms were proposed to explain the risk of malignancy in inflammatory chronic and autoimmune diseases, with the involvement of both immune dysregulation and immunosuppressive therapies: chronic inflammation and tissue damage, increased cellular replication, altered apoptotic and DNA repair pathways, and impaired tumor surveillance [121, 122]. Diak et al. [123] published in 2010 the results of 2008 FDA black box warning about the FDA's AE Reporting System (AERS) to identify malignancies associated with the use of antitumor necrosis factor agents such as infliximab, etanercept, and adalimumab in children that had started therapy between 0 and 18 years of age. Half of the malignancies reported were lymphomas (both Hodgkin's and non-Hodgkin's lymphoma), while the remaining reported cases were leukemia, melanoma, and solid organ cancers, and in 88% of the reported cases, anti-TNF blockers were used concomitantly with other immunosuppressants. The reporting rates for all malignancies were higher compared with the general pediatric population, but Diak et al. [123] recognized several biases that could have confounded and limited the interpretation of their results as the underreporting rate of spontaneous communication to the AERS database, the co-occurrence with other diseases (with different associations with cancer occurrence), and the previous or concomitant treatment with other immunosuppressive drugs. Their conclusions were that although TNF blockers might increase the risk of malignancy, a convincing relationship could not be founded [123, 124].

Prognosis

More recent studies seem to suggest that JIA itself is (weakly) associated with malignancy and that treatment with TNF blockers does not increase this risk. Safety information regarding drugs different from anti-TNF are very limited. A case of acute lymphoblastic leukemia was reported in the study which enrolled 190 patients in the open-label phase, but no cases of malignancy were reported in the double-blind phase [125] or in a long-term open-label follow-up study of the participants in the trial ($n = 153$) with abatacept [126]. No cases of malignancy have been reported in the studies with anti-IL-1 or anti-IL-6 inhibitors [127–133]. It is necessary to have information about long-term studies in JIA patients treated with drugs different from anti-TNF.

However, since both cancer and JIA in childhood are rare, a very large group of patients from all (inter-) national registries needs to be analyzed for a long period of time before a firm conclusion can be drawn.

Cardiovascular Disease

Background

Cardiovascular disease (CVD) might clinically manifest itself as hypertension, myocardial infarction, cerebrovascular accidents, and congestive heart failure. Early atherosclerosis can be measured noninvasively by flow-mediated dilatation (FMD), carotid intima-media thickness (cIMT), and pulse wave velocity.

Epidemiology

Anderson et al. studied cohort 1 consisting of 41 patients with JIA and follow-up ≥30 years of age in comparison to 41 age and sex matched controls [25]. Three patients (7%) had CVD, compared to one control (2%, $p = 0.31$). They also studied cohort 2 comprising 170 patients with JIA and a median of 29 years of follow-up since disease onset in comparison to 91 age and sex controls. Two patients (2%) had CVD, compared to none of the controls ($p = 0.29$). The presence of CVD risk factors was also found to be increased in the JIA group compared to the controls in three categories: family history of CVD (cohort 1), hypertension (cohort 2), and ever smokers (cohorts 2) [25].

Pathogenesis

Recent studies have confirmed that chronic inflammation plays a crucial role in the development and progression of atherosclerosis in adults affected by inflammatory and immune disorders such as systemic lupus erythematosus (SLE) and rheumatoid arthritis (RA), or in ankylosing spondylitis [134, 135], where there is a 48% increased risk of incident cardiovascular disease (CVD), including myocardial infarction, cerebrovascular accidents, and congestive heart failure, in comparison to the general population [136].

The last three decades have seen a marked change in the management of JIA shifting from NSAIDs and corticosteroids (systemic and intra-articular) to the use of several DMARDS and since 2000, the biological agents [137]. Recent studies suggest that NSAIDs [138] as well as glucocorticoids are associated with an increased risk of CVD in adults [139]. To date, there are no studies considering the impact of steroid therapy in children or adults with JIA on future cardiovascular risk. Otherwise data in pediatric population with JIA are few and preliminary. JIA is a heterogeneous disease with clinical course and prognosis variable. Since sustained systemic inflammation is known to accelerate atherosclerosis, children with JIA and in particular those with persistent inflammation may be at increased risk of CVD. Traditional cardiovascular risk factors have been investigated in JIA as dyslipidemia, but data on the lipid profile in JIA patients are conflicting [140–144], maybe the variability in lipid profiles might be due to the variable disease subtypes and the levels of disease activity, which may impact the composition of lipid fractions in the blood [145]. Satija et al. [146] did not find a significant difference in endothelial function studied by cIMT between JIA patients and controls. Their patients had a low disease activity and lower disease duration and had not received steroids or any disease-modifying antirheumatic drug. Furthermore there was no significant difference in FMD between cases and controls [146]. In contrast to this, the study by Vlahos et al. [147] showed increased cIMT in JIA patients compared to controls mostly in systemic arthritis than oligoarthritis or polyarthritis. They also demonstrated a FMD significantly lower in 30 JIA as compare to 33 matched controls [147]. Breda et al. demonstrated an increased cIMT only in prepubertal children with JIA [140]. Similar to what was reported by Pietrewicz et al. [148], JIA patients had increased c-IMT compared to control group (higher IMT in polyarthritis group compared to oligoarthritis in their study), with also significant correlation between IMT and disease duration.

Prognosis

Breda et al. [149] considered the potential effect of anti-TNF therapy on cardiovascular indices in children with JIA: of the 38 patients, 22 received NSAID alone or in combination with a DMARD (mainly MTX) and 16 (all with polyarticular JIA) were treated with etanercept. Both groups showed a significant improvement in cIMT after 12 months of therapy, mostly in the etanercept-treated patients.

Larger population-based studies or JIA registries are necessary to characterize the role of traditional risk factors related to cardiovascular disease in JIA. It could be useful also to increase the population data studies to support evidence for aggressive management with DMARDs and biological agents in JIA patients with a higher risk of cardiovascular events and advice patients in their lifestyle choices.

Conclusions

Juvenile idiopathic arthritis is a chronic inflammatory disease of children which might persist into adulthood, so it is important to plan prevention or screening strategies for other comorbidities and integrated follow-up once comorbidity exists. Early diagnosis and optimal disease control are essential in order to facilitate normal adolescent development and minimize long-term disease sequelae, even more so in the context of comorbidity. Uveitis, asthma/atopic diseases, and diabetes mellitus are prevalent comorbidities in JIA with 11.6–30%, 10.8%, and 3.5%, respectively. More information is needed on the long-term development of malignancies and cardiovascular diseases and the role of anti-inflammatory drugs in JIA patients. The influence of a co-existing chronic disease in a patient with juvenile idiopathic arthritis should be taken into account in treating and advising JIA patients. The recognition of the extra disease burden might provide a strategy in the optimal management of these patients. A multidisciplinary team that includes a psychologist and a social worker must be offered to these patients and their family to guide them and prevent severe psychological consequences of such a complex disease.

References

1. Wolff JL, Starfield B, Anderson G. Prevalence, expenditures, and complications of multiple chronic conditions in the elderly. Arch Intern Med. 2002;162:2269–76.
2. Valderas JM, Starfield B, Sibbald B, et al. Defining comorbidity: implications for understanding health and health services. Ann Fam Med. 2009;7:357–63. doi:10.1370/afm.983.Martin.
3. Feinstein AR. The pre-therapeutic classification of co-morbidity in chronic disease. J Chronic Dis. 1970;23:455–68.
4. Piette JD, Kerr EA. The impact of comorbid chronic conditions on diabetes care. Diabetes Care. 2006;29:725–31. doi:10.2337/diacare.29.03.06.dc05-2078.
5. Gabriel SE, Michaud K. Epidemiological studies in incidence, prevalence, mortality, and comorbidity of the rheumatic diseases. Arthritis Res Ther. 2009;11:229. doi:10.1186/ar2669.
6. Summary health statistics for the U.S. population: National Health Interview Survey, 2012. Natl Cent Heal Stat Centers Dis Control Prev. 2013.
7. The power of prevention. Centers Dis Control Prev. 2009. https://www.cdc.gov/chronicdisease/pdf/2009-power-of-prevention.pdf.
8. The Lancet. Tackling the burden of chronic diseases in the USA. Lancet. 2009;373:185. doi:10.1016/S0140-6736(09)60048-9.
9. Chartbook on trends in the health of Americans. Limitation of activity: children. Centers Dis Control Prev Natl Cent Heal Stat. 2007. http://www.nationalhealthcouncil.org/sites/default/files/NHC_Files/Pdf_Files/AboutChronicDisease.pdf.
10. Gerteis J, Izrael D, Deitz D, et al. Multiple chronic conditions chartbook: 2010 medical expenditure panel survey data. Agency Healthc Res Qual. 2014. https://www.ahrq.gov/sites/default/files/wysiwyg/professionals/prevention-chronic-care/decision/mcc/mccchartbook. pdf
11. DeVol R, Bedroussian A. An unhealthy America: the economic burden of chronic disease. *Milken Inst.* 2007. http://www.milkeninstitute.org/publications/view/321.
12. Baillet A, Gossec L, Carmona L, et al. Points to consider for reporting, screening for and preventing selected comorbidities in chronic inflammatory rheumatic diseases in daily practice: a EULAR initiative. Ann Rheum Dis. 2016:1–9. doi:10.1136/annrheumdis-2016-209233.
13. Oen KG, Cheang M. Epidemiology of chronic arthritis in childhood. Semin Arthritis Rheum. 1996;26:575–91. doi:10.1016/S0049-0172(96)80009-6.
14. Petty RE, Southwood TR, Manners P, et al. International league of associations for rheumatology classification of juvenile idiopathic arthritis: second revision, Edmonton, 2001. Rheumatol. 2004;31:390–2.
15. Ravelli A, Martini A. Juvenile idiopathic arthritis. Lancet. 2007;369:767–78. doi:10.1016/S0140-6736(07)60363-8.
16. Angelis A, Kanavos P, López-Bastida J, et al. Socioeconomic costs and health-related quality of life in juvenile idiopathic arthritis: a cost-of-illness study in the United Kingdom. BMC Musculoskelet Disord. 2016;17:321. doi:10.1186/s12891-016-1129-1.
17. Kuhlmann A, Schmidt T, Treskova M, et al. Social/economic costs and health-related quality of life in patients with juvenile idiopathic arthritis in Europe. Eur J Health Econ. 2016;17:79–87. doi:10.1007/s10198-016-0786-1.
18. Barnett K, Mercer SW, Norbury M, et al. Epidemiology of multimorbidity and implications for health care, research, and medical education: a cross-sectional study. Lancet. 2012;380:37–43. doi:10.1016/S0140-6736(12)60240-2.
19. Diederichs C, Berger K, Bartels DB. The measurement of multiple chronic diseases – a systematic review on existing multimorbidity indices. J Gerontol A Biol Sci Med Sci. 2011;66(A):301–11. doi:10.1093/gerona/glq208.
20. Fortin M, Stewart M, Poitras M, et al. A systematic review of prevalence studies on Multimorbidity: toward a more Uni- form methodology. Ann Fam Med. 2012;10:142–51. doi:10.1370/afm.1337.

21. Angeles-Han ST, Pelajo CF, Vogler LB, et al. Risk markers of juvenile idiopathic arthritis-associated uveitis in the Childhood Arthritis and Rheumatology Research Alliance (CARRA) registry. J Rheumatol. 2013;40:2088–96. doi:10.3899/jrheum.130302.
22. Rudolf MC, Genel M, Tamborlane WV, Jr DJ. Juvenile rheumatoid arthritis in children with diabetes mellitus. J Pediatr. 1981;99:519–24.
23. Barthel D, Ganser G, Kuester R-M, et al. Inflammatory bowel disease in juvenile idiopathic arthritis patients treated with biologics. J Rheumatol. 2015;42:2160–5. doi:10.3899/jrheum.140472.
24. Zahedi Niaki O, Clarke AE, Ramsey-Goldman R, et al. Malignancy incidence in 5294 patients with juvenile arthritis. RMD open. 2016;2:e000212. doi:10.1136/rmdopen-2015-000212.
25. Anderson JH, Anderson KR, Aulie HA, et al. Juvenile idiopathic arthritis and future risk for cardiovascular disease: a multicenter study. *Scand J Rheumatol.* 2016;45:1–5. doi:10.3109/03009742.2015.1126345.
26. Deschenes J, Murray PI, Rao NA, et al. International Uveitis Study Group (IUSG): clinical classification of uveitis. Ocul Immunol Inflamm. 2008;16:1–2. doi:10.1080/09273940801899822.
27. Jabs DA, Nussenblatt RB, Rosenbaum JT. Standardization of uveitis nomenclature for reporting clinical data. Results of the First International Workshop. Am J Ophthalmol. 2005;140:509–16. doi:10.1016/j.ajo.2005.03.057.
28. Clarke SL, Sen ES, Ramanan AV. Juvenile idiopathic arthritis-associated uveitis. Pediatr Rheumatol Online J. 2016;14:27.
29. Hoeve M, Kalinina Ayuso V, Schalij-Delfos NE, et al. The clinical course of juvenile idiopathic arthritis-associated uveitis in childhood and puberty. Br J Ophthalmol. 2012;96:852–6. doi:10.1136/bjophthalmol-2011-301023.
30. Sabri K, Saurenmann RK, Silverman ED, et al. Course, complications, and outcome of juvenile arthritis-related uveitis. J AAPOS. 2008;12:539–45. doi:10.1016/j.jaapos.2008.03.007.
31. Chia A, Lee V, Graham EM, et al. Factors related to severe uveitis at diagnosis in children with juvenile idiopathic arthritis in a screening program. Am J Ophthalmol. 2003;135:757–62. doi:10.1016/S0002-9394(03)00225-3.
32. Giannini EH, Malagon CN, Van Kerckhove C, et al. Longitudinal analysis of HLA associated risks for iridocyclitis in juvenile rheumatoid arthritis. J Rheumatol. 1991;18:1394–7.
33. Melin-Aldana H, Giannini EH, Taylor J, et al. Human leukocyte antigen-DRB1*1104 in the chronic iridocyclitis of pauciarticular juvenile rheumatoid arthritis*. J Pediatr. 1992;121:56–60. doi:10.1016/S0022-3476(05)82541-7.
34. Du L, Kijlstra A, Yang P. Immune response genes in uveitis. Ocul Immunol Inflamm. 2009;17:249–56. doi:10.1080/09273940902999356.
35. Kalinina Ayuso V, Makhotkina N, van Tent-Hoeve M, et al. Pathogenesis of juvenile idiopathic arthritis associated uveitis: the known and unknown. Surv Ophthalmol. 2014;59:517–31. doi:10.1016/j.survophthal.2014.03.002.
36. Skarin A, Elborgh R, Edlund E, et al. Long-term follow-up of patients with uveitis associated with juvenile idiopathic arthritis: a cohort study. Ocul Immunol Inflamm. 2009;17:104–8. doi:10.1080/09273940802650398.
37. Kotaniemi K, Arkela-Kautiainen M, Haapasaari J, et al. Uveitis in young adults with juvenile idiopathic arthritis: a clinical evaluation of 123 patients. Ann Rheum Dis. 2005;64:871–4. doi:10.1136/ard.2004.026955.
38. Carvounis PE, Herman DC, Cha S, et al. Incidence and outcomes of uveitis in juvenile rheumatoid arthritis, a synthesis of the literature. Graefes Arch Clin Exp Ophthalmol. 2006;244:281–90. doi:10.1007/s00417-005-0087-3.
39. Kotaniemi K, Sihto-Kauppi K, Salomaa P, et al. The frequency and outcome of uveitis in patients with newly diagnosed juvenile idiopathic arthritis in two 4-year cohorts from 1990–1993 and 2000–2003. Clin Exp Rheumatol. 2014;32:143–7.
40. Bolt IB, Cannizzaro E, Seger R, et al. Risk factors and longterm outcome of juvenile idiopathic arthritis-associated uveitis in Switzerland. J Rheumatol. 2008;35:703–6.
41. Haasnoot AJ, Vernie LA, Rothova A, V D Doe P, Los LI, Schalij-Delfos NE, de Boer JH. Impact of juvenile idiopathic arthritis associated uveitis in early adulthood. PLoS One. 28(supl 1): 2016;S79–83.

42. Gregory AC, Kempen JH, Daniel E, et al. Risk factors for loss of visual acuity among patients with uveitis associated with juvenile idiopathic arthritis: the systemic immunosuppressive therapy for eye diseases study. Ophthalmology. 2013;120:186–92. doi:10.1016/j.ophtha.2012.07.052.
43. Edelsten C, Lee V, Bentley CR, et al. An evaluation of baseline risk factors predicting severity in juvenile idiopathic arthritis associated uveitis and other chronic anterior uveitis in early childhood. Br J Ophthalmol. 2002;86:51–6. doi:10.1136/bjo.86.1.51.
44. Ayuso VK, ten Cate HAT, van der Does P, et al. Male gender and poor visual outcome in uveitis associated with juvenile idiopathic arthritis. Am J Ophthalmol. 2010;149:987–93. doi:10.1016/j.ajo.2010.01.014.
45. Zannin ME, Buscain I, Vittadello F, et al. Timing of uveitis onset in oligoarticular juvenile idiopathic arthritis (JIA) is the main predictor of severe course uveitis. Acta Ophthalmol. 2012;90:91–5. doi:10.1111/j.1755-3768.2009.01815.x.
46. Heiligenhaus A, Michels H, Schumacher C, et al. Evidence-based, interdisciplinary guidelines for anti-inflammatory treatment of uveitis associated with juvenile idiopathic arthritis. Rheumatol Int. 2012;32:1121–33. doi:10.1007/s00296-011-2126-1.
47. Simonini G, Paudyal P, Jones GT, et al. Current evidence of methotrexate efficacy in childhood chronic uveitis: a systematic review and meta-analysis approach. Rheumatol (United Kingdom). 2013;52:825–31. doi:10.1093/rheumatology/kes186.
48. Simonini G, Cantarini L, Bresci C, et al. Current therapeutic approaches to autoimmune chronic uveitis in children. Autoimmun Rev. 2010;9:674–83. doi:10.1016/j.autrev.2010.05.017.
49. Sharma SM, Dick AD, Ramanan AV. Non-infectious pediatric uveitis: an update on immunomodulatory management. Pediatr Drugs. 2009;11:229–41. doi:10.2165/00148581-200911040-00002.
50. Sen ES, Ramanan AV. New age of biological therapies in paediatric rheumatology. Arch Dis Child. 2014;99:679–85. doi:10.1136/archdischild-2013-304396.
51. Smith JA, Thompson DJS, Whitcup SM, et al. A randomized, placebo-controlled, double-masked clinical trial of etanercept for the treatment of uveitis associated with juvenile idiopathic arthritis. Arthritis Care Res. 2005;53:18–23. doi:10.1002/art.20904.
52. Tynjälä P, Lindahl P, Honkanen V, et al. Infliximab and etanercept in the treatment of chronic uveitis associated with refractory juvenile idiopathic arthritis. Ann Rheum Dis. 2007;66:548–50. doi:10.1136/ard.2006.058248.
53. Schmeling H, Horneff G. Etanercept and uveitis in patients with juvenile idiopathic arthritis. Rheumatology (Oxford). 2005;44:1008–11. doi:10.1093/rheumatology/keh658.
54. Saurenmann RK, Levin AV, Feldman BM, et al. Risk of new-onset uveitis in patients with juvenile idiopathic arthritis treated with anti-TNFalpha agents. J Pediatr. 2006;149:833–6. doi:10.1016/j.jpeds.2006.08.044.
55. Lim LL, Fraunfelder FW, Rosenbaum JT. Do tumor necrosis factor inhibitors cause uveitis? A registry-based study. Arthritis Rheum. 2007;56:3248–52. doi:10.1002/art.22918.
56. Simonini G, Druce K, Cimaz R, et al. Current evidence of anti-tumor necrosis factor ?? Treatment efficacy in childhood chronic uveitis: a systematic review and meta-analysis approach of individual drugs. Arthritis Care Res 2014;66:1073–84. doi:10.1002/acr.22214.
57. Simonini G1, Taddio A, Cattalini M, Caputo R, De Libero C, Naviglio S, Bresci C, Lorusso M, Lepore L, Cimaz R. Prevention of flare recurrences in childhood-refractory chronic uveitis: an open-label comparative study of adalimumab versus infliximab. Arthritis Care Res (Hoboken). 2011;63:612–8.
58. Barker JM. Type 1 diabetes-associated autoimmunity: natural history, genetic associations, and screening. J Clin Endocrinol Metab. 2006;91:1210–7. doi:10.1210/jc.2005-1679.
59. Smyth DJ, Plagnol V, Walker NM, et al. Shared and distinct genetic variants in type 1 diabetes and celiac disease. N Engl J Med. 2008;359:2767–77. doi:10.1056/NEJMoa0807917.
60. Stagi S, Giani T, Simonini G, et al. Thyroid function, autoimmune thyroiditis and coeliac disease in juvenile idiopathic arthritis. Rheumatol. 2005;44:517–20. doi:10.1093/rheumatology/keh531.

61. Freeman HJ. Endocrine manifestations in celiac disease. World J Gastroenterol. 2016;22:8472. doi:10.3748/wjg.v22.i38.8472.
62. Pohjankoski H, Kautiainen H, Korppi M, et al. Simultaneous juvenile idiopathic arthritis and diabetes mellitus type 1 – a Finnish nationwide study. J Rheumatol. 2012;39:377–81. doi:10.3899/jrheum.110654.
63. Minden K, Niewerth M. Juvenile idiopathic arthritis – clinical subgroups and classification. Z Rheumatol. 2008;67:100, 102–6, 108–10. doi:10.1007/s00393-007-0246-5
64. Hermann G, Thon A, Mönkemöller K, et al. Comorbidity of type 1 diabetes and juvenile idiopathic arthritis. J Pediatr. 2015;166:930–5.e3. doi:10.1016/j.jpeds.2014.12.026.
65. Castleman BMB. Case records of the Massachusetts General Hospital, case 44. N Engl J Med. 1968;279:987–9.
66. Agrawal S, Desai MP. Simultaneous occurrence of type I diabetes mellitus and juvenile rheumatoid arthritis. Indian Pediatr. 2003;40(6):568–71.
67. Nagy KH, Lukacs K, Sipos P, et al. Type 1 diabetes associated with Hashimoto's thyroiditis and juvenile rheumatoid arthritis: a case report with clinical and genetic investigations. Pediatr Diabetes. 2010;11:579–82. doi:10.1111/j.1399–5448.2010.00676.x; 10.1111/j.1399–5448.2010.00676.x.
68. Hinks A, Martin P, Flynn E, Eyre S, Packham JBA. Investigation of type 1 diabetes and coeliac disease susceptibility loci for association with juvenile idiopathic arthritis. Ann Rheum Dis. 2010;69:2169–72. doi:10.1136/ard.2009.126938.
69. De Maddi F, Pellegrini F, Raffaele CGL, et al. Celiac disease and juvenile idiopathic arthritis: a still enigmatic crossover. Scand J Gastroenterol. 2013;48:511–2. doi:10.3109/00365521.2013.772232.
70. Thierry S, Fautrel B, Lemelle I, et al. Prevalence and incidence of juvenile idiopathic arthritis: a systematic review. Joint Bone Spine. 2014;81:112–7. doi:10.1016/j.jbspin.2013.09.003.
71. Lepore L, Martelossi S, Pennesi M, et al. Prevalence of celiac disease in patients with juvenile chronic arthritis. J Pediatr. 1996;129:311–3. doi:10.1016/S0022-3476(96)70262-7.
72. Prahalad S, McCracken CE, Ponder LA, et al. Familial autoimmunity in the childhood arthritis and rheumatology research alliance registry. Pediatr Rheumatol. 2016;14:1–7. doi:10.1186/s12969-016-0075-7.
73. Onengut-Gumuscu S, Chen W-M, Burren O, et al. Fine mapping of type 1 diabetes susceptibility loci and evidence for colocalization of causal variants with lymphoid gene enhancers. Nat Genet. 2015;47:381–6. doi:10.1038/ng.3245.
74. Thompson SD, Sudman M, Ramos PS, et al. The susceptibility loci juvenile idiopathic arthritis shares with other autoimmune diseases extend to PTPN2, COG6, and ANGPT1. Arthritis Rheum. 2010;62:3265–76. doi:10.1002/art.27688.
75. Albers HM, Kurreeman FAS, Stoeken-Rijsbergen G, et al. Association of the autoimmunity locus 4q27 with juvenile idiopathic arthritis. Arthritis Rheum. 2009;60:901–4. doi:10.1002/art.24296.
76. Alpigiani MG, Cerboni M, Bertini I, et al. Endocrine autoimmunity in young patients with juvenile chronic arthritis. Clin Exp Rheumatol. 2002;20:565–8.
77. Neuhausen SL, Steele L, Ryan S, et al. Co-occurrence of celiac disease and other autoimmune diseases in celiacs and their first-degree relatives. J Autoimmun. 2008;31:160–5. doi:10.1016/j.jaut.2008.06.001.
78. Van Dijken TD, Vastert SJ, Gerloni VM, et al. Development of inflammatory bowel disease in patients with juvenile idiopathic arthritis treated with Etanercept development of inflammatory bowel disease in patients with juvenile idiopathic arthritis treated with etanercept. J Rheumaol. 2011;38:1441–6. doi:10.3899/jrheum.100809.
79. Wiegering V, Morbach H, Dick A, et al. Crohn's disease during etanercept therapy in juvenile idiopathic arthritis: a case report and review of the literature. Rheumatol Int. 2010;30:801–4. doi:10.1007/s00296-009-0991-7.
80. Gerloni V, Pontikaki I, Gattinara M, et al. Focus on adverse events of tumour necrosis factor alpha blockade in juvenile idiopathic arthritis in an open monocentric long-term prospective study of 163 patients. Ann Rheum Dis. 2008;67:1145–52. doi:10.1136/ard.2007.069484.

81. Pichler J, Ong C, Shah N, et al. Histopathological features of gastrointestinal mucosal biopsies in children with juvenile idiopathic arthritis. Pediatr Res. 2016;79:895–901. doi:10.1038/pr.2016.27.
82. Jose FA, Garnett EA, Vittinghoff E, et al. Development of extraintestinal manifestations in pediatric patients with inflammatory bowel disease. Inflamm Bowel Dis. 2009;15:63–8. doi:10.1002/ibd.20604.
83. Diefenbach KA, Breuer CK. Pediatric inflammatory bowel disease. World J Gastroenterol. 2006;12:3204–12.
84. Cardile S, Romano C. Current issues in pediatric inflammatory bowel diseaseassociated arthropathies. World J Gastroenterol. 2014;20:45–52. doi:10.3748/wjg.v20.i1.45.
85. Wordsworth P. Arthritis and inflammatory bowel disease. Curr Rheumatol Rep. 2000;2:87–8.
86. Sawczenko A, Sandhu B, Logan R, et al. Prospective survey of childhood inflammatory bowel disease in the British Isles. Lancet. 2001;357:1093–4. doi:10.1016/S0140-6736(00)04309-9.
87. Katsicas MM, Russo R. Biologic agents in juvenile spondyloarthropathies. Pediatr Rheumatol Online J. 2016;14:17. doi:10.1186/s12969-016-0076-6.
88. De Vos M. Joint involvement associated with inflammatory bowel disease. Dig Dis. 2009;27:511–5. doi:10.1159/000233290.
89. Rodríguez-Reyna TS, Martínez-Reyes C, Yamamoto-Furusho JK. Rheumatic manifestations of inflammatory bowel disease. World J Gastroenterol. 2009;15:5517–24. doi:10.3748/wjg.15.5517.
90. Zou J, Rudwaleit M, Brandt J, et al. Up regulation of the production of tumour necrosis factor alpha and interferon gamma by T cells in ankylosing spondylitis during treatment with etanercept. Ann Rheum Dis. 2003;62:561–4. doi:10.1136/ard.62.6.561.
91. Toussirot É, Houvenagel É, Goëb V, et al. Development of inflammatory bowel disease during anti-TNF-(alpha) therapy for inflammatory rheumatic disease: a nationwide series. Jt Bone Spine. 2012;79:457–63. doi:10.1016/j.jbspin.2011.10.001.
92. Di Paola M, Cavalieri D, Albanese D, et al. Alteration of fecal microbiota profiles in juvenile idiopathic arthritis. Associations with HLA-B27 allele and disease status. Front Microbiol. 2016;7:1703. doi:10.3389/fmicb.2016.01703.
93. Arvonen M, Berntson L, Pokka T, et al. Gut microbiota-host interactions and juvenile idiopathic arthritis. Pediartr Rheumatol. 2016;14:1–9. doi:10.1186/s12969-016-0104-6.
94. Lin C-H, Lin C-L, Shen T-C, et al. Epidemiology and risk of juvenile idiopathic arthritis among children with allergic diseases: a nationwide population-based study. Pediatr Rheumatol Online J. 2016;14:15. doi:10.1186/s12969-016-0074-8.
95. Murray CJL, Vos T, Lozano R, et al. Disability-adjusted life years (DALYs) for 291 diseases and injuries in 21 regions, 1990–2010: a systematic analysis for the Global Burden of Disease Study 2010. Lancet. 2012;380:2197–223. doi:10.1016/S0140-6736(12)61689-4.
96. Rabin RL, Levinson AI. The nexus between atopic disease and autoimmunity: a review of the epidemiological and mechanistic literature. Clin Exp Immunol. 2008;153:19–30. doi:10.1111/j.1365-2249.2008.03679.x.
97. Shah A. The pathologic and clinical intersection of atopic and autoimmune disease. Curr Allergy Asthma Rep. 2012;12:520–9. doi:10.1007/s11882-012-0293-0.
98. Gor DO, Rose NR, Greenspan NS. TH1-TH2: a procrustean paradigm. Nat Immunol. 2003;4:503–5. doi:10.1038/ni0603-503.
99. Schubert K, von Bonnsdorf H, Burke M, et al. A comprehensive candidate gene study on bronchial asthma and juvenile idiopathic arthritis. Dis Markers. 2006;22:127–32.
100. Heinzmann A, Gerhold K, Ganter K, et al. Association study of polymorphisms within interleukin-18 in juvenile idiopathic arthritis and bronchial asthma. Allergy Eur J Allergy Clin Immunol. 2004;59:845–9. doi:10.1111/j.1398-9995.2004.00538.x.
101. Boissier MC, Assier E, Falgarone G, et al. Shifting the imbalance from Th1/Th2 to Th17/treg: the changing rheumatoid arthritis paradigm. Joint Bone Spine. 2008;75:373–5. doi:10.1016/j.jbspin.2008.04.005.
102. Guo R, Cao L, Kong X, et al. Atopy in children with the enthesitis-related arthritis (ERA) subtype of juvenile idiopathic arthritis is associated with a worse outcome. Eur J Pediatr. 2015;174:1441–50. doi:10.1007/s00431-015-2553-1.

103. Zhang W-M, Xu L-Y, Lu Y, et al. Atopy in children with systemic onset juvenile idiopathic arthritis (SoJIA) is associated with a worse outcome. Immunopharmacol Immunotoxicol. 2014;36:176–81. doi:10.3109/08923973.2014.898068.
104. Ruperto N, Martini A. Juvenile idiopathic arthritis and malignancy. Rheumatology (Oxford). 2014;53:968–74. doi:10.1093/rheumatology/ket318.
105. Nordstrom BL, Mines D, Gu Y, et al. Risk of malignancy in children with juvenile idiopathic arthritis not treated with biologic agents. Arthritis Care Res (Hoboken). 2012;64:1357–64. doi:10.1002/acr.21709.
106. Simard JF, Neovius M, Hagelberg S, et al. Juvenile idiopathic arthritis and risk of cancer: a nationwide cohort study. Arthritis Rheum. 2010;62:3776–82. doi:10.1002/art.27741.
107. Beukelman T, Haynes K, Curtis JR, et al. Rates of malignancy associated with juvenile idiopathic arthritis and its treatment. Arthritis Rheum. 2012;64:1263–71. doi:10.1002/art.34348.
108. Bernatsky S, Rosenberg AM, Oen KG, et al. Malignancies in juvenile idiopathic arthritis: a preliminary report. J Rheumatol. 2011;38:760–3. doi:10.3899/jrheum.100711.
109. Burmester GR, Panaccione R, Gordon KB, et al. Adalimumab: long-term safety in 23 458 patients from global clinical trials in rheumatoid arthritis, juvenile idiopathic arthritis, ankylosing spondylitis, psoriatic arthritis, psoriasis and Crohn's disease. Ann Rheum Dis. 2013;72:517–24. doi:10.1136/annrheumdis-2011-201244.
110. Mannion ML, Beukelman T. What is the background incidence of malignancy in children with rheumatic disease? Curr Rheumatol Rep. 2013;15:310. doi:10.1007/s11926-012-0310-2.
111. Swart JF, de Roock S, Wulffraat NM. What are the immunological consequences of long-term use of biological therapies for juvenile idiopathic arthritis? Arthritis Res Ther. 2013;15:213. doi:10.1186/ar4213.
112. Horneff G, Klein A, Oommen PT, et al. Update on malignancies in children with juvenile idiopathic arthritis in the German BIKER Registry. *Clin Exp Rheumatol.* Published Online First: 2016. http://www.ncbi.nlm.nih.gov/pubmed/27749226.
113. Barth S, Schlichtiger J, Hartmann B, et al. Incidence of malignancies in patients with juvenile idiopathic arthritis: a retrospective single-center cohort study in Germany. Mod Rheumatol. 2016;7595:1–6. doi:10.1080/14397595.2016.1204711.
114. Klotsche J, Niewerth M, Haas J-P, et al. Long-term safety of etanercept and adalimumab compared to methotrexate in patients with juvenile idiopathic arthritis (JIA). Ann Rheum Dis. 2016;75:855–61. doi:10.1136/annrheumdis-annrheumdis-2014-206747.
115. Constantin T, Foeldvari I, Vojinovic J, et al. Two-year efficacy and safety of etanercept in pediatric patients with extended oligoarthritis, enthesitisrelated arthritis, or psoriatic arthritis. J Rheumatol. 2016;43:816–24. doi:10.3899/jrheum.150430.
116. Ruperto N, Martini A. Networking in paediatrics: the example of the Paediatric Rheumatology International Trials Organisation (PRINTO). Arch Dis Child. 2011;96:596–601. doi:10.1136/adc.2010.188946.
117. Mantovani A, Mantovani A, Allavena P, et al. Cancer-related inflammation. Nature. 2008;454:436–44. doi:10.1038/nature07205.
118. Baecklund E, Iliadou A, Askling J, et al. Association of chronic inflammation, not its treatment, with increased lymphoma risk in rheumatoid arthritis. Arthritis Rheum. 2006;54:692–701. doi:10.1002/art.21675.
119. Simon TA, Thompson A, Gandhi KK, et al. Incidence of malignancy in adult patients with rheumatoid arthritis: a meta-analysis. Arthritis Res Ther. 2015;17:212. doi:10.1186/s13075-015-0728-9.
120. Ramiro S, Gaujoux-Viala C, Nam JL, et al. Safety of synthetic and biological DMARDs: a systematic literature review informing the 2013 update of the EULAR recommendations for management of rheumatoid arthritis. Ann Rheum Dis. 2014;73:529–35. doi:10.1136/annrheumdis-2013-204575.
121. Franks AL, Slansky JE. Multiple associations between a broad spectrum of autoimmune diseases, chronic inflammatory diseases and cancer. Anticancer Res. 2012;32:1119–36.
122. Onel KB, Onel K. Anti-tumor necrosis factor therapy and cancer risk in patients with autoimmune disorders. Arthritis Care Res (Hoboken). 2010;62:1024–8. doi:10.1002/acr.20228.

123. Diak P, Siegel J, La Grenade L, et al. Tumor necrosis factor alpha blockers and malignancy in children: forty-eight cases reported to the Food and Drug Administration. Arthritis Rheum. 2010;62:2517–24. doi:10.1002/art.27511.
124. Lehman TJA. Should the food and drug administration warning of malignancy in children receiving tumor necrosis factor alpha blockers change the way we treat children with juvenile idiopathic arthritis? Arthritis Rheum. 2010;62:2183–4. doi:10.1002/art.27506.
125. Ruperto N, Lovell DJ, Quartier P, et al. Abatacept in children with juvenile idiopathic arthritis: a randomised, double-blind, placebo-controlled withdrawal trial. Lancet (London, England). 2008;372:383–91. doi:10.1016/S0140-6736(08)60998-8.
126. Ruperto N, Lovell DJ, Quartier P, et al. Long-term safety and efficacy of abatacept in children with juvenile idiopathic arthritis. Arthritis Rheum. 2010;62:1792–802. doi:10.1002/art.27431.
127. Ruperto N, Quartier P, Wulffraat N, et al. A phase II, multicenter, open-label study evaluating dosing and preliminary safety and efficacy of canakinumab in systemic juvenile idiopathic arthritis with active systemic features. Arthritis Rheum. 2012;64:557–67. doi:10.1002/art.33342.
128. Quartier P, Allantaz F, Cimaz R, et al. A multicentre, randomised, double-blind, placebo-controlled trial with the interleukin-1 receptor antagonist anakinra in patients with systemic-onset juvenile idiopathic arthritis (ANAJIS trial). Ann Rheum Dis. 2011;70:747–54. doi:10.1136/ard.2010.134254.
129. Ruperto N, Brunner HI, Quartier P, et al. Two randomized trials of canakinumab in systemic juvenile idiopathic arthritis. N Engl J Med. 2012;367:2396–406. doi:10.1056/NEJMoa1205099.
130. Yokota S, Imagawa T, Mori M, et al. Efficacy and safety of tocilizumab in patients with systemic-onset juvenile idiopathic arthritis: a randomised, double-blind, placebo-controlled, withdrawal phase III trial. Lancet. 2008;371:998–1006. doi:10.1016/S0140-6736(08)60454-7.
131. De Benedetti F, Brunner HI, Ruperto N, et al. Randomized trial of tocilizumab in systemic juvenile idiopathic arthritis. N Engl J Med. 2012;367:2385–95. doi:10.1056/NEJMoa1112802.
132. Ilowite N, Porras O, Reiff A, et al. Anakinra in the treatment of polyarticular-course juvenile rheumatoid arthritis: safety and preliminary efficacy results of a randomized multicenter study. Clin Rheumatol. 2009;28:129–37. doi:10.1007/s10067-008-0995-9.
133. Tarkiainen M, Tynjälä P, Vähäsalo P, et al. Occurrence of adverse events in patients with JIA receiving biologic agents: long-term follow-up in a real-life setting. Rheumatology (Oxford). 2015;54:1170–6. doi:10.1093/rheumatology/keu457.
134. Hollan I, Meroni PL, Ahearn JM, et al. Cardiovascular disease in autoimmune rheumatic diseases. Autoimmun Rev. 2013;12:1004–15. doi:10.1016/j.autrev.2013.03.013.
135. Han C, Robinson DWJ, Hackett MV, et al. Cardiovascular disease and risk factors in patients with rheumatoid arthritis, psoriatic arthritis, and ankylosing spondylitis. J Rheumatol. 2006;33:2167–72.
136. Avina-Zubieta JA, Thomas J, Sadatsafavi M, et al. Risk of incident cardiovascular events in patients with rheumatoid arthritis: a meta-analysis of observational studies. Ann Rheum Dis. 2012;71:1524–9. doi:10.1136/annrheumdis-2011-200726.
137. Coulson EJ, Ng W-F, Goff I, et al. Cardiovascular risk in juvenile idiopathic arthritis. Rheumatology (Oxford). 2013;52:1163–71. doi:10.1093/rheumatology/ket106.
138. Solomon DH, Avorn J, Sturmer T, et al. Cardiovascular outcomes in new users of coxibs and nonsteroidal antiinflammatory drugs: high-risk subgroups and time course of risk. Arthritis Rheum. 2006;54:1378–89. doi:10.1002/art.21887.
139. Greenberg JD, Kremer JM, Curtis JR, et al. Tumour necrosis factor antagonist use and associated risk reduction of cardiovascular events among patients with rheumatoid arthritis. Ann Rheum Dis. 2011;70:576–82. doi:10.1136/ard.2010.129916.
140. Breda L, Di Marzio D, Giannini C, et al. Relationship between inflammatory markers, oxidant-antioxidant status and intima-media thickness in prepubertal children with juvenile idiopathic arthritis. Clin Res Cardiol. 2013;102:63–71. doi:10.1007/s00392-012-0496-3.

141. Ilowite NT, Samuel P, Beseler L, et al. Dyslipoproteinemia in juvenile rheumatoid arthritis. J Pediatr. 1989;114:823–6.
142. Tselepis AD, Elisaf M, Besis S, et al. Association of the inflammatory state in active juvenile rheumatoid arthritis with hypo-high-density lipoproteinemia and reduced lipoprotein-associated platelet-activating factor acetylhydrolase activity. Arthritis Rheum. 1999;42:373–83. doi:10.1002/1529-0131(199902)42:2<373::AID-ANR21>3.0.CO;2-3.
143. Bakkaloglu A, Kirel B, Ozen S, et al. Plasma lipids and lipoproteins in juvenile chronic arthritis. Clin Rheumatol. 1996;15:341–5.
144. Marangoni RG, Hayata AL, Borba EF, et al. Decreased high-density lipoprotein cholesterol levels in polyarticular juvenile idiopathic arthritis. Clinics (Sao Paulo). 2011;66:1549–52.
145. Dursunoglu D, Evrengul H, Polat B, et al. Lp(a) lipoprotein and lipids in patients with rheumatoid arthritis: serum levels and relationship to inflammation. Rheumatol Int. 2005;25:241–5. doi:10.1007/s00296-004-0438-0.
146. Satija M, Yadav TP, Sachdev N, et al. Endothelial function, arterial wall mechanics and intima media thickness in juvenile idiopathic arthritis. Clin Exp Rheumatol. 2014;32:432–9. http://www.ncbi.nlm.nih.gov/pubmed/24564946.
147. Vlahos AP, Theocharis P, Bechlioulis A, et al. Changes in vascular function and structure in juvenile idiopathic arthritis. Arthritis Care Res (Hoboken). 2011;63:1736–44. doi:10.1002/acr.20613.
148. Pietrewicz E, Urban M. Early atherosclerosis changes in children with juvenile idiopathic arthritis. Pol Merkur Lek. 2007;22:211–4.
149. Breda L, Di Marzio D, Giannini C, et al. Relationship between inflammatory markers, oxidant–antioxidant status and intima-media thickness in prepubertal children with juvenile idiopathic arthritis. Clin Res Cardiol. 2012:63–71. doi:10.1007/s00392-012-0496-3.

Chapter 14
Targeting Comorbidity in Routine Rheumatology Care

Tuulikki Sokka

Targeting Outcomes in Rheumatology Care

Management of rheumatic diseases and patient monitoring was described in the 1980s as "Clinicians may all too easily spend years writing 'doing well' in the notes of a patient who has become progressively crippled before their eyes..." [1]. Although clinical picture of rheumatology patients has changed over the decades and outcomes have improved in many countries, measuring and documenting of outcomes does not appear to be routine practice in most clinics around the world. Similarly, screening, preventing and reporting of comorbidities needs more attention and should be an essential part of the infrastructure of the clinic.

More Attention Needed for Management of Comorbidities

Awareness has increased over the past two decades of the fact that general risk factors and comorbidities may not be adequately identified or addressed in patients with chronic diseases [2]. A study from 2007 indicated that in patients with rheumatoid arthritis (RA), rheumatologists managed obesity, high blood pressure and lipids significantly less often than did primary care physicians [3]. Further, primary care physicians addressed obesity least often among patients with RA, compared to diabetes mellitus, or individuals with no chronic conditions; the corresponding percentages were 31%, 68% and 46%, respectively [3]. These and similar observations concerning other health issues lead to the development of international and national

T. Sokka (✉)
Department of Rheumatology, Jyväskylä Central Hospital, Jyväskylä 40620, Finland

University of Eastern Finland, Faculty of Health Sciences, Kuopio, Finland
e-mail: tuulikki.sokka-isler@ksshp.fi

Y. El Miedany (ed.), *Comorbidity in Rheumatic Diseases*,
DOI 10.1007/978-3-319-59963-2_14

recommendations and their updates, for the management of comorbidities in patients with rheumatic diseases [4–7].

Patients with rheumatic diseases meet health professionals regularly. Many patients may not meet any other health professionals except the rheumatologist and the rheumatology nurse although, officially, management of other than rheumatic diseases may have been assigned to the primary care. In many cases, the rheumatology clinic is in a key position to recognize patient's health issues and presence of risk factors for cardiovascular disease, osteoporosis, infections and other common comorbidities. The rheumatology clinic may not be able to fully manage a large variety of comorbid conditions and referrals to other specialist may be needed – or back to the primary care. Nevertheless, the rheumatology clinic is in an important position to recognize patients' health-related issues in general.

Which Comorbidities to Target?

All other diseases that coexist with a disease of interest are called comorbidities [8, 9]. Therefore, diseases that are most prevalent in the background population are also most prevalent in patients with rheumatic diseases. Similarly, diseases that are rare in population may also occur in some patients with rheumatic diseases. Lifestyle such as smoking or physical inactivity contributes to comorbidity in any individual. In rheumatic diseases, likelihood of certain comorbidities increases, due to persistent inflammatory activity and organ damage, as well as due to the use of antirheumatic medications.

The EULAR initiative for the points to consider for reporting, screening and preventing comorbidities lists cardiovascular diseases, kidney diseases, lung diseases, infections, malignancies, osteoporosis, gastrointestinal diseases and depression as comorbidities of interest [5]. In addition, fibromyalgia is possibly one of the most prevalent and most under-recognized health problems in patients with rheumatic diseases and may interfere with the evaluation of disease activity of other rheumatic diseases [10, 11]. The variety of comorbidities in rheumatic and any chronic diseases is rather wide including any diagnoses related and unrelated to the disease in question.

Points to Consider in Comorbidities

The EULAR recommendations [5] include a detailed list of points to consider for reporting or detecting prevalent comorbidities and screening for comorbidity or for risk factors and treatments/vaccination and are presented here in Table 14.1. These recommendations also suggest a standardized reporting form for reporting ischaemic cardiovascular diseases, for risk factors and treatments [5]. Other similar and more comprehensive comorbidity lists have been suggested, as part of research programmes such as COMORA [12] and QUEST-RA [13].

Table 14.1 Overarching principles and points to consider for reporting or detecting prevalent comorbidities and screening for comorbidity or for risk factors and treatments/vaccination

	Overarching principles
A	Comorbidities such as cardiovascular diseases, malignancies, infections, osteoporosis, peptic ulcer and depression should be carefully assessed and managed in patients with chronic inflammatory rheumatic diseases
B	All clinicians including health professionals such as nurses, treating general practitioners and rheumatologists and patients through self-administered questionnaires and self-management programmes play a key role in the screening and detection of comorbidities
C	Comorbidities should be subject to a systematic, standardized periodical review (e.g. at least every 5 years) for those with a chronic inflammatory rheumatic disease
	Points to consider
	Cardiovascular diseases
1	History of myocardial infarction, pectoris angina, stent, stroke, transient ischaemic attack, heart failure and lower limb peripheral arterial disease should be documented
2	Cardiovascular risk factors such as smoking status, body mass index, history of hypertension, hypercholesterolaemia, renal insufficiency and HEART-SCORE index should be documented
3	Current cardiovascular treatments such as antihypertensive therapy, antiplatelet therapy, diabetes insulin or non-insulin therapies, lipid-lowering agents and anticoagulants should be documented
	Malignancies
4	History of malignancies should be documented
5	Screening procedures for malignancy (including mammography, pap smear, visit to a dermatologist, faecal occult blood test, colonoscopy) and for malignancy risk factors (including family history of breast or colon cancer and personal history of inflammatory bowel disease) should be documented
	Infections
6	History of tuberculosis should be documented including prior results of chest X-ray, tuberculin skin test, interferon-γ release assay and BCG vaccination
7	History of serious infections, opportunistic infections and chronic viral infections should be documented
8	Vaccination status for infections including influenza, *Streptococcus pneumoniae*, herpes zoster, human papillomavirus, poliomyelitis, diphtheria, tetanus and hepatitis B should be documented
	Peptic ulcer
9	History of gastroscopy-proven peptic ulcer should be documented
10	Risk factors for peptic ulcer such as age > 65 years, proton-pump inhibitor intake, personal history of complicated ulcer, *Helicobacter pylori* infection, current use of aspirin, non-steroidal anti-inflammatory drugs, corticosteroids and anticoagulants should be documented
	Osteoporosis
11	History of osteoporotic fracture should be documented
12	Risk factors for osteoporosis including body mass index <19, physical inactivity, glucocorticoid exposure, alcohol intake, family history of femoral neck fracture, secondary osteoporosis and bone mineral density should be collected, and the FRAX global risk should be calculated where applicable
13	Current or prior osteoporosis treatments including calcium/vitamin D supplementation, bisphosphonates, strontium ranelate, raloxifene, teriparatide and denosumab should be documented
	Depression
14	History of depression, current depression and prior screening for depression should be documented
15	Current treatments for depression should be collected

From Baillet et al. [5] with permission

Infrastructure of the Clinic to Review and Manage Rheumatic Diseases and Comorbidities

The work load in rheumatology clinics and private practices is known to be overwhelming. Therefore, any extra work is not welcome to the nurse or to the rheumatologist. User-friendly IT solutions may be used in the review of comorbidities, with data entry by the patient him-/herself or by a dedicated monitoring specialist. Possibly the only approach to review and manage comorbidities consistently is to build it into the infrastructure of the rheumatology clinic, as an automatic procedure. An example of such an infrastructure is provided here (text adapted from [14]).

Vision

The vision of the clinical model is based on a "Finnish treat to target" manifest from the 1970s, "We are treating not only the actual inflammation of the joints but also the quality of the patient's life for many decades in the future" [15]. In this model, treatment target is early and permanent remission in inflammatory rheumatic diseases. The model aims at an informed patient and an informed health professional so that treatment decisions would not be based on the beliefs of the patient or the doctor.

Setting

Jyväskylä Central Hospital is Finland's biggest nonuniversity hospital, covering the secondary level health care for 250,000 inhabitants. The rheumatology clinic model has its roots in the development of rheumatology care and its scientific reporting, which started many decades ago [16]. The goal was to enhance the patient "journey" through rheumatology services by providing all necessary education, treatment and care, avoiding unnecessary visits and optimizing the overall quality of care provided.

The Patient Monitoring Tool, GoTreatIT

An electronic monitoring tool for continuing treatment data collection via software GoTreatIT is integrated into the everyday clinical work since 2007. The program is developed by rheumatologists with a Norwegian company DiaGraphIT and is used to support systematic collection of data at every visit and during the entire course of the patient's illness [17].

Patient Self-Report

Upon arrival to the clinic at every visit, the patient signs in to GoTreatIT with his/her unique ID, to complete a questionnaire, before seeing the nurse or the doctor. The questionnaire comprises of questions aimed at identifying the patient's current performance status, quality of life, the level of pain, fatigue, disease activity, psychological items, comorbidities and certain medications. Patient self-report items are collected in Table 14.2.

Table 14.2 Items to be selected for the patient self-report in GoTreatIT monitoring tool

Self-report category	Question/questionnaire
Functional status	HAQ, mHAQ, MD-HAQ, HAQ-II
	cHAQ Parent, cHAQ child
	ROAD
	BASFI
Disease activity	Disease activity VAS
	BASDAI
Symptoms	Pain VAS
	Fatigue VAS
	Patient global assessment VAS
	Duration of morning stiffness in joints
	Self-reported joint count for painful joints
	RAID
Acceptance of symptom level	PASS
Psychological status	Sleep
	Stress
	Anxiety
	Depression
Lifestyle/risk factors	Weight – automatic BMI calculated
	Physical exercise: times per week
	Smoking
Socio-/demographics	Living alone/together with someone
	Work status
	Years of education
Recent events over half-year	Surgery
	Hospitalization
	New diagnosis or trauma
	New symptoms
	Side effects from medications
	Change is marital status
	Change in work status
Quality of life	SF-36/RAND
	EQ5D
Others	WPAI:RA
Comorbidities and risk factors	List of comorbidities and risk factors of special interest provided
Medications	List of medications with special interest provided

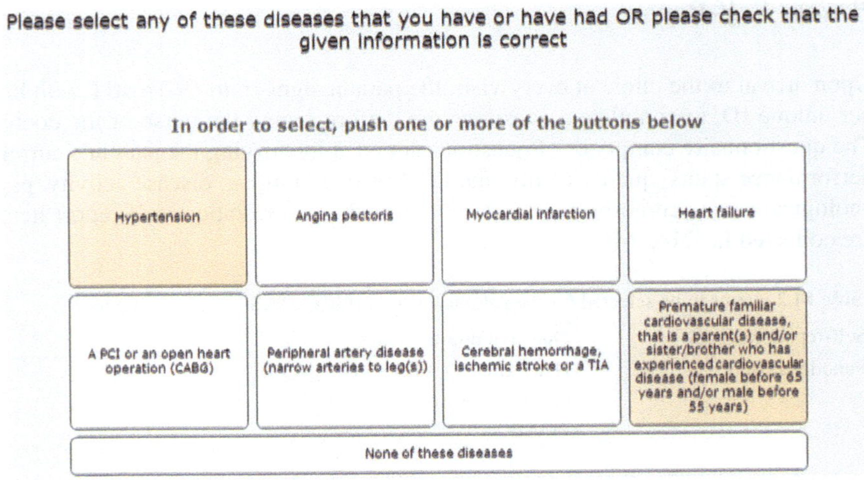

Fig. 14.1 A screenshot view of the patient self-report for cardiovascular disease/risk factors on GoTreatIT monitoring tool

Several touch-screen stations and tablets are reserved for patient self-report, to ensue availability of devices at the arrival of the patient. The number of questions varies between the patients. The set of questions is predefined, depending on the diagnosis and patient's capacities. For example, a young person with axial and peripheral symptoms completes a maximal number of questions, and an old person with memory problems completes a short one. Some questionnaires are only used for the documentation in clinical trials such as generic quality of life questionnaires. An example of screenshot of patient self-report for cardiovascular disease/risk factors is presented in Fig. 14.1 and an example of screenshot for self-reported medications in Fig. 14.2.

Using the questionnaire completed by patient and current laboratory values and joint status completed by doctor, the program generates commonly used comparable values such as Health Assessment Questionnaire (HAQ), 28-joint count Disease Activity Score (DAS28) and Bath Ankylosing Spondylitis Functional Index (BASFI) and BMI for every visit.

Remote Patient Monitoring with GoTreatIT

In patients who are in stable remission, remote monitoring is a potential option. At certain intervals such as every half a year, a reminder, such as a text message or an e-mail, is sent to the patient to complete GoTreatIT self-report and to get laboratory tests taken. Results are being reviewed by the rheumatology nurse or the rheumatologist, with comparison to patient's previous values. If self-reported disease activity/symptoms are higher than earlier or other problems are found, remote monitoring will lead to a telephone contact and/or patient visit to the clinic.

a

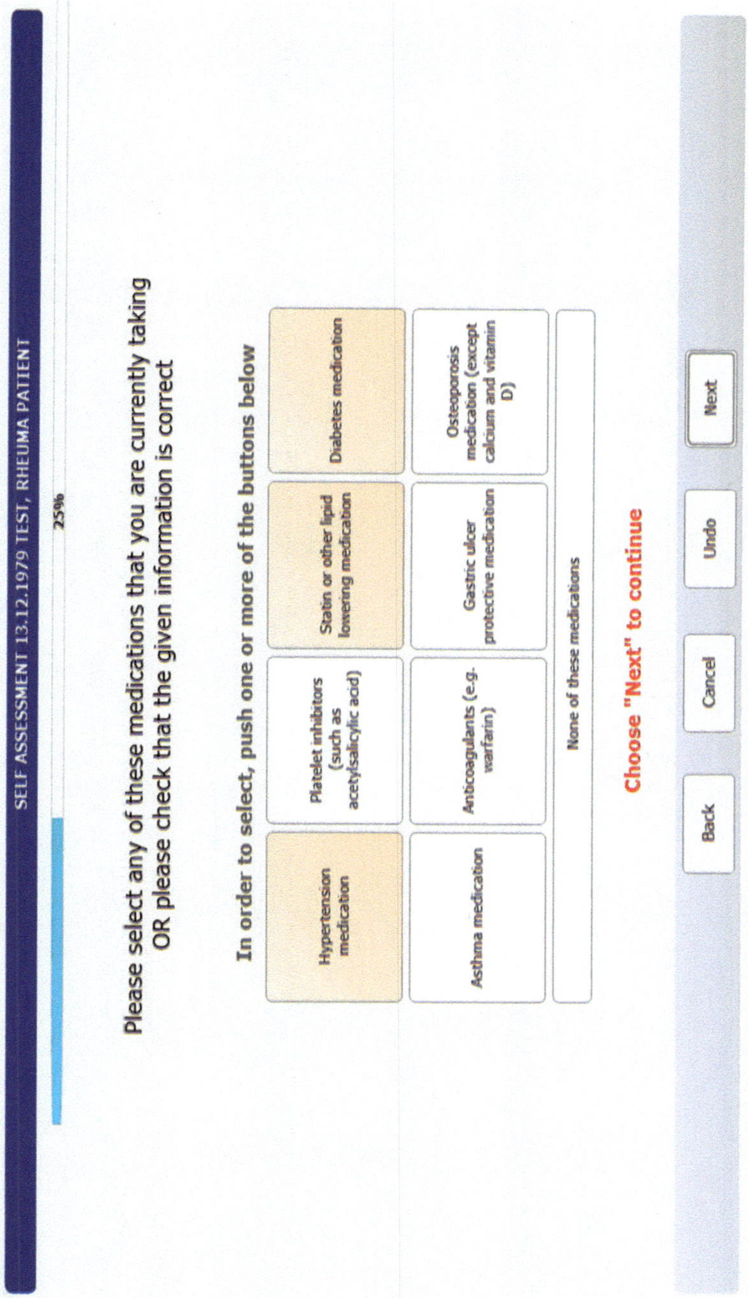

Fig. 14.2 **(a, b)** Screenshot views for the patient self-report for medications on GoTreatIT monitoring tool

b

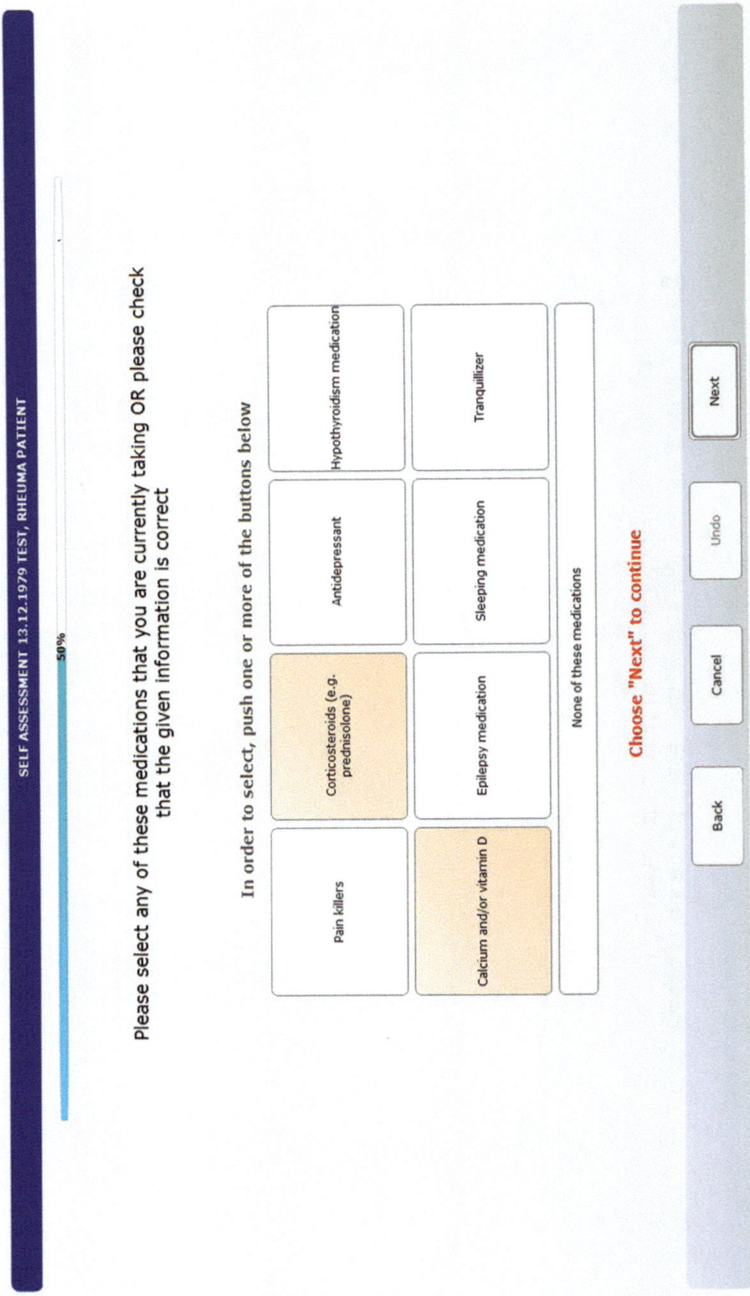

Fig. 14.2 (continued)

Review of Data

The electronic monitoring system enables a quick review of the individual patient's history of presentation, medication used, examination findings, comorbidities, joint surgeries, values of patient self-report, disease activity measures and any other patient or disease-related details in a table or a graph for individual patients (Fig. 14.3).

Data for comorbidities are confirmed and updated by the monitoring specialist with information from the medical records, for time (month and year) of the diagnosis of the comorbidity. Any changes in the type and dose of medications during the course of the disease and reasons for that including any adverse events are indicated in GoTreatIT, allowing the doctor to see the complete history of medications used at a glance. The automatically generated view in Table 14.3 is available with one keystroke only. Reviewing patient comorbidity data is made fast, easy and helpful in a busy clinic. Data are confirmed by the monitoring specialist with the date and electronic signature, to ensure accuracy of the data.

Responses for patient self-report can also be reviewed one by one and compared to the previous responses. Patient self-report is available, while patient is working on it, and can be reviewed and compared to values of previous visits before the patient enters to the doctor's room. A review of patient self-report directs doctor's attention to the current problem. For example, patient self-report seen in Fig. 14.4, reviewed before patient visit, is very helpful and suggests of fibromyalgia.

Multidisciplinary Care

At every clinical visit, patient is seen by the rheumatologist and the nurse specialist, which have predefined tasks. The physical therapist is involved in certain treatment paths, and other therapists can be consulted if needed such as an occupational therapist, nutritionist, social worker, podiatrist, etc.

Doctor Review

The doctor review is conducted over 30–60 min. Prior to the visit, doctor reviews patient self-report values, comparing to the previous values, to identify current problems if any.

At every visit, the doctor undertakes a complete joint assessment, denoting on GoTreatIT all tender and swollen joints and any intra-articular injections completed using a visual map of joints. In the same way, doctor can easily compare current joint status to that of previous visits. Entering the data to the system is simple and takes less than half a minute.

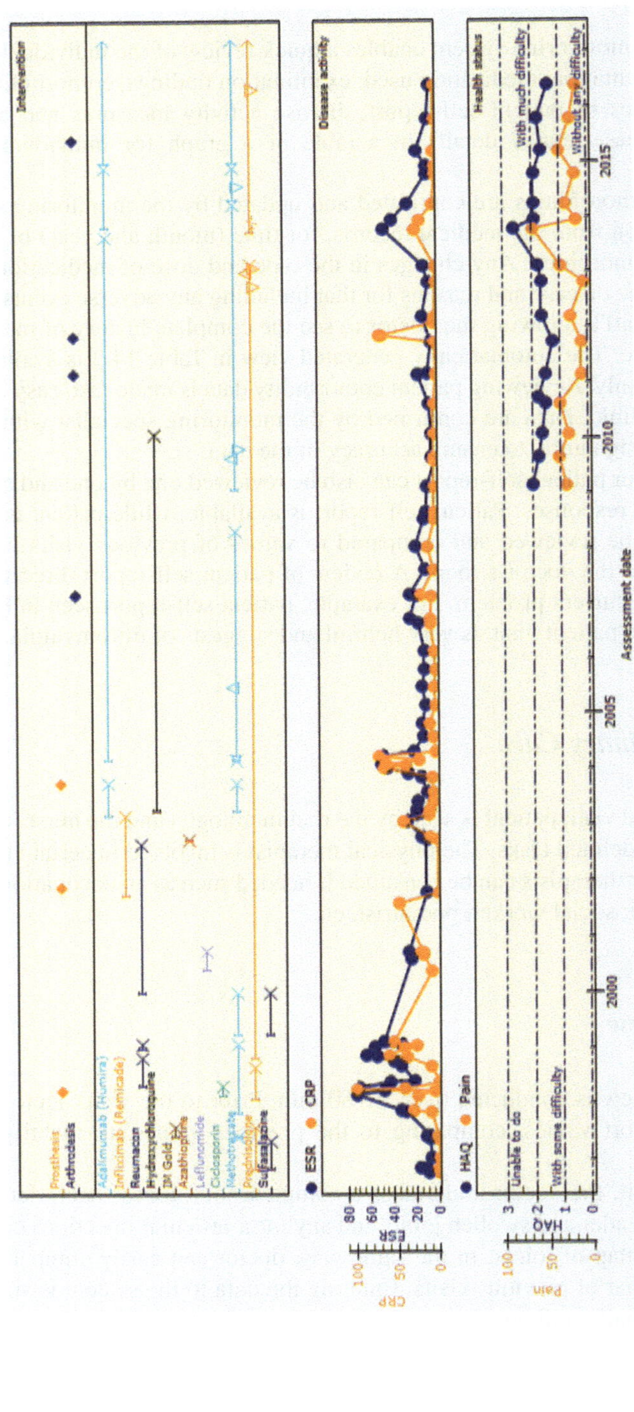

Fig. 14.3 A graphic presentation of patient data from the GoTreatIT monitoring tool including joint surgery, medications, disease activity and patient-reported outcomes

Table 14.3 An automatic flow sheet of patient data from the GoTreatIT monitoring tool

Data extracted	25.08.2015
ID	Case 1
Age, gender	68, female
Work status	Pensioner since diagnosis
Diagnosis	Rheumatoid arthritis
Diagnosis criteria	Symptoms: 1.1996
	Clinical diagnosis of RA: 10.1996
Highest RF (IgM)	Negative (9) 3.2012
Highest (aCCP)	Negative (4) 8.2009
aCarP	Negative 7.2015
HLA-B27	Positive
Smoking	Non-smoking, past history of smoking
Medications (used) TRUNCATED	
Medications (now)	Methotrexate 1.2015
	7,50 mg subcutaneous once a week
	Adalimumab (Humira) 1.2015
	40,00 mg subcutaneous every 2 weeks
	Prednisolone 10.2013
	5,00 mg peroral every day
Comorbidity	Vertebral fracture 10.2005
	Herpes zoster infection 9.2002
	Arm fracture, not wrist 8.2001
	Osteopenia by DXA 2001
	Cholelithiasis 3.1998
	Arterial hypertension 11.1996
	Fibromyalgia 7.1990
	Lumbago/dorsalgia/sciatica 1980
	Migraine – before rheuma diagnosis
Surgery	Left ankle arthrodesis 11.2011
	Right ankle arthrodesis 3.2011
	Left MTP arthrodesis 3.2007
	Right MTP arthrodesis 3.2007
	Left knee arthroplasty 10.2003
	Left knee synovectomy 5.2003
	Right knee arthroscopy and synovectomy 10.2002
	Right knee rearthroplasty 12.2001
	Right knee arthroplasty 4.1998
	Right knee other surgery 8.1996
Confirmed by	25.08.2015 (miina_l)

(continued)

Table 14.3 (continued)

Latest scores					
Date	13.12.2013	02.04.2014	20.10.2014	08.12.2014	17.03.2015
Health status					
Pain	16	28	17		35
Fatigue	19	12	18		6
Patient global	35	28	29		30
Morning stiffness	2.50	0.75	0.50		0.50
Rheumatic activity	21	26	15		15
Physical exercise	Cannot	Do not	Do not		Do not
M-HAQ (0–3)	1.25	0.63	0.75		0.38
MDHAQ (FN) (0–3)	2.2	1.5	1.6		1.2
MDHAQ (PS) (0–3)	0.5	0.5	0.25		0
HAQ (0–3)	1.88	1.88	1.88		1.63
Raw HAQ (0–24)	14	13	12		10
Disease act.					
Inv. global	33	15	8		
ESR	38	24	8	8	16
CRP	19	3	1	1	2
TJC 28/32	7/7	5/5	2/2		2/2
SJC 28/32	3/3	1/1	0/0		1/1
TJC 46	7	5	2		2
SJC 46	3	1	0		1
DAS28(4)	5	4.1	2.7		3.4
DAS28(3)	5	4.2	2.6		3.4
DAS28-CRP(4)	4.5	3.4	2.4		2.8
DAS28-CRP(3)	4.5	3.4	2.3		2.8
CDAI	16.8	10.3	5.7		
Anthr.data					
Weight	93	98	98		100
BMI	33	34.7	34.7		35.4

A Full Clinical Examination at Every Visit

After discussions of the current situation, whether a first or a follow-up visit, a full clinical examination is performed. Patient dresses off including shoes and socks, wearing only light underwear. Examination includes listening to the lungs and the heart, observing the skin including skin mobility in scleroderma, palpation of the thyroid gland and abdomen and search for lymph nodes. Lining of the mouth and tongue is checked. Joints are checked for the range on motion, passive flexion of the arm (to observe rigidity), tenderness and swelling. When needed, reflects will be checked. Extremities are checked for warmth, sweating and colour. Nails and nail

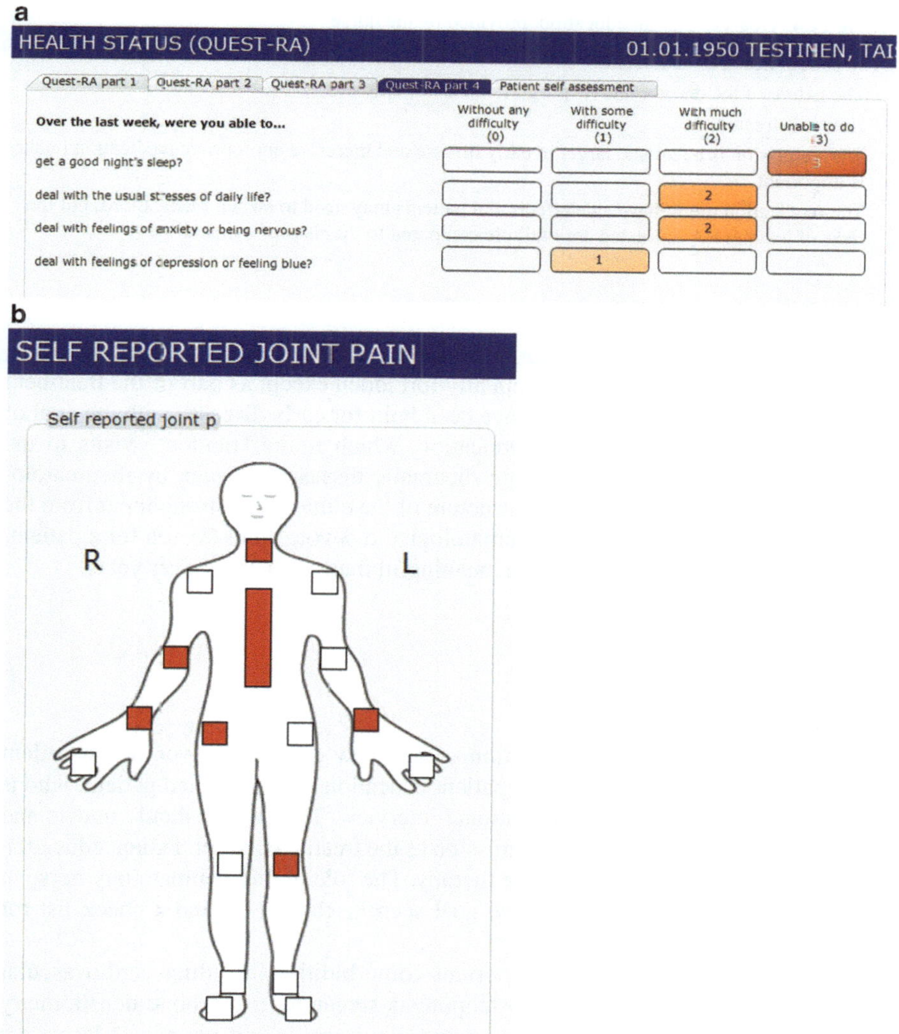

Fig. 14.4 (**a, b**) Patient self-report suggests of fibromyalgia, screenshots from GoTreatIT monitoring tool

beds are checked. In case of axial disease, physical tests include cervical rotation, modified Schober, occiput-to-wall distance, lateral spinal flexion and chest expansion, with documentation in GoTreatIT. Walking barefoot, normal, on toes and with heels is observed. Squatting is observed, as well as patient's posture and musculature. A careful examination may reveal underlying comorbidities in any organ examined.

Table 14.4 Goals of patient education, provided by the nurse

The patient needs to understand:
The nature of the disease and its progression if left untreated
How it is treated
That remission is a realistic target in early disease and therefore appropriate medication intake is important
The medication might have side effects and patients may need to switch medications, but the risks of leaving RA untreated are multiple compared to the risks of medications

Every doctor's visit should be meaningful with long-haul treatment decisions; "see you back in 3 months" is practically forbidden except as part of the treatment paths. Structured treatment paths have been built for early diseases with the goal of remission and scheduled patient education, which limits "random" visits to the clinic. Patients with stabile systemic rheumatic diseases are seen by rheumatologists once a year. The prespecified structure of the clinic and a strong input from the rheumatology nurse allows the rheumatologist to devote up to 60 min for a patient, which, in a long term, may be more meaningful than 6 × 10 min over years.

Nurse Review

The nurse provides detailed education on any new diagnoses given to the patient and treatments started. The goal of patient education is an informed patient, who is provided with methods of a motivational interview. The patient should understand the natural course of disease and remission as the treatment target. Patient education facilitates patient's adherence to the therapy. The role of the rheumatology nurse in patient education is crucial with the goal seen in Table 14.4 and a check list for specific items in Table 14.5.

The patient is assessed for important comorbidities including cardiovascular disease and related risk factors. Osteoporosis screening using bone densitometry can be arranged if needed. Blood pressure, lipid profile and vitamin D levels are screened and recorded on a routine basis with follow-up instructions as necessary.

The nurse independently provides patient education to the patient, e.g. concerning prevention of CV disease. If doctor's input is needed, the issue is discussed with the rheumatologist or the nurse may suggest close monitoring of the finding, e.g. high blood pressure, with the nurse in the general practice.

The review of comorbidities and risk factors is most detailed at baseline at the time of the diagnosis of a rheumatic disease. Points to consider are identified and documented and based on these data, and patient education continues at every visit to the rheumatology unit over time.

Table 14.5 Item in patient education, review of comorbidities/risk factors by the nurse

Use GoTreatIT self-report for review of patient's
Symptoms
Functional capacity
Work status
Sleep, psychological aspects
Provide detailed information of the prescribed medications
Purpose
Efficacy
How to administer
Side effects
Lab monitoring
How to take in special situations such as operation, infection pregnancy, etc.
Provide education of self-management for
Pain management
Pain medications
Glucocorticoid pills
Adherence to medications
Calcium, vitamin D supplementation
Vaccinations
Nutrition
Weight management
Attention to mouth, teeth
Attention to skin
Attention to eyes
Attention to feet, check need for podiatrist
Attention to possible infections
Pregnancy
Birth control
Operations
Travelling
Emphasize healthy lifestyle
Alcohol
Smoking
Exercise
Check for CV risk
Family history
Measure blood pressure
Cholesterol
Glucose
BMI (readily available in GoTreatIT)
Waist circumference
Check lab values for
Vitamin D
Cholesterol
Blood glucose if needed

Physiotherapist

The treatment path for inflammatory joint and axial disease includes consultation to a physiotherapist at the baseline. Patients with inflammatory joint diseases have follow-up visits to the physiotherapist also at the 1- and 2-year visits, according to the treatment path. At the physiotherapy visit, patients' aerobic performance capacity as well as muscle strength is tested, and patients receive basic education on healthy exercise habits accordingly. Patients are advised to perform physical exercises according to recommendations to all adults: aerobic exercises at least 2.5 h a week and muscle strength exercises at least two times a week. The goal is to prevent physical inactivity in patients with inflammatory musculoskeletal diseases and to improve health by improving aerobic and musculoskeletal capacity.

Discussion

In this presentation we provide a practical view to patient monitoring including comorbidities, to busy rheumatology clinics. First, the vision of the clinic needs to be defined: is it to make money and to roll as many patients as possible with the highest revenue or is the vision to make 1 day after another to do a good job? Or, as we think: "We are treating not only the actual inflammation of the joints but also the quality of the patient's life for many decades in the future" [15] with a view of long-lasting benefits to the patient.

Second, the structure of the clinic needs to be optimal, including treatment paths to known diagnoses and multidisciplinary care. It is important that each health professional performs the tasks that belong to that job: rheumatologist makes the diagnosis and is responsible for providing the best medications to the disease, the nurse provides all patient education devoting enough time to each patient and the physical therapist is responsible for advice for physical training to the patient. Special attention is needed to the content of the rheumatologist's visit: how many times it is discussion only without a through physical examination of the patient. Indeed, patient needs to be examined carefully to discover comorbidities in other organs than in joints. Content of patient education and review of risk factors are crucial with a check list, such as described in this presentation, including physical tests for blood pressure and waist circumference and laboratory tests such as lipids and glucose. Physiotherapist plays a major role in giving advice of healthy lifestyle.

Third, a proper automatic clinical monitoring tool is an essential part of patient monitoring. It is practically impossible to organize documentation of comorbidities without a well-working user-friendly IT solution that provides data as easy as one keystroke, as seen in tables.

The model described in this presentation is applicable to any modern healthcare service. It necessitates a certain amount of staff, resources and expertise to implement. However, as an infrastructure of the clinic, it leads to successful patient monitoring including targeting comorbidities.

Declaration of Conflicting Interests This research received no specific grant from any funding agency in the public, commercial or not-for-profit sectors. Tuulikki Sokka: honoraria, consultation fees, support for travel, research grants from Abbott, Abbvie, BMS, Celgene, DiaGraphIT, Eli Lilly, GSK, Hospira, Medac, MSD, Muikkusäätiö, Mundipharma, Novo Nordisk, Orion Pharma, Pfizer, Roche, UCB and Academy of Finland.

References

1. Smith T. Questions on clinical trials (editorial). Br Med J. 1983;287:569.
2. Redelmeier DA, Tan SH, Booth GL. The treatment of unrelated disorders in patients with chronic medical diseases. N Engl J Med. 1998;338:1516–20.
3. Desai SS, Myles JD, Kaplan MJ. Suboptimal cardiovascular risk factor identification and management in patients with rheumatoid arthritis: a cohort analysis. Arthritis Res Ther. 2012;14:R270.
4. Agca R, Heslinga SC, Rollefstad S, Heslinga M, McInnes IB, Peters MJ, et al. EULAR recommendations for cardiovascular disease risk management in patients with rheumatoid arthritis and other forms of inflammatory joint disorders: 2015/2016 update. Ann Rheum Dis. 2016;76(1):17–28.
5. Baillet A, Gossec L, Carmona L, Wit M, van Eijk-Hustings Y, Bertheussen H, et al. Points to consider for reporting, screening for and preventing selected comorbidities in chronic inflammatory rheumatic diseases in daily practice: a EULAR initiative. Ann Rheum Dis. 2016;75:965–73.
6. Strehl C, Bijlsma JW, de Wit M, Boers M, Caeyers N, Cutolo M, et al. Defining conditions where long-term glucocorticoid treatment has an acceptably low level of harm to facilitate implementation of existing recommendations: viewpoints from an EULAR task force. Ann Rheum Dis. 2016;75:952–7.
7. Cordeiro I, Duarte AC, Ferreira JF, Goncalves MJ, Meirinhos T, Rocha TM, et al. Recommendations for vaccination in adult patients with systemic inflammatory rheumatic diseases from the portuguese society of rheumatology. Acta Reumatol Port. 2016;41(2):112–30.
8. Michaud K, Wolfe F. Comorbidities in rheumatoid arthritis. Best Pract Res Clin Rheumatol. 2007;21:885–906.
9. Gabriel SE, Michaud K. Epidemiological studies in incidence, prevalence, mortality, and comorbidity of the rheumatic diseases. Arthritis Res Ther. 2009;11:229.
10. Haliloglu S, Carlioglu A, Akdeniz D, Karaaslan Y, Kosar A. Fibromyalgia in patients with other rheumatic diseases: prevalence and relationship with disease activity. Rheumatol Int. 2014;34:1275–80.
11. Inanc N, Yilmaz-Oner S, Can M, Sokka T, Direskeneli H. The role of depression, anxiety, fatigue, and fibromyalgia on the evaluation of the remission status in patients with rheumatoid arthritis. J Rheumatol. 2014;41:1755–60.
12. Dougados M, Soubrier M, Antunez A, Balint P, Balsa A, Buch MH, et al. Prevalence of comorbidities in rheumatoid arthritis and evaluation of their monitoring: results of an international, cross-sectional study (COMORA). Ann Rheum Dis. 2014;73:62–8.
13. Naranjo A, Sokka T, Descalzo MA, Calvo-Alen J, Horslev-Petersen K, Luukkainen RK, et al. Cardiovascular disease in patients with rheumatoid arthritis: results from the QUEST-RA study. Arthritis Res Ther. 2008;10:R30.
14. Vare P, Nikiphorou E, Hannonen P, Sokka T. Delivering a one-stop, integrated, and patient-centered service for patients with rheumatic diseases. SAGE Open Med. 2016;4:2050312116654404.
15. Luukkainen R, Kajander A, Isomäki H. Treatment of rheumatoid arthritis (letter). Br Med J. 1978;2:1501.

16. Oka M, Rekonen A, Ruotsi A, Kuikka J. Measurement of systemic inflammatory activity in rheumatoid arthritis by the 99mTc method. Scand J Rheumatol. 1973;2:101–7.
17. Sokka T, Haugeberg G, Pincus T. Assessment of quality of rheumatoid arthritis care requires joint count and/or patient questionnaire data not found in a usual medical record: examples from studies of premature mortality, changes in clinical status between 1985 and 2000, and a QUEST-RA global perspective. Clin Exp Rheumatol. 2007;25:86–97.

Chapter 15
Comorbidity and Physical Therapy

Nadia El Aroussy and Yasser El Miedany

Outpatient physical therapy and rehabilitation provides services for a wide variety of medical and surgical conditions as well as disabilities. This includes a diversity of musculoskeletal conditions such as spinal, joint, and soft tissue pains, a wide range of injuries, medical conditions, or postsurgical rehabilitation programs. Having a baseline information about these patients referred for physical therapy and starting their rehabilitation courses help in guiding the therapist to set the most appropriate management plan for the patient, avoid strenuous exercises which might have negative impact on the patient, and assist in monitoring the patient's condition and response to therapy. Considering a full profile for the patient helps also in setting the appropriate patient education program tailored to the patient condition/needs and setting up patients' group therapy services. On the research level, such data helps researchers in reclassifying the outpatient subpopulations, provides outpatient clinics direction concerning these patients, and evaluates the outcomes of physical therapy professional programs considering what to emphasize in musculoskeletal and orthopedic courses.

Though comorbidities vary from patient to another and some patients may have more than one comorbidity at the same time, majority of the studies carried out to assess comorbidity in patients referred for physiotherapy included patients referred mainly for specific musculoskeletal conditions such as low back pain and arthritis [1]. This chapter will discuss the prevalence of comorbid conditions in physical therapy population as well as the association between physical therapy and comorbidity. It will also review the impact of comorbidities on physiotherapy programs, setting up targeted

N. El Aroussy (✉)
Department of Rheumatology and Rehabilitation, Ain Shams University, Cairo, Egypt

Y. El Miedany
King's College, London, London, UK

Rheumatology and Rehabilitation, Ain Shams University, Cairo, Egypt

Department of Rheumatology, Darent Valley Hospital, Dartford, Kent, UK

Y. El Miedany (ed.), *Comorbidity in Rheumatic Diseases*,
DOI 10.1007/978-3-319-59963-2_15

rehabilitation programs for patients with comorbidity in addition to the barriers to comprehensive patient management and treatment of comorbidities.

Prevalence of Comorbid Conditions in Physical Therapy Population

Identifying comorbidities and the potential impact of such comorbid conditions on the patient care are mandatory for physical and occupational therapists to implement appropriate strategies, aiming at minimizing the consequences of the comorbidity, and establish a reasonable prognosis. However, in standard clinical practice, it is not entirely clear how the patients with comorbidities are assessed or treated [1]. In 1999, Boissonnault [2] conducted multicentral study for comorbidities reported by patients receiving physiotherapy in 177 therapy clinics located in 20 states within the physiotherapy association organization. Results revealed that headache, hypertension, arthritis, depression, heart disease, chronic obstructive pulmonary diseases, and diabetes were the most common comorbidities observed. In another vignette study [3], the authors reported that comorbidities could force physiotherapist to deviate from guidelines. The work assessed whether the physical therapists considered the baseline comorbidities the patient might have and could make reasoned adaptations to the standard treatment program of the index disease when comorbidity(ies) is present. Results revealed that most physical therapists had to make such adaptations when comorbidity was present. However, these adaptations varied towards better or worse as it was noticed that the same patient was treated in various ways by different physiotherapists. This highlights the importance of the referral process identifying the presence of comorbidities and its impact on the patient's rehabilitation program. Therefore, in a trial to tackle such challenge, perhaps the first step is to consider the referral format and the decision-making process of physical therapists, followed by exploring the possible approaches to unravel the complexity of treating multi-diseased patients. Figure 15.1 shows an example of an online referral format including the patient's diagnosis, the expected targets of physical therapy, the impact of the disease on the patient, as well as the associated comorbidities for this particular patient.

The Association Between Comorbidity and Physical Therapy

While in some cases, physiotherapy programs might have a positive impact on the patients' primary disease and its associated comorbidities, it may cause untoward complications in other cohort of patients. Therefore, it is mandatory to consider pretreatment assessment of the patient to consider the consequences of the classic physiotherapy/rehabilitation programs on patients with variable comorbidities and identify the most appropriate rehabilitation course.

Physiotherapy Referral Form

Diagnosis:
- Hypermobility □ Fibromyalgia □
- Rheumatoid arthritis □ Ankylosing Spondylitis □
- Chronic fatigue syndrome □ Low Back Pain □
- Other: ....
- **Status:** Inpatient: □ Outpatient: □
- **Priority:** Urgent: □ Routine: □
- **Date:** / /20

Required service:
- Hydrotherapy □
- Acupuncture □
- Back to fitness □
- Mechanical back pain □
- US □
- Manipulation/ manual therapy □
- Gym Rehab □
- Women's health □
- Post operative shoulder rehab □
- Joint replacement Rehab □
- Fatigue self management □
- Sleep self management □
- Other... □
- **Clinical details -Targets – Recommendations:**

....

....

Duration of symptoms: < 2weeks □; 2-6 weeks □; 6-12 weeks □; > 12 weeks □

Is the patient off work: Yes □; No □; Not employed □

Is Sleep Disturbed: Yes □; No □

Has the patient's functional ability been affected? Yes □; No □; Disabled □

Comorbidities: Asthma □ Diabetes □; Hypertension □ Cancer □; Rheumatoid Arthritis □ COPD □; Angina □ Epilepsy □; Myocardial infarction □ Vasculitis □; Other: ....

None □

Fig. 15.1 An example of physical therapy online referral form showing the patient's diagnosis, the main physical therapy targets, impact on the patient's life, and associated comorbidities

Earlier studies indicated that physical exercise can reduce the incidence of coronary artery disease [4], lower blood pressure [5], decrease inflammation [6], lower the serum triglyceride concentration [7], and decrease the fasting blood glucose concentration [8]. Thus, it can be hypothesized that physiotherapy programs, for example, for osteoarthritic joint pain treatment, such as hot packing/ultrasound with transcutaneous electrical nerve stimulation around bilateral knee joint for 10 min, and followed by quadriceps muscle strengthening and aerobic exercise for 20 min, 3–5 times per week, may increase aerobic fitness levels and weight loss during treatment programs. These programs also decrease the immobility in daily life by eliminating pain. So, physiotherapy may have the potential to reduce the incidence of coronary artery disease, diabetes mellitus, or dyslipidemia in patients with mechanically disabling joint pains. Furthermore, the evidence shows that physiotherapy modalities, including exercise, ultrasound, or whole-body vibration, can increase bone density [9, 10]. These physiotherapy modalities can be prescribed to patients with osteoarthritis or osteopenic patients with high falls risk [11]. Physiotherapy may also reduce the use of analgesics, as well as lower the incidence of gastrointestinal tract ulcers, gastrointestinal tract bleeding, or renal failure.

On the other hand, physiotherapy outcomes as well as programs can be negatively linked to the associated comorbidity(ies). In a study carried out by Di Fabio and Boissonnault [12], the patients with spinal impairments who were depressed at the time they received physical therapy had poorer outcomes in both the physical and psychologic health domains. Furthermore, in some cases, patients might complain of headache while they do their physiotherapy program. Though headache is a common complaint in the general population, it may be the presenting symptoms of serious intracranial pathologic conditions (less than 1%) such as ischemia, aneurysm, arteriovenous malformation, meningitis, sinusitis, hypertension, and ocular sources. Similarly, patients with coronary heart disease or heart failure should avoid the effect of physical exertion and to modify their rehabilitation program to avoid the risk of cardiac decompensation [13]. In concordance, type II diabetic patients may show autonomic neuropathy which makes them highly prone to falls with its negative consequence. This may be the result of decreased cardiovascular response to exercise, impaired thermoregulation, response to dehydration, or postural hypotension. Therefore, baseline, heart rate, and blood glucose level should be estimated before and after management, and the physiotherapist should adjust the type of exercise and its duration according to the patient status [14].

Similarly, while in cases of chronic non-specific pain or low back pain, the therapist has to provide a graded activity program; in patients with COPD with disturbed oxygen transport in the lungs, the therapist has to reduce the training intensity in warm climatic conditions, to take care if there is fear of exercise due to breathlessness, and to reduce the body weight if there is marked obesity [15].

Knowledge of the commonly prescribed interventions (medications, surgery, etc.) is necessary, because the treatment of comorbid conditions may be clinically significant. For example, beta-adrenergic blocking agents are commonly prescribed for hypertension. These adrenergic blocking agents dampen the expected cardiac response to physical exertion [16]. If the therapist is planning to initiate a conditioning exercise program for a patient taking a beta-adrenergic blocking agents, clinical measures other than heart rate and blood pressure must be monitored during the activity to assess the individual's cardiovascular status.

By all means, when the therapist is in doubt or suspect an associated comorbidity, discussing the patient's symptoms with the referring physiatrist or physician is important to assess for possible underlying pathology.

Impact of Comorbidities on Physiotherapy Programs

How patients with comorbidities are treated in daily practice remains a challenge. Understanding the decision-making process of physical therapists and exploring the treatment of comorbid patients in daily practice might be a first step to unravel the complexity of treating multi-diseased patients. Adding comorbidities to the equation raise some points which need tackling: (1) Has the patient been assessed for comorbidities prior to setting up the treatment program? (2) Are reasoned adaptations to evidence-based treatment recommendations made when comorbidity influences the initial treatment of the index disease? (3) What are the tools which can help in identifying and monitoring the comorbidities the patient might have?

A second concern is that comorbidities are often not classified by severity but grouped together and considered the same. Few studies have examined comorbidity rates in this manner [17, 18, 32]. When setting up a physiotherapy program, the presence of severe comorbidities may negatively impact the prognosis of a patient and require significant changes in the treatment plan compared to the presence of non-severe comorbidities. These results support the need to examine rates of different types of comorbidity. Unfortunately, focused screening for comorbidities and its severity for patients seen in outpatient physical therapy clinics has not been assessed thoroughly in the literature, and further research is highly needed.

The department of epidemiology and CAPHRI School for Public Health and Primary Care, Maastricht University, the Netherlands, carried out a study [20], to assess whether physiotherapists considered the impact of comorbidities on the primary disease as well as the patients' physical status/needs, hence amended the treatment program. The study revealed that 30% of the physical therapists did not adjust treatment despite comorbidity while another 30% partly adapted the treatment plan when comorbidity was added to the vignette. The presence of comorbidity induced 40% of the therapists to abandon guideline recommendations and to create an individualized treatment plan based on the health needs of the patient. However, the study showed that, for better or for worse, the majority of physiotherapists made adaptations to evidence-based recommendations when comorbidity is present, but not leading to uniformity. This was evidenced by the finding that the same patient was treated in various ways by different physiotherapists.

The next section will present the red flags amongst patients who have comorbidities and referred for physiotherapy. The aim is to highlight for the treating doctor or therapist what are the vital parameters which require close monitoring while the patient is receiving his treatment program.

Impact of Comorbidities on Physiotherapy Programs: Red Flags

Patients with Cardiovascular Manifestations

- Hypertension:

In patients with hypertension, it is contraindicated to participate in the program of rehabilitation if resting systolic blood pressure is 200 mm Hg or more or diastolic blood pressure is 115 mm Hg or higher.

Blood pressure lowering medication should be checked, and physiotherapy program can be started with low to moderate intensity strength training exercises [21].

- Coronary disease and heart failure:

It is contraindicated for participation in the training program if the patient showed progressive increase in heart failure symptoms such as dyspnea while speaking, increased respiratory frequency of more than 30 breaths/min, heart rate at rest more than 110 bpm, and Vo_2 max 10 ml/kg/min. Also it is contraindicated in fever, acute systemic diseases, recent pulmonary embolism (3 months ago), thrombophlebitis, acute pericarditis or myocarditis, aortic stenosis, mitral valve stenosis, unstable angina, atrial fibrillation, and myocardial infarction (less than 3 month) [14].

Therapists can use maximum or symptom-limited exercise test to calculate the individual aerobic exercise intensity in patients with cardiac problems.

The warming up and cooling down sessions can be prolonged to decrease the risk of decompensation of the heart. The therapist has to terminate the exercise sessions if there is angina, impaired pump function in the form of shortness of breath, abnormal fatigue, increased peripheral edema, arrhythmias, abnormal increase or decrease of blood pressure, fainting, and dizziness [15].

Patients with Pulmonary Affection

Patients with COPD and pneumonia with ventilator limitation or disturbed oxygen transport in the lungs have to start with interval training. O_2 saturation level should remain 90% during exercising and chest expansion exercise, and other breathing exercises are recommended. The patient must be coached while exercising if the patient was breathless or gave history of breathlessness during activity [22].

Patients with Musculoskeletal Affection

Patients with chronic non-specific pain or low back pain may be more affected if they participated in normal training program. It should be clarified to the patient that the primary goal of the treatment is to improve the function and not to relieve the pain. Short-term and long-term goals should be set for each activity. Adaptation of the starting position of exercises and reduction of training intensity should be done in case of acute/subacute low back pain in order to stay active [13]. The patients have to follow gradually increasing scheme and should neither underperform nor overperform. Performance charts should be used to record the performance. Interruption of the gradual increase of activities may occur if concomitant active inflammation was diagnosed.

Endocrinal Causes

Diabetes may cause autonomic neuropathy with decreased cardiovascular response to exercise, impaired thermoregulation, and response to dehydration due to impaired skin blood flow and sweating. The therapist has to avoid intensive resistance training and to monitor blood glucose level before and after training. The patients should be checked regularly for wounds and sensory defects [23].

Hearing or Visual Impairment

Patients with hearing or visual impairments should have special program of rehabilitation as they need more manual guidance, good lighting, and proper sound for communications. They may be in need also for balancing training to avoid falling. The therapist may be in need for sign language to understand those patients or give instructions. The therapist should check whether the patient understands the information in case of hearing impairments.

The training environment should be checked for using the proper lighting system and avoiding background noise. Balancing exercises are important for such cases. Coaching patients is highly advised to reduce fear of falling.

Psychological Diseases

Depression anxiety may interfere with the performance of physiotherapy. The patients are in need for enough time to express their feelings to the therapist, to stimulate positive attitudes towards the extra attention to provide positive feedback. No appointments early in the morning as they are usually in fatigue during this period [24].

Osteoporosis

Theoretically, physiotherapy may reduce the risk of osteoporosis through several pathways, such as resistance and weight-bearing exercises which can increase bone density [25]. Some physical agents, such as vibratory platforms low-intensity electrical stimulation, laser therapy, and ultrasound, may also exert positive effects on osteoporotic tissue [26, 27]. However, treating patients with osteoporotic vertebral fractures warrants amending the physiotherapy program to minimize the risk of pain or developing another fracture. Furthermore, when treating a patient with skin, breast, lung, or prostate cancer, the therapist should recognize that there is a high incidence of spinal metastasis, and the patient may develop pain over areas of axial skeleton which could reflect pathological fracture [28, 29].

Development of Comorbidity-Adapted Protocols

When dealing with comorbidity, a patient-centered rather than a disease-oriented approach, in which the process of decision making should be based on clinical reasoning, is preferred. The Hypothesis-Oriented Algorithm for Clinicians (HOAC) II [30] describes a framework for clinical decision making, bearing in mind the patient's medical and physical status, in physical therapy; it addresses examination, evaluation, diagnosis, prognosis, and intervention in a specific patient. Although the HOAC II gives general direction in clinical reasoning, specific advice concerning comorbidity-adapted exercise therapy through comorbidity guidance might not be available for different diseases in the literature.

This paved the way and highlighted the need for comorbidity-adapted protocols. These protocols are expected to improve the application of the disease-specific exercise therapy, help to avoid adverse events, and improve the outcomes of the physical therapy program. Because of specific difficulties in developing, identifying, documenting, and reproducing the intervention, the evaluation of complex interventions requires a phased approach. de Rooij and his colleagues [13] reported five steps to develop comorbidity-adapted protocols. First is based on identifying the comorbidities that (1) are common (present in 5% or more) and (2) have impact on pain and/or affect daily functioning. Common examples include: cardiac diseases, hypertension, type 2 diabetes, obesity, COPD, low back pain, chronic pain, depression, and visual or hearing impairments [31]. Second is a literature search in the PubMed database to make an inventory of restrictions and contraindications for exercise therapy in patients with highly prevalent comorbidities. Third is a preliminary version of the protocols to be developed: based on the results of the first two steps, comorbidity-related adaptations to the diagnosis and treatment to be considered. Guidelines on exercise therapy in each comorbidity (e.g., cardiac disease, diabetes, COPD, and non-specific low back pain) are to be assessed [32, 33]. If there was no exercise therapy guideline available for a specific comorbidity, an available medical guideline can be used (e.g., guidelines for depression or anxiety) [23, 34]. The principles described in these guidelines are to be incorporated into the adapted protocols based on the patient's condition. Fourth, the preliminary versions of the protocols should be discussed with clinical experts in the fields of each comorbid disease and, subsequently, based on their feedback, further improvements of the physical therapy protocol can be implemented. Advice should also include options for the treatment of each comorbidity and on how the principles of physical therapy and training of the comorbid diseases should be incorporated into the final program. After optimizing the protocols, the clinical experts should be consulted also for the collection of feedback and to gain final consensus on the protocols. Fifth, the draft protocols should be field-tested in a pilot study in patients with the target comorbidities. Thereafter, the protocols are further improved, based on the feedback from therapists and patients, leading to a final version of the protocols.

Assessment and Testing for Comorbidity

As patients with multiple long-term conditions are becoming the norm rather than the exception and the number of people with comorbidities is set to increase, it became essential to identify these specific populations for targeted interventions and personalized care plans. There are at least two key populations with comorbidities requiring a different emphasis of action: those who have comorbidities mostly due to increased life expectancy and longer exposure to risk factors over time and those who have comorbidities mostly from more intense exposure to risk factors, particularly smoking, obesity, alcohol, and physical inactivity due to challenging personal, occupational, and societal factors throughout the life course. These patients are likely to face complex physical, social, and emotional problems. Therefore, identifying such comorbidities is mandatory, while strategies are considered to set up a physical therapy course aiming at improving the patient's ability and maintaining everyday functioning and quality of life.

Comorbidity generally is measured by medical record abstraction; however, this approach imposes limitations, such as the availability of medical records and the quality of documentation. Moreover, reliance on trained chart abstractors is expensive and time consuming. It may also be unnecessary in some settings. Research has shown that patients can accurately assess their current [35] and past medical conditions [36, 37], including comorbidities [38, 39].

On the other hand, the patient is an attractive source of data on comorbid conditions because, after all, the patient is the principal source of this information in his/her medical record. Prior research has indicated that the patient can accurately and reliably report coexisting diseases, particularly for specific conditions such as cardiac, respiratory, and musculoskeletal or for surgical procedures [35]. Greenfield et al. have developed a measure of case mix for office practice that uses patients' report on symptoms and diseases, as well as patients' self-perceived disease severity [39]. This measure of overall disease burden accounts for severity of 15 different disease groups. The instrument had a statistically significant association with health status as measured by the SF-36. Sangha et al. [40] published a self-administered comorbidity questionnaire for clinical and health services. Electronic comorbidity questionnaire was recently published [41]. It offered a specific and dynamic approach tailored to the patient's needs, which is applicable in standard practice. Patient-reported e-comorbidity outperformed the standard medical recording systems and can have a role in healthcare management and research. On another front, recent patient-reported outcome measures [42, 43] included comorbidity assessment in addition to scores rated by the patient for pain, global assessment, fatigue, morning stiffness, as well as functional disability and quality of life. Such tools not only help in assessment of the disease activity status or comorbidity, but it also offers a way to monitor the patient's response to therapy whether medical or physical. This also helps the treating therapist adapt the physical therapy program to meet the patient's requirements. An example of the multidimensional patient-reported outcome measures questionnaire for musculoskeletal disorders [44] which can be used in standard clinical practice, to have a baseline for the patient's physical status as well as comorbidity screen, is shown in Fig. 15.2.

Poor Adherence and Barriers to Comprehensive Patient Management

Poor adherence to treatment can have negative effects on effectiveness, outcomes, as well as healthcare cost. Therefore, studies were carried out to assess for the barriers to treatment adherence both medically as well as within physiotherapy. The extent of non-adherence within physical therapy treatment varied from one study to another. Vasey and his colleagues [45] found that 14% of physiotherapy patients did not return for follow-up outpatient appointments. Another study carried out by Sluijs et al. [46] suggested that non-adherence to treatment and exercise performance could be as high as 70%.

Multi-Dimensional Questionnaire for Patient Reported Outcome Measures-Musculoskeletal

This questionnaire includes information not available from blood tests, X-rays, or any source other than you. Please try to answer each question. There is **no right or wrong answer**. Please answer exactly as **YOU** think or feel.

1.We are interested in learning how your illness affects your ability to function in daily life. Please tick (√) the ONE best answer that describes your usual abilities OVER THE PAST WEEK:

Over the LAST WEEK, were you able to	Without ANY Difficulty	With SOME Difficulty	With MUCH Difficulty	Unable TO DO	Not Applicable
1. Get on and off the toilet?	....	....	....	....	
2. Use your grip strength e.g. open previously opened Jars Or lift a saucepan during cooking?	....	....	....	....	
3. Dress yourself, including tying shoelaces & doing buttons?	....	....	....	....	
4. Stand up from a chair without arms?	....	....	....	....	
5. Wait in a line for 15 minutes?	....	....	....	....	
6. Reach and get down a 5-pounds-object (such as a bag of sugar) from just above your head?	....	....	....	....	
7. Walk outdoors on a flat ground?	....	....	....	....	
8. Go Up 2 or more flights of stairs?	....	....	....	....	
9. Do house work / DIY jobs around the house?	....	....	....	....	
10. Move heavy objects?	....	....	....	....	
1. Get a good night's sleep?	....	....	....	....	....
2. Deal with the usual stresses of daily life?	....	....	....	....	....
3. Cope with social/ family activities?	....	....	....	....	....
4. Deal with feelings of anxiety or being nervous?	....	....	....	....	....
5. Deal with feelings of low self esteem or feeling blue?	....	....	....	....	....
6. Get going in the morning?	....	....	....	....	....
7. Do your work as you used to do?	....	....	....	....	....
8. Deal with any worries about your future?	....	....	....	....	....
9. Continue doing things you used to do, despite tiredness?	....	....	....	....	....
10. Continue your relationship with your partner (husband/wife)?	....	....	....	....	....

Fn. Dis.

QoL

2. How much PAIN have you had because of your arthritis/ joint or body ache OVER THE PAST WEEK? Please put a circle around the number that best indicates your level of pain:

Pain

NO PAIN 0 5 10 15 20 25 30 35 40 45 50 55 60 65 70 75 80 85 90 95 100 PAIN As Bad As It Could Be

3. Considering all the ways your arthritis/ joint or body ache may be affecting you AT THIS TIME Please put a circle around the number that best indicates how well you are doing:

PGA

VERY WELL 0 5 10 15 20 25 30 35 40 45 50 55 60 65 70 75 80 85 90 95 100 VERY POORLY

4. How much of a problem has UNUSUAL FATIGUE or tiredness been for you OVER THE PAST WEEK? (please put a circle around the number that best indicates your fatigue)

Fatigue

FATIGUE No Problem 0 5 10 15 20 25 30 35 40 45 50 55 60 65 70 75 80 85 90 95 100 A MAJOR Problem

5. OVER THE LAST WEEK when you awakened in the morning, did you feel stiff?

MS

YES: ☐ Please indicate the number of **minutes** ...., or **hours** .... until you are as limber as you will be for the day.

No: ☐

Fig. 15.2 An example of multidimensional patient-reported outcome measures questionnaire for musculoskeletal disorders including the patient's rates for his/her pain, stiffness, comorbidity, motivation, as well as functional ability and quality of life

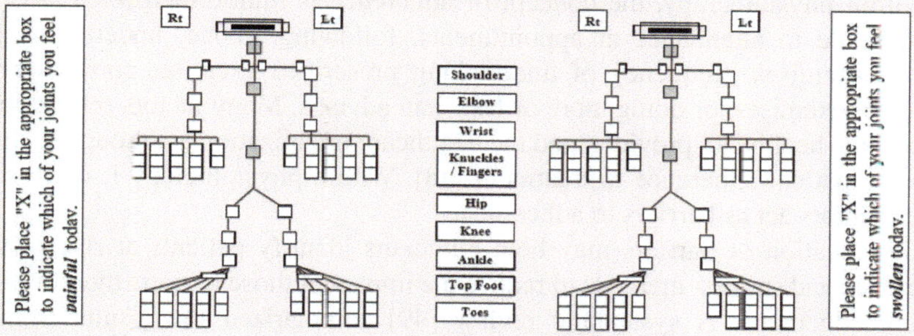

7. Please tick (√) if you have experienced any of the following OVER THE LAST MONTH:

Fever		Dry Eye		Gynecological problem		Cardiovascular Risk Assessment	
Weight Loss (> 10 lbs)		Dry Mouth		Short plans for having a baby		Age > 50 years old	
Loss of appetite		Other eye problems		Sexual Relationship Problems		High Blood pressure	
Trouble swallowing		Headache		Problems with erection (for men)		High Cholesterol	
Soreness in the mouth		Shortness of breath		I am Registered Disabled		Current Smoker	
Bleeding/inflammation of the gum		Wheezing / asthma		Absent from work due to joint pain		Ischemic Heart Disease	
Psoriasis		Cough		> 3 Alcoholic drinks per day		Stroke	
Unusual bruising or bleeding		Heartburn		Lost Height		Irregular Heart beats	
Numbness or tingling		Feeling Sickly / Nausea		Had a recent fracture		Diabetes Mellitus	
Loss of hair		Constipation		Falls Risk Assessment			
Swollen Glands		Diarrhea		Loss of your balance		Take steroids> 5mg/day	
Problems with hearing		Dark or bloody stools		Problems with your sight		Ulcer or stomach problem	
Thyroid Disease		Problems with urination		Weakness of your grip strength		Lung Disease	
Diagnosed to have cancer		Kidney problems		>1 Fall in the last year		Admitted cos of infection	
Muscle pain, ache or weakness		Pulmonary Embolism / DVT		Change in Gait / Slow walking speed		Liver Disease	

8. The statements below concern your personal beliefs. Please circle the number that best describes how do you feel about the statement. 0 = Not at all; 10 = Strongly Agree

Pt. Motivation

1. I understand the nature of my condition, the reasons for the symptoms, the course it runs and the consequences if left untreated.	0 1 2 3 4 5 6 7 8 9 10
2. I am aware of the different treatment options available to me, understand how each medication can help and feel able to share in making the decision regarding my management.	0 1 2 3 4 5 6 7 8 9 10
3. Overall I understand I am in charge of managing my condition and I feel confident I would know when to seek medical advice.	0 1 2 3 4 5 6 7 8 9 10
4. I am aware of my role in my own care, and feel able to manage the disease symptoms from interfering with my everyday activities.	0 1 2 3 4 5 6 7 8 9 10
5. I have the confidence to discuss any questions I may have or raise any concerns regarding my condition or treatment with my Doctor/nurse.	0 1 2 3 4 5 6 7 8 9 10
6. I am confident I am able to take any tablet and/or administer any injection prescribed for me.	0 1 2 3 4 5 6 7 8 9 10
7. I am able to self-manage my disease, ease the symptoms and overcome some of the difficulties associated with my condition.	0 1 2 3 4 5 6 7 8 9 10
8. I feel confident and able to manage any new symptom related to my condition	0 1 2 3 4 5 6 7 8 9 10
9. I am able to maintain life style changes like diet and exercise and feel confident I can continue these during difficult times.	0 1 2 3 4 5 6 7 8 9 10
10. I am confident I can find reliable sources of information about my condition and health choices	

□ I consent to my clinical data being used for research/audit. Signature: Date: / /20

Fig. 15.2 (continued)

Within physiotherapy, the concept of adherence is multidimensional [47] and could relate to attendance at appointments, following advice, undertaking prescribed exercises, frequency of undertaking prescribed exercise, correct performance of exercises, or doing more or less than advised. Many factors related to the patient, the healthcare provider, and the healthcare organization are thought to influence the patient adherence to treatment [48]. Within physiotherapy it is not clear which factors act as barriers to adherence.

Identification of barriers may help clinicians identify patients at risk of nonadherence and suggest methods to reduce the impact of those barriers thereby maximizing adherence. A systematic review [49] summarized the results from 20 high-quality studies and found strong evidence that low levels of physical activity at baseline or in previous weeks, low in-treatment adherence with exercise, low self-efficacy, depression, anxiety, helplessness, poor social support or activity, greater perceived number of barriers to exercise, and increased pain levels during exercise are barriers to treatment adherence. Identification of these barriers during patient assessments may be important, in order to adopt appropriate management strategies which help to counteract their effects and improve treatment outcomes. Physiotherapists should be concerned about the attitudes, beliefs, and barriers facing their patients and act collaboratively with their patients to design realistic treatment plans which are customized to the patient's life circumstances. The addition of coping plans may help patients to overcome difficulties that may arise and allow them to maintain the treatment program [50].

Conclusion

In conclusion, in physical therapy, the impact of coexisting comorbidities, other than the primary disease the patients are treated for (index disease), on the treatment and the outcomes of physiotherapy programs for individual patient, has become more recognized nowadays. However, how patients with comorbidities are treated in daily practice remain not clear and subject to the therapist's experience and knowledge. Understanding the decision-making process of physical therapy and exploring the treatment of comorbid patients in daily practice might be the first step to unravel the complexity of treating multi-diseased patients. Comorbidity (e.g., diabetes mellitus) may require adaptations in intervention strategies, as comorbidity negatively affects treatment results of the index disease (e.g., COPD or rheumatoid arthritis) or treatment for one disease (e.g., cardiopulmonary endurance training). Furthermore, comorbidity may negatively interact with the treatment or natural course of a coexisting disease (e.g., severe osteoarthritis of the knee). Therefore, insight of considerations required when applying physical therapy in comorbid patients and suggestions to enhance and accelerate clinical reasoning may be helpful for healthcare providers to obtain optimal treatment and outcomes. Dealing with comorbidity in standard patients' management needs a patient-centered rather than a disease-oriented approach, in order to obtain optimal treatment and results. Physical therapists should improve their skills and knowledge of high prevalent comorbidities, be fully informed, monitor more than the index disease outcomes alone, and adequately adjust interventions. General practitioners and physicians can improve the level of information given in their referral of a patient to a physical therapist, by providing information on all coexisting diseases and related medication.

References

1. Yeh H, Chou Y, Yang N, Cheng C, Huang N. Association between physical therapy and risk of coronary artery disease and dyslipidemia among osteoarthritis patients: a nationwide database study. Arch Phys Med Rehabil. 2016;97:8–16.
2. Boissonnault W. Prevalence of comorbid conditions, surgeries, and medication use in a physical therapy outpatient population: a multicentered study. J Orthop Sports Phys Ther. 1999;29(9):506–25.
3. Dörenkamp S, Mesters I, Teijink J, de Bie R. Comorbidities force physiotherapist to deviate from guidelines: a vignette study. https://www.epidemiologie.nl/weon/abstract-doerenkamp.html.
4. Naci H, Ioannidis JP. Comparative effectiveness of exercise and drug interventions on mortality outcomes: metaepidemiological study. BMJ. 2013;347:f5577.
5. Fagard RH. Exercise characteristics and the blood pressure response to dynamic physical training. Med Sci Sports Exerc. 2001;33(6 Suppl):S484–92. discussion S493 e84.
6. Colombo CM, de Macedo RM, Fernandes-Silva MM, et al. Short-term effects of moderate intensity physical activity in patients with metabolic syndrome. Einstein (Sao Paulo). 2013;11:324–30.
7. Shaw I, Shaw BS. Relationship between resistance training and lipoprotein profiles in sedentary male smokers. Cardiovasc J Afr. 2008;19(4):194–7.
8. Conceicao MS, Bonganha V, Vechin FC, et al. Sixteen weeks of resistance training can decrease the risk of metabolic syndrome in healthy postmenopausal women. Clin Interv Aging. 2013;8:1221–8.
9. Hojan K, Milecki P, Molinska-Glura M, Roszak A, Leszczynski P. Effect of physical activity on bone strength and body composition in breast cancer premenopausal women during endocrine therapy. Eur J Phys Rehabil Med. 2013;49:331–9.
10. Andrade Gomes do Nascimento LE, Sant'anna EF, Carlos de Oliveira Ruellas A, Issamu Nojima L, Goncalves Filho AC, Antonio Pereira Freitas S. Laser versus ultrasound on bone density recuperation after distraction osteogenesis da cone-beam computer tomographic analysis. J Oral Maxillofac Surg. 2013;71:921–8.
11. Park YG, Kwon BS, Park JW, et al. Therapeutic effect of whole body vibration on chronic knee osteoarthritis. Ann Rehabil Med. 2013;37:505–15.
12. Di Fabio R, Boissonnault W. Physical therapy and health-related outcomes for patients with common orthopaedic diagnoses. J Orthop Sports Phys Ther. 1998;27(3):219–30.
13. de Rooij M, van der Leeden M, Avezaat E, Häkkinen A, Klaver R, Maas T, et al. Development of comorbidity-adapted exercise protocols for patients with knee osteoarthritis. Clin Interv Aging. 2014;9:829–42.
14. Lavie CJ, Thomas RJ, Squires RW, Allison TG, Milani RV. Exercise training and cardiac rehabilitation in primary and secondary prevention of coronary heart disease. Mayo Clin Proc. 2009;84(4):373–83.
15. Myers JN, Brubaker PH. Chronic heart failure. In: Durstine JL, Moore GE, Painter PL, et al., editors. ACSM's exercise management for persons with chronic diseases and disabilities. 3rd ed. Champaign: Human Kinetics; 2009. p. 92–7.

16. McArdle W, Katch F, Katch V. Exercise physiology, energy nutrition and Human performance. 3rd ed. Philadelphia: Lea and Febiger; 1993.
17. Holm LW, Carroll LJ, Cassidy JD, Ahlbom A. Factors influencing neck pain intensity in whiplash associated disorders. Spine (Phila Pa 1976). 2006;31:E98–104. http://dx.doi.org/10.1097/01. brs.0000199901.52053.8
18. Piccirillo JF, Tierney RM, Costas I, Grove L, Spitznagel EL Jr. Prognostic importance of comorbidity in a hospital-based cancer registry. JAMA. 2004;291:2441–7. http://dx.doi.org/10.1001/jama.291.20.2441
19. Struijs JN, Baan CA, Schellevis FG, Westert GP, van den Bos GA. Comorbidity in patients with diabetes mellitus: impact on medical health care utilization. BMC Health Serv Res. 2006;6:84. http://dx.doi.org/10.1186/1472-6963-6-84
20. DörenkampS, MestersI, Teijink J, de Bie R. Comorbidities force physiotherapists to deviate from guidelines: a vignette study. https://www.epidemiologie.nl/weon/abstract-doerenkamp.html.
21. Achttien RJ, Staal JB, Merry AHH, et al. KNGF-richtlijn hartre¬validatie [KNGF–Guideline for Cardiac Rehabilitation], The Royal Dutch Society for Physical Therapy (KNGF). Dutch Journal of Physical Therapy. 2011;121(4):1–61 Supplement. URL Available from http://www.fysionetevidencebased.nl/images/pdfs/guidelines_in_english/cardiac_rehabilitation_practice_guidelines_2011.pdf. Accessed November 20, 2016.
22. Gosselink RA, Langer D, Burtin C, et al. KNGF-richtlijn chronisch obstructieve longziekte [KNGF-guideline for physical therapy in chronic obstructive pulmonary disease]. Royal Dutch Society for Physical Therapy. 2008;118(4):1–60. URL Available from http://www.fysionet-evidencebased.nl/index.php/kngf-guidelines-in-english. Accessed February 20, 2014.
23. van Marwijk HWJ, Grundmeijer HGLM, van Gelderen MG, et al. NHG-Standaard Depressieve stoornis (depressie). Huisarts Wet. 2003;46(11):614–33. Dutch.
24. Axford J, Butt A, Heron C, et al. Prevalence of anxiety and depression in osteoarthritis: use of the hospital anxiety and depression scale as a screening tool. Clin Rheumatol. 2010;29:1277–83.
25. Balsamo S, Mota LM, Santana FS, et al. Resistance training versus weight-bearing aquatic exercise: a cross-sectional analysis of bone mineral density in postmenopausal women. Rev Bras Reumatol. 2013;53:193–8.
26. Ritzmann R, Kramer A, Bernhardt S, Gollhofer A. Whole body vibration training improving balance control and muscle endurance. PLoS One. 2014;9:e89905.
27. Ligouri GC, Shoepe TC, Almstedt HC. Whole body vibration training is osteogenic at the spine in college-age men and women. J Hum Kinet. 2012;31:55–68.
28. Lirani-Galvao AP, Lazaretti-Castro M. Physical approach for prevention and treatment of osteoporosis. Arq Bras Endocrinol Metabol. 2010;54:171–8.
29. Friedman RJ, Rigel DS, Silverman MK, Kopf AW, Vossaert KA. Malignant melanoma in the 1990s: the continued importance of early detection and the role of physician examination and self-examination of the skin. CA Cancer J Clin. 1991;41:201–26.
30. Echternach JL, Riddle DL. The hypothesis-oriented algorithm for clinicians II (HOAC II): a guide for patient management. Phys Ther. 2003;83(5):455–70.
31. Reeuwijk KG, de Rooij M, van Dijk GM, Veenhof C, Steultjens MP, Dekker J. Osteoarthritis of the hip or knee: which coexisting disorders are disabling? Clin Rheumatol. 2010;29(7):739–47.
32. Achttien RJ, Staal JB, Merry AHH, et al. KNGF-richtlijn hartrevalidatie [KNGF–Guideline for Cardiac Rehabilitation], The Royal Dutch Society for Physical Therapy (KNGF). Dutch Journal of Physical Therapy. 2011;121(3):1–61 Supplement. URL Availble from http://www.fysionet-evidencebased.nl/images/pdfs/guidelines_in_english/cardiac_rehabilitation_practice_ guidelines_2011.pdf.
33. Bekkering GE, Hendriks HJM, Koes BW, et al. KNGF-richtlijn lage rugpijn [KNGF-guideline low back pain], The Royal Dutch Society for Physical Therapy (KNGF). 2001;111(3). Available from Bekkering GE, Hendriks HJM, Koes BW, et al. KNGF-richtlijn lage rugpijn [KNGFguideline low back pain], The Royal Dutch Society for Physical Therapy (KNGF). Dutch Journal of Physical Therapy. 2013;123 Supplement.

34. Walma EP, Thomas S, Prins A, Grundmeijer HGLM, Laan van der JR, Wiersma TJ. NHG-Standaard Hypertensie. Huisarts Wet. 2003;46:435–49.
35. Mechanic D The experiences and reporting of common physical complaints. J Health Soc Behav. 1980 21:146–55.
36. Linet M, Harlow S, McLaughlin JK, McCaffrey LD. A comparison of interview data and medical records for previous medical conditions and surgery. J Clin Epidemiol. 1989;42:1207–13.
37. Colditz GA, Martin P, Stampfer MJ, Willett WC, Sampson L, Rosner B, et al. Validation of questionnaire information on risk factors and disease outcomes in a prospective cohort study of women. Am J Epidemiol. 1986;123:894–900.
38. Katz JN, Chang LC, Sangha O, Fossel AH, Bates DW. Can comorbidity be assessed by questionnaire rather than medical record review? Med Care. 1996;34:73–84.
39. GreenfieldS SL, DukesKA SR, D'AgostinoR KSH. Development and testing of a new measure of case mix for use in office practice. Med Care. 1995;33:AS47–55.
40. Sangha O, Stucki G, Liang M, Fossel A, Katz J. The self-administered comorbidity questionnaire: a new method to assess comorbidity for clinical and health services research. Arthritis Care Res. 2003;49(2):156–63.
41. El Miedany Y, El Gaafary M, Youssef S, Bahlas S, Hegazi H, Ahmed I. E-comorbidity: evaluation of the validity of electronic comorbidity assessment in identifying comorbid conditions among patients with rheumatoid and psoriatic arthritis. Arthritis Rheumatol. 2016; 68(suppl 10). Abstract number 1555.
42. El Miedany Y. PROMs in inflammatory arthritis: moving from static to dynamic. Clin Rheumatol. 2013;32(6):735–42.
43. El Miedany Y. Adopting patient-centered care in standard practice: PROMs moving toward disease-specific era. Clin Exp Rheumatol. 2014;32(5 Suppl 85):S-40–6.
44. El Miedany Y, El Gaafary M, Youssef SS, Palmer D. Incorporating patient reported outcome measures in clinical practice: development and validation of a questionnaire for inflammatory arthritis. Clin Exp Rheumatol. 2010;28(5):734–44.
45. Vasey L. DNAs and DNCTs – why do patients fail to begin or complete a course of physiotherapy treatment? Physiotherapy. 1990;76:575–8.
46. Sluijs EM, Kok GJ, van der Zee J. Correlates of exercise compliance in physical therapy. Phys Ther. 1993;73(11):771–82.
47. Kolt GS, Brewer BW, Pizzari T, Schoo AMM, Garrett N. The sport injury rehabilitation adherence scale: a reliable scale for use in clinical physiotherapy. Physiotherapy. 2007;93(1):17–22.
48. Miller NH, Hill M, Kottke T, Ockene IS. The multilevel compliance challenge: recommendations for a call to action. A statement for healthcare professionals. Circulation. 1997;95(4):1085–90.
49. Jack K, McLean S, Moffett J, Gardinerc E. Barriers to treatment adherence in physiotherapy outpatient clinics: a systematic review. Man Ther. 2010;15(3–2):220–8
50. KhlGohner W, Schlicht W. Preventing chronic back pain: evaluation of a theory-based cognitive-behavioural training programme for patients with subacute back pain. Patient Educ Couns. 2006;64(1–3):87–95.

Chapter 16
Comorbidity Index

Yasser El Miedany

Though the treatment paradigm for chronic inflammatory arthritic conditions has changed dramatically over the last 15 years, with more effective interventions introduced, able to prevent joint damage and functional impairment, managing the complexity of rheumatic diseases in clinical practice remains as a great challenge. Meta-analyses revealed that, while the long-term prognosis of inflammatory arthritic conditions has improved significantly following the introduction of new diagnostic and management guidelines, the life span of rheumatic patients has not improved accordingly [1–3]. This higher mortality rate has been attributed to associated comorbidities. By definition, comorbidity refers to the coexistence of other chronic diseases in patients with an index disease [4]. In inflammatory arthritic conditions, the chronic active inflammatory process may predispose to the development of some of these comorbidities (e.g., increased prevalence of cardiovascular disease, a greater incidence of infections, and the development of certain malignancies [5–9]). However, medications used to treat the arthritic conditions (e.g., steroids and nonsteroidal anti-inflammatory medications [8]) have been linked also to the occurrence of further comorbidities. Therefore, it has become essential to consider the synergism of treating the index disease and comorbid conditions concomitantly. Calculating the patient risk before commencing therapy would have a positive impact on the way these patients are managed as it would make care fit for arthritic patients.

Comorbidities can be assessed via two approaches: either recording each comorbidity separately (e.g., cardiovascular, osteoporosis, infection, malignancy, diabetes mellitus, etc.) or summing the comorbidity risk into a single score which provides a single measure for multiple comorbidities (e.g., comorbidity indices). In real-life

Y. El Miedany (✉)
King's College, London, UK

Rheumatology and Rehabilitation, Ain Shams University, Cairo, Egypt

Department of Rheumatology, Darent Valley Hospital, Dartford, Kent, UK
e-mail: yasser_elmiedany@yahoo.com

Y. El Miedany (ed.), *Comorbidity in Rheumatic Diseases*,
DOI 10.1007/978-3-319-59963-2_16

practice, the advantage of comorbidity indices is that by reducing all coexistent illnesses and the severity of those into a single numeric score, monitoring of the patient as well as comparison of comorbidity between patients is possible, whereas in scientific research, the greatest advantage of these indices is to adjust multivariate analysis in observational studies giving a single and highly informative score. Comorbidity indices can be classified according to the outcome of interest such as mortality/hospitalization, physical function, or quality of life or the source of data, such as administrative, e.g., International Classification of Diseases such as ICD-9/ICD-10, or self-administered questionnaires (Table 16.1).

In this chapter, commonly used comorbidity indices and self-administered comorbidity questionnaires will be discussed with their implication onto standard rheumatology clinical practice as well as on the patients' management.

Comorbidity Indices

Comorbidity indices are tools developed to enable the physician to quantify the total comorbidity burden which contributes to the patient's overall illness. Comorbidity indices have several clinical and research benefits, including the identification of patients (or research participants) with worse prognosis in terms of declines in health-related quality of life, functional ability, risk of hospitalization or mortality [10]. The simplest method to measure comorbidity is to use the summation of each comorbid illness to generate a total value of comorbidity, often termed as "comorbidity counts." However, not all comorbid diseases have the same impact on the outcome of interest. Thus, more complex comorbidity indices were created to select and weight specific comorbid illnesses to measure more accurately the burden and impact of overall comorbidity [11–16]. Table 16.1 shows a list of the most comorbidity indices used in rheumatology research which will be discussed in this chapter.

Charlson Comorbidity Index (CCI)

The Charlson Comorbidity Index (CCI) [11], published in 1987, was based on the mortality rates of 607 patients admitted to the general internal medicine service for 1-month period. The aim was to develop a prospective measure which can be applied to classify comorbidities, which might alter the mortality risk, for use in longitudinal studies. Seventeen diseases were included in this index, with different weights, and were selected and weighted based on the strength of their association with mortality (Table 16.2). All weights are summed to obtain a numeric comorbidity score (range, 0–33) for any particular patient.

Table 16.1 Comparison of the basic criteria of the comorbidity indices

Criteria	CCI	ECM	FCI	RDCI	MMI	RACI	PsACI
Data collection	Administrative	Administrative	Administrative	Patient questionnaire administrative	Administrative	Patient questionnaire administrative (ICD-9)	Patient questionnaire administrative (ICD-10)
Scoring	Weighted	Count	Count	Weighted	Count	Weighted	Weighted
Disease duration at inclusion	Variable	Variable	Variable	Variable	Variable	<6 months	<12 months
Data fixed at baseline	√	√	√	√	√		
Follow-up						√ (10 years)	√ (10 years)
Outcome of interest	Mortality	Hospital resource use/ in-hospital mortality	Physical function	Direct medical costs, work disability, social security disability, Health Assessment Questionnaire (HAQ) functional disability, hospitalization, and death	Eur-QoL	Functional disability, QoL, complications from treatment, hospitalization, and death	Functional disability, QoL, complications from treatment, hospitalization, and death
Content validity	√	√	√	√	√	√	√
Construct validity	√	√	√	√	√	√	√
Criteria validity	√	√	√	√	√	√	√
Reliability	√	√	√	√	√	√	√
External validation	√	√	√	√	√	√	√
Not-rheumatology specific	√	√	√				
Rheumatology specific				√	√		
Disease specific						√	√

Table 16.2 Charlson Comorbidity Index

Disease	Points
Myocardial infarction	1
Congestive heart failure	1
Peripheral vascular disease	1
Cerebrovascular disease	1
Dementia	1
COPD	1
Connective tissue disease	1
Peptic ulcer disease	1
Diabetes mellitus	1 point if uncomplicated
	2 points if end-organ damage
Moderate to severe CKD	2
Hemiplegia	2
Leukemia	2
Malignant lymphoma	2
Solid tumor	2 points
	6 points if metastatic
Liver disease	1 point if mild
	3 points if moderate to severe
AIDS	6 points

From Charlson et al. [11], with permission
Calculation: Add all items of the comorbidity score. The total score is the Charlson Comorbidity Index. Range, 0–36
COPD chronic obstructive pulmonary disease, *CKD* chronic kidney disease

CCI Characteristics

The CCI was developed to predict 1-year patient mortality using comorbidity data obtained from hospital chart review. Later on, comorbidities of patients were categorized based on the International Classification of Diseases (ICD) diagnosis codes found in administrative data (such as hospital abstracts or medical services data). Each comorbidity category has an associated weight (from 1 to 6), based on the adjusted risk of mortality or resource use, and the sum of all the weights results in a single comorbidity score for a patient. A score of zero indicates no comorbidities in the list. The higher the score, the more likely the predicted outcome will result in mortality or higher resource use.

Clinical conditions and associated scores are as follows:

- 1 point each: myocardial infarct, congestive heart failure, peripheral vascular disease, dementia, cerebrovascular disease, chronic lung disease, connective tissue disease, ulcer, chronic liver disease, diabetes
- 2 points each: hemiplegia, moderate or severe kidney disease, diabetes with end-organ damage, tumor, leukemia, lymphoma
- 3 points each: moderate or severe liver disease
- 6 points each: malignant tumor, metastasis, AIDS

Regarding the content validity (the completeness and relevance of the items content to measuring what they claimed to measure [17]) of the CCI, the items and the weights included were statistically derived by the relative risk estimates of the proportional regression model to predict mortality using clinical data. As far as construct validity (which refers to the degree to which a test measures what it claims, or purports, to be measuring), in the study carried out by Kiefe et al. [18], outcomes suggested a good construct validity of the CCI. Criterion validity refers to the correlation of a scale with some other measure of the disorder under study, ideally, a gold standard that has been used and accepted in the field [19]. However, as there is no gold standard that exists for measuring comorbidity, another comorbidity measure is usually used for comparison. Earlier studies revealed that CCI presented moderate to good correlation with other comorbidity indices [20–22], as well as other outcome criteria such as disability, mortality, and length of stay [19, 23]. Lastly, the reliability of the CCI (which refers to the overall consistency of a measure and also has been defined as the extent to which repeated measurements of a stable phenomenon by different people, at different times and places, get similar results and are usually assessed by the intra-class correlation coefficient (ICC) in case of several assessors [24]) was reported to be moderate to very good indicating good reliability of the CCI [25, 26].

Development and Changes to the CCI

Over time, there have been changes to the original index. A summary of these variations includes:

- The original index was developed with 19 categories [11] but has been modified to 17 categories published by Deyo et al. in 1992 [27].
- The list of specific ICD diagnosis codes that are used to identify different categories of comorbidity has been modified as reported in the Romano et al. study published in 1993 [28] and updated from ICD-9-CM to work with ICD-10 coding as reported in the Halfon et al. study (2002) [29] and then in the Quan et al. study (2005) [30].
- The original weights developed for use with the index have also been modified (Schneeweiss et al. 2003) [31].

Critical Analysis of the CCI

The Charlson Comorbidity Index (CCI) is the most widely used comorbidity index. CCI has been adapted and verified as applicable and valid tool for predicting the outcome and risk of death from many comorbid diseases [32, 33]. However, while the CCI was created to predict death in a sample of hospitalized patients, it has been widely used outside its originally intended scope. A systematic review of the CCI using Canadian administrative databases was carried out by Needham et al. (2005)

[34] with a perspective on risk adjustment in critical care research. Results revealed lower predictive ability of the CCI in comparison to Acute Physiology and Chronic Health Evaluation (APACHE), yet the study highlighted the advantages of using the CCI instrument for population-based research. Another study reported that some comorbidities collected in other indices, such as alcoholism, were not included in the CCI [35]. Rheumatology-wise, in the current RA management context, the CCI can be considered as outdated. Being developed in 1987, most (if not all) of the rheumatoid arthritis or other connective disease patients included in the CCI, most likely, have not been treated according to the treatment protocols approved in the last 20 years. Furthermore, it is worth noting that some diseases such as fibromyalgia have not been included in the comorbidity index.

Elixhauser Comorbidity Measure (ECM)

The Elixhauser Comorbidity Measure (ECM) [16] is a method of categorizing comorbidities of patients based on the International Classification of Diseases (ICD) diagnosis codes found in administrative data, such as hospital abstracts data. Each comorbidity category is dichotomous, i.e., it is either present or absent. The index can be used to predict hospital resource use and in-hospital mortality. The ECM was developed using administrative data from a state-wide California inpatient database (n = 1,779,167). Its original aim was to identify a list of 30 comorbidities (the 17 from the CCI + 13 new ones), relying on the ICD-9-CM, that had a major impact on short-term outcomes in acute hospital inpatients (Table 16.3). Elixhauser et al. [16] treated conditions separately or as a count. The comorbidities identified in the ECM were significantly associated with in-hospital mortality and include both acute and chronic conditions.

ECM Characteristics

Regarding its content validity, the ECM comprises a larger number of items compared to the CCI. In addition to the empirical-generated items (that were also included in the CCI), 13 additional judgmental items were added, based on a systematic literature review. On the other hand, no weight was given to the comorbidities included, implicitly assuming that all conditions are equally important in their relationship to outcomes, which is unlikely to be true. There were no studies published to evaluate the construct validity of the ECM. Interestingly, assessment of the ECM criterion validity revealed that when ECM was compared to CCI, in most of the studies ECM tended to outperform the CCI tool [36–39], while in others performances were similar [40]. In concordance, a systematic review and comparative analysis showed that, among various comorbidity indices, the Elixhauser index predicts the risk better, especially beyond 30 days of hospitalization [41]. ECM also tended to perform better, when compared to other illness indicators, such as

Table 16.3 Elixhauser Comorbidity Measure

Comorbidity
Congestive heart failure
Valvular disease
Pulmonary circulation disorders
Peripheral vascular disorders
Hypertension
Paralysis
Other neurological disorders
COPD
Diabetes uncomplicated
Diabetes complicated
Hypothyroidism
Renal failure
Liver disease
Peptic ulcer excluding bleeding
AIDS
Lymphoma
Metastatic cancer
Solid tumor without metastasis
Rheumatoid arthritis/collagen vascular diseases
Coagulopathy
Obesity
Weight loss
Fluid and electrolyte disorders
Blood loss anemia
Deficiency anemia
Alcohol abuse
Drug abuse
Psychosis
Depression

From Elixhauser et al. [16], with permission
Calculation: 1 point per comorbidity; add all items. The total score is the Elixhauser Comorbidity Measure. Range, 0–18.
COPD chronic obstructive pulmonary disease, *AIDS* acquired immunodeficiency syndrome

"previous years expenditures" [42]. As far as reliability, no data were available on the ECM. However, the inter-rater reliability may appear less relevant since it uses administrative data. Furthermore, its developers highlighted the fact that diagnoses from administrative data may be less accurate than those from physicians, although diagnoses from physicians are not perfectly accurate.

Development and Changes to the ECM

Over time, there have been changes to the ECM index based on different research studies. A summary of these variations includes:

- While the original index was developed including 30 categories [16], Garland et al. 2012 [43] suggested increasing them to 31 categories.
- The list of specific ICD diagnosis codes used to identify different categories of comorbidity has been modified and updated from ICD-9-CM to work with ICD-10 coding. Results were published in the Quan et al. study (2005) [30].
- In the study carried out by van Walraven et al. (2009), a weighting algorithm was developed, based on the association between comorbidity and death, in order to produce an overall score for the Elixhauser Total Score (ETS) [44].

Critical Analysis of the ECM

Generally, one of the ECM limitations is that the index has been designed for use with very specific ICD coding (up to 5-digit ICD-9-CM codes and 7-digit ICD-10 codes) found in the hospital abstracts data. This is due to the specificity required to distinguish between diagnoses that should/should not be included in the index and to be able to properly identify and place codes into the appropriate category. Therefore, using only 3-digit ICD codes to calculate the ECM is not recommended as they lack the specificity required to properly categorize diagnoses in the Elixhauser Comorbidity Index.

Rheumatology-wise, similar to the CCI, ECM index has been applied in situations extending beyond its intended scope, and, in the current RA management context, Elixhauser indices can be also considered as outdated. Being developed in 1998, the majority of the RA patients included in the ECM original study, most likely, have missed the biologic therapy era or are treated according to the management protocols approved in the last 18 years. Furthermore, ECM uses a comorbidity count and not weights. The use of comorbidity counts is discouraged because they vary in the number and types of conditions included, and wide variability in predictive ability should be expected.

The Functional Comorbidity Index (FCI)

Prior comorbidity indices have been developed primarily to predict mortality or administrative outcomes such as length of stay in acute care or disease-specific populations [13, 45]. These indices typically include diagnoses, often asymptomatic, such as hypertension, that are important in predicting mortality, and exclude diagnoses, such as arthritis, that impact physical function but are unlikely to result in short-term mortality. Research using indices designed to predict mortality have concluded that comorbid illnesses have little relationship with physical disability [46, 47], a finding that seems intuitively false but underscores the need to consider the purpose for which an index was designed. This paved the way to develop new indices with different outcomes of interest such as physical function or quality of life.

The Functional Comorbidity Index [48] was developed using two databases: a cross-sectional, simple random sample of 9423 Canadian adults and a sample of 28,349 US adults seeking treatment for spine ailments. The purpose was to develop a self-administered, general population index of comorbid diseases with physical function, assessed by the physical function subscale of the SF-36, as the outcome of interest. The underlying premise was that diagnoses associated with impairments in physical function would be, at least in part, different from those associated with mortality, and therefore, an index designed with physical function as the outcome would perform better in the previous context—i.e., spinal problems—than indices designed with mortality as the outcome of interest.

The FCI Characteristics

Multiple linear regression identified 18 variables that were associated with the SF-36 physical function score (Table 16.4) [48]. The FCI was scored as both a simple count (yes/no) and a weighted count of the diagnoses. "Weights" were derived from the standardized beta coefficients from the regression analysis. A score of "0" indicates no comorbid illnesses, and a score of "18" indicates the highest number of comorbid illnesses. The weighted count did not perform significantly better, and therefore, it is not used. Simple counts are clearly easier to score and use. The FCI scores correlated weak to moderate with both the SF-36 physical function and role physical subscale scores (−.53 and −.31, respectively). When the SF-36 physical function subscale score was dichotomized into "high" and "low," the FCI simple count correctly classified 76.6% of people, whereas using a weighted count, the FCI correctly classified 77.0%. Compared with the CCI [11] and the Kaplan-Feinstein index [13], the FCI accounted for more variation in the physical function subscale scores (R^2 = 0.29, 0.18, and 0.07%, respectively).

Critical Analysis of the FCI

The Functional Comorbidity Index was developed specifically for use in the general population with physical function, not mortality, as the outcome of interest. The Functional Comorbidity Index contains conditions such as visual impairment, osteoporosis, and arthritis, which do not appear in the most widely used indices, namely, the CCI or the Kaplan-Feinstein index. However, the FCI does not take into consideration the severity of the diagnoses, an important factor to be considered when dealing with diseases such as inflammatory arthritis. Severity ratings are likely to provide better adjustment. Furthermore, the FCI study relied mainly on secondary data sources for development and thus may have overlooked some diagnoses associated with functional status. For example, HIV/AIDS was not explicitly collected in either database and may contribute significantly to functional disability.

Table 16.4 The Functional Comorbidity Index

1. Arthritis (rheumatoid and osteoarthritis)
2. Osteoporosis
3. Asthma
4. Chronic obstructive pulmonary disease (COPD), acquired respiratory distress syndrome (ARDS), or emphysema
5. Angina
6. Congestive heart failure (or heart disease)
7. Heart attack (myocardial infarct)
8. Neurological disease (such as multiple sclerosis or Parkinson's)
9. Stroke or TIA
10. Peripheral vascular disease
11. Diabetes types I and II
12. Upper gastrointestinal disease (ulcer, hernia, reflux)
13. Depression
14. Anxiety or panic disorders
15. Visual impairment (such as cataracts, glaucoma, macular degeneration)
16. Hearing Impairment (very hard hearing, even with hearing aids)
17. Degenerative disc disease (back disease, spinal stenosis, or severe chronic back pain)
18. Obesity and/or body mass index >30 (weight in kg/height in meters^2) Height_____________________(cm or inches?) Weight_____________________(kg or lbs?) BMI =

From Grolla et al. [48], with permission
Calculation: 1 point per comorbidity; add all items. The total score is the Elixhauser Comorbidity Measure. Range, 0–18
Abbreviations: *TIA* transient ischemic attack

The Rheumatic Disease Comorbidity Index (RDCI)

The RDCI [49] was created from self-report questionnaires from patients with RA, osteoarthritis, systemic lupus erythematosus, or fibromyalgia. The RDCI is characterized by having multiple outcomes of interest. Comorbid illnesses were assessed for impact on six outcomes: direct medical costs, work disability, social security disability, Health Assessment Questionnaire (HAQ) functional disability, hospitalization, and death.

The RDCI Characteristics

While 22 comorbid illnesses were assessed, the final score encompasses 11 comorbid illnesses (Table 16.5); the range is 0–9. The RDCI was compared to six comorbidity indices: the Charlson-Deyo Index (CDI), Functional Comorbidity Index (FCI), Elixhauser Comorbidity Measure (ECM), Elixhauser Point System (EPS), and a simple comorbidity count (COUNT) using a US cohort of rheumatoid arthritis patients [10]. Relative to other common comorbidity indices, the

Table 16.5 The Rheumatic Disease Comorbidity Index

Comorbidity	Point
Lung disease	2
Heart attack, other CV, *or* stroke	2
Hypertension	1
Fracture	1
Depression	1
Diabetes	1
Cancer	1
Ulcer or stomach problem	1

From Michaud and Wolfe [49], with permission
Calculation: Add all items. The total score is the Rheumatic Disease Comorbidity Index score (range 0–9)

RDCI and ECM Score were superior indices for predicting death and physical disability in an administrative data set composed of individuals with RA. The RDCI predicted physical disability with self-report data from a clinic questionnaire. In contrast to the Elixhauser Comorbidity Measure (ECM) which is composed of 30 different comorbidities, the RDCI relies on only 11 comorbidities. The RDCI may also be used as a foundation to tailor to a specific outcome of interest. For example, if death from myocardial infarction is being studied, additional predictive power is obtained by adding certain binary comorbid conditions (previous myocardial infarction, hypertension, and hyperlipidemia) to the RDCI [10]. In contrast to other indices such as CCI and FCI which perform optimally only for one outcome, RDCI can perform well in multiple outcomes.

Critical Analysis

The RDCI is the first comorbidity index addressing diseases commonly associated to rheumatic diseases specifically. The RDCI can be used with administrative data sets as well as with patient-reported data. This ability to use both sources allows the index to be more widely applicable and to serve as a standardized measure of comorbidity within rheumatology. Furthermore, the RDCI relies on relatively smaller number of comorbidities (only 11) and was assessed for variable relevant outcomes of interest. However, the RDCI has some limitations. First, the index was fixed at baseline values for analysis, thus removing the chronological component of comorbidity during the follow-up period. This reduces the predictive power of comorbidity indices [50]. Additionally, the ICD-9-CM codes were collected from outpatient visits, which rely on the providers to maintain an accurate list of comorbid conditions. There is usually a delay in data recording, which represents a significant limitation to the index (in the RDCI validation study mortality data collected through the National Death Index had approximately a 2-year delay; thus, deaths collected through the National Death Index from 2008 to 2010 may have been missed and not included in the analysis). Thirdly, the population in the RDCI administrative data set was composed entirely of individuals with RA and was predominantly male. Thus, generalizability of the results to other populations may not be appropriate.

The Multimorbidity Index (MMI)

The notion of multimorbidity was introduced based on the fact that rheumatology patients are typically afflicted by more than one disease; therefore, considering multimorbidity is vital when deciding on diagnostic or therapeutic strategies. Furthermore, multimorbidity can cause polypharmacy, an increasing treatment burden, which might also impact patients' overall HRQoL. Therefore, the concept was that developing an index reflecting multimorbidity that is based on HRQoL might be helpful to better address the disease-related aspects of patients' overall well-being, which could also be useful for application in both clinical trials and epidemiological studies.

The MMI [51] was developed based on health-related quality of life (HRQoL) in an observational RA cohort. The MMI identified quality of life as the main outcome, associated with physical function, pain, and global health. The hypothesis was that, incorporating a multidimensional patient-centered concept, quality of life reflects patients' overall well-being and can be considered a main treatment target. This was supported by the findings of an earlier study which reported that an increasing number of morbidities lead to a decrease of HRQoL [52].

The MMI Characteristics

The index includes 40 morbidities, all identified using ICD-9 codes (Table 16.6). MMIs of two types were calculated: one by enumerating morbidities (MMI count) and the other by weighting morbidities based on their association with HRQoL as assessed by the European Quality of Life – 5 dimensions (EQ-5D) questionnaire in multiple linear regression analysis. Criterion validity was assessed by comparing the MMI to CCI and FCI indices as well as HRQoL, all measured at the baseline visit. Both MMI count and MMI weight indices were more strongly associated with EQ-5D than CCI (Spearman: MMI count = −0.20, MMI weight = −0.26, and CCI = −0.10; $p < 0.01$). R^2 obtained by linear regression using EQ-5D as a dependent variable and the various indices as independent variables, adjusted for age and gender, was the highest for MMI (R^2: MMI count = 0.05, MMI weight = 0.11, and CCI = 0.02). When accounting for clinical disease activity index (CDAI), R^2 increased (MMI count = 0.18, MMI weight = 0.22, and CCI = 0.17), still showing higher values of MMI compared with CCI but in any case rather small. External validation in different RA cohorts [51] showed good performance of both Indices. In view of this, and considering that not much improvement was gained by weighting, the authors endorsed a simple MMI count

Table 16.6 The Multimorbidity Index

Comorbidity	Point	Comorbidity	Point
Glaucoma	1	Psoriasis eczema coronary heart disease	1
Irritable bowel syndrome	1	Hearing loss	1
Schizophrenia bipolar disorder	1	Stroke/transient ischemic attack	1
Learning disability	1	Peripheral vessel disease	1
Anorexia/bulimia	1	Chronic kidney disease	1
Migraine	1	Inflammatory bowel disease	1
Prostate disorders, diverticulitis	1	Thyroid disorders	1
Chronic sinusitis hypertension	1	Asthma	1
Cancer	1	Obesity	1
Diabetes	1	Chronic liver disease	1
Atrial fibrillation	1	Heart failure	1
Constipation	1	Bronchiectasis	1
Multiple sclerosis	1	Depression	1
Substance misuse osteoporosis	1	Anxiety/neurotic disorders	1
Hepatitis	1	Alcohol abuse	1
Epilepsy	1	Blind or low vision	1
Dementia	1	Parkinson	1
Dyspepsia	1	Chronic obstructive pulmonary disease (COPD)	1

From Rander et al. [51], with permission
Calculation: 1 point per comorbidity; add all items. The total score is the multimorbidity measure. Range, 0–40

index for its use in the assessment of multimorbidity in RA patients and its impact on the patients' overall well-being.

Critical Analysis

Similar to the FCI which considered physical function as the main outcome, the MMI addressed the patients' overall well-being (QoL) as the main outcome. This comes in contrast to the earlier existing indices such as CCI and ECM which are based on other specific outcomes, such as mortality, costs, or hospitalization. However, for the MMI, the diseases were selected as either recommended as a core for any multimorbidity measure by a systemic literature review or defined as chronic (long-term) disorders with important impact as proposed by the National Health Service Scotland. These selection criteria may be the explanation for the long list of comorbidities, a good number of which are not commonly reported in inflammatory arthritic conditions. This may, in turn, explain the poor criterion validity shown in the study and why the average range of the multimorbidity count ranged from 1 to 16 only, while the total score is 40. This, also, may elucidate the low correlation of the MMI count when compared with the FCI despite both of them used HRQoL as the outcome of interest. Furthermore, the MMI was developed in a disease-specific cohort, namely, RA patients, yet it has not been assessed in non-RA patients.

Self-administered Comorbidity Questionnaires

Self-administered comorbidity questionnaires for assessing comorbidities have been introduced [53, 54] as an alternative to medical records or administrative data approach. The self-administered comorbidity questionnaire (SCQ), which was first published by Sangha et al. in 2003 [54], requires the patients to indicate whether they suffer at the moment from 12 medical conditions in addition to the index disease (Table 16.7). The comorbidities listed were selected by an expert panel based on the ones captured by the CCI. The score of the SCQ ranges from 0 to 45 points. Construct validity was assessed by the correlation between SCQ and CCI and was moderate (0.55). Test-retest reliability was very good (ICC 0.94 [95%CI 0.72–0.99]). Criterion validity was evaluated through the correlation of SCQ with SF-36 and was weak to fair (from $r = 0.03$ to 0.39 depending on the SF-36 subscale, with better correlations observed for physical-related subscales) and fairly correlated with the number of prescriptions in a year ($r = 0.37$). Stolwijk et al. [55] have published a validation study for SCQ in patients with ankylosing spondylitis (AS), where criterion validity was assessed by the agreement between the SCQ answers and

Table 16.7 Self-administered comorbidity questionnaire

Problem	Do you have the problem		Do you receive treatment for it		Does it limit your activities	
Heart disease	No ☐	Yes ☐	No ☐	Yes ☐	No ☐	Yes ☐
High blood pressure	No ☐	Yes ☐	No ☐	Yes ☐	No ☐	Yes ☐
Lung disease	No ☐	Yes ☐	No ☐	Yes ☐	No ☐	Yes ☐
Diabetes	No ☐	Yes ☐	No ☐	Yes ☐	No ☐	Yes ☐
Ulcer or stomach disease	No ☐	Yes ☐	No ☐	Yes ☐	No ☐	Yes ☐
Kidney disease	No ☐	Yes ☐	No ☐	Yes ☐	No ☐	Yes ☐
Liver disease	No ☐	Yes ☐	No ☐	Yes ☐	No ☐	Yes ☐
Anemia or other heart disease	No ☐	Yes ☐	No ☐	Yes ☐	No ☐	Yes ☐
Cancer	No ☐	Yes ☐	No ☐	Yes ☐	No ☐	Yes ☐
Depression	No ☐	Yes ☐	No ☐	Yes ☐	No ☐	Yes ☐
Pain and swelling in joints other than the back	No ☐	Yes ☐	No ☐	Yes ☐	No ☐	Yes ☐
Osteoporosis	No ☐	Yes ☐	No ☐	Yes ☐	No ☐	Yes ☐
Fractures	No ☐	Yes ☐	No ☐	Yes ☐	No ☐	Yes ☐
Other medical problems (please write)						
1.	No ☐	Yes ☐	No ☐	Yes ☐	No ☐	Yes ☐
2.	No ☐	Yes ☐	No ☐	Yes ☐	No ☐	Yes ☐
3.	No ☐	Yes ☐	No ☐	Yes ☐	No ☐	Yes ☐

From Sangha et al. [54], with permission

Instructions: The following is a list of common health problems. Please indicate (circle correct answer) if you currently have the problem in the first column. If you do not have the problem, skip to the next problem. If you do have the problem, please indicate in the second column if you receive medications or some other type of treatment for the problem. Also, indicate in that case in the third column if the problem limits any of your activities. Finally, indicate also medical conditions that are not listed under "other medical problems" at the end of the list comorbidities identified in medical records and was moderate to perfect for most conditions (κ 0.47–1.00), except for ulcer disease, depression, and OA. Other validation studies using this questionnaire in other pathologies are currently on going.

Disease-Specific Comorbidity Indices

In view of the recent developments in the diagnosis and management of inflammatory arthritic conditions and the reports showing variable comorbidity patterns in patients suffering from different rheumatic diseases [56], there has been an unmet need for new comorbidity indices addressing these points. The recently published Rheumatoid Arthritis Comorbidity Index (RACI) [57] and Psoriatic Arthritis Comorbidity Index (PsACI) [58] were created from self-report questionnaires completed by patients with early rheumatoid and psoriatic arthritis. Both indices are disease specific and are characterized by having multiple outcomes of interest. In both RACI and PsACI, comorbid illnesses were assessed for impact on four outcomes: functional disability, quality of life, medication-associated comorbidities, and hospitalization and death.

The RACI and PsACI Characteristics

Original studies for both questionnaires [57, 58] revealed that the patients included were suffering from early inflammatory as well as psoriatic arthritis (disease duration <6 months and <12 months, respectively). The patients were monitored over 10-year period and received treatment in the form of DMARDs and biologic therapy according to the recently published guidelines; hence, both indices were not fixed to baseline data. Furthermore, each index addressed its specific disease activity. The development of both RACI and PsACI was based on patient self-administered questionnaire as well as ICD-10 data record. Results revealed variation of the comorbidity prevalence over the 10-year study period. While depression and anxiety were more prevalent in the first few years of the disease course, other comorbidities including cardiovascular, osteoporosis, and medication-associated comorbidities were more prevalent at later stages of the disease course. Thirty-one comorbidities were identified in the RACI with a score ranging between 0 and 36 (Table 16.8), whereas the PsACI included 29 items with a score ranging between 0 and 36 (Table 16.9). Criterion validity was evaluated through the index correlation with both functional disability and quality of life. Multivariate linear regression analysis for functional disability score prediction using RACI adjusted for age and gender revealed significant correlations at 1, 3, 5, and 10 years (R^2, 0.743, 0.767, 0.908, and 0.835, respectively). Similarly PsACI showed significant correlation with the functional disability score (R^2, 0.725, 0.773, 0.847, and 0.872 at 1, 3, 5, and 10 years, respectively). Construct validity was assessed by studying the correlation between

Table 16.8 Rheumatoid Arthritis Comorbidity Index (RACI)

Comorbidity	Point	Comorbidity	Point
DAS-28 > 3.6	5	Osteoporosis	1
Fracture	2	Falls risk	1
Ischemic heart disease	2	Liver disease	1
Myocardial infarction	2	Renal disease	1
Depression	2	GIT disease	1
Diabetes mellitus	2	Endocrine disease	1
Hypertension	1	Pulmonary disease	1
Hyperlipidemia	1	Tumor	1
Metabolic syndrome	1	Periodontitis	0.5
Peripheral vascular disease	1	Osteoarthritis	0.5
Cerebrovascular disease	1	Fibromyalgia	0.5
Arrhythmia	1	Atlantoaxial subluxation	0.5
Infection	1	Carpal tunnel syndrome	0.5
Anxiety	1	Vasculitis	0.5
Smoking	1	Amyloidosis	0.5
		Eye inflammation/cataract	0.5

From El Miedany et al. [57], with permission
Calculation: add all items. The total score is the Rheumatoid Arthritis Comorbidity Index (RACI). Range, 0–36. Score ≥ 8 indicates high comorbidity risk

Table 16.9 Psoriatic Arthritis Comorbidity Index (PsACI)

Comorbidity	Point	Comorbidity	Point
Disease severity (3/5)	5	Osteoporosis	1
Metabolic syndrome	2	Falls risk	1
Ischemic heart disease	2	Liver disease	1
Myocardial infarction	2	Renal disease	1
Depression	2	GIT disease	1
Diabetes mellitus	2	Endocrine disease	1
Hypertension	1	Pulmonary disease	1
Hyperlipidemia	1	Tumor	1
Fracture	2	Periodontitis	0.5
Peripheral vascular disease	1	Osteoarthritis	0.5
Cerebrovascular disease	1	Fibromyalgia	0.5
Arrhythmia	1	Vasculitis	0.5
Infection	1	Amyloidosis	0.5
Anxiety	1	Eye inflammation/cataract	0.5
Smoking	1		

From El Miedany et al. [58], with permission
Calculation: add all items. The total score is the Psoriatic Arthritis Comorbidity Index (PsACI). Range, 0–36. Score ≥ 8 indicates high comorbidity risk

the RACI and four comorbidity indices: the CCI, FCI, RDCI, and MMI. Relative to other comorbidity indices, the RACI and RDCI showed high correlation for predicting death and physical disability in data set composed of individuals with RA (1 year, 0.963; 3 years, 0.598; 5 years, 0.966; 10 years,0.919). Similarly, PsACI was compared to the CCI, FCI, RDCI, and MMI. In concordance with the RACI, both PsACI and RDCI had the highest correlations at 1 year ($r = 0.863$), 3 years (0.798), 5 years (0.886), and 10 years (0.916). Test-retest reliability for both RACI and PsACI was very good (ICC 0.97 and 0.96, respectively). Receiver operating characteristic (ROC) illustrating the discriminating ability of the RACI revealed that a score of 8/36 gave an area under the curve (AUC) of 0.967, whereas in the PsACI a score of 8/36 gave an AUC of 0.987. External validation studies for both RACI and PsACI revealed that both indices were able to predict outcomes of physical disability, quality of life, as well as hospitalization/death and showed significant correlation with all the other comorbidity indices (CCI, FCI, RDCI, and MMI).

Critical Analysis

Both RACI and PsACI are the first disease-specific comorbidity indices which include disease activity as a comorbid factor with the highest weight in contrast to the other disease-associated comorbidities. Similarly, both indices are the first to address medication-associated comorbidities as an outcome of interest. Both the RACI and PsACI were able to predict outcomes of physical disability, quality of life, as well as hospitalization/death. Both indices outperformed CCI, which is commonly used but not validated for outcomes such as health-related quality of life (HRQoL). Both comorbidity indices can be measured with either patient-reported questionnaire (part of a patient-reported outcome measure) or administrative data (ICD-9 or ICD-10) for comorbidity assessment and management.

Comorbidity Indices in Standard Practice and Research

Though guidelines such as NICE [59] and EULAR [60] have stressed on the importance of screening inflammatory arthritic patients regularly for associated comorbidities, assessment of these in standard clinical practice has yet to be widely implemented. The Comorbidities in Rheumatoid Arthritis (COMORA) study [61], which included 3920 patients from 17 countries around the world, revealed that the management of comorbidities in RA patients is far from optimum and that there have been disparities in the screening process in different countries. Furthermore, the studies used to assess the associated comorbidity risk, for example, the cardiovascular risk, were based on cohorts assembled in 1955–1973 [62–65]. Longitudinal studies which included RA patients diagnosed and treated before the introduction of methotrexate into clinical practice in 1986 [66] would bias the results toward poor outcomes as they will not be representative of the modern disease management or the current clinical presentation of RA. In addition, the inclusion of RA disease duration >10 years as a risk factor for cardiovascular risk may undermine its risk assessment earlier in the disease course when the disease activity is at its peak.

The findings that the occurrence of comorbidities varies across rheumatic diseases and that separate patterns of comorbidity may be identified in patients who have rheumatoid arthritis, psoriatic arthritis, systemic lupus, as well as fibromyalgia syndrome highlighted the unmet need for systems to assess specific comorbidity risk in these patients [56]. To date, no gold standard exists on how to measure comorbidity. This was supported by the outcomes of a systematic literature review [67] on assessing comorbidity and multimorbidity, which identified 39 different indices showing heterogeneity in terms of types and numbers of conditions included and outcomes the indices are based on. Perhaps that is the reason why comparisons of comorbidity indices in rheumatic diseases are limited. Gabriel et al. [21] showed that the CCI and the Index of Coexistent Disease (designed mainly for patients on hemodialysis [68]) were both highly statistically significant predictors of death in an administrative data set of 450 RA and 441 OA patients. In another study, both RDCI and ETS were reported to best predict death in RA patients [49]. These results are similar to those previously published in myocardial infarction and cancer, which showed that ECM outperforms CDI in predicting death when the source was administrative data [37, 69]. As for physical disability, the FCI was found to predict MDHAQ best in RA with considerable support. In a random sampling of Canadian adults and a sample of US adults seeking treatment for spine ailments, Groll et al. [12] showed the FCI outperformed CCI in correlating with physical function, as measured by the physical function subscale of the Short Form 36 Health Survey. The most recently published comorbidity indices specific for RA and psoriatic arthritis pave the way for a new approach to comorbidity risk assessment and management tailored to the individual patient's status.

There has been a misconception in that, clinically, comorbidity indices have limited use. The window of opportunity and treat to target approaches highlighted the importance of assessing for the comorbid conditions or its risk on regular basis when managing the disease or prescribing therapeutics. The comorbid conditions important for these roles in standard clinical practice may not always be applicable in research settings, as highlighted by the recently published EULAR points to consider for reporting, screening for, and preventing selected comorbidities in chronic inflammatory rheumatic diseases [70].

Several important steps should be considered when selecting a comorbidity index for research. First, one must determine the outcome of interest. While some indices like ETS and RDCI can perform well in multiple outcomes, other indices such as CDI and FCI may only perform optimally for a single outcome. Second, investigators must determine the source of data. Many of the indices can only be used in administrative data sets with ICD-9-CM codes (CDI, ETS, EPS). Furthermore, one must consider the data available for model construction as evidenced by the robust improvement in model fit with the administrative and clinical models. Last, the comorbid conditions available must be considered. Many indices require a substantial number of comorbid conditions, but if these are not available, a comorbidity count can be used, though with less predictive ability. Use of a comorbidity count is discouraged because comorbidity counts vary in the number and types of conditions included, and wide variability in predictive ability have been reported [10]. Therefore, it is strongly recommend that researchers use a standardized and validated comorbidity index in rheumatology analysis for improved comparability and reproducibility.

In conclusion, considering the recent developments in the diagnosis and management of inflammatory arthritic conditions, there is a still a need for systems to assess for comorbidity in standard clinical settings. Periodic assessment for comorbidities should be carried out by the treating healthcare physician as one of the management outcome measures. Electronic comorbidity calculators would be a step forward toward implementing comorbidity screening in the day-to-day patient management. This should be carried out in collaboration with primary care providers and other specialists. Developing a disease-specific comorbidity index able to predict morbidity, mortality, cost, and hospitalization would be a step forward on the way to achieve full disease remission.

Acknowledgment Special thanks to Dr. Loreto Carmona, MD, PhD, Research Director, Instituto de Salud Musculoesquelética, Madrid, Spain, for peer reviewing this chapter.

References

1. Wolfe F, Mitchell DM, Sibley JT, et al. The mortality of rheumatoid arthritis. Arthritis Rheum. 1994;37:481–94.
2. Gabriel SE, Michaud K. Epidemiological studies in incidence, prevalence, mortality, and comorbidity of the rheumatic diseases. Arthritis Res Ther. 2009;11:229.
3. Gabriel SE. Why do people with rheumatoid arthritis still die prematurely? Ann Rheum Dis. 2008;67:30–4.
4. Feinstein AR. The pre-therapeutic classification of co-morbidity in chronic disease. J Chronic Dis. 1970;23(7):455–68.
5. Avina-Zubieta JA, Choi HK, Sadatsafavi M, et al. Risk of cardiovascular mortality in patients with rheumatoid arthritis: a meta-analysis of observational studies. Arthritis Rheum. 2008;59:1690–7.
6. Lindhardsen J, Ahlehoff O, Gislason GH, et al. The risk of myocardial infarction in rheumatoid arthritis and diabetes mellitus: a Danish nationwide cohort study. Ann Rheum Dis. 2011;70:929–34.
7. Listing J, Gerhold K, Zink A. The risk of infections associated with rheumatoid arthritis, with its comorbidity and treatment. Rheumatology (Oxford). 2013;52:53–61.
8. Wotton CJ, Goldacre MJ. Risk of invasive pneumococcal disease in people admitted to hospital with selected immune-mediated diseases: record linkage cohort analyses. J Epidemiol Community Health. 2012;66:1177–81.
9. Uresson C, Matteson EL. Malignancy as a comorbidity in rheumatic diseases. Rheumatology (Oxford). 2013;52:5–14.
10. England B, Sayles H, Mikuls TED, Johnson D, Michaud A. Validation of the rheumatic disease comorbidity index. Arthritis Care Res. 2015;67(6):865–72.
11. Charlson ME, Pompei P, Ales KL, MacKenzie CR. A new method of classifying prognostic comorbidity in longitudinal studies: development and validation. J Chronic Dis. 1987;40:373–83.

12. Groll DL, To T, Bombardier C, Wright JG. The development of a comorbidity index with physical function as the outcome. J Clin Epidemiol. 2005;58:595–602.
13. Kaplan MH, Feinstein AR. The importance of classifying initial co-morbidity in evaluating the outcome of diabetes mellitus. J Chronic Dis. 1974;27:387–404.
14. Miller MD, Paradis CF, Houck PR, Mazumdar S, Stack JA, Rifai AH, et al. Rating chronic medical illness burden in geropsychiatric practice and research: application of the cumulative illness rating scale. Psychiatry Res. 1992;41:237–48.
15. Von Korff M, Wagner EH, Saunders K. A chronic disease score from automated pharmacy data. J Clin Epidemiol. 1992;45:197–203.
16. Elixhauser A, Steiner C, Harris DR, Coffey RM. Comorbidity measures for use with administrative data. Med Care. 1998;36:8–27.
17. Hall SF. A user's guide to selecting a comorbidity index for clinical research. J Clin Epidemiol. 2006;59:849–55.
18. Kiefe CI, Funkhouser E, Fouad MN, May DS. Chronic disease as a barrier to breast and cervical cancer screening. J Gen Intern Med. 1998;13:357–65.
19. Streiner DL, Norman GR. Health measurement scales. A practical guide to their development and use, vol. 2. Oxford: Oxford University Press; 1995. p. 1–230.
20. Rochon PA, Katz JN, Morrow LA, et al. Comorbid illness is associated with survival and length of hospital stay in patients with chronic disability. A prospective comparison of three comorbidity indices. Med Care. 1996;34:1093–101.
21. Gabriel SE, Crowson CS, O'Fallon WM. A comparison of two comorbidity instruments in arthritis. J Clin Epidemiol. 1999;52:1137–42.
22. Kieszak SM, Flanders WD, Kosinski AS, Shipp CC, Karp H. A comparison of the Charlson comorbidity index derived from medical record data and administrative billing data. J Clin Epidemiol. 1999;52:137–42.
23. Poses RM, McClish DK, Smith WR, Bekes C, Scott WE. Prediction of survival of critically ill patients by admission comorbidity. J Clin Epidemiol. 1996;49:743–7.
24. Fletcher RH, Fletcher SW, WAGNER EH. Clinical epidemiology: the essentials. 3rd ed. Baltimore: Williams & Wilkins; 1996.
25. de Groot V, Beckerman H, Lankhorst GJ, Bouter LM. How to measure comorbidity. A critical review of available methods. J Clin Epidemiol. 2003;56:221–9.
26. Katz JN, Chang LC, Sangha O, Fossel AH, Bates DW. Can comorbidity be assessed by questionnaire rather than medical record review ? Med Care. 1996;34:73–84.
27. Deyo RA, Cherkin DC, Ciol MA. Adapting a clinical comorbidity index for use with ICD-9-CM administrative databases. J Clin Epidemiol. 1992;45(6):613–9.
28. Romano PS, Roos LL, Jollis JG. Adapting a clinical comorbidity index for use with ICD-9-CM administrative data: differing perspectives. J Clin Epidemiol. 1993;46(10):1075–9.
29. Halfon P, Eggli Y, van Melle G, Chevalier J, Wasserfallen JB, Burnand B. Measuring potentially avoidable hospital readmissions. J Clin Epidemiol. 2002;55(6):573–87.
30. Quan H, Sundararajan V, Halfon P, Fong A, Burnand B, Luthi JC, Saunders LD, Beck CA, Feasby TE, Ghali WA. Coding algorithms for defining comorbidities in ICD-9-CM and ICD-10 administrative data. Med Care. 2005;43(11):1130–9.
31. Schneeweiss S, Wang PS, Avorn J, Glynn RJ. Improved comorbidity adjustment for predicting mortality in Medicare populations. Health Serv Res. 2003;38(4):1103–20.
32. Sarfati D, Tan L, Blakely T, et al. Comorbidity among patients with colon cancer in New Zealand. N Z Med J. 2011;124(1338):76–88.
33. Mnatzaganian G, Ryan P, Norman PE, et al. Accuracy of hospital morbidity data and the performance of comorbidity scores as predictors of mortality. J Clin Epidemiol. 2012;65(1):107–15.
34. Needham DM, Scales DC, Laupacis A, Pronovost PJ. A systematic review of the Charlson comorbidity index using Canadian administrative databases: a perspective on risk adjustment in critical care research. J Crit Care. 2005;20(1):12–9.
35. Moltó A, Dougados M. Comorbidity indices. Clin Exp Rheumatol. 2014;32(Suppl. 85):S131–4.
36. Condon JR, You J, McDonnell J. Performance of comorbidity indices in measuring outcomes after acute myocardial infarction in Australian indigenous and non-indigenous patients. Intern Med J. 2012;42:e165–73.

37. Southern DA, Quan H, Ghali WA. Comparison of the Elixhauser and Charlson/Deyo methods of comorbidity measurement in administrative data. Med Care. 2004;42:355–60.
38. Menendez ME, Neuhaus V, van Dijk CN, Ring D. The Elixhauser comorbidity method outperforms the Charlson index in predicting inpatient death after orthopaedic surgery. Clin Orthop Relat Res. 2014;472:2878–86.
39. Dominick KL, Dudley TK, Coffman CJ, Bosworth HB. Comparison of three comorbidity measures for predicting health service use in patients with osteoarthritis. Arthritis Rheum. 2005;53:666–72.
40. Antoniou T, Ng R, Glazier RH, Kopp A, Austin PC. Comparison of comorbidity classification methods for predicting outcomes in a population-based cohort of adults with human immunodeficiency virus infection. Ann Epidemiol. 2014;24:532–7.
41. Gandjour A, Ku-Goto MH, Ho V. Comparing the validity of different measures of illness severity: a hospital-level analysis for acute myocardial infarction. Health Serv Manag Res. 2012;25:138–43.
42. Sharabiani M, Aylin P, Bottle A. Systematic review of comorbidity indices for administrative data. Med Care. 2012;50(12):1109–18.
43. Garland A, Fransoo R, Olafson K, Ramsey C, Yogendran M, Chateau D, McGowan K. The epidemiology and outcomes of critical illness in Manitoba. Winnipeg: Manitoba Centre for Health Policy; 2012.
44. Van Walraven C, Austin PC, Jenings A, Quan H, Forster AJ. A modification of the Elixhauser comorbidity measures into a point system for hospital death using administrative data. Med Care. 2009;47(6):626–33.
45. Linn BS, Linn MW, Gurel L. Cumulative illness rating scale. J Am Geriatr Soc. 1968;16:622–6.
46. Extermann M, Overcash J, Lyman G, Parr J, Balducci L. Comorbidity and functional status are independent in older cancer patients. J Clin Oncol. 1998;16(4):1582–7.
47. Repetto L, Fratino L, Audisio RA, Venturino A, Gianni W, Vercelli M, Parodi S, Dal Lago D, Gioia F, Monfardini S, Aapro MS, Serrainc D, Zagonel V. Comprehensive geriatric assessment adds information to Eastern Cooperative Oncology Group performance status in elderly cancer patients: an Italian Group for Geriatric Oncology Study. J Clin Oncol. 2002;20(2):494–502.
48. Grolla D, Tob T, Bombardierc C, Wrightd J. The development of a comorbidity index with physical function as the outcome. J Clin Epidemiol. 2005;58:595–602.
49. Michaud K, Wolfe F. Comorbidities in rheumatoid arthritis. Best Pract Res Clin Rheumatol. 2007;21:885–906.
50. Chang TI, Paik J, Greene T, Miskulin DC, Chertow GM. Updated comorbidity assessments and outcomes in prevalent hemodialysis patients. Hemodial Int. 2010;14:478–85.
51. Rander H, Yoshida K, Mjaavatten M, Aletaha D, et al. Development of a multimorbidity index: impact on quality of life using a rheumatoid arthritis cohort. Semin Arth Rheumatsim. 2015;45(2):167–73.
52. Radner H, Smolen JS, Aletaha D. Comorbidity affects all domains of physical function and quality of life in patients with rheumatoid arthritis. Rheumatology (Oxford). 2010;50:381–8.
53. Frenkel WJ, Jongerius EJ, Mandjes-van Uitert MJ, van Munster BC, de Rooij SE. Validation of the Charlson comorbidity index in acutely hospitalized elderly adults a prospective cohort study. J Am Geriatr Soc. 2014;62:342–6.
54. Sangha O, Stucki G, Liang M, Fossel AH, Katz JN. The self-administered comorbidity questionnaire: a new method to assess comorbidity for clinical and health services research. Arthritis Rheum. 2003;49:156–63.
55. Stolwijk C, van Tubergen A, Ramiro S, et al. Aspects of validity of the self-administered comorbidity questionnaire in patients with ankylosing spondylitis. Rheumatology (Oxford). 2014;53:1054–64.
56. El Miedany Y. Co-morbidity index in rheumatoid arthritis: time to think. Clin Rheumatol. 2015;34(12):1995–2000.
57. El Miedany Y, El Gaafary M, Youssef S, Bahlas S, Ahmed I, Hegazi M. Rheumatoid arthritis comorbidity index: development and validation of a new specific tool for classifying prognostic comorbidity in rheumatoid arthritis patients. Ann Rheum Dis. 2016;75(Suppl2):154.

58. El Miedany Y, El Gaafary M, Youssef S, Bahlas S, Hegazi M. Psoriatic arthritis comorbidity index: development and validation of a new specific tool for classifying prognostic comorbidity in psoriasis and psoriatic arthritis patients. Rheumatol Orthop Med. 2017;2 doi: 10.15761/ROM.1000117.
59. NICEguidelines [CG79]. Rheumatoidarthritis:the management of rheumatoid arthritis in adults. http://www.nice.org.uk/guidance/cg79. 2009.
60. Smolen J, Landewé R, Breedveld F, et al. EULAR recommendations for the management of rheumatoid arthritis with synthetic and biological disease-modifying antirheumatic drugs: 2013 update. Ann Rheum Dis. 2014;73(3):492–509. doi:10.1136/annrheumdis-2013204573.
61. Dougados M, Soubrier M, Antunez A, et al. Prevalence of comorbidities in rheumatoid arthritis and evaluation of their monitoring: results of an international, cross-sectional study (COMORA). Ann Rheum Dis. 2013;1:1–7. doi:10.1136/annrheumdis2013-204223.
62. Jacobsson LT, Knowler WC, Pillemer S, et al. Rheumatoid arthritis and mortality. A longitudinal study in pima Indians. Arthritis Rheum. 1993;36:1045–53.
63. Turesson C, McClelland RL, Christianson TJ, et al. Severe extra-articular disease manifestations are associated with an increased risk of first ever cardiovascular events in patients with rheumatoid arthritis. Ann Rheum Dis. 2007;66:70–5.
64. Nicola PJ, Maradit-Kremers H, Roger VL, et al. The risk of congestive heart failure in rheumatoid arthritis: a population-based study over 46 years. Arthritis Rheum. 2005;52:412–20.
65. Gabriel SE, Crowson CS, Kremers HM, et al. Survival in rheumatoid arthritis: a population-based analysis of trends over 40 years. Arthritis Rheum. 2003;48:54–8.
66. Weinblatt ME, Coblyn JS, Fox DA, et al. Efficacy of lowdose methotrexate in rheumatoid arthritis. N Engl J Med. 1985;312:818–22.
67. Radner H, Yoshida K, Smolen J, Solomon D. Multimorbidity and rheumatic conditions—enhancing the concept of comorbidity. Nat Rev Rheumatol. 2014;10:252–6.
68. Miskulin DC, Athienites NV, Yan G, Martin AA, Ornt DB, et al. Comorbidity assessment using the index of coexistent diseases in a multicenter clinical trial. Kidney Int. 2001;60(4):1498–510.
69. Lieffers JR, Baracos VE, Winget M, Fassbender K. A comparison of Charlson and Elixhauser comorbidity measures to predict colorectal cancer survival using administrative health data. Cancer. 2011;117:1957–65.
70. Baillet A, Gossec L, Carmona L, de Wit M, et al. Points to consider for reporting, screening for and preventing selected comorbidities in chronic inflammatory rheumatic diseases in daily practice: a EULAR initiative. Ann Rheum Dis. 2014;73(3):492–509. doi:10.1136/annrheumdis-2016-209233.

Chapter 17
Anti-Rheumatic Therapy and Comorbidity

J. Steuart Richards, Sharon Dowell, and Mercedes Quinones

Therapy for rheumatic diseases may be classified as immunosuppressive agents, synthetic chemical compound disease-modifying anti-rheumatic drugs (csDMARDs) or biologic disease-modifying anti-rheumatic drugs (bDMARDs). The improved quality of life, reduced morbidity and mortality, of patients with rheumatic disease validates the efficacy of these agents [1, 2].

Rheumatic diseases are, for the most part, chronic illnesses with patients dying with, rather than from them. The excess mortality reported for rheumatoid arthritis is often attributed to concomitant comorbidity; however, greater disease activity is a contributing factor [3, 4]. This argues for greater control of disease activity, necessitating the use of anti-rheumatic medications in patients with rheumatic disease despite comorbid illness. Selecting not only the most efficacious but least harmful options can be challenging for rheumatologists as randomized clinical trials restrict enrollment of patients with complex comorbidities. The short duration of clinical trials, 6–12 months, precludes judgment on the long-term safety of anti-rheumatic medications. Biologic registries or observational studies, typically of longer duration, should provide evidence on the use of anti-rheumatic medications in patients with comorbid disease; however, preselection of younger, healthier patients for bDMARDs or more potent csDMARDs limits the interpretation of results. An overlooked consideration is the potential benefit these drugs have on non-rheumatic disease including the reduction of serum insulin and insulin: glucose index as well as myocardial infarction with tumor necrosis factor-α (TNF-α) inhibitors [5–7].

J.S. Richards (✉)
Medical Service Line, Division of Rheumatology, Veterans Affairs Pittsburgh Healthcare System, Pittsburgh, PA, USA
e-mail: john.richards1@va.gov

S. Dowell • M. Quinones
Department of Internal Medicine, Division of Rheumatology, Howard University Hospital, Washington, DC, USA
e-mail: Sharon.dowell@howard.edu; Mercedes.quinones@howard.edu

Y. El Miedany (ed.), *Comorbidity in Rheumatic Diseases*,
DOI 10.1007/978-3-319-59963-2_17

Therapeutic guidelines serve as a manual for the appropriate selection of anti-rheumatic drugs or strategies based on the stage and severity of the disease, frequently without consideration for comorbidity [8].

In this chapter we will discuss the use of anti-rheumatic medications in patients with chronic infections, cardiovascular disease, cancer, lung disease, diabetes mellitus, renal disease, and pregnancy.

Liver Disease

There is an increased incidence of hepatotoxicity in rheumatic patients with chronic viral hepatitis and concomitant use of anti-rheumatic medications (Table 17.1). The risk of hepatotoxicity is increased in patients with normal baseline liver function as well as those with elevated transaminases at baseline, being more pronounced in the latter [9]. In addition to this, some DMARDs are hepatotoxic in their own right. In the following paragraphs, we discuss the use of anti-rheumatic medications in patients with chronic viral hepatitis or other chronic liver disease.

Chronic Viral Hepatitis

Several of the csDMARDs have been implicated in the occurrence of hepatotoxicity in patients with chronic viral hepatitis (CVH). Acute liver disease may be precipitated or exacerbated by both a direct hepatotoxic effect of the drug itself and by inducing viral replication and subsequent liver injury. Azathioprine and combination DMARD therapy have further been associated with hepatic injury through reactivation of hepatitis B, a mechanism most popularly associated with bDMARDs and the newer small-molecule therapies.

Hydroxychloroquine and sulfasalazine have rarely been associated with hepatotoxicity in CVH, with no contraindication to the use of either in these patients [9–13]. Conversely, methotrexate may potentiate severe hepatic damage in the presence of CVH via a synergistic effect and is associated with hepatitis B virus (HBV) reactivation in hepatitis B surface antigen (HBsAg)-positive and HBsAg-negative/anti-hepatitis B core (anti-HBc)-positive patients. Its true impact on HBV reactivation is unclear due to frequent coadministration of glucocorticoid therapy [14–17]. However, methotrexate discontinuation can lead to fulminant hepatic failure in HBsAg-positive patients via resurgent T-cell-mediated destruction of infected hepatocytes [18]. It is hence best avoided in patients with untreated HBV. Institutional guidelines recommend screening for chronic viral hepatitis in all patients prior to initiation of methotrexate therapy [19, 20], although some argue that screening should be targeted to endemic populations or other identified risks such as concomitant glucocorticoid use [16, 17, 21].

Table 17.1 Recommendations for the use anti-rheumatic drugs in patients with chronic infections

Recommendations	Level of evidence[a]
Hepatitis B (HBV)	
Hydroxychloroquine and sulfasalazine do not require screening for HBV prior to treatment	IV
Screen for HBV before the start of treatment with azathioprine, methotrexate, leflunomide, MMF, tofacitinib, and bDMARDs (EMA)	IV
Do not use azathioprine, methotrexate, leflunomide, MMF, tofacitinib, or bDMARDs in patients with chronic untreated HBV or treated HBV with liver dysfunction (Child-Pugh class B or higher) (ACR, EMA) [12–14]	III
Monitor viral loads and transaminases of HBSAg-positive patients starting methotrexate, leflunomide, azathioprine, or MMF [69]	IV
Start antiviral prophylaxis with entecavir, tenofovir, or adefovir 1 week before and continue for 52 weeks after TNF-α inhibitors, abatacept, or rituximab in HBsAg-positive patients [72]	III
Start antiviral prophylaxis before rituximab in HBsAg-negative/HBcAb-positive patients	III
Monitor viral loads and transaminases of HBsAg-negative/HBcAb-positive patients starting methotrexate, leflunomide, azathioprine, MMF, or TNF-alpha inhibitors [71]	IV
Hepatitis C (HCV)	
Hydroxychloroquine and sulfasalazine do not require screening for HBC prior to treatment Screen for HCV before the starting azathioprine, methotrexate, leflunomide, MMF, tofacitinib, and bDMARDs (based on regional prevalence; AR)	II
Etanercept can be used in patients with HCV (ACR) [33]	II
Do not use azathioprine, methotrexate, leflunomide, MMF, tofacitinib, or bDMARDs in patients with chronic untreated HCV or treated HCV with liver dysfunction (Child-Pugh class B or higher) (AR)	IV
HIV	
Hydroxychloroquine and sulfasalazine do not require HIV screening	IV
Screen for HIV before azathioprine, methotrexate, leflunomide, MMF, tofacitinib, and bDMARDs on the basis of risk factors and national guidelines (AR)	IV
Monitor HIV viral loads and CD4 counts for patients treated with immunosuppressants and bDMARDs	IV
Tuberculosis	
Hydroxychloroquine and sulfasalazine use does not require prescreening for TNB	IV
Follow local guidelines for screening for TB prior to starting azathioprine, methotrexate, leflunomide, MMF, or tofacitinib	IV
Screen for latent tuberculosis with TST or IGRA before starting bDMARDs (ACR, EMA, CRA) [126, 127] Follow a positive TST or IGRA test by repeat testing or chest radiography based on national/regional guidelines (EMA)	II (TNF-α inhibitor), IV (rituximab, abatacept) IV

(continued)

Table 17.1 (continued)

Recommendations	Level of evidence[a]
Complete at least 1 month of treatment for latent tuberculosis before starting bDMARDs	III
Rituximab is first-line bDMARD if chemoprophylaxis is contraindicated or for patients living in regions endemic for tuberculosis (EULAR) [128]	IV

Abbreviations: *AR* authors' recommendations, *ACR* 2012 update of the American College of Rheumatology recommendations, *CRA* Canadian Rheumatology Association recommendations for the pharmacological management of rheumatoid arthritis, *EMA* European Medicines Agency approved summary of product characteristics, *EULAR* European League against Rheumatism, *HBsAg* hepatitis B surface antigen, *HBcAg* hepatitis B core antibody, *MMF* mycophenolate mofetil, *TNF-alpha* tumor necrosis factor alpha

[a]Levels of evidence I = meta-analyses, systematic reviews of randomized controlled trials (RCTs), or individual RCTs; II = meta-analysis of systemic reviews of observational studies, case control studies; III = case series and case reports; IV = expert opinion

Similarly to methotrexate, cases of viral reactivation of HBV or hepatitis C virus (HCV) have been documented with use of mycophenolate mofetil (MMF). Data is predominantly from the transplant literature, where MMF is used as part of a multi-drug immunosuppressive regimen. Interestingly, in one analysis of renal transplant patients with HBV infection, less use of MMF was associated with an increased risk of HBV reactivation. It was proposed that this could be due to its potent immunosuppressive effect as well as a possible inhibitory effect on HBV replication [22–24].

Reports of azathioprine-induced reactivation of HBV are rare and, in reported cases, it occurs in the presence of combination immunosuppressive therapy [9, 25, 26]. Leflunomide has been associated with severe hepatotoxicity and is not recommended in patients with acute or chronic HCV or HBV. Performing baseline liver function tests as well as screening for viral hepatitis is recommended prior to the start of therapy with methotrexate, MMF, azathioprine, and leflunomide [8, 12, 20, 27]. Patients who are HBsAg positive are considered at low risk of reactivation when starting monotherapy with methotrexate or azathioprine. These patients, in addition to those with natural immunity from prior exposure to HBV (anti-HBc Ab positive/anti hepatitis B surface antibody (HBsAb) positive/HBsAg negative) with normal liver function tests, should have regular monitoring of the HBV viral load at least every 6–12 months [28]. The use of combination DMARD therapy or concomitant systemic glucocorticoids leads to a moderate risk of reactivation, and antiviral prophylaxis should be considered on an individual basis. Patients with chronic untreated HBV or HCV should be referred to a hepatologist for appropriate antiviral therapy prior to starting immunosuppressive therapy with methotrexate, MMF, and azathioprine [8]. There are no reports of HBV or HCV reactivation with apremilast, and this medication may be safely used in CVH.

Tumor necrosis factor (TNF) alpha levels are elevated in patients with HBV, and TNF alpha plays a role in clearing and controlling viral replication. Several cases of reactivation of HBV have hence been reported with use of the TNF-alpha inhibitors [29, 30]. Infliximab was the most frequently implicated TNF-alpha inhibitor, while etanercept and adalimumab are thought to be safer, although there have been case reports of HBV reactivation with these agents as well [31, 32]. The implementation of routine screening for HBV prior to the start of biologic therapy and prophylaxis with antiviral therapy in high-risk patients has led to a fall in the number of reported cases of HBV reactivation. Conversely, TNF alpha is instrumental in chronic HCV infection, and TNF-alpha inhibitors have been used successfully in these patients. Etanercept was found to be a powerful adjunct to antiviral therapy for chronic HCV infection in one randomized control trial [33–35]. Reactivation of HBV and increased HCV viral loads also occur with rituximab therapy in patients with rheumatic diseases [36–40]. Rituximab leads to a decrease in titers of HBsAb, and rates of reactivation have ranged from 3.4% to 80% and 1.5% to 23.8%, respectively, in HBsAg-positive and HBsAg-negative lymphoma patients on rituximab-based chemotherapy [36]. In patients with HCV, the occurrence of liver dysfunction did not usually lead to a change in treatment regimen or further clinical consequences although there are few reports of severe hepatotoxicity with rituximab-based chemotherapy [41, 42]. Rituximab induces increased HCV replication, and on completion of therapy, reconstitution of the immune system may result in cell-mediated hepatocellular injury and necrosis [43, 44]. Despite this, it has been used successfully in patients with HCV-associated cryoglobulinemic vasculitis and is generally thought to be safe in rheumatology patients with HCV [27, 45, 46]. Abatacept has rarely been associated with HBV reactivation in HBsAg-positive and HBsAg-negative/HBcAb-positive patients [47–49]. Data on abatacept and chronic HCV are limited, but mild fluctuations in HCV viral loads have been reported in two patients [50].

There are no reported cases of HBV reactivation in patients treated with tocilizumab, and it has been used successfully in two patients with chronic HBV with concomitant prophylactic antiviral therapy [49–51]. There is a single report of increased HCV viral load and transaminitis leading to the discontinuation of tocilizumab with no other reports of exacerbation of HCV [51, 52]. Given the potential protective role of interleukin-6 in hepatocyte regeneration and proliferation and raised levels in chronic HCV, cirrhosis, and hepatocellular cancer, more long-term data on tocilizumab are needed [51, 53].

HBV reactivation and new HBV infection have been occasionally reported with tofacitinib, and patients should be screened for viral hepatitis prior to initiation of therapy [54, 55].

There have been rare reports of reactivation of HBV and increased HCV viral loads with ustekinumab [56–58]. Interestingly, these cases of HBV reactivation have been mild and self-limited and rarely associated with symptoms or elevations of transaminases. The newly released secukinumab has not been associated with HBV or HCV, although its immunomodulating effect suggests this may be possible [59–61].

There have been no reports of reactivation of HBV or exacerbation of liver injury in patients with chronic viral hepatitis treated with belimumab, anakinra, rilonacept, or canakinumab [62–68].

The use of prophylactic antiviral therapy in HBV decreases the risk of viral reactivation and is hence recommended for high-risk patients. This group includes HBsAg-positive patients starting rituximab or systemic glucocorticoid therapy >20 mg/day for >4 weeks and HBcAb positive-/HBsAg-negative patients starting rituximab [19, 20, 28]. HBSAg-positive patients on non-rituximab bDMARD therapy are considered at moderate risk for HBV reactivation and can either receive prophylactic antiviral therapy or can be followed with close monitoring of viral loads and transaminases [69]. The issue of viral resistance has led to caution with recommending widespread use of antiviral therapy in all patients with prior HBV exposure [70], with particular reference to the cohort of HBsAg-negative, HBcAb-positive patients who are also at risk of viral reactivation [31]. Patients with positive viral serologies should be managed in concert with a hepatologist [71]. It is generally agreed that antiviral prophylaxis in HBsAg-positive patients should start 1–2 weeks before immunosuppressive therapy and should be continued for 6–12 months after completion of therapy [72]. Patients with HCV should not be treated differently than unexposed patients, but management in concert with a hepatologist is desirable, especially with the recent advent of highly effective antiviral therapy for HCV.

Hepatotoxicity

Transaminitis and rare hepatotoxicity have been noted with the use of most DMARDs; however, the greatest risk of severe liver injury occurs during therapy with methotrexate and leflunomide.

There have been isolated cases of hepatotoxicity with the use of hydroxychloroquine, but given the rarity and unpredictability of these events, routine screening for hepatic dysfunction is unnecessary prior to its use [10]. Sulfasalazine-associated hepatotoxicity requiring withdrawal of therapy occurs in an estimated 0.4–0.5% of patients [11, 73]. It may cause a severe hypersensitivity reaction characterized by fever, rash, and markedly elevated transaminases. Baseline hepatic function is recommended, followed by hepatic function tests every 2–4 weeks for 3 months, then every 3 months [12, 13]. Azathioprine, too, may cause a mild transient transaminitis but rarely results in severe hepatotoxicity. There are case reports of acute idiosyncratic hepatitis (cholestatic or hepatocellular) as well as an increased risk of chronic non-cirrhotic portal hypertension with long-term use [25]. Liver function tests should be done prior to starting azathioprine, and it should be used with caution in patients with baseline hepatic dysfunction, with frequent monitoring of liver function tests, and dose reduction or discontinuation of therapy with hepatotoxicity [74]. Transaminitis without fatal hepatotoxicity has been reported with tofacitinib. Serial monitoring of liver function tests is recommended, and a dose reduction by 50% is advised in patients with moderate hepatic impairment, with total avoidance in patients with severe liver failure. Apremilast and MMF have not been associated with hepatotoxicity, and there is no contraindication or dosage adjustment necessary when using these drugs in patients with chronic liver disease.

Chronic low-dose methotrexate can induce hepatic injury ranging from mild transaminitis to hepatic fibrosis and cirrhosis. The mechanism of hepatic injury with methotrexate is unclear, but hepatic folate stores are depleted during its use, and folic acid supplementation reduces the incidence of transaminitis [75, 76]. Concomitant alcohol use, obesity, hyperlipidemia, psoriasis, or psoriatic arthritis is associated with an increased risk of methotrexate-induced hepatotoxicity [77, 78]. Patients with psoriasis have a higher prevalence of metabolic syndrome and nonalcoholic hepatic steatosis compared to patients with rheumatoid arthritis [78–80]. Alcohol use should be avoided, and patients should have serial monitoring of liver function tests at 2–4 week intervals for the first 3 months after initiation of therapy and then at 8–12 week intervals thereafter [27]. An increase in methotrexate dose or combination therapy with known hepatotoxic agents (leflunomide, sulfasalazine, azathioprine) would require more frequent and vigilant monitoring. Patients on methotrexate with persistent elevations in 5/9 aspartate aminotransferase levels over 12 months or decreased serum albumin levels should be referred for a liver biopsy. A liver biopsy prior to initiation of therapy may be needed in patients with a known history of chronic alcohol use, persistently elevated transaminases, or chronic viral hepatitis. Given the higher risk of hepatotoxicity in patients with psoriasis, the American Academy of Dermatology recommends that a liver biopsy should be done in low-risk patients (no comorbidities) with psoriasis after a cumulative dose of 3.5–4 g of methotrexate, with consideration for subsequent biopsies after a further cumulative dose of 1.5 g. Patients at high risk (diabetes, obesity, abnormal liver function tests, hazardous alcohol intake, and chronic liver disease) should be considered for a liver biopsy after 6 months of methotrexate therapy and subsequent biopsies after cumulative doses of 1–1.5 g [27, 81].

There is no absolute contraindication for the use of methotrexate in patients with chronic liver disease, although a dose reduction by 75% has been suggested in patients with a bilirubin level of 3.1–5 mg/dL or transaminases >3 times ULN, and complete avoidance in patients with a bilirubin >5 mg/dl. Patients with chronic liver disease should be referred to a hepatologist for guidance prior to initiating therapy with methotrexate. Both alcoholic liver disease and steatohepatitis have been identified as underlying conditions which significantly increase the risk of methotrexate hepatotoxicity, and it would be prudent to consider alternative therapeutic options in these patients [82].

Leflunomide has been associated with hepatotoxicity since its emergence as a csDMARD in 1998. There were 49 reported cases of severe liver failure between 2002 and 2009 prompting a black box warning by the United States Food and Drug Administration in 2011 [83]. More than 90% of these cases were associated with preexisting liver disease and/or concomitant use of another hepatotoxic agent (methotrexate, alcohol). Currently, leflunomide may be used in patients where prior transaminitis has normalized but is not recommended in patients with preexisting liver disease [27]. Hepatic function should be monitored every 4 weeks for 3 months after initiation of therapy and then at least every 3 months for the duration of therapy [84]. In cases of ALT elevation >2ULN, leflunomide should be discontinued and cholestyramine washout begun.

There is no known direct hepatotoxic effect associated with the TNF-alpha inhibitors, but warnings have been issued for possible severe liver failure with infliximab unrelated to viral hepatitis. Infliximab is associated with transient elevations of transaminases with repeated infusions, cholestatic hepatitis, and an autoimmune hepatitis marked by the presence of autoantibodies. Both etanercept and adalimumab may cause mild transient elevations of transaminases and rarely, clinically apparent liver injury which may be immune mediated.

Belimumab and ustekinumab have been associated with rare instances of transaminases elevation, without reports of serious or fatal hepatotoxicity. These events did not require discontinuation of either drug [85]. There are no contraindications to the use of TNF-alpha inhibitors, belimumab, or ustekinumab in patients with chronic liver disease.

HIV

Logically, it would seem that immunosuppressive therapy in a patient with HIV would increase the risk of opportunistic infections or lead to exacerbation of underlying infection. However, several DMARDs have been safely used in patients with HIV. Academic organizations recommend that immunomodulating therapy should only be used in HIV-positive patients with a stable CD4 count of $>200 \times 10^6$/L.

Hydroxychloroquine and sulfasalazine appear to be safe and well tolerated in patients with HIV, and the antimalarials have antiviral properties mediated by intracellular inhibition of posttranslational modification of gp120. Hydroxychloroquine has been evaluated in the treatment of HIV infection and the associated immune reconstitution syndrome. The results of clinical trials have been variable, attributed to the varying doses of hydroxychloroquine used, as the antiviral effect is thought to be dose dependent [86–89]. For patients on highly active antiretroviral therapy (HAART), there are no major drug interactions with hydroxychloroquine. Prior to the routine use of antiretroviral therapy, there were case reports of fatal opportunistic infections in patients with concomitant HIV infection and methotrexate therapy; however, it appears safe for use in patients with stable HIV infection on therapy [90–92]. MMF, cyclosporine, azathioprine, and leflunomide have also been used successfully in patients with HIV, and all have antiviral properties. MMF and cyclosporine inhibit HIV replication by decreasing the numbers of activated CD4 + lymphocytes, needed for active viral replication, and additionally MMF inhibits reverse transcriptase. Both MMF and leflunomide have been evaluated in clinical trials as adjuncts to antiretroviral therapy with generally favorable but variable results. In one clinical trial, leflunomide was found to be superior to MMF in suppressing in vitro viral replication [93–98].

There is limited data available on apremilast and tofacitinib in patients with HIV. The Janus activating kinase-signal transducer and activator of transcription (JAK-STAT) pathway is activated early in HIV-1 infection and promotes viral replication and HIV-associated inflammation and has been proposed as a new target in the treatment of HIV infection. [99].

TNF alpha has been implicated in the pathogenesis and progression of HIV infection, and, theoretically, TNF-alpha inhibitors should have little effect on the progression of HIV disease. The TNF-alpha inhibitors have been used safely in patients with HIV who have stable CD4 counts above 200 × 10^6/L, with a single report of recurrent polymicrobial infections in those with lower counts [100, 101]. In patients with HIV-associated lymphoma, rituximab does not seem to increase the risk of opportunistic infection [102]. Ustekinumab has been safely used in patients with psoriasis and HIV [103, 104]. Data on the use of other bDMARDs in patients with HIV are limited.

It is recommended that patients should be screened for HIV before they start treatment with DMARDs. Most immunosuppressive therapies seem to be safe in patients with HIV who have a stable CD4 count of >200 × 10^6/L. Decisions with respect to therapy should be made together with the patient and infectious disease specialists. Patients should have regular monitoring of CD4 counts and HIV viral loads while taking DMARDs.

Latent Tuberculosis

Patients with rheumatic diseases have an increased risk of developing infection with mycobacterium tuberculosis (TB) [105–107], and this risk may be potentiated by immunosuppressive therapy such as corticosteroids and DMARDs. The risk is exponentially higher with bDMARDs compared to csDMARDs, with one study quoting a RR of 1.5 (95 % CI 1.1–1.9) with bDMARDs and 1.2 with csDMARDs (95 % CI 1.0–1.5) [105]. Pulmonary TB was more commonly noted in patients on bDMARDs than non-pulmonary TB. The risk of reactivation of TB in patients with hydroxychloroquine and sulfasalazine is considered low, and hydroxychloroquine is most often associated with non-TB mycobacterial infection [108]. Methotrexate, however, has been occasionally implicated in both the occurrence of primary TB and reactivation of TB [109, 110]. There are also reports of reactivation of TB occurring in the presence of therapy with leflunomide, MMF, and azathioprine, although the true impact of these medications is unclear due to concomitant use of glucocorticoids [111–113]. There are no reports of reactivation with belimumab or apremilast, and the occurrence of opportunistic infections with anakinra is rare [114, 115]. There have been a few isolated cases of TB reactivation with ustekinumab but no reports of this with secukinumab during clinical trials or since its approval [60, 116, 117].

The risk of TB reactivation seems to be highest with TNF-alpha inhibitors, with reported rates four times that seen in patients with rheumatoid arthritis not treated with these agents [118]. TNF-alpha inhibitors are also associated with increased rates of nontuberculous mycobacterial infections [119]. The risk of reactivating TB seems to be greatest with infliximab and lowest with etanercept [118, 120]. Reports of TB reactivation with abatacept, tocilizumab, and rituximab are rare, and rituximab is considered safer than the other bDMARDs [121–125].

Patients should be screened for latent TB before starting treatment with a bDMARD, and although there is insufficient data to mandate screening for TB before treatment with rituximab, its use is not recommended in the presence of opportunistic infections [126, 127]. Rituximab is suggested as the first-line bDMARD if TB chemoprophylaxis is contraindicated and for patients from endemic regions [128]. Patients should be screened for latent TB infection according to regional guidelines with either the tuberculin skin test (TST) or interferon gamma release assay (IGRA). Indeterminate IGRA tests should either be repeated or should be followed by a TST. Expert opinion is divided on the superiority of either test, and both are reported to perform similarly in immunocompromised people [129]. Patients with positive results (TST or IGRA) should have a chest radiograph to exclude active tuberculosis and, if negative, begin treatment for latent tuberculosis infection at least 1 month prior to starting bDMARD therapy [126]. The value of serial tuberculosis screening thereafter, in the absence of known exposure or high risk, is unclear [44, 129].

Cancer

Rheumatic disease affects the incidence of certain malignancies. Patients with scleroderma have an increased risk of lung cancer, while lymphoma is increased in Sjögren's syndrome and rheumatoid arthritis, particularly active disease for the latter [130]. Advances in the treatment of cancer by inducing remission or slowing tumor growth and spread have improved the prognosis for many patients. Consequently cancer has become a chronic disease. Anti-rheumatic medications, by impairing tumor surveillance, may inadvertently awaken previously dormant malignant cells (Table 17.2). Thus suppressing the activity of a rheumatic disease without stimulating the regrowth of a cancer presents a challenge.

Hydroxychloroquine is a weaker immunosuppressant and hence not expected to promote the growth of malignant cells. In fact, the inhibitory effect of hydroxychloroquine on autophagy has prompted its experimental use as an adjuvant to the chemotherapy of certain cancers [131]. Hydroxychloroquine is tolerated by most patients; however, side effects include hemolysis, particularly in patients with glucose-6-phosphae dehydrogenase (G-6PD) deficiency. Screening cancer patients for this enzyme deficiency prior to beginning treatment with hydroxychloroquine is recommended. If the patient should consequently develop anemia, cancer chemotherapy is the likely culprit provided G-6PD levels were previously normal. There are no published reports of sulfasalazine promoting the de novo occurrence of cancer or its recurrence; similar to hydroxychloroquine sulfasalazine is being investigated as an adjuvant agent in the treatment of cancers [132].

Methotrexate was first used in childhood leukemia as an antimetabolite by inhibiting folic acid function. However, as a csDMARD low-dose methotrexate may function via other mechanisms including increasing cytoplasmic adenosine or blocking cyclooxygenase and lipoxygenase enzymes. However, low-dose methotrexate is

Table 17.2 Recommendations for the use of anti-rheumatic medications in patients with rheumatoid arthritis and specific comorbidities

Recommendation	Level of evidence[a]
Cancer	
Age-appropriate cancer screening as per national guidelines if not previously performed (AR)	IV
Hydroxychloroquine and sulfasalazine may be used with most cancers provided no interaction with chemotherapy (AR)	IV
Methotrexate, azathioprine, and MMF should be avoided or used with caution in patients with a history of lymphoma (AR)	IV
Hold or delay bDMARDs in patients with active cancer while receiving chemotherapy or radiotherapy (CRA)	IV
TNF-alpha inhibitors are not recommended or should be used with caution in patients with treated lymphoma (CRA, ACR) [126, 159]	III
Consider rituximab in patients with treated lymphoma (CRA, ACR)	IV
Patients with a treated solid cancer >5 years earlier may receive a bDMARD (ACR), or these drugs may be used with caution (CRA) [126, 159]	II
Cardiovascular disease	
Optimum management of traditional cardiovascular disease risk factors (AR)	IV
Hydroxychloroquine, methotrexate, sulfasalazine, azathioprine, methotrexate, leflunomide, and MMF may be used in patients with CAD (AR)	IV
Clinical monitoring for symptoms of heart failure in patients taking TNF-alpha inhibitors	IV
TNF-alpha inhibitors are contraindicated inpatients with class III or class IV heart failure (ACR, CRA, EMA) [126]	III
Rituximab is contraindicated in class IV heart failure or uncontrolled CAD(EMA) [170]	IV
Interstitial lung disease	
Hydroxychloroquine, sulfasalazine, azathioprine, MMF, and cyclophosphamide may be used with clinical monitoring of patients (AR)	IV
Methotrexate and leflunomide should be avoided in patients with active ILD	IV
Patients should have PFT with DLCO and consultation with a pulmonologist before starting bDMARDs [204]	IV
Chronic obstructive pulmonary disease (COPD)	
TNF-alpha inhibitors recommended [208]	II
Avoid abatacept in patients with symptomatic COPD [209]	II
Diabetes	
Hydroxychloroquine, sulfasalazine, azathioprine, and MMF do not worsen glycemic control	IV
Methotrexate requires careful monitoring of liver function in diabetics [212, 213]	IV
bDMARDs recommended [135, 136]	II
Monitor patients with brittle diabetes who start a TNF-alpha inhibitor for hypoglycemia [137]	III

(continued)

Table 17.2 (continued)

Recommendation	Level of evidence[a]
Renal	
Hydroxychloroquine appears to be the safest drug	IV
Avoid methotrexate if creatinine clearance <50 ml/min/1.73m^2 [217]	IV
Azathioprine, cyclophosphamide, and MMF may require a decreased dose and careful monitoring of blood counts	IV
bDMARDs may be used with caution	IV
Pregnancy	
Methotrexate, MMF, and leflunomide are contraindicated	II
Azathioprine, sulfasalazine, and hydroxychloroquine use requires discussion of risks to fetus with obstetrician and patient	IV
bDMARDs not recommended during pregnancy (EMA)	IV
Given the absence of evidenced-based data, a discussion between patient, obstetrician, and rheumatologist is recommended before planning a pregnancy [143]	III

Abbreviations: *AR* authors' recommendations, *ACR* 2012 update of the American College of Rheumatology recommendations, *CRA* Canadian Rheumatology Association recommendations for the pharmacological management of rheumatoid arthritis, *EMA* European Medicines Agency approved summary of product characteristics, *EULAR* European League against Rheumatism, *HBsAg* hepatitis B surface antigen, *HBcAg* hepatitis B core antibody, *MMF* mycophenolate mofetil, *TNF-alpha* tumor necrosis factor alpha

[a]Levels of evidence I = meta-analyses, systematic reviews of randomized controlled trials (RCTs), or individual RCTs; II = meta-analysis of systemic reviews of observational studies, case control studies; III = case series and case reports; IV = expert opinion

associated with lymphoproliferative and possibly other malignancies in patients with rheumatoid arthritis and Sjögren's syndrome. These lymphomas are often associated with Epstein-Barr virus and regress after withdrawal of methotrexate [133, 134]. This increased risk, however, is not solely due to the drug and is in part caused by the under lying rheumatic disease. Supporting this is a report from the Swedish National Patient Register which found no increased risk for lymphoma in patients with psoriatic arthritis treated with methotrexate [135]. Other cancers may be increased with methotrexate, specifically melanoma, in patients with rheumatoid arthritis and nonmelanoma skin cancer in psoriasis [136]. The effect methotrexate may have on solid tumors is not clearly defined.

Given the current data, it appears prudent to discontinue methotrexate regardless of the underlying rheumatic disease if the patient develops a new lymphoma or melanoma even if they were on treatment with a concomitant tumor necrosis factor alpha inhibitor. Recommendations for patients with solid tumors are less clear, but regardless a discussion with the patient's oncologist is warranted.

Leflunomide was first used in 1998 in the treatment of rheumatoid arthritis, and there are no reported associations with lymphoma or nonmelanoma skin cancer [137]. This drug should be avoided if patients are to be treated with other drugs that may suppress the bone marrow, precluding its use in patients receiving many chemotherapeutic regimens [138]. Leflunomide and its active metabolites have a prolonged half-life and may take up to 2 years to achieve low serum concentrations.

If chemotherapy that is likely to suppress the bone marrow is to be administered, an enhanced removal of leflunomide may be performed with cholestyramine, 8 g, three times daily for 11 days.

Azathioprine, similar to methotrexate, is associated with an increased risk of lymphoproliferative malignancies [139]. However, much of the evidence comes from the transplant literature, where azathioprine is used in combination regimens; an increased risk of squamous cell skin cancer has been reported [140]. The associations between azathioprine and cancer render it a less than ideal choice for rheumatic patients with current or a recent cancer diagnosis.

Cyclophosphamide is a chemotherapeutic drug that has found use for some of the most severe and life-threatening rheumatic diseases, specifically lupus nephritis and antineutrophil cytoplasmic antibody-associated vasculitis. Bladder cancer is associated with the use of cyclophosphamide in a dose-dependent relationship [141]. However, a number of other malignancies including squamous cell skin cancer, leukemia, and lymphoma are associated with cyclophosphamide [141]. The side effects of cyclophosphamide include bone marrow suppression, and frequent monitoring of cell counts is required with its use in rheumatic diseases. Ideally this agent should not be utilized for the treatment of rheumatic diseases in patients with malignancies; however, given that it is reserved for the most severe often life-threatening situations, other options may be limited; a careful and frank discussion with the patient and oncologist is imperative. Patients also require monitoring of their urine for red blood cells after being treated with cyclophosphamide. If microscopic or gross hematuria occurs, cystoscopy to rule out bladder cancer should be performed. MMF is used in combination immunosuppression post-solid organ transplantation, clouding interpretation of its malignancy risk. A report of solid organ transplant recipients noted an increased risk for colorectal cancer associated with cyclosporine and azathioprine but not for MMF and tacrolimus [142]. However an association with lymphoproliferative disease specifically CNS lymphoma was noted in renal transplant recipients treated with MMF [143]. Thus like most of the immunosuppressive agents, MMF should be avoided in patients with a history of lymphoma.

Apremilast is a selective inhibitor of phosphodiesterase 4 that increases intracellular cyclic adenosine and is approved for the treatment of psoriatic skin and joint disease. It is well tolerated; however because of reports of suicidal ideation, it should be used with caution in patients with cancer who are prone to the development of depression. These patients should be monitored clinically for the development of symptoms suggestive of melancholy. Apremilast may also interact with chemotherapeutic agents that are inducers of CYP3A4 and should be avoided if these drugs are required.

Tofacitinib is an oral-selective Janus kinase inhibitor used to control symptomatic rheumatoid arthritis. An analysis of pooled data from phase II and phase III clinical trials and two long-term extension studies reported an expected rate of malignancy for lymphoma, solid tumors, and nonmelanoma skin cancer [144]. The American College of Rheumatology, however, recommends the use of csDMARDs over tofacitinib for patients with prior treated or untreated melanoma or nonmelanoma skin cancer [8].

TNF alpha has a paradoxical effect on malignant cells; high doses may be cytotoxic to some tumor cells, but other cancers may produce TNF alpha that stimulates their growth. The body's own tumor surveillance system includes $CD8^+$ T cells and natural killer cells that utilize TNF alpha against immunogenic tumor cells [145, 146]. Randomized controlled trials of TNF-alpha inhibitors compared with placebo reported a safety concern related to malignancies [146]. Disparate results are reported from two meta-analyses and the acknowledgement of the prolonged latency period, years for most cancers, stressed the need for long-term data to study the safety of TNF-alpha inhibitors and other bDMARDs under development.

National registries and chronic disease cohorts for rheumatic diseases have provided a resource for analyzing the risk for developing cancer. A US observational study compared cancer rates with data from the US National Cancer Institute Surveillance, Epidemiology, and End Results (SEER) database [148]. The study pooled results for three TNF-alpha inhibitors, infliximab, etanercept, and adalimumab, and the IL1 receptor antagonist, anakinra. These bDMARDs were associated with an increased risk for nonmelanoma skin cancer but not for solid tumors, and after controlling for the severity of rheumatoid arthritis, there was no increased risk of lymphoma. However, this study did not examine the risk of recurrence in patients with a prior cancer history.

Reports from three European biologic registries have sought to answer this question. There was no increased risk of solid tumors or lymphoma associated with TNF-alpha inhibitors in patients with prior malignancies reported from the German biologic and British biologic registries [149, 150]. Additionally a case control study examining the risk for recurrence of breast cancer, which was performed utilizing data from the Swedish biologic registry (ARTIS), reported similar recurrence rates for patients treated with TNF-alpha inhibitors and non-TNF-alpha inhibitors [151, 152]. This data should be interpreted with caution as the interval between the diagnosis of cancer and initiation of the TNF-alpha inhibitors was greater than 5 years in both the German and British registries. Both the American College of Rheumatology and the Canadian Rheumatology Association do not recommend the use of TNF-alpha inhibitors in patients with current or recent (< 5 years) solid tumors or skin cancer. They are best avoided in patients with a prior lymphoma.

An analysis of pooled data for patients who were entered into long-term extension studies for tocilizumab in rheumatoid arthritis and had a mean of 4 years of follow-up reported an expected rate of malignancies [153]. This information, while reassuring, does not apprise us on the effect of tocilizumab on current or recent cancers. It should be noted, however, that tocilizumab has been used successfully in the management of multi-centric Castleman's disease, a lymphoproliferative disorder [154]. Abatacept has not been reported to have any cancer associations in clinical trials; however, reports of eruptive squamous cell skin cancer have tempered any enthusiasm regarding its safety in patients with prior malignancies [152, 155]. There are reports from two registries, the German psoriasis biologics registry PsoBest and the Psoriasis Longitudinal Assessment and Registry (PSLOAR), that reported no increased malignancy signal with ustekinumab [156, 157].

Rituximab, although utilized in the treatment of lymphoma, has an unknown effect on solid and cutaneous malignancies. Pooled data from eight randomized and two long-term extension studies did not discern an increased risk for any malignancies associated with rituximab in patients with rheumatoid arthritis [158]. Both the American College of Rheumatology and the Canadian Rheumatology Association recommend the use of rituximab in patients with a prior history of lymphoma, solid tumors, nonmelanoma skin cancer, and melanoma within the past 5 years over TNF-alpha inhibitors [126, 159]. A study of pooled data from a phase II and two phase III clinical trials of belimumab in patients with SLE did not report an increased risk for malignancy [160].

Treating rheumatic diseases in patients with cancer is challenging. Rheumatologists must seek out not only the type (lymphoproliferative, solid, melanoma, or nonmelanoma skin cancer) but also the stage, presence of metastases, prognosis, and type of treatment. Only then can a frank discussion take place to determine goals of care for the rheumatic disease, symptom control and prevention of major organ damage, or tight control of disease activity. Selection of appropriate anti-rheumatic therapy requires an assessment of the oncogenic potential of the drug but also its side effects, bone marrow suppression, for example, and potential interactions with current or planned chemotherapy. Low-dose prednisone should not be forgotten when symptom control is the primary goal of treatment.

Cardiovascular Disease

The inherent inflammatory nature of certain rheumatologic diseases like rheumatoid arthritis increases the risk of cardiovascular disease (atherosclerosis, cerebrovascular disease, coronary artery disease, heart failure, myocardial infarction) beyond that attributable to traditional risk factors.

Hydroxychloroquine has myriad beneficial effects in addition to its anti-rheumatic properties including a less atherogenic lipid profile, antithrombotic properties, and a decreased risk of diabetes. In addition, a recent study showed that its use was associated with a 72% decrease in the risk of incident cardiovascular disease (CVD) in rheumatoid arthritis patients (hazard ratio [HR] 0.28) [161]. Incident CVD was defined as a composite of coronary artery disease (CAD), stroke, transient ischemic attack, sudden cardiac death, and peripheral artery disease with arterial revascularization procedure. Patients on hydroxychloroquine should be monitored for the possible development of a drug-induced cardiomyopathy due to an acquired lysosomal storage disorder. Hydroxychloroquine-related cardiomyopathy is characterized by concentric hypertrophy and conduction abnormalities [162]. Most clinical manifestations of this entity occur after 3 years of exposure, but there is a wide range of variability in this regard. It is imperative to recognize this entity as it is potentially reversible if identified in its early stages. Although no formal recommendations are in place, annual electrocardiograms should be considered, with further testing, i.e., cardiac MRI, echocardiogram, and endomyocardial biopsy, to be pursued depending on any abnormal results [162].

Based on outcomes of randomized controlled trials (RCTs) to evaluate the efficacy of etanercept and infliximab (ATTACH) in treating heart failure, TNF-α inhibitors are contraindicated in patients with New York Heart Association (NYHA) class III–IV heart failure and to be used with caution in those with NYHA class II heart failure [163–165]. According to 2012 ACR guidelines, TNF-alpha inhibitors are not recommended in patients with NYHA class III–IV heart failure who have an ejection fraction of 50% or less [126]. In those patients without a history of heart failure, baseline screening echocardiograms prior to starting TNF-alpha inhibitors are not recommended [166]. Although limited by various factors, clinical registry data from Germany found no significant risk for exacerbation of or new onset of heart failure with TNF-alpha inhibitors versus csDMARDs [167].

Prospective data from the British Society of Rheumatology Biologics Register (BSRBR) showed an incidence rate ratio (IRR) of 1.44 for initial myocardial infarction (MI) in patients treated with TNF-alpha inhibitors versus those treated with csDMARDs. However, they also showed an IRR for initial MI of 0.36 in "responder" patients treated with TNF-alpha inhibitors (response within 6 months of treatment) versus those whom were "nonresponders" [6]. Overall, evidence does not support that TNF-alpha inhibitors are contraindicated in patients with previous CAD or MI. In fact, a retrospective US study showed that use of TNF-alpha inhibitors was associated with a 55% reduction in the risk of incident CAD events (coronary revascularization procedure, MI, unstable angina) versus use of csDMARDs (excluding methotrexate) with a HR of 0.45 [168].

With regard to abatacept, cardiovascular events are uncommon, and the presence of stable CVD does not preclude its use [169]. With regard to rituximab, it is contraindicated in patients with NYHA class IV heart failure or uncontrolled CAD [170]. With regard to tocilizumab, it is known that it is associated with induction of an atherogenic lipid profile, but this does not necessarily translate into increased CVD events [125, 171]. This effect, i.e., changes in lipid profile, is not usually seen in patients treated with TNF-alpha inhibitors. Serious adverse event rates, including cardiac deaths, serious MIs, and serious strokes, were similar in post-marketing tocilizumab data sets as compared to those seen in tocilizumab clinical trials and users of TNF-alpha inhibitors [172]. Despite an elevation in lipid levels seen with tofacitinib, studies with this medication to date have not shown that this translates into an increase in major adverse cardiac events (MACEs) [173].

Anakinra, in addition to standard therapy, has been shown to be effective in preventing left ventricular remodeling and the development of heart failure in the post-MI period [174]. Improved exercise performance has been shown in patients with heart failure whom were given a 14-day course of anakinra [174]. Improved cardiac contractility was shown in rheumatoid arthritis patients getting anakinra, even within a few hours of a single dose [174]. In patients with diastolic heart failure, those given a 14-day course of anakinra showed increased peak oxygen consumption [174].

With regard to IL-12/23 blocking agents, namely, ustekinumab, there has been varying results with regard to its association with MACEs. Two meta-analyses of RCTs regarding its use in patients with psoriasis showed no statistically significant increased risk of MACEs and a statistically significant increased odds ratio (OR) for MACEs of 4.23, respectively [175]. Data with regard to this imbalance in MACEs is less compelling in patients using ustekinumab for treatment of psoriatic arthritis. An important consideration to take into account as a clinician is that patients with more severe psoriasis and psoriatic arthritis are at increased risk of MACEs independent of traditional risk factors. It is advisable that modifiable cardiovascular risk factors be optimized in patients with psoriasis and psoriatic arthritis [175]. A recent study looking at the use of bDMARDs for treatment of severe psoriasis, including ustekinumab, showed that patients treated with bDMARDs had reduced CAD progression as assessed by contrast-enhanced coronary CT angiography and non-contrast coronary artery calcium CT at baseline and after 13 months of follow-up [176].

There is insufficient data to contraindicate the use of bDMARDs in patients with previous cerebrovascular disease.

Rheumatic patients with a higher risk for cardiovascular disease should have optimum management of all traditional risk factors coupled with tight control of their inflammatory disease.

Interstitial Lung Disease

Interstitial lung disease (ILD) occurs with varying frequencies in many rheumatic diseases. The absence of a biomarker and presentations that may be mistaken for infection, asthma, or heart failure delays recognition. Its management is complicated by imprecise tools, high-resolution computerized tomography of the chest, or pulmonary function tests for monitoring treatment response or disease progression. Complicating this situation is the association of many anti-rheumatic medications with ILD.

Methotrexate-induced ILD was reported in leukemia, psoriasis, and rheumatoid arthritis albeit at a lower dose in the latter [177–179]. The typical presentation is that of an acute or subacute hypersensitivity pneumonitis with granuloma formation and bronchiolitis or diffuse alveolar damage from a toxic drug reaction. The clinical presentation is nonspecific and includes dyspnea and nonproductive cough with or without fever. Symptoms may resolve with discontinuation of the drug or progress to respiratory failure. Chronic interstitial lung disease secondary to methotrexate is reported, but given the nonspecific presentation that can mimic lung disease associated with many of the connective tissue disorders, its existence as a distinct syndrome is questioned. A study of rheumatoid arthritis patients followed prospectively with serial pulmonary function tests and high-resolution computerized tomographic scans of the chest over 2 years reported no evidence of low-dose methotrexate associated chronic interstitial lung disease [180]. Supporting this was a report of clinical trials for psoriasis, psoriatic arthritis, and inflammatory bowel disease where no increased risk of methotrexate lung toxicity was reported [181].

The diagnosis of methotrexate-induced lung disease is clinical; usually patients will have used the methotrexate for less than a year, but hypersensitivity pneumonitis may occur in patients who have been using the drug for longer. Diagnostic imaging is nonspecific with chest radiographs and computerized tomography scans revealing patchy, diffuse, or focal infiltrates, but high resolution scanning may reveal ground-glass infiltrates, findings that may be seen with rheumatoid arthritis, scleroderma, and other connective tissue diseases. Improvement in symptoms with drug withdrawal supports the diagnosis of methotrexate-induced ILD. Rechallenging is not recommended.

Methotrexate remains an integral part of the management of patients with rheumatic diseases, even in the presence of lung disease [182]. In fact, given the prevalence of ILD in many rheumatic diseases including rheumatoid arthritis, patients with asymptomatic lung disease are treated with methotrexate without adverse respiratory events [180]. Given the current availability of alternative drugs, patients who have presumed ILD secondary to methotrexate should not be rechallenged. Use of methotrexate in patients with ILD secondary to their underlying rheumatic disease remains controversial. Serial monitoring of pulmonary function tests has not been uniformly recommended given their variable ability to predict pneumonitis [183, 184]. Patients at greatest risk of methotrexate-induced lung injury include older patients, diabetics, pleural-pulmonary involvement secondary to rheumatoid arthritis, prior use of DMARDs, and hypoalbuminemia.

Shortly after the release of leflunomide in Japan, several reports of ILD secondary to this drug were published in 2004 [185]. Further reports describe a more consistent clinical picture with acute lung disease occurring within 20 weeks of initiating the drug. Computerized tomography of the chest revealed diffuse ground-glass alveolar opacities, but cryptogenic organizing pneumonia was also reported [186]. Further studies of a large cohort reported that there was no increased risk for hospitalization secondary to ILD associated with leflunomide for patients without a prior history of lung disease and who had not been previously treated with methotrexate [187]. The authors concluded that the apparent increased rate of ILD associated with leflunomide was the result of channeling patients at high risk for developing ILD to that drug. We recommend that leflunomide not be used in patients with preexisting ILD or methotrexate-induced ILD, even if the patient has made a full recovery. Methotrexate should also not be used concurrently with leflunomide [188].

MMF and cyclophosphamide have both been reported to be efficacious in patients with scleroderma-associated ILD [189]. Similarly azathioprine, hydroxychloroquine, and sulfasalazine are not reported to be associated with pulmonary toxicity and are relatively safe in patients with ILD. However, patients should be informed of rare or idiosyncratic reactions affecting the lungs with many medications; there is a report of nonspecific interstitial pneumonia associated with MMF [190].

TNF-alpha has a complex and sometimes opposing role in lung pathology. This cytokine has a central role in granuloma formation whether combating infectious agents such as mycobacteria or in granulomatous diseases like sarcoidosis. TNF-alpha may be pro-fibrotic and have a pathogenic role in idiopathic pulmonary fibrosis [191]. Despite apparent success in small studies, TNF-alpha inhibitors were not successful in larger trials of idiopathic pulmonary fibrosis [192]. Notwithstanding TNF-alpha inhibitors were used with success in the treatment of other fibrotic and granulomatous pulmonary diseases including scleroderma, sarcoidosis, and RA-associated ILD [193–195]. Hence it was surprising to see reports of TNF-alpha inhibitors linked to rheumatoid arthritis-associated ILD exacerbations and sarcoidosis [196, 197]. Because ILD may occur in rheumatoid arthritis without the use of TNF-alpha inhibitors or csDAMRDs, the information from these case reports and case series is difficult to interpret. Supporting a lack of association is an analysis of data from a US cohort of greater than 8000 patients with rheumatoid arthritis that were followed for more than 10 years and reported no association between ILD and TNF-alpha inhibitors [198].

Reports supporting a link between TNF-alpha inhibitors and the development or progression of ILD have noted the onset of respiratory symptoms within 6 months of beginning therapy. Other potential factors include concomitant therapy with methotrexate, prior use of csDMARDs, and older age [196].

Rituximab is utilized in the treatment of a number of rheumatic diseases with lung involvement. Rituximab was associated with an increase in carbon monoxide pulmonary diffusing capacity in patients with scleroderma-associated ILD in a small study [199]. These results were supported by similar outcomes from the European Scleroderma Trial and Research (EUSTAR) cohort [200].

There are case reports of exacerbations of ILD in patients treated with tocilizumab and abatacept [201, 202]. An analysis of combined data from the Medicare supplemental and commercial claims and encounter databases examined the incidence of ILD in users of abatacept, rituximab tocilizumab, and TNF-alpha inhibitors and did not find any difference in the incidence of ILD for any of these agents [203].

ILD occurs in many rheumatic diseases, and with the difficulty of its evaluation, assigning cause to underlying disease, anti-rheumatic medication, or opportunistic infection is challenging. Prior to beginning anti-rheumatic medications, patients should be questioned and examined for pulmonary disease. Those with unexplained shortness of breath or chronic cough should be evaluated by pulmonary function testing, and if the carbon monoxide pulmonary diffusing capacity is below 70%, a high-resolution computerized tomography is recommended [204]. The selection of the csDMARD or bDMARD will depend on the underlying disease and prior therapy. Although MMF and rituximab appear to be the agents least associated with progression of ILD, rare pulmonary adverse events have been reported. Whichever agent is chosen, it appears best to avoid combination therapy if possible and monitor the patients for symptomatic progression or with serial carbon monoxide pulmonary diffusing capacity [204].

Asthma and Chronic Obstructive Pulmonary Disease

Asthma and chronic obstructive pulmonary disease are common ailments and though unrelated may accompany many rheumatic diseases. More severe cases are corticosteroid-dependent and immunosuppressant drugs including methotrexate and azathioprine, were used to successfully lower the corticosteroid dose [205, 206]. Biologic agents specifically TNF-alpha inhibitors have been studied as therapeutic agents for both COPD and asthma with mixed results, a disappointing outcome given the pathogenic role of TNF-alpha in both diseases [207]. Patients with rheumatoid arthritis prescribed etanercept had a decreased risk for hospitalization for COPD on review of a North American claims database [208]. However, not all biologics were found to be without risk of exacerbation of respiratory symptoms. One of the early trials of abatacept in rheumatoid arthritis enrolled 54 patients (4%) with COPD, 37 of whom received abatacept, the remainder placebo [209]. Respiratory complications occurred nearly twice as frequently in the abatacept group compared with the placebo group. Ustekinumab on the other hand was reported to improve not only psoriatic skin disease in one patient but she was also able to taper off all of the maintenance medications for her asthma [210]. Although most immunosuppressive agents and biologics appear to be well tolerated in patients with asthma and COPD, these respiratory diseases are susceptible to external triggers, and any new medication could trigger bronchospasm. Abatacept is best used with caution in patients with COPD and avoided if the disease is uncontrolled.

Diabetes Mellitus

Diabetes mellitus is a metabolic disease characterized by hyperglycemia, inadequate insulin secretion, and insulin resistance. Many chronic rheumatic diseases are associated with inflammation that impairs glucose handling and increases insulin resistance that can be ameliorated with control of the disease activity [211]. However, high doses or chronic use of prednisone may offset any beneficial glycemic effect because of steroid-induced diabetes. Apart from prednisone and related corticosteroids, other anti-rheumatic medications do not directly increase the glycemic index. However, patients with diabetes are at risk for the development of coronary artery disease and infections. These potential complications should be considered when selecting anti-rheumatic medications.

Hepatotoxicity is a major complication associated with chronic methotrexate therapy. In early studies diabetes mellitus was reported as a risk factor for hepatotoxicity from methotrexate in patients with psoriasis and rheumatoid arthritis [212, 213]. Subsequently on further review, many of these patients were obese, a contributing factor to the development of steatohepatitis. It is thus prudent to follow methotrexate monitoring guidelines for patients with diabetes. Other potential hepatotoxic drugs particularly alcohol must be avoided. Other anti-rheumatic drugs including hydroxychloroquine, sulfasalazine, azathioprine, and MMF are not reported to worsen glycemic control.

Infliximab improved insulin resistance in nondiabetic patients with rheumatoid arthritis [7]. Along these lines tocilizumab was reported to improve glycosylated hemoglobin values in patients with rheumatoid arthritis and type 2 diabetes, while none of their nondiabetic counterparts experienced hypoglycemic episodes [214]. There is one report of a patient with type I diabetes mellitus developing a severe hypoglycemic episode within 12 h of starting adalimumab [215]. Although there are concerns regarding infections both in diabetic patients and patients on TNF-alpha inhibitors, one study evaluating the long-term safety of etanercept in patients with comorbidities included 265 patients with diabetes who were followed for a mean of 3.5 years and reported no increased risk of infections [216]. All diabetic patients on anti-rheumatic drugs should be observed for infections.

Renal Disease

Methotrexate is primarily eliminated via the kidneys with active tubular secretion playing a role. Weak acids may impair excretion. Biliary secretion accounts for less than 10% of the removal of methotrexate from the body. Methotrexate is often the first csDMARD selected in treating rheumatoid arthritis and psoriatic arthritis, two rheumatic diseases where kidney disease is not a major manifestation. Renal impairment in patients with these diseases is usually secondary to hypertension, diabetes mellitus, or other comorbid illnesses and may be slowly progressive. Rheumatologists may be less inclined to monitor renal function deferring this to the patients' internist, risking inappropriate dosing of methotrexate in these patients. Patients with chronic kidney disease are at greater risk for the development of pancytopenia secondary to methotrexate. Methotrexate should not be used for treating chronic rheumatic diseases in patients with serum creatinine greater than 2.0 mg/dl (152.5 μmol/L) or creatinine clearance <50 ml/min/1.73 m^2 [217].

Although leflunomide is excreted in the feces and also urine, the European Medicines Agency recommends that moderate to severe renal impairment is a contraindication because of insufficient data in this population. Recently leflunomide has been studied as a therapeutic option for patients with lupus nephritis and, one review reported comparable efficacy to cyclophosphamide [218]. In a recent cross-sectional study of patients with rheumatoid arthritis and ESRD, hydroxychloroquine was the most frequently used csDMARD and appears relatively safe in that population [219].

Azathioprine, cyclophosphamide, and MMF are potent immunosuppressive agents that are used in the treatment of glomerulonephritis associated with SLE and ANCA-associated vasculitis. Despite the efficacy of these agents for inducing or maintaining remission, patients with reduced renal function need to be carefully monitored for bone marrow suppression or mucositis. Adjustment to a lower dose may be needed to prevent those side effects.

TNF-alpha inhibitors appear safe in patients with reduced estimated glomerular filtration rate (eGFR). One study reported that rheumatoid arthritis patients on TNF-alpha inhibitors had a slower decline in eGFR compared with patients in their cohort not on TNF-alpha inhibitors Tocilizumab and ustekinumab are reported to be safe and effective in rheumatoid and psoriatic arthritis patients, respectively, with renal disease [220, 221]. Rituximab has been used successfully in the treatment of ANCA-associated vasculitis including patients with significant renal disease and remains an option for active rheumatic diseases in patients with poor kidney function [222].

Pregnancy and Lactation

Rheumatologic diseases can affect women of child-bearing age; thus the use of csDMARDs and bDMARDs before conception, during pregnancy, in the postpartum period, and during breastfeeding is an important consideration.

It is well known that csDMARDs including leflunomide and methotrexate are FDA Pregnancy Category "X" meaning that studies in animals or humans have demonstrated fetal abnormalities and/or there is positive evidence of human fetal risk based on adverse reaction data from investigational or marketing experience, and the risks involved in using these drugs in pregnant woman clearly outweigh potential benefits. Spontaneous abortions and birth defects are linked to the use of methotrexate postconception. "Methotrexate embryopathy" characterized by cranial abnormalities, growth deficiency, hydrocephaly, limb hypoplasia, meningomyelocele, microcephaly, and micrognathia has been described [223]. Breastfeeding is generally not advised while on methotrexate, especially on the day that the dose is taken. In women who are planning to become pregnant, it is advisable that they discontinue methotrexate at least 3 months prior to conception [223]. If a woman becomes pregnant while on leflunomide, cholestyramine needs to be administered for drug "washout" given its long half-life (dose: 8 g orally three times a day until serum leflunomide level is undetectable <0.02 mg/mL) [223]. Breastfeeding is also generally not advised while on leflunomide because there are no data about its levels in breast milk. Congenital malformations have been linked to cyclophosphamide and MMF in addition to leflunomide and methotrexate. Cyclophosphamide should be discontinued at least 3 months prior to conception due to the following being associated with its use during pregnancy, especially in the first trimester: craniosynostosis, growth deficiency, limb defects, microcephaly, miscarriages, and oral clefts [223]. Breastfeeding is contraindicated while on this medication because it is excreted in breast milk and can cause cytopenia, i.e., neutropenia and thrombocytopenia, in nursing infants [223]. "Mycophenolate mofetil embryopathy" characterized by auditory canal atresia, hypertelorism, micrognathia, microtia, and orofacial clefts has been described [223]. Breastfeeding is also generally not advised while on mycophenolate mofetil because there are no data about its levels in breast milk. This medication should be discontinued at least 6 weeks prior to conception [223].

Safer csDMARD options during pregnancy include the use of azathioprine, hydroxychloroquine, and sulfasalazine. Azathioprine is FDA Pregnancy Category

"D" meaning that there is positive evidence of human fetal risk based on adverse reaction data from investigational or marketing experience or studies in humans, but potential benefits may warrant use of the drug in pregnant women despite potential risks. Hydroxychloroquine is FDA Pregnancy Category "C" meaning that animal reproduction studies have shown an adverse effect on the fetus, and there are no adequate and well-controlled studies in humans, but potential benefits may warrant their use in pregnant women despite potential risks. Sulfasalazine is FDA Pregnancy Category "B" meaning that animal reproduction studies have failed to demonstrate a risk to the fetus, and there are no adequate and well-controlled studies in pregnant women. Azathioprine is teratogenic in animal studies but reassuringly not so in humans with no increased risk for fetal malformations [223]. Although it is minimally transferred into breast milk, no adverse effects have been observed. Overall, azathioprine is an attractive option during pregnancy due to its favorable safety profile and steroid-sparing properties. Although hydroxychloroquine crosses the placenta, no fetal defects have been observed [223]. Likewise, although its levels are detected in breast milk, no adverse effects have been observed. Because sulfasalazine has certain antifolate drug properties, folate supplementation is needed prior to conception and during pregnancy [223]. Despite concern that this drug may lead to neonatal jaundice, cases of kernicterus have not been reported [223]. Mothers taking sulfasalazine whom are breast feeding should do so with caution since there has been a report of bloody diarrhea in an infant, and it is detectable in breast milk [223].

Reasonable options for transitioning medications in a woman who is planning to become pregnant include the following: hydroxychloroquine or sulfasalazine in lieu of leflunomide or methotrexate and azathioprine in lieu of mycophenolate mofetil.

A careful discussion is warranted between the patient and rheumatologist about the use of bDMARDs during pregnancy, especially since safety data is either limited or not available for certain agents including abatacept, anakinra, belimumab, tocilizumab, tofacitinib, and ustekinumab [223].

All TNF-alpha inhibitors are FDA Pregnancy Category "B" (see above). Abatacept, rituximab, and tocilizumab are FDA Pregnancy Category "C" (see above) [224]. Among the TNF-alpha inhibitors, certolizumab is thought to have the least placental transfer as compared to adalimumab and infliximab [225]. It is reasonable to discontinue monoclonal antibody TNF-alpha inhibitors, i.e., adalimumab, golimumab, and infliximab, in the third trimester, i.e., 30th week of pregnancy, in order to decrease the risk of neonatal immunosuppression. More robust data in patients with inflammatory bowel disease has suggested that it is safe to maintain and even start treatment with TNF-alpha inhibitors during pregnancy. Limited data indicates no adverse outcomes in breast-fed infants of mothers who continue to use TNF-alpha inhibitors [226]. With regard to rituximab, cases of congenital malformations, miscarriages, and prematurity have been reported [227]. Also, due to its mechanism of action, much is unknown about the effects of in utero and neonatal B-cell depletion. For these reasons, it is generally recommended that effective methods of contraception be used and pregnancy be avoided for 6–12 months after exposure. Although it is not confirmed that rituximab is present in human breast milk, breastfeeding is not advisable [170]. Lack of data with regard to abatacept, belimumab, tocilizumab, tofacitinib, and ustekinumab suggests that no recommendations can be made regarding their use in pregnancy and/or lactation, and, thus, alternative and safer therapies should be used instead.

With regard to use of bDMARDs in pregnancy, it seems that the use of TNF-alpha inhibitors, at least based on observational data, seems to be the safest option. Additional implications include delaying live vaccinations, i.e., BCG, measles, polio (oral), rotavirus, and yellow fever, for at least 6 months after birth in infants who have been exposed to TNF-α inhibitors in utero, especially if they were continued in the third trimester of pregnancy [228].

Conclusion

Anti-rheumatic medications improve disease outcomes and the quality of life of patients. However, their unique pharmacodynamic properties can potentially exacerbate certain comorbidities. The exclusion of this patient population from clinical trials and the channeling of healthier patients to more "high-risk" drugs obfuscate interpretation of data. However, to properly attribute the effect of an anti-rheumatic drug on a comorbidity, either positive or negative merely the presence or absence of the comorbid disease is insufficient information. Rheumatologists managing rheumatic diseases must strive to garner more information about their patients' non-rheumatic disease. This information needs to be collected concurrently along with the disease activity and organ involvement of the rheumatic disease. A frank discussion with the patient about their aspirations for the treatment of their rheumatic and comorbid disease may help individualize therapy to achieve these goals. Hopefully this approach will lead to more evidenced-based strategies for managing rheumatic diseases in patients with other chronic medical conditions.

References

1. Mathias SD, Colwell HH, Miller DP, Moreland LW, Buatti M, Wanke L. Health-related quality of life and functional status of patients with rheumatoid arthritis randomly assigned to receive etanercept or placebo. Clin Ther. 2000;22(1):128–39.
2. Alarcon GS, McGwin G, Bertoli AM, Fessler BJ, Calvo-Alen J, Bastian HM, et al. Effect of hydroxychloroquine on the survival of patients with systemic lupus erythematosus: data from LUMINA, a multiethnic US cohort (LUMINA L). Ann Rheum Dis. 2007;66(9):1168–72.
3. Tiippana-Kinnunen T, Kautiainen H, Paimela L, Leirisalo-Repo M. Co-morbidities in Finnish patients with rheumatoid arthritis: 15-year follow-up. Scand J Rheumatol. 2013;42(6):451–6.
4. Mikuls TR, Fay BT, Michaud K, Sayles H, Thiele GM, Caplan L, et al. Associations of disease activity and treatments with mortality in men with rheumatoid arthritis: results from the VARA registry. Rheumatology (Oxford). 2011;50(1):101–9.
5. Feig DI, Soletsky B, Johnson RJ. Effect of allopurinol on blood pressure of adolescents with newly diagnosed essential hypertension: a randomized trial. JAMA. 2008;300(8):924–32.
6. Dixon WG, Watson KD, Lunt M, Hyrich KL, Silman AJ, Symmons DP. Reduction in the incidence of myocardial infarction in patients with rheumatoid arthritis who respond to

anti-tumor necrosis factor alpha therapy: results from the British Society for Rheumatology Biologics Register. Arthritis Rheum. 2007;56(9):2905–12.
7. Gonzalez-Gay MA, De Matias JM, Gonzalez-Juanatey C, Garcia-Porrua C, Sanchez-Andrade A, Martin J, et al. Anti-tumor necrosis factor-alpha blockade improves insulin resistance in patients with rheumatoid arthritis. Clin Exp Rheumatol. 2006;24(1):83–6.
8. Singh JA, Saag KG, Bridges SL, Akl EA, Bannuru RR, Sullivan MC, et al. 2015 American College of Rheumatology guideline for the treatment of rheumatoid arthritis. Arthritis Care Res (Hoboken). 2016;68(1):1–25.
9. Mok MY, Ng WL, Yuen MF, Wong RW, Lau CS. Safety of disease modifying anti-rheumatic agents in rheumatoid arthritis patients with chronic viral hepatitis. Clin Exp Rheumatol. 2000;18(3):363–8.
10. Sontheimer RD. Questions answered and a $1 million question raised concerning lupus erythematosus tumidus: is routine laboratory surveillance testing during treatment with hydroxychloroquine for skin disease really necessary. Arch Dermatol. United States. 2000;136:1044–9.
11. Jobanputra P, Amarasena R, Maggs F, Homer D, Bowman S, Rankin E, et al. Hepatotoxicity associated with sulfasalazine in inflammatory arthritis: a case series from a local surveillance of serious adverse events. BMC Musculoskelet Disord. 2008;9:48.
12. Chakravarty K, McDonald H, Pullar T, Taggart A, Chalmers R, Oliver S, et al. BSR/BHPR guideline for disease-modifying anti-rheumatic drug (DMARD) therapy in consultation with the British Association of Dermatologists. Rheumatology (Oxford). 2008;47(6):924–5.
13. Jobanputra P. BSR DMARD monitoring guidelines: sulfasalazine. Rheumatology (Oxford). England. 2008;47:1587–8.
14. Watanabe K, Takase K, Ohno S, Ideguchi H, Nozaki A, Ishigatsubo Y. Reactivation of hepatitis B virus in a hepatitis B surface antigen-negative patient with rheumatoid arthritis treated with methotrexate. Mod Rheumatol. 2012;22(3):470–3.
15. Gwak GY, Koh KC, Kim HY. Fatal hepatic failure associated with hepatitis B virus reactivation in a hepatitis B surface antigen-negative patient with rheumatoid arthritis receiving low dose methotrexate. Clin Exp Rheumatol. 2007;25(6):888–9.
16. Tan J, Zhou J, Zhao P, Wei J. Prospective study of HBV reactivation risk in rheumatoid arthritis patients who received conventional disease-modifying antirheumatic drugs. Clin Rheumatol. 2012;31(8):1169–75.
17. Xuan D, Yu Y, Shao L, Wang J, Zhang W, Zou H. Hepatitis reactivation in patients with rheumatic diseases after immunosuppressive therapy--a report of long-term follow-up of serial cases and literature review. Clin Rheumatol. 2014;33(4):577–86.
18. Ito S, Nakazono K, Murasawa A, Mita Y, Hata K, Saito N, et al. Development of fulminant hepatitis B (precore variant mutant type) after the discontinuation of low-dose methotrexate therapy in a rheumatoid arthritis patient. Arthritis Rheum. 2001;44(2):339–42.
19. Lok AS, McMahon BJ. Chronic hepatitis B. Hepatology. 2007;45(2):507–39.
20. Lok AS, McMahon BJ. Chronic hepatitis B: update 2009. Hepatology. 2009;50(3):661–2.
21. Laohapand C, Arromdee E, Tanwandee T. Long-term use of methotrexate does not result in hepatitis B reactivation in rheumatologic patients. Hepatol Int. 2015;9(2):202–8.
22. Gong ZJ, De Meyer S, Clarysse C, Verslype C, Neyts J, De Clercq E, et al. Mycophenolic acid, an immunosuppressive agent, inhibits HBV replication in vitro. J Viral Hepat. 1999;6(3):229–36.
23. Wu J, Xie HY, Jiang GP, Xu X, Zheng SS. The effect of mycophenolate acid on hepatitis B virus replication in vitro. Hepatobiliary Pancreat Dis Int. 2003;2(3):410–3.
24. Emori CT, Perez RM, Matos CA, Uehara SN, Pereira Pda S, Feldner AC, et al. Acute exacerbation of chronic hepatitis B virus infection in renal transplant patients. Braz J Infect Dis. 2014;18(6):625–30.
25. Meggitt SJ, Anstey AV, Mohd Mustapa MF, Reynolds NJ, Wakelin S. British Association of Dermatologists' guidelines for the safe and effective prescribing of azathioprine 2011. Br J Dermatol. 2011;165(4):711–34.
26. Bessone F, Dirchwolf M. Management of hepatitis B reactivation in immunosuppressed patients: an update on current recommendations. World J Hepatol. 2016;8(8):385–94.

27. Saag KG, Teng GG, Patkar NM, Anuntiyo J, Finney C, Curtis JR, et al. American College of Rheumatology 2008 recommendations for the use of nonbiologic and biologic disease-modifying antirheumatic drugs in rheumatoid arthritis. Arthritis Rheum. 2008;59(6):762–84.
28. Tavakolpour S, Alavian SM, Sali S. Hepatitis B reactivation during immunosuppressive therapy or cancer chemotherapy, management, and prevention: a comprehensive review-screened. Hepat Mon. 2016;16(4):e35810.
29. Carroll MB, Bond MI. Use of tumor necrosis factor-alpha inhibitors in patients with chronic hepatitis B infection. Semin Arthritis Rheum. 2008;38(3):208–17.
30. Michel M, Duvoux C, Hezode C, Cherqui D. Fulminant hepatitis after infliximab in a patient with hepatitis B virus treated for an adult onset still's disease. J Rheumatol. 2003;30(7):1624–5.
31. Montiel PM, Solis JA, Chirinos JA, a Casis B, Sanchez F, Rodriguez S. Hepatitis B virus reactivation during therapy with etanercept in an HBsAg-negative and anti-HBs-positive patient. Liver Int. England. 2008;28:718–20.
32. Verhelst X, Orlent H, Colle I, Geerts A, De Vos M, Van Vlierberghe H. Subfulminant hepatitis B during treatment with adalimumab in a patient with rheumatoid arthritis and chronic hepatitis B. Eur J Gastroenterol Hepatol. 2010;22(4):494–9.
33. Zein NN. Etanercept as an adjuvant to interferon and ribavirin in treatment-naive patients with chronic hepatitis C virus infection: a phase 2 randomized, double-blind, placebo-controlled study. J Hepatol. 2005;42(3):315–22.
34. Brunasso AM, Puntoni M, Gulia A, Massone C. Safety of anti-tumour necrosis factor agents in patients with chronic hepatitis C infection: a systematic review. Rheumatology (Oxford). 2011;50(9):1700–11.
35. Cavazzana I, Ceribelli A, Cattaneo R, Franceschini F. Treatment with etanercept in six patients with chronic hepatitis C infection and systemic autoimmune diseases. Autoimmun Rev. 2008;8(2):104–6.
36. Kim SJ, Hsu C, Song YQ, Tay K, Hong XN, Cao J, et al. Hepatitis B virus reactivation in B-cell lymphoma patients treated with rituximab: analysis from the Asia Lymphoma Study Group. Eur J Cancer. 2013;49(16):3486–96.
37. Pyrpasopoulou A, Douma S, Vassiliadis T, Chatzimichailidou S, Triantafyllou A, Aslanidis S. Reactivation of chronic hepatitis B virus infection following rituximab administration for rheumatoid arthritis. Rheumatol Int. 2011;31(3):403–4.
38. Ghrenassia E, Mekinian A, Rouaghe S, Ganne N, Fain O. Reactivation of resolved hepatitis B during rituximab therapy for rheumatoid arthritis. Joint Bone Spine. France. 2012;79:100–1.
39. Nosotti L, D'Andrea M, Pitidis A, Pimpinelli F, Dessanti ML, Pisani F, et al. Hepatitis C virus infection prevalence and liver dysfunction in a cohort of B-cell non-Hodgkin's lymphoma patients treated with immunochemotherapy. Scand J Infect Dis. 2012;44(1):70–3.
40. Lin KM, Lin JC, Tseng WY, Cheng TT. Rituximab-induced hepatitis C virus reactivation in rheumatoid arthritis. J Microbiol Immunol Infect. 2013;46(1):65–7.
41. Ennishi D, Maeda Y, Niitsu N, Kojima M, Izutsu K, Takizawa J, et al. Hepatic toxicity and prognosis in hepatitis C virus-infected patients with diffuse large B-cell lymphoma treated with rituximab-containing chemotherapy regimens: a Japanese multicenter analysis. Blood. 2010;116(24):5119–25.
42. Coppola N, Pisaturo M, Guastafierro S, Tonziello G, Sica A, Iodice V, et al. Increased hepatitis C viral load and reactivation of liver disease in HCV RNA-positive patients with onco-haematological disease undergoing chemotherapy. Dig Liver Dis. 2012;44(1):49–54.
43. Yazici O, Sendur MA, Aksoy S. Hepatitis C virus reactivation in cancer patients in the era of targeted therapies. World J Gastroenterol. 2014;20(22):6716–24.
44. Richards JS, Dowell SM, Quinones ME, Kerr GS. How to use biologic agents in patients with rheumatoid arthritis who have comorbid disease. BMJ. 2015;351:h3658.
45. Roccatello D, Baldovino S, Rossi D, Giachino O, Mansouri M, Naretto C, et al. Rituximab as a therapeutic tool in severe mixed cryoglobulinemia. Clin Rev Allergy Immunol. 2008;34(1):111–7.
46. Ferri C, Cacoub P, Mazzaro C, Roccatello D, Scaini P, Sebastiani M, et al. Treatment with rituximab in patients with mixed cryoglobulinemia syndrome: results of multicenter cohort study and review of the literature. Autoimmun Rev. 2011;11(1):48–55.

47. Kim PS, Ho GY, Prete PE, Furst DE. Safety and efficacy of abatacept in eight rheumatoid arthritis patients with chronic hepatitis B. Arthritis Care Res (Hoboken). 2012;64(8):1265–8.
48. Germanidis G, Hytiroglou P, Zakalka M, Settas L. Reactivation of occult hepatitis B virus infection, following treatment of refractory rheumatoid arthritis with abatacept. J Hepatol. England. 2012;56:1420–1.
49. Tsuboi H, Tsujii A, Nampei A, Yoshihara H, Kawano K, Takeuchi E, et al. A patient with rheumatoid arthritis treated with tocilizumab together with lamivudine prophylaxis after remission of infliximab-reactivated hepatitis B. Mod Rheumatol. 2011;21(6):701–5.
50. Kishida D, Okuda Y, Onishi M, Takebayashi M, Matoba K, Jouyama K, et al. Successful tocilizumab treatment in a patient with adult-onset Still's disease complicated by chronic active hepatitis B and amyloid A amyloidosis. Mod Rheumatol. 2011;21(2):215–8.
51. Nagashima T, Minota S. Long-term tocilizumab therapy in a patient with rheumatoid arthritis and chronic hepatitis B. Rheumatology (Oxford). England. 2008;47:1838–40.
52. Dragonas C, Ehrenstein B, Fleck M. Tocilizumab treatment in a patient suffering from rheumatoid arthritis and concomitant chronic hepatitis C infection. Rheumatology (Oxford). England. 2012;51:1520–1.
53. Streetz KL, Luedde T, Manns MP, Trautwein C. Interleukin 6 and liver regeneration. Gut. 2000;47(2):309–12.
54. Cutolo M. The kinase inhibitor tofacitinib in patients with rheumatoid arthritis: latest findings and clinical potential. Ther Adv Musculoskelet Dis. 2013;5(1):3–11.
55. Cohen S, Radominski SC, Gomez-Reino JJ, Wang L, Krishnaswami S, Wood SP, et al. Analysis of infections and all-cause mortality in phase II, phase III, and long-term extension studies of tofacitinib in patients with rheumatoid arthritis. Arthritis Rheumatol. 2014;66(11):2924–37.
56. Chiu HY, Chen CH, Wu MS, Cheng YP, Tsai TF. The safety profile of ustekinumab in the treatment of patients with psoriasis and concurrent hepatitis B or C. Br J Dermatol. 2013;169(6):1295–303.
57. Navarro R, Vilarrasa E, Herranz P, Puig L, Bordas X, Carrascosa JM, et al. Safety and effectiveness of ustekinumab and antitumour necrosis factor therapy in patients with psoriasis and chronic viral hepatitis B or C: a retrospective, multicentre study in a clinical setting. Br J Dermatol. 2013;168(3):609–16.
58. Motaparthi K, Stanisic V, Van Voorhees AS, Lebwohl MG, Hsu S. From the Medical Board of the National Psoriasis Foundation: recommendations for screening for hepatitis B infection prior to initiating anti-tumor necrosis factor-alfa inhibitors or other immunosuppressive agents in patients with psoriasis. J Am Acad Dermatol. 2014;70(1):178–86.
59. Secukinumab (Cosentyx) for psoriasis. Med Lett Drugs Ther. 2015;57(1465):45–7.
60. van de Kerkhof PC, Griffiths CE, Reich K, Leonardi CL, Blauvelt A, Tsai TF, et al. Secukinumab long-term safety experience: a pooled analysis of 10 phase II and III clinical studies in patients with moderate to severe plaque psoriasis. J Am Acad Dermatol. 2016;75(1):83–98.e4.
61. Drug Record Secukinumab. LiverTox 2015 [cited]; Available from: https://livertox.nlm.nih.gov/Secukinumab.htm.
62. Furie R, Stohl W, Ginzler EM, Becker M, Mishra N, Chatham W, et al. Biologic activity and safety of belimumab, a neutralizing anti-B-lymphocyte stimulator (BLyS) monoclonal antibody: a phase I trial in patients with systemic lupus erythematosus. Arthritis Res Ther. 2008;10(5):R109.
63. Navarra SV, Guzman RM, Gallacher AE, Hall S, Levy RA, Jimenez RE, et al. Efficacy and safety of belimumab in patients with active systemic lupus erythematosus: a randomised, placebo-controlled, phase 3 trial. Lancet. 2011;377(9767):721–31.
64. Merrill JT, Ginzler EM, Wallace DJ, McKay JD, Lisse JR, Aranow C, et al. Long-term safety profile of belimumab plus standard therapy in patients with systemic lupus erythematosus. Arthritis Rheum. 2012;64(10):3364–73.
65. Diallo A, Mekinian A, Boukari L, Mouas H, Zamy M, Nahon P, et al. Severe hepatitis in a patient with adult-onset Still's disease treated with anakinra. Rev Med Interne. 2013;34(3):168–70.

66. Taylor SA, Vittorio JM, Martinez M, Fester KA, Lagana SM, Lobritto SJ, et al. Anakinra-induced acute liver failure in an adolescent patient with Still's disease. Pharmacotherapy. 2016;36(1):e1–4.
67. Canna S, Frankovich J, Higgins G, Narkewicz MR, Nash SR, Hollister JR, et al. Acute hepatitis in three patients with systemic juvenile idiopathic arthritis taking interleukin-1 receptor antagonist. Pediatr Rheumatol Online J. 2009;7:21.
68. Ruperto N, Brunner HI, Quartier P, Constantin T, Wulffraat N, Horneff G, et al. Two randomized trials of canakinumab in systemic juvenile idiopathic arthritis. N Engl J Med. 2012;367(25):2396–406.
69. Hwang JP, Lok AS. Management of patients with hepatitis B who require immunosuppressive therapy. Nat Rev Gastroenterol Hepatol. 2014;11(4):209–19.
70. Hann HW, Gregory VL, Dixon JS, Barker KF. A review of the one-year incidence of resistance to lamivudine in the treatment of chronic hepatitis B: lamivudine resistance. Hepatol Int. 2008;2(4):440–56.
71. Bae SC, Gun SC, Mok CC, Khandker R, Nab HW, Koenig AS, et al. Improved health outcomes with Etanercept versus usual DMARD therapy in an Asian population with established rheumatoid arthritis. BMC Musculoskelet Disord. 2013;14(1):13.
72. Mori S, Fujiyama S. Hepatitis B virus reactivation associated with antirheumatic therapy: risk and prophylaxis recommendations. World J Gastroenterol. 2015;21(36):10274–89.
73. Box SA, Pullar T. Sulphasalazine in the treatment of rheumatoid arthritis. Br J Rheumatol. 1997;36(3):382–6.
74. Gisbert JP, Gonzalez-Lama Y, Mate J. Thiopurine-induced liver injury in patients with inflammatory bowel disease: a systematic review. Am J Gastroenterol. 2007;102(7):1518–27.
75. Prey S, Paul C. Effect of folic or folinic acid supplementation on methotrexate-associated safety and efficacy in inflammatory disease: a systematic review. Br J Dermatol. 2009;160(3):622–8.
76. van Ede AE, Laan RF, Rood MJ, Huizinga TW, van de Laar MA, van Denderen CJ, et al. Effect of folic or folinic acid supplementation on the toxicity and efficacy of methotrexate in rheumatoid arthritis: a forty-eight week, multicenter, randomized, double-blind, placebo-controlled study. Arthritis Rheum. 2001;44(7):1515–24.
77. Schmajuk G, Miao Y, Yazdany J, Boscardin WJ, Daikh DI, Steinman MA. Identification of risk factors for elevated transaminases in methotrexate users through an electronic health record. Arthritis Care Res (Hoboken). 2014;66(8):1159–66.
78. Psoriasis-liver-methotrexate interactions. Arch Dermatol. 1973;108(1):36–42.
79. Helliwell PS, Taylor WJ. Treatment of psoriatic arthritis and rheumatoid arthritis with disease modifying drugs – comparison of drugs and adverse reactions. J Rheumatol. 2008;35(3):472–6.
80. Menter A, Korman NJ, Elmets CA, Feldman SR, Gelfand JM, Gordon KB, et al. Guidelines of care for the management of psoriasis and psoriatic arthritis: section 4. Guidelines of care for the management and treatment of psoriasis with traditional systemic agents. J Am Acad Dermatol. 2009;61(3):451–85.
81. Kalb RE, Strober B, Weinstein G, Lebwohl M. Methotrexate and psoriasis: 2009 National Psoriasis Foundation Consensus conference. J Am Acad Dermatol. 2009;60(5):824–37.
82. Lewis JH. The rational use of potentially hepatotoxic medications in patients with underlying liver disease. Expert Opin Drug Saf. 2002;1(2):159–72.
83. van Roon EN, Jansen TL, Houtman NM, Spoelstra P, Brouwers JR. Leflunomide for the treatment of rheumatoid arthritis in clinical practice: incidence and severity of hepatotoxicity. Drug Saf. 2004;27(5):345–52.
84. Arava (leflunomide) tablets. Medwatch 2014 [cited 2016]; Available from: http://www.fda.gov/safety/medwatch/safetyinformation/ucm230245.htm.
85. Gottlieb A, Menter A, Mendelsohn A, Shen YK, Li S, Guzzo C, et al. Ustekinumab, a human interleukin 12/23 monoclonal antibody, for psoriatic arthritis: randomised, double-blind, placebo-controlled, crossover trial. Lancet. 2009;373(9664):633–40.

86. Paton NI, Goodall RL, Dunn DT, Franzen S, Collaco-Moraes Y, Gazzard BG, et al. Effects of hydroxychloroquine on immune activation and disease progression among HIV-infected patients not receiving antiretroviral therapy: a randomized controlled trial. JAMA. 2012;308(4):353–61.
87. Sperber K, Chiang G, Chen H, Ross W, Chusid E, Gonchar M, et al. Comparison of hydroxy-chloroquine with zidovudine in asymptomatic patients infected with human immunodeficiency virus type 1. Clin Ther. 1997;19(5):913–23.
88. Savarino A, Gennero L, Sperber K, Boelaert JR. The anti-HIV-1 activity of chloroquine. J Clin Virol. 2001;20(3):131–5.
89. Romanelli F, Smith KM, Hoven AD. Chloroquine and hydroxychloroquine as inhibitors of human immunodeficiency virus (HIV-1) activity. Curr Pharm Des. 2004;10(21):2643–8.
90. Maurer TA, Zackheim HS, Tuffanelli L, Berger TG. The use of methotrexate for treatment of psoriasis in patients with HIV infection. J Am Acad Dermatol. 1994;31(2 Pt 2):372–5.
91. Galeazzi M, Giannitti C, Manganelli S, Benucci M, Scarpato S, Bazzani C, et al. Treatment of rheumatic diseases in patients with HCV and HIV infection. Autoimmun Rev. 2008;8(2):100–3.
92. Yao Q, Frank M, Glynn M, Altman RD. Rheumatic manifestations in HIV-1 infected in-patients and literature review. Clin Exp Rheumatol. 2008;26(5):799–806.
93. Garcia F, Plana M, Arnedo M, Brunet M, Castro P, Gil C, et al. Effect of mycophenolate mofetil on immune response and plasma and lymphatic tissue viral load during and after interruption of highly active antiretroviral therapy for patients with chronic HIV infection: a randomized pilot study. J Acquir Immune Defic Syndr. 2004;36(3):823–30.
94. Rizzardi GP, Harari A, Capiluppi B, Tambussi G, Ellefsen K, Ciuffreda D, et al. Treatment of primary HIV-1 infection with cyclosporin A coupled with highly active antiretroviral therapy. J Clin Invest. 2002;109(5):681–8.
95. Chamberlain FE, Dinani N, Jagjit Singh GK, Bower M, Nelson M. Azathioprine can be safely used in HIV-infected individuals. AIDS. England. 2014;28:447–8.
96. Adizie T, Moots RJ, Hodkinson B, French N, Adebajo AO. Inflammatory arthritis in HIV positive patients: a practical guide. BMC Infect Dis. 2016;16:100.
97. Schlapfer E, Fischer M, Ott P, Speck RF. Anti-HIV-1 activity of leflunomide: a comparison with mycophenolic acid and hydroxyurea. AIDS. 2003;17(11):1613–20.
98. Newton L, van Halsema C, Snowden N. HIV and rheumatology: a practical guide. Topical Rev. Issue 5, Autumn 2014.
99. Gavegnano C, Detorio M, Montero C, Bosque A, Planelles V, Schinazi RF. Ruxolitinib and tofacitinib are potent and selective inhibitors of HIV-1 replication and virus reactivation in vitro. Antimicrob Agents Chemother. 2014;58(4):1977–86.
100. Aboulafia DM, Bundow D, Wilske K, Ochs UI. Etanercept for the treatment of human immunodeficiency virus-associated psoriatic arthritis. Mayo Clin Proc. 2000;75(10):1093–8.
101. Cepeda EJ, Williams FM, Ishimori ML, Weisman MH, Reveille JD. The use of anti-tumour necrosis factor therapy in HIV-positive individuals with rheumatic disease. Ann Rheum Dis. 2008;67(5):710–2.
102. Boue F, Gabarre J, Gisselbrecht C, Reynes J, Cheret A, Bonnet F, et al. Phase II trial of CHOP plus rituximab in patients with HIV-associated non-Hodgkin's lymphoma. J Clin Oncol. 2006;24(25):4123–8.
103. Saeki H, Ito T, Hayashi M, Fukuchi O, Umezawa Y, Nobeyama Y, et al. Successful treatment of ustekinumab in a severe psoriasis patient with human immunodeficiency virus infection. J Eur Acad Dermatol Venereol. 2015;29(8):1653–5.
104. Paparizos V, Rallis E, Kirsten L, Kyriakis K. Ustekinumab for the treatment of HIV psoriasis. J Dermatolog Treat. 2012;23(6):398–9.
105. Brassard P, Kezouh A, Suissa S. Antirheumatic drugs and the risk of tuberculosis. Clin Infect Dis. United States. 2006;43:717–22.
106. Arkema EV, Jonsson J, Baecklund E, Bruchfeld J, Feltelius N, Askling J. Are patients with rheumatoid arthritis still at an increased risk of tuberculosis and what is the role of biological treatments? Ann Rheum Dis. 2015;74(6):1212–7.

107. Wolfe F, Michaud K, Anderson J, Urbansky K. Tuberculosis infection in patients with rheumatoid arthritis and the effect of infliximab therapy. Arthritis Rheum. 2004;50(2):372–9.
108. Danza A, Ruiz-Irastorza G. Infection risk in systemic lupus erythematosus patients: susceptibility factors and preventive strategies. Lupus. 2013;22(12):1286–94.
109. Binymin K, Cooper RG. Late reactivation of spinal tuberculosis by low-dose methotrexate therapy in a patient with rheumatoid arthritis. Rheumatology (Oxford). 2001;40(3):341–2.
110. di Girolamo C, Pappone N, Melillo E, Rengo C, Giuliano F, Melillo G. Cavitary lung tuberculosis in a rheumatoid arthritis patient treated with low-dose methotrexate and steroid pulse therapy. Br J Rheumatol. 1998;37(10):1136–7.
111. Jenks KA, Stamp LK, O'Donnell JL, Savage RL, Chapman PT. Leflunomide-associated infections in rheumatoid arthritis. J Rheumatol. 2007;34(11):2201–3.
112. Hocevar A, Rozman B, Praprotnik S, Lestan B, Erzen D, Petric V, et al. Leflunomide-associated tuberculosis? Rheumatology (Oxford). England. 2006;45:228–9.
113. Brode SK, Jamieson FB, Ng R, Campitelli MA, Kwong JC, Paterson JM, et al. Increased risk of mycobacterial infections associated with anti-rheumatic medications. Thorax. 2015;70(7):677–82.
114. Cantarini L, Lopalco G, Caso F, Costa L, Iannone F, Lapadula G, et al. Effectiveness and tuberculosis-related safety profile of interleukin-1 blocking agents in the management of Behcet's disease. Autoimmun Rev. 2015;14(1):1–9.
115. Dinarello CA, Simon A, van der Meer JW. Treating inflammation by blocking interleukin-1 in a broad spectrum of diseases. Nat Rev Drug Discov. 2012;11(8):633–52.
116. Tsai TF, Chiu HY, Song M, Chan D. A case of latent tuberculosis reactivation in a patient treated with ustekinumab without concomitant isoniazid chemoprophylaxis in the PEARL trial. Br J Dermatol. 2013;168(2):444–6.
117. Tsai T-F, Blauvelt A, Gong Y, et al. Secukinumab treatment shows no evidence for reactivation of previous or latent TB infection in subjects with psoriasis: a pooled phase 3 safety analysis. J Am Assoc Dermatol. 2015;72(5):AB251–1.
118. Askling J, Fored CM, Brandt L, Baecklund E, Bertilsson L, Coster L, et al. Risk and case characteristics of tuberculosis in rheumatoid arthritis associated with tumor necrosis factor antagonists in Sweden. Arthritis Rheum. 2005;52(7):1986–92.
119. Winthrop KL, Chang E, Yamashita S, Iademarco MF, LoBue PA. Nontuberculous mycobacteria infections and anti–tumor necrosis factor-α therapy. Emerg Infect Dis. 2009;15(10):1556–61.
120. Gomez-Reino JJ, Carmona L, Valverde VR, Mola EM, Montero MD. Treatment of rheumatoid arthritis with tumor necrosis factor inhibitors may predispose to significant increase in tuberculosis risk: a multicenter active-surveillance report. Arthritis Rheum. 2003;48(8):2122–7.
121. Pehlivan Y, Kisacik B, Bosnak VK, Onat AM. Rituximab seems to be a safer alternative in patients with active rheumatoid arthritis with tuberculosis. BMJ Case Rep 2013;1–3.
122. Salliot C, Dougados M, Gossec L. Risk of serious infections during rituximab, abatacept and anakinra treatments for rheumatoid arthritis: meta-analyses of randomised placebo-controlled trials. Ann Rheum Dis. 2009;68(1):25–32.
123. Ottaviani S, Tiendrebeogo J, Choudat L, Gill G, Palazzo E, Meyer O, et al. Knee tuberculosis under rituximab therapy for rheumatoid arthritis. Joint Bone Spine. 2013;80(4):435–6.
124. Souto A, Maneiro JR, Salgado E, Carmona L, Gomez-Reino JJ. Risk of tuberculosis in patients with chronic immune-mediated inflammatory diseases treated with biologics and tofacitinib: a systematic review and meta-analysis of randomized controlled trials and long-term extension studies. Rheumatology (Oxford). 2014;53(10):1872–85.
125. Schiff MH, Kremer JM, Jahreis A, Vernon E, Isaacs JD, van Vollenhoven RF. Integrated safety in tocilizumab clinical trials. Arthritis Res Ther. 2011;13(5):R141.
126. Singh JA, Furst DE, Bharat A, Curtis JR, Kavanaugh AF, Kremer JM, et al. 2012 update of the 2008 American College of Rheumatology recommendations for the use of disease-modifying antirheumatic drugs and biologic agents in the treatment of rheumatoid arthritis. Arthritis Care Res (Hoboken). 2012;64(5):625–39.

127. Furst DE, Keystone EC, So AK, Braun J, Breedveld FC, Burmester GR, et al. Updated consensus statement on biological agents for the treatment of rheumatic diseases, 2012. Ann Rheum Dis. 2013;72(Suppl 2):ii2–34.
128. Smolen JS, Landewe R, Breedveld FC, Buch M, Burmester G, Dougados M, et al. EULAR recommendations for the management of rheumatoid arthritis with synthetic and biological disease-modifying antirheumatic drugs: 2013 update. Ann Rheum Dis. 2014;73(3):492–509.
129. Hatemi G, Yazici H. Tuberculosis screening before and during treatment with tumor necrosis factor antagonists: something old, something new. J Rheumatol. Canada. 2013;40:1938–40.
130. Bielefeld P, Meyer P, Caillot D, Dalac S, Camus P, Tavernier C, et al. Systemic scleroderma and cancers: 21 cases and review of the literature. Rev Med Interne. 1996;17(10):810–3.
131. Chi KH, Ko HL, Yang KL, Lee CY, Chi MS, Kao SJ. Addition of rapamycin and hydroxychloroquine to metronomic chemotherapy as a second line treatment results in high salvage rates for refractory metastatic solid tumors: a pilot safety and effectiveness analysis in a small patient cohort. Oncotarget. 2015;6(18):16735–45.
132. Ma MZ, Chen G, Wang P, Lu WH, Zhu CF, Song M, et al. Xc-inhibitor sulfasalazine sensitizes colorectal cancer to cisplatin by a GSH-dependent mechanism. Cancer Lett. 2015;368(1):88–96.
133. Georgescu L, Quinn GC, Schwartzman S, Paget SA. Lymphoma in patients with rheumatoid arthritis: association with the disease state or methotrexate treatment. Semin Arthritis Rheum. 1997;26(6):794–804.
134. Dawson TM, Starkebaum G, Wood BL, Willkens RF, Gown AM. Epstein-Barr virus, methotrexate, and lymphoma in patients with rheumatoid arthritis and primary Sjogren's syndrome: case series. J Rheumatol. 2001;28(1):47–53.
135. Hellgren K, Smedby KE, Backlin C, Sundstrom C, Feltelius N, Eriksson JK, et al. Ankylosing spondylitis, psoriatic arthritis, and risk of malignant lymphoma: a cohort study based on nationwide prospectively recorded data from Sweden. Arthritis Rheumatol. 2014;66(5):1282–90.
136. Krathen MS, Gottlieb AB, Mease PJ. Pharmacologic immunomodulation and cutaneous malignancy in rheumatoid arthritis, psoriasis, and psoriatic arthritis. J Rheumatol. 2010;37(11):2205–15.
137. Chakravarty EF, Michaud K, Wolfe F. Skin cancer, rheumatoid arthritis, and tumor necrosis factor inhibitors. J Rheumatol. 2005;32(11):2130–5.
138. Chan J, Sanders DC, Du L, Pillans PI. Leflunomide-associated pancytopenia with or without methotrexate. Ann Pharmacother. 2004;38(7–8):1206–11.
139. Pasternak B, Svanstrom H, Schmiegelow K, Jess T, Hviid A. Use of azathioprine and the risk of cancer in inflammatory bowel disease. Am J Epidemiol. 2013;177(11):1296–305.
140. Jiyad Z, Olsen CM, Burke MT, Isbel NM, Green AC. Azathioprine and risk of skin cancer in organ transplant recipients: systematic review and meta-analysis. Am J Transplant. 2016;16:3490–503.
141. Knight A, Askling J, Granath F, Sparen P, Ekbom A. Urinary bladder cancer in Wegener's granulomatosis: risks and relation to cyclophosphamide. Ann Rheum Dis. 2004;63(10):1307–11.
142. Safaeian M, Robbins HA, Berndt SI, Lynch CF, Fraumeni JF Jr, Engels EA. Risk of colorectal cancer after solid organ transplantation in the United States. Am J Transplant. 2016;16(3):960–7.
143. Crane GM, Powell H, Kostadinov R, Rocafort PT, Rifkin DE, Burger PC, et al. Primary CNS lymphoproliferative disease, mycophenolate and calcineurin inhibitor usage. Oncotarget. 2015;6(32):33849–66.
144. Curtis JR, Lee EB, Kaplan IV, Kwok K, Geier J, Benda B, et al. Tofacitinib, an oral Janus kinase inhibitor: analysis of malignancies across the rheumatoid arthritis clinical development programme. Ann Rheum Dis. 2016;75(5):831–41.
145. Balkwill F. Tumour necrosis factor and cancer. Nat Rev Cancer. 2009;9(5):361–71.
146. Bongartz T, Sutton AJ, Sweeting MJ, Buchan I, Matteson EL, Montori V. Anti-TNF antibody therapy in rheumatoid arthritis and the risk of serious infections and malignancies:

systematic review and meta-analysis of rare harmful effects in randomized controlled trials. JAMA. 2006;295(19):2275–85.
147. Michaud TL, Rho YH, Shamliyan T, Kuntz KM, Choi HK. The comparative safety of TNF inhibitors in rheumatoid arthritis – a meta-analysis update of 44 randomized controlled trials. Am J Med. 2014;127(12):1208–32.
148. Wolfe F, Michaud K. Biologic treatment of rheumatoid arthritis and the risk of malignancy: analyses from a large US observational study. Arthritis Rheum. 2007;56(9):2886–95.
149. Strangfeld A, Hierse F, Rau R, Burmester GR, Krummel-Lorenz B, Demary W, et al. Risk of incident or recurrent malignancies among patients with rheumatoid arthritis exposed to biologic therapy in the German biologics register RABBIT. Arthritis Res Ther. 2010;12(1):R5.
150. Dixon WG, Watson KD, Lunt M, Mercer LK, Hyrich KL, Symmons DP. Influence of anti-tumor necrosis factor therapy on cancer incidence in patients with rheumatoid arthritis who have had a prior malignancy: results from the British Society for Rheumatology Biologics Register. Arthritis Care Res (Hoboken). 2010;62(6):755–63.
151. Raaschou P, Frisell T, Askling J. TNF inhibitor therapy and risk of breast cancer recurrence in patients with rheumatoid arthritis: a nationwide cohort study. Ann Rheum Dis. 2015;74(12):2137–43.
152. Lopez-Olivo MA, Tayar JH, Martinez-Lopez JA, Pollono EN, Cueto JP, Gonzales-Crespo MR, et al. Risk of malignancies in patients with rheumatoid arthritis treated with biologic therapy: a meta-analysis. JAMA. 2012;308(9):898–908.
153. Rubbert-Roth A, Sebba A, Brockwell L, Kelman A, Porter-Brown B, Pulley J, et al. Malignancy rates in patients with rheumatoid arthritis treated with tocilizumab. RMD Open. 2016;2(1):e000213.
154. Nagao A, Nakazawa S, Hanabusa H. Short-term efficacy of the IL6 receptor antibody tocilizumab in patients with HIV-associated multicentric Castleman disease: report of two cases. J Hematol Oncol. 2014;7(1):10.
155. Corcorran MA, Olson JM, Hecht C, Knezevich S, Vary JC. Eruptive squamous cell carcinoma in a patient receiving abatacept for rheumatoid arthritis. J Am Acad Dermatol. 2013;69(4):e178–9.
156. Reich K, Mrowietz U, Radtke MA, Thaci D, Rustenbach SJ, Spehr C, et al. Drug safety of systemic treatments for psoriasis: results from The German Psoriasis Registry PsoBest. Arch Dermatol Res. 2015;307(10):875–83.
157. Papp K, Gottlieb AB, Naldi L, Pariser D, Ho V, Goyal K, et al. Safety surveillance for ustekinumab and other psoriasis treatments from the Psoriasis Longitudinal Assessment and Registry (PSOLAR). J Drugs Dermatol. 2015;14(7):706–14.
158. van Vollenhoven RF, Emery P, Bingham CO 3rd, Keystone EC, Fleischmann RM, Furst DE, et al. Long-term safety of rituximab in rheumatoid arthritis: 9.5-year follow-up of the global clinical trial programme with a focus on adverse events of interest in RA patients. Ann Rheum Dis. 2013;72(9):1496–502.
159. Bombardier C, Hazlewood GS, Akhavan P, Schieir O, Dooley A, Haraoui B, et al. Canadian Rheumatology Association recommendations for the pharmacological management of rheumatoid arthritis with traditional and biologic disease-modifying antirheumatic drugs: part II safety. J Rheumatol. 2012;39(8):1583–602.
160. Wallace DJ, Navarra S, Petri MA, Gallacher A, Thomas M, Furie R, et al. Safety profile of belimumab: pooled data from placebo-controlled phase 2 and 3 studies in patients with systemic lupus erythematosus. Lupus. 2013;22(2):144–54.
161. Sharma TS, Wasko MC, Tang X, Vedamurthy D, Yan X, Cote J, et al. Hydroxychloroquine use is associated with decreased incident cardiovascular events in rheumatoid arthritis patients. J Am Heart Assoc. 2016;5(1):e002867.
162. Yogasundaram H, Putko BN, Tien J, Paterson DI, Cujec B, Ringrose J, et al. Hydroxychloroquine-induced cardiomyopathy: case report, pathophysiology, diagnosis, and treatment. Can J Cardiol. 2014;30(12):1706–15.
163. Chung ES, Packer M, Lo KH, Fasanmade AA, Willerson JT. Randomized, double-blind, placebo-controlled, pilot trial of infliximab, a chimeric monoclonal antibody to tumor necrosis

factor-alpha, in patients with moderate-to-severe heart failure: results of the anti-TNF Therapy Against Congestive Heart Failure (ATTACH) trial. Circulation. 2003;107(25):3133–40.
164. Coletta AP, Clark AL, Banarjee P, Cleland JG. Clinical trials update: RENEWAL (RENAISSANCE and RECOVER) and ATTACH. Eur J Heart Fail. Netherlands. 2002;4:559–61.
165. Cacciapaglia F, Navarini L, Menna P, Salvatorelli E, Minotti G, Afeltra A. Cardiovascular safety of anti-TNF-alpha therapies: facts and unsettled issues. Autoimmun Rev. 2011;10(10):631–5.
166. Khanna D, McMahon M, Furst DE. Anti-tumor necrosis factor alpha therapy and heart failure: what have we learned and where do we go from here? Arthritis Rheum. 2004;50(4):1040–50.
167. Listing J, Strangfeld A, Kekow J, Schneider M, Kapelle A, Wassenberg S, et al. Does tumor necrosis factor alpha inhibition promote or prevent heart failure in patients with rheumatoid arthritis? Arthritis Rheum. 2008;58(3):667–77.
168. Bili A, Tang X, Pranesh S, Bozaite R, Morris SJ, Antohe JL, et al. Tumor necrosis factor alpha inhibitor use and decreased risk for incident coronary events in rheumatoid arthritis. Arthritis Care Res (Hoboken). 2014;66(3):355–63.
169. Pham T, Bachelez H, Berthelot JM, Blacher J, Claudepierre P, Constantin A, et al. Abatacept therapy and safety management. Joint Bone Spine. France: 2012 Elsevier Masson SAS; 2012. p. 3–84.
170. Pham T, Fautrel B, Gottenberg JE, Goupille P, Hachulla E, Masson C, et al. Rituximab (MabThera) therapy and safety management. Clinical tool guide. Joint Bone Spine. France. 2008;75:S1–99.
171. Atzeni F, Turiel M, Caporali R, Cavagna L, Tomasoni L, Sitia S, et al. The effect of pharmacological therapy on the cardiovascular system of patients with systemic rheumatic diseases. Autoimmun Rev. 2010;9(12):835–9.
172. Curtis JR, Perez-Gutthann S, Suissa S, Napalkov P, Singh N, Thompson L, et al. Tocilizumab in rheumatoid arthritis: a case study of safety evaluations of a large postmarketing data set from multiple data sources. Semin Arthritis Rheum. 2015;44(4):381–8.
173. Charles-Schoeman C, Gonzalez-Gay MA, Kaplan I, Boy M, Geier J, Luo Z, et al. Effects of tofacitinib and other DMARDs on lipid profiles in rheumatoid arthritis: implications for the rheumatologist. Semin Arthritis Rheum. 2016;46(1):71–80.
174. Cavalli G, Dinarello CA. Treating rheumatological diseases and co-morbidities with interleukin-1 blocking therapies. Rheumatology (Oxford). 2015;54(12):2134–44.
175. Dommasch ED, Troxel AB, Gelfand JM. Major cardiovascular events associated with anti-IL 12/23 agents: a tale of two meta-analyses. J Am Acad Dermatol. 2013;68(5):863–5.
176. Hjuler KF, Bottcher M, Vestergaard C, Botker HE, Iversen L, Kragballe K. Association between changes in coronary artery disease progression and treatment with biologic agents for severe psoriasis. JAMA Dermatol. 2016;152(10):1114–21.
177. Filip DJ, Logue GL, Harle TS, Farrar WH. Pulmonary and hepatic complications of methotrexate therapy of psoriasis. JAMA. 1971;216(5):881–2.
178. Sostman HD, Matthay RA, Putman CE, Smith GJ. Methotrexate-induced pneumonitis. Medicine (Baltimore). 1976;55(5):371–88.
179. Carson CW, Cannon GW, Egger MJ, Ward JR, Clegg DO. Pulmonary disease during the treatment of rheumatoid arthritis with low dose pulse methotrexate. Semin Arthritis Rheum. 1987;16(3):186–95.
180. Dawson JK, Graham DR, Desmond J, Fewins HE, Lynch MP. Investigation of the chronic pulmonary effects of low-dose oral methotrexate in patients with rheumatoid arthritis: a prospective study incorporating HRCT scanning and pulmonary function tests. Rheumatology (Oxford). 2002;41(3):262–7.
181. Conway R, Low C, Coughlan RJ, O'Donnell MJ, Carey JJ. Methotrexate use and risk of lung disease in psoriasis, psoriatic arthritis, and inflammatory bowel disease: systematic literature review and meta-analysis of randomised controlled trials. BMJ. 2015;350:h1269.
182. Baughman RP, Winget DB, Lower EE. Methotrexate is steroid sparing in acute sarcoidosis: results of a double blind, randomized trial. Sarcoidosis Vasc Diffuse Lung Dis. 2000;17(1):60–6.

183. Cottin V, Tebib J, Massonnet B, Souquet PJ, Bernard JP. Pulmonary function in patients receiving long-term low-dose methotrexate. Chest. 1996;109(4):933–8.
184. Khadadah ME, Jayakrishnan B, Al-Gorair S, Al-Mutairi M, Al-Maradni N, Onadeko B, et al. Effect of methotrexate on pulmonary function in patients with rheumatoid arthritis--a prospective study. Rheumatol Int. 2002;22(5):204–7.
185. McCurry J. Japan deaths spark concerns over arthritis drug. Lancet. England. 2004;363:461.
186. Sakai F, Noma S, Kurihara Y, Yamada H, Azuma A, Kudoh S, et al. Leflunomide-related lung injury in patients with rheumatoid arthritis: imaging features. Mod Rheumatol. 2005;15(3):173–9.
187. Suissa S, Hudson M, Ernst P. Leflunomide use and the risk of interstitial lung disease in rheumatoid arthritis. Arthritis Rheum. 2006;54(5):1435–9.
188. Alarcon GS, Kremer JM, Macaluso M, Weinblatt ME, Cannon GW, Palmer WR, et al. Risk factors for methotrexate-induced lung injury in patients with rheumatoid arthritis. A multicenter, case-control study. Methotrexate-Lung Study Group. Ann Intern Med. 1997;127(5):356–64.
189. Shenoy PD, Bavaliya M, Sashidharan S, Nalianda K, Sreenath S. Cyclophosphamide versus mycophenolate mofetil in scleroderma interstitial lung disease (SSc-ILD) as induction therapy: a single-centre, retrospective analysis. Arthritis Res Ther. 2016;18(1):123.
190. Tull TJ, Toma T, Menage HP. Reversible interstitial lung disease following treatment of atopic dermatitis with mycophenolate mofetil. Clin Exp Dermatol. 2016;41(6):702–3.
191. Piguet PF, Ribaux C, Karpuz V, Grau GE, Kapanci Y. Expression and localization of tumor necrosis factor-alpha and its mRNA in idiopathic pulmonary fibrosis. Am J Pathol. 1993;143(3):651–5.
192. Raghu G, Brown KK, Costabel U, Cottin V, du Bois RM, Lasky JA, et al. Treatment of idiopathic pulmonary fibrosis with etanercept: an exploratory, placebo-controlled trial. Am J Respir Crit Care Med. 2008;178(9):948–55.
193. Bargagli E, Galeazzi M, Bellisai F, Volterrani L, Rottoli P. Infliximab treatment in a patient with systemic sclerosis associated with lung fibrosis and pulmonary hypertension. Respiration. 2008;75(3):346–9.
194. Baughman RP, Drent M, Kavuru M, Judson MA, Costabel U, du Bois R, et al. Infliximab therapy in patients with chronic sarcoidosis and pulmonary involvement. Am J Respir Crit Care Med. 2006;174(7):795–802.
195. Antoniou KM, Mamoulaki M, Malagari K, Kritikos HD, Bouros D, Siafakas NM, et al. Infliximab therapy in pulmonary fibrosis associated with collagen vascular disease. Clin Exp Rheumatol. 2007;25(1):23–8.
196. Nakashita T, Ando K, Kaneko N, Takahashi K, Motojima S. Potential risk of TNF inhibitors on the progression of interstitial lung disease in patients with rheumatoid arthritis. BMJ Open. 2014;4(8):e005615.
197. O'Shea FD, Marras TK, Inman RD. Pulmonary sarcoidosis developing during infliximab therapy. Arthritis Rheum. 2006;55(6):978–81.
198. Herrinton LJ, Harrold LR, Liu L, Raebel MA, Taharka A, Winthrop KL, et al. Association between anti-TNF-alpha therapy and interstitial lung disease. Pharmacoepidemiol Drug Saf. 2013;22(4):394–402.
199. Daoussis D, Liossis SN, Tsamandas AC, Kalogeropoulou C, Kazantzi A, Sirinian C, et al. Experience with rituximab in scleroderma: results from a 1-year, proof-of-principle study. Rheumatology (Oxford). 2010;49(2):271–80.
200. Jordan S, Distler JH, Maurer B, Huscher D, van Laar JM, Allanore Y, et al. Effects and safety of rituximab in systemic sclerosis: an analysis from the European Scleroderma Trial and Research (EUSTAR) group. Ann Rheum Dis. 2015;74(6):1188–94.
201. Nakashita T, Ando K, Takahashi K, Motojima S. Possible effect of abatacept on the progression of interstitial lung disease in rheumatoid arthritis patients. Respir Investig. 2016;54(5):376–9.
202. Akiyama M, Kaneko Y, Yamaoka K, Kondo H, Takeuchi T. Association of disease activity with acute exacerbation of interstitial lung disease during tocilizumab treatment in patients with rheumatoid arthritis: a retrospective, case-control study. Rheumatol Int. 2016;36(6):881–9.

203. Curtis JR, Sarsour K, Napalkov P, Costa LA, Schulman KL. Incidence and complications of interstitial lung disease in users of tocilizumab, rituximab, abatacept and anti-tumor necrosis factor alpha agents, a retrospective cohort study. Arthritis Res Ther. 2015;17:319.
204. Jani M, Hirani N, Matteson EL, Dixon WG. The safety of biologic therapies in RA-associated interstitial lung disease. Nat Rev Rheumatol. 2014;10(5):284–94.
205. Knarborg M, Hilberg O, Hoffmann HJ, Dahl R. Methotrexate as an oral corticosteroid-sparing agent in severe asthma: the emergence of a responder asthma endotype. Eur Clin Respir J. 2014;1–8
206. Bush A, Pedersen S, Hedlin G, Baraldi E, Barbato A, de Benedictis F, et al. Pharmacological treatment of severe, therapy-resistant asthma in children: what can we learn from where? Eur Respir J. 2011;38(4):947–58.
207. Matera MG, Calzetta L, Cazzola M. TNF-alpha inhibitors in asthma and COPD: we must not throw the baby out with the bath water. Pulm Pharmacol Ther. 2010;23(2):121–8.
208. Suissa S, Ernst P, Hudson M. TNF-alpha antagonists and the prevention of hospitalisation for chronic obstructive pulmonary disease. Pulm Pharmacol Ther. 2008;21(1):234–8.
209. Weinblatt M, Combe B, Covucci A, Aranda R, Becker JC, Keystone E. Safety of the selective costimulation modulator abatacept in rheumatoid arthritis patients receiving background biologic and nonbiologic disease-modifying antirheumatic drugs: a one-year randomized, placebo-controlled study. Arthritis Rheum. 2006;54(9):2807–16.
210. Amarnani A, Rosenthal KS, Mercado JM, Brodell RT. Concurrent treatment of chronic psoriasis and asthma with ustekinumab. J Dermatolog Treat. 2014;25(1):63–6.
211. Svenson KL, Pollare T, Lithell H, Hallgren R. Impaired glucose handling in active rheumatoid arthritis: relationship to peripheral insulin resistance. Metabolism. 1988;37(2):125–30.
212. Zachariae H, Kragballe K, Sogaard H. Methotrexate induced liver cirrhosis. Studies including serial liver biopsies during continued treatment. Br J Dermatol. 1980;102(4):407–12.
213. Shergy WJ, Polisson RP, Caldwell DS, Rice JR, Pisetsky DS, Allen NB. Methotrexate-associated hepatotoxicity: retrospective analysis of 210 patients with rheumatoid arthritis. Am J Med. 1988;85(6):771–4.
214. Ogata A, Morishima A, Hirano T, Hishitani Y, Hagihara K, Shima Y, et al. Improvement of HbA1c during treatment with humanised anti-interleukin 6 receptor antibody, tocilizumab. Ann Rheum Dis. England. 2011;70:1164–5.
215. Boulton JG, Bourne JT. Unstable diabetes in a patient receiving anti-TNF-alpha for rheumatoid arthritis. Rheumatology (Oxford). England. 2007;46:178–9.
216. Weisman MH, Paulus HE, Burch FX, Kivitz AJ, Fierer J, Dunn M, et al. A placebo-controlled, randomized, double-blinded study evaluating the safety of etanercept in patients with rheumatoid arthritis and concomitant comorbid diseases. Rheumatology (Oxford). 2007;46(7):1122–5.
217. MacKinnon SK, Starkebaum G, Willkens RF. Pancytopenia associated with low dose pulse methotrexate in the treatment of rheumatoid arthritis. Semin Arthritis Rheum. 1985;15(2):119–26.
218. Cao H, Rao Y, Liu L, Lin J, Yang H, Zhang X, et al. The efficacy and safety of leflunomide for the treatment of lupus nephritis in Chinese patients: systematic review and meta-analysis. PLoS One. 2015;10(12):e0144548.
219. Paudyal S, Yang FM, Rice C, Chen CC, Skelton M, Bethel M, et al. End-stage renal disease in patients with rheumatoid arthritis. Semin Arthritis Rheum. 2016;46:418–22. pii: S0049-0172(16)30158-5
220. Mori S, Yoshitama T, Hidaka T, Hirakata N, Ueki Y. Effectiveness and safety of tocilizumab therapy for patients with rheumatoid arthritis and renal insufficiency: a real-life registry study in Japan (the ACTRA-RI study). Ann Rheum Dis. England. 2015;74:627–30.
221. Nimmannitya K, Tateishi C, Mizukami Y, Hamamoto K, Yamada S, Goto H, et al. Successful treatment with ustekinumab of psoriasis vulgaris in a patient undergoing hemodialysis. J Dermatol. 2016;43(1):92–4.
222. Jones RB, Tervaert JW, Hauser T, Luqmani R, Morgan MD, Peh CA, et al. Rituximab versus cyclophosphamide in ANCA-associated renal vasculitis. N Engl J Med. 2010;363(3):211–20.

223. Levy RA, de Jesus GR, de Jesus NR, Klumb EM. Critical review of the current recommendations for the treatment of systemic inflammatory rheumatic diseases during pregnancy and lactation. Autoimmun Rev. 2016;15(10):955–63.
224. Krause ML, Amin S, Makol A. Use of DMARDs and biologics during pregnancy and lactation in rheumatoid arthritis: what the rheumatologist needs to know. Ther Adv Musculoskelet Dis. 2014;6(5):169–84.
225. Mahadevan U, Wolf DC, Dubinsky M, Cortot A, Lee SD, Siegel CA, et al. Placental transfer of anti-tumor necrosis factor agents in pregnant patients with inflammatory bowel disease. Clin Gastroenterol Hepatol. 2013;11(3):286–92. quiz e24
226. Berthelsen BG, Fjeldsoe-Nielsen H, Nielsen CT, Hellmuth E. Etanercept concentrations in maternal serum, umbilical cord serum, breast milk and child serum during breastfeeding. Rheumatology (Oxford). England. 2010;49:2225–7.
227. Hyrich KL, Verstappen SM. Biologic therapies and pregnancy: the story so far. Rheumatology (Oxford). 2014;53(8):1377–85.
228. Hyrich KL, Symmons DP, Watson KD, Silman AJ. Pregnancy outcome in women who were exposed to anti-tumor necrosis factor agents: results from a national population register. Arthritis Rheum. 2006;54(8):2701–2.

Chapter 18
Comorbidity and Patient-Reported Outcomes

Deborah Palmer and Yasser El Miedany

The recognition that patients have unique knowledge of their own health and are experts in terms of their illness and its impact on their lives led to the recent concept of "patient-centred care" which has been endorsed as the best model of care for patient presenting with chronic inflammatory arthritic conditions. In 2010, the Affordable Care Act created the Patient-Centered Outcomes Research Institute (PCORI), which stresses the importance of patient-centeredness care [1]. Patient-centred care refers to the need to address patient views, characteristics, functional ability and quality of life, comorbidities, preferences as well as decision-making needs. This was emphasised by the improvement associated with treatment outcomes and treatment satisfaction when patients' perspectives are taken into consideration [2, 3].

In the past decade, there have been significant developments in the management of inflammatory arthritic conditions. The introduction of biologic therapy, intensive new treatment policies such as window of opportunity and treat to target, as well as the regularly updated guidelines led to significant developments and high expectations of the disease management outcomes. However, the patients' mortality and morbidity remained significantly impaired, which was attributed to comorbidities. Consequently, clinical and research interest in comorbidities have increased. A widely accepted definition of comorbidity is "the existence or occurrence of any distinct additional entity during the clinical course of a patient who has the index disease under study" [4]. In addition to the high prevalence of comorbidities in

D. Palmer
Department of Rheumatology, North Middlesex University Hospital, London, UK
e-mail: cnsdebspalmer@yahoo.co.uk

Y. El Miedany, MD, FRCP (✉)
King's College, London, UK

Ain Shams University, Cairo, Egypt

Department of Rheumatology, Darent Valley Hospital, Dartford, Kent, UK
e-mail: yasser_elmiedany@yahoo.com

Y. El Miedany (ed.), *Comorbidity in Rheumatic Diseases*,
DOI 10.1007/978-3-319-59963-2_18

patients with chronic inflammatory arthritic conditions (the average patient with rheumatoid arthritis (RA) has 1.6 comorbid conditions, and the number of these conditions increases with age, disease duration and/or disease activity) [5–7], comorbidities were reported to have a negative impact on the patients' health, as they reduce function and work productivity, decrease quality of life, and might shorten life expectancy [8–10]. As most of these parameters are mainly reported by the patients, the interaction between comorbidities and patient-reported outcomes (PROs) attracted the attention of the clinicians as well as researchers, and questions were raised regarding the best ways to endorse such relation in standard clinical practice. This chapter will discuss the interplay between comorbidities and patient-reported outcomes as well as its impact on the patients' management.

The Interplay Between Comorbidities and Patient-Reported Outcomes

To better understand the interplay between the patients and their reported outcomes, the chronic inflammatory arthritic conditions, and comorbidities, it is important to conceptualise the index relative to other comorbid health conditions that patients may have (Fig. 18.1). Some of the associations between comorbid conditions and PROs can be endogenous. For example, it is uncertain whether diabetes causes patients to experience negative PROs such as physical limitations and depression or whether physical limitations and depression predispose patients to behavioural risk factors for diabetes [11]. On the other hand, such association can be exogenous. In this model, no index disease is defined, and all morbidities are regarded of equal importance including the arthritic condition. Such approach constitutes a more generic, patient-centred-based concept, where both the inflammatory disease and comorbidities are considered at equal distance with the patient in the core of the model. This was defined as "multimorbidity", which is the "coexistence of two or more chronic diseases in the same individual", irrespective of whether the disease started before or after onset of the index disease" [12].

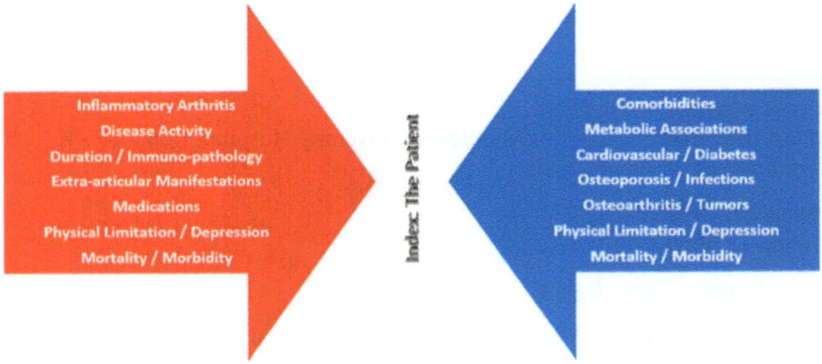

Fig. 18.1 The index of patient disease relative to other comorbid health conditions

Resolving the interplay between inflammatory arthritic conditions, comorbidities, and its determinants is challenging. While the occurrence of "emerging" comorbidities is more common in chronic arthritic diseases such as RA, spondyloarthritis (SpA) or lupus (SLE), the clinical consequences of comorbidity are also more severe in these patients as compared to controls. Despite this observation, comorbidity is often under-recognised and undertreated in standard clinical practice [13, 14]. Furthermore, guidelines and outcome measures focus on the index inflammatory arthritic condition as a single disease and consider the presence of comorbidity and its impact later in the disease course. This has been compounded by the fact that, in contrast to many chronic diseases, where a single *gold standard* measure, such as blood pressure in hypertension, haemoglobin A_1C in diabetes, and lipid profile in hyperlipidaemia, is applicable to diagnosis, management, prognosis, and analyses of outcomes in all individual patients in clinical trials, clinical care, and long-term databases, in inflammatory arthritic conditions (excluding gouty arthritis), there is not a single gold standard measure to assess outcomes. This is applicable both in short-term trials such as joint and laboratory measures and in long-term studies such as radiographic progression, comorbidities, disability and death. The absence of such a gold standard measure highlighted the need for pooled indices as a valid tool [15–17]. However, so far, these tend to be complex, expensive and currently used in clinical trials but not in clinical care.

Adding other factors, such as ageing, to the equation may add to the complexity of this interplay. By 2030, about one in four inhabitants of the European Union will be above the age of 65 [18]. The relevance of ageing is becoming more and more apparent in industrialised countries as, in parallel to an increase in life expectancy, birth rates are decreasing. In an ageing population, it is expected that the number of patients with inflammatory as well as noninflammatory arthritic conditions will grow proportionally. Several studies showed that both ageing and comorbidity may independently alter commonly used patient outcome measures, including joint scores, remission and response criteria as well as functional disability assessments [19–23]. In another study, ageing was an independent predictor for higher scores on both the pain VAS and global assessment VAS [24]. However, the challenge is that the inclusion of patients in most of the RCTs which included arthritic patients is usually restricted by stringent criteria. Therefore, patients included in these trials often do not resemble the spectrum of patients treated in the "real world", i.e. elderly patients who often face comorbidity and polypharmacy.

Looking globally, the effect magnitude of ageing and comorbidity on outcome measures and management remains largely unknown. For many of the comorbidities, it is equally unclear whether they should be managed similarly in middle-aged versus older patients. It seems clear that elderly RA patients who also face comorbidity will need a different management approach since the needs of these patients are more than just the sum of needs in relation to single diseases [25]. The symptoms of inflammatory arthritis such as RA or Sjogren's syndrome and comorbidities may be overlapping, treatments may interact, underlying pathophysiology may be shared and the course of all diseases may be altered. As a consequence, the current treatment strategies might not be directly translatable to elderly patients with comorbidity [26]. Research should focus on the impact of comorbidities on screening, diagnosis, and outcome measurement of patients with chronic inflammatory arthritis. While, nowadays, elderly patients with comorbidities are often excluded from intervention studies [27], future clinical trials should take the complex treatment reality of these patients into consideration by developing, for example, comprehensive comorbidity measures in order to correct for confounding and effect modification in clinical trials [28, 29]. This may ultimately result in the development of recommendations which can guide the complex management decisions that need to be made in the case of an ageing arthritic patient who faces comorbidity. In doing so, a goal-oriented approach should be prioritised above a disease-centred approach. Maintaining maximal functional status and active social participation is an essential component of a goal-oriented approach. Avoiding inefficient healthcare utilisation and medication side effects (e.g. suffering more from the treatment than from the disease) is important [30].

Comorbidity as Predictors of Patient Outcomes

The relation between comorbidity and patient-reported outcomes is quite variable in course. This is subject to the disease stage, disease activity and response to therapy (Fig. 18.2). Several published studies have described a cross-sectional relationship between the comorbidities and a reduced probability of remission [23, 31, 32]. A large multinational cross-sectional study of 5848 RA patients demonstrated that the number of comorbidities is independently associated with the clinical disease activity index "CDAI" [odds ratio (OR) 0.75, CI 0.68, 0.83] [23]. Burmester et al. [8] evaluated 6610 active RA patients who were treated with adalimumab for 3 months for predictors of achieving remission. Patients with one or no comorbidity had an OR of 0.86 of

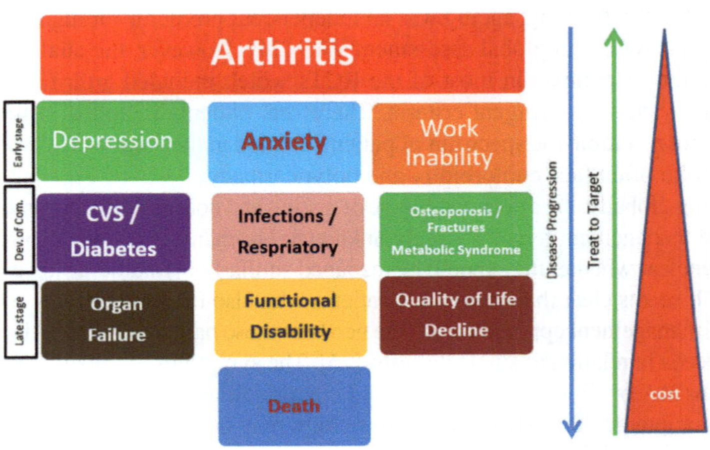

Fig. 18.2 Relationship between comorbidity and patient-reported outcomes

attaining DAS-28 remission compared with those with more than one. Krishnan et al. [23] studied a random sample of 1530 Finnish patients in the general population and demonstrated that age and comorbidities correlated with pain and patient global VAS. In a later article, Sokka et al. [32] suggested that only 15% of non-RA patients, >50 years of age, met ACR remission criteria. This suggests that even in a non-RA population, a population where remission should be easier to attain, comorbidities may play a substantial role in negatively impacting the ability to achieve remission.

On another front, several studies have examined the relationship between comorbidities and worsening functional disability [33, 34, 36, 37, 73]. Functional disability is an important outcome measure in inflammatory arthritic conditions. In 1991 Verbrugge et al. [37] evaluated chronic conditions in general in RA patients and showed a strong relationship between the number of comorbidities and functional disability in a cross-sectional and longitudinal cohort. In a more recent study, Radner et al. [35] evaluated the impact of comorbidities on the components of the HAQ in a cross section of 380 RA patients; they suggest that comorbidities may partly account for a portion of irreversible disability. Michaud et al. [38] recently reported that age and comorbidities were independently associated with the loss of functional status in RA in a cohort of 18,485 patients in the US National Data Bank for Rheumatic Diseases.

Interestingly, such associations of different comorbidity measures with patient-reported outcomes are not limited to patients with inflammatory arthritic conditions, but expand also to involve patients with osteoarthritis (OA). Data were from a recent study [11], carried out on 300 patients with OA hip and knee joints, revealed that comorbid conditions exacerbated the symptoms of OA (including pain and physical limitations, feeling down, fatigue and insomnia) and complicated or even compromise its management. This was supported by the outcomes of other studies. Perruccio and colleagues identified that 68% of patients with OA undergoing elective joint replacement surgery reported at least one other comorbid health condition, while nearly 10% of patients reported three or more other comorbid health conditions [39, 40]. In another study which included a community-based cohort of patients with symptomatic knee OA, the average number of additional self-reported comorbid health conditions was 1.73 [41]. This is particularly important given the high prevalence of OA in contrast to the other chronic inflammatory arthritic conditions and the high likelihood of multiple comorbid health conditions among aged older adults [42–44].

Impact of Inflammatory Arthritis Treatment on Comorbidities

This pro-inflammatory environment in patients with chronic inflammatory arthritis may, together with the development of self-reactive T and B cells, promote the development of other comorbidities such as cardiovascular comorbidity. Since both RA and atherosclerosis are inflammatory diseases, it was hypothesised that anti-rheumatic therapy may also inhibit various inflammatory pathways responsible for atherosclerosis. This was supported by the change in the lipid profile and lipid paradox and in active RA patients who received treatment with biologic therapy and achieved remission [45]. However, such possible beneficial effects of antirheumatic treatment on concomitant cardiovascular disease (CVD) has not been addressed in prospective randomised controlled trials, as usually patients with comorbidities are often excluded from these trials. Recent research studies focussed on RA patients and addressed the question whether antirheumatic therapy may prevent the occurrence of cardiovascular events. While the exact mechanism remains unknown, the beneficial effect on macrophage cholesterol metabolism and lipoprotein functions has been reported [46]. A recent meta-analysis of 28 observational studies reported that the risk of CV events can be reduced by using TNF-inhibitors (RR 0.7; 95% -CI 0.5–0.9; $p = 0.005$) and methotrexate (RR 0.7; 95% -CI 0.6–0.9; $p = 0.007$) [47]. In concordance, changes in bone mineral content showed similar positive impact. In the study carried out by Sakthiswary and his colleagues [48], it was reported that TNF inhibitors prevented further generalised bone loss by inhibiting bone resorption and development of osteoporosis. However, in most of these short-term and open-label trials, TNF inhibitors were prescribed in combination with methotrexate. Therefore, it needs to be assessed whether this protective effect can be attributed to the use of TNF inhibitors on its own or the use of the combination therapy and hence better RA disease control. In addition, no fracture data are currently available. Interestingly, in early RA patients, short-term use of steroids early in the disease course may have a positive impact on the bone mineral density, which was attributed to the steroids' potent anti-inflammatory effect. In a randomised, placebo-controlled, double-blind 2-year study by van der Goes et al. [49], addition of 10 mg prednisone daily to a methotrexate-based tight control strategy did not result in a negative effect on bone mineral density in early RA patients on bisphosphonates. Few studies have prospectively assessed the impact of antirheumatic medications on the body composition [50–54]. In a randomised study, carried out by Engvall et al. [24], which included 40 patients monitored over 21 month, the use of TNF inhibitors was associated with an increase in body fat mass (+3.8 (1.6–5.9) kg in the TNF inhibitor group vs +0.4 (−1.5–2.2) kg ($p = 0.04$) in the conventional synthetic DMARD group). There were no changes in muscle mass or lipid profile. Other studies with a shorter follow-up duration did not show a change in body composition [55, 56]. Therefore, there is an unmet need to determine whether these possible body composition changes can be confirmed in other research studies and, if so, whether they are associated with development of cardiovascular disease on the long term. In a recent systematic review and meta-analysis, the effect of TNF-inhibitors on anxiety as well as depression was evaluated [57]. Overall, the effects were to be small or not significant. However, several studies have shown that antirheumatic therapy improves important patient-reported outcomes including general well-being, fatigue and quality of life [58]. Similar findings were reported in patients with spondyloarthritis. Patient-reported outcome measures revealed variance among patients that was significantly correlated to the stage of the disease course and the disease activity status. Early in the disease process, though symptoms may be unrecognised, patients' priorities included difficulty to have good night sleep, worries about the future, as well as feelings of anxiety or depression. Late in the disease process, the psychometric priorities included disability at work, sexual dysfunction, difficulty to deal with stresses of daily life as well as social family activities. In addition, there were additional priorities for consideration in the late disease process patients, such as the need for surgery and other major interventions, comorbidities (cardiovascular and falls), non-articular organ involvement (mainly respiratory) and medication toxicities. The majority of patients had fatigue for the majority of the time. Self-helplessness, functional disability as well as quality of life scores correlated significantly ($p < 0.01$) with the disease activity (ASDAS >3.5, BASDAI and BASFI >4) as well as presence of comorbidities and responded well to treatment with biologic therapy [59, 60].

Impact of Comorbidity Treatment on Inflammatory Arthritis

Earlier studies showed some evidence that medication regularly prescribed for comorbidities, such as statins, might also lower inflammatory markers and have a positive effect on RA disease activity measures [55, 56]. In addition to their lipid lowering effects, statins also exert an anti-inflammatory action, which is held responsible for the beneficial impact on RA disease activity. In the randomised, placebo-controlled trial of atorvastatin in rheumatoid arthritis (TARA), it was reported that addition of atorvastatin to standard antirheumatic therapy significantly improved the DAS-28 as compared to placebo (treatment group: −0.50, 95% -CI −0.8 to −0.3; placebo group: +0.03, 95% -CI −0.2 to 0.3) [57]. In a recent cohort study by Schoenfeld et al. [59], it was reported that statin use was independently associated with a 21% lower risk of all-cause mortality among RA patients (HR 0.8, 95% -CI 0.7–0.9). There is some evidence that denosumab, a human monoclonal antibody against the receptor activator of nuclear factor kappa B ligand and used in the treatment of osteoporosis, may inhibit the development of joint erosions in patients with RA [61, 62, 63]. However, denosumab had no effect on joint space narrowing or on RA disease activity. Although selective serotonin reuptake inhibitors have been reported to exhibit anti-inflammatory effects in addition to their antidepressant effects, there is currently insufficient evidence that treatment of depression positively or negatively influences RA disease-specific outcome measures and other clinical outcomes [64, 65]. In addition, the evidence to routinely prescribe antidepressants as analgesics in patients with inflammatory arthritis is also inconclusive [66].

Comorbidity Impact on Prescription Trends

It is increasingly recognised that comorbid conditions play a pivotal role in inflammatory arthritis outcomes. These comorbid conditions also have an impact on the patients' treatment choices. On the other hand, some medications may also interact with the patient comorbidities, hence get contraindicated and cannot be used all together. Therefore, screening arthritic patients for their comorbidities prior to starting new medications become mandatory. NSAIDs are the most common medication used for patients with joint pains in general. NSAIDs have been advocated to exacerbate preexisting high blood pressure [67]. This was attributed to different mechanisms, e.g. sodium and water retention, renin–angiotensin–aldosterone system activation and inhibition of renal vasodilator prostaglandins [68–71]. Subsequently, it was advised to avoid these agents in patients with hypertension. However, NSAIDs with nitric oxide-promoting properties can help RA patients with high blood pressure. In a similar manner, in patients at a high risk of bleeding (e.g. those with peptic ulcer, gastrointestinal risk factors), alternative therapy has been advised. Taking NSAIDs with low-dose aspirin (taken for its anti-platelet effect) was also reported to double the risk of gastrointestinal bleeding. If NSAID therapy is necessary, cyclooxygenase (COX)-2 inhibitors with misoprostol or proton pump inhibitors (PPI) can be used [72]. Questionnaires have been published to help identify the patients at high risk of developing complications or have contraindication to NSAID use (Fig. 18.3).

Patients suffering from inflammatory arthritis are prone to develop insulin resistance [73, 74]. This was supported by the results of other studies showing that controlling inflammation reduces insulin resistance [75]. Studies showed that the anti-TNFα biologic therapy reduces the risk of developing diabetes mellitus in patients with inflammatory arthritis [74]. On the other hand, steroids (e.g. prednisolone) are known to cause hyperglycaemia and thus should be used with caution or better avoided in patients with risk factors or already have hyperglycaemia/diabetes mellitus. Similarly, steroids should be used cautiously in inflammatory arthritis patients at risk of osteoporosis. Careful consideration of the patient risk factors of osteoporosis, assessment of the bone mineral density and employment of primary prevention techniques and secondary treatment approaches are recommended when long-term steroid therapy is planned. In concordance, steroid-induced dyslipidaemia has been extensively studied [76, 77]. This finding, in addition to the recent publications reporting lipid profile changes induced by the inflammatory arthritic process itself [45], highlights the importance of screening for comorbidities by the treating rheumatologist before commencing long-term steroid therapy.

When disease modifying drugs (DMARDs) are considered, the patient should be screened for baseline liver and kidney functions as well as full blood count. Obesity, diabetes, fatty liver as well as viral and alcoholic hepatitis can deteriorate the condition of patients taking DMARDs [77]. Similarly, patients due to start biologic therapy should be screened initially for history of infections such as tuberculosis, or recurrent infections. Also malignancy and multiple sclerosis are contraindications to such treatment. Figure 18.4 shows a prebiologic therapy screening questionnaire which can be used in standard clinical practice. The recent American College of Rheumatology recommendations entailed that RA patients know to have hepatitis B and C can be treated using etanercept [78].

In conclusion, the available data in the literature regarding the interaction of comorbidities and the patients' medical management highlights the importance of the "patient-centred care" approach, and not the disease-targeted approach, when

NARAQ
(Non-Steroidal Anti-Inflammatory Risk Assessment Questionnaire)

PATIENT DETAILS	
Name :	Date : / /201
D.O.B. :	Age : years
Hospital No:	GP:

Dear Patient :
As you may be aware, there has been some concern regarding the safety of anti-inflammatory tablets for some patients. Anti-inflammatory therapy is the most commonly used medication for patients presenting with joint pains.
To help us choose the most appropriate medication for you, please would you spend few minutes answering this questionnaire.

Please answer the following questions by ticking the appropriate box			*For Official Use Only*
Do you smoke?	Yes □	No □	Smoking □
Do you have high blood pressure?	Yes □	No □	Uncontrolled B.P. □
Do you take tablets for high blood pressure?	Yes □	No □	
Is your blood pressure controlled with treatment?	Yes □	No □	
Have you ever had angina?	Yes □	No □	C.V.S. Risk □
Have you ever had heart attack?	Yes □	No □	
Have you ever had deep venous thrombosis (e.g. D.V.T. / blood clot) / peripheral artery disease ?	Yes □	No □	
Have you ever had heart failure?	Yes □	No □	
Have you ever had a stroke?	Yes □	No □	
Do you have any impairment of your kidney function?	Yes □	No □	Reno-vascular Affection □
Have you had any swelling in the legs from the knee down/ or around the ankles?	Yes □	No □	
Have you ever had gastric (stomach) bleeding?	Yes □	No □	Upper GI Risk □
Do you have heart burn?	Yes □	No □	
Do you take any treatment for peptic ulcer? (e.g. P.P.I.)	Yes □	No □	
Have you received treatment for *H. Pylori* in the past year? (a bug that affects the stomach)	Yes □	No □	
Do you have inflammatory bowel disease? (e.g. ulcerative colitis, Crohn's disease or diverticulitis)	Yes □	No □	Lower GI Risk □
Do you have irritable bowel syndrome?	Yes □	No □	
Have you ever had bleeding from the back passage?	Yes □	No □	
Do you have asthma?	Yes □	No □	AERD □
Is your asthma sensitive to *aspirin*?	Yes □	No □	
Do you take *warfarin*? (a drug to thin your blood)	Yes □	No □	Warfarin □
Do you take *aspirin* regularly?	Yes □	No □	Aspirin □
Do you have sensitivity to *sulpha*? (antibiotic)	Yes □	No □	Sulpha □

Fig. 18.3 NARAQ questionnaire (Data from Ref. [140])

managing inflammatory arthritic patients. To successfully manage inflammatory arthritis patients, comorbidities should be carefully considered, and they should be treated. Using questionnaires could be a valid tactic to keep a documented record of the patient's status prior to commencing medical therapy.

Pre-Biologic Therapy Assessment Proforma

Patient Name:

Hospital Number:

Diagnosis: **Rheumatoid Arthritis:** ☐
Ankylosing Spondylitis: ☐
Psoriatic Arthritis: ☐
IBD: ☐

Current Medications:

Biologic Naïve ☐	**Biologic Therapy Switch** ☐
Past DMARD Therapy (Dose, Reason for stopping): **- MTX:** ☐ **- SZP:** ☐ **- Arava:** ☐ **- HCQ:** ☐ **-Other:**	**Past Biologic Therapy (reason for stopping):** **- Anti-TNF:** ☐ **- Abatacept:** ☐ **- Rituximab:** ☐ **- Tocilizumab:** ☐ **- Other:**

To be completed by the patient **Clinic Date: / /201**

Please read carefully the following statements and tick the appropriate box that matches your condition

Please do not hesitate to discuss any of these questions that are unclear to you with the rheumatology doctor / nurse

Questions regarding your health status	**Yes**	**No**	**NA**
I had TB infection at some stage of my life	☐	☐	☐
I have a close relative who was diagnosed with TB	☐	☐	☐
I have a history of malignancy/ cancer	☐	☐	☐
My last cervical smear result came as clear	☐	☐	☐
I had a mammogram to assess for breast cancer	☐	☐	☐
I was diagnosed to have breast cancer	☐	☐	☐
I suffer from heart failure	☐	☐	☐
I suffer from Liver disease	☐	☐	☐
I suffer from a condition affecting the central nervous system, e.g Multiple Sclerosis	☐	☐	☐
I am pregnant	☐	☐	☐
I am breast feeding	☐	☐	☐
I suffer from recurrent/frequent infections e.g. chest/ skin/ urinary tract	☐	☐	☐
I was diagnosed to have hepatitis at some stage of my life (Which Heptatitis? A / B / C)	☐	☐	☐
I was diagnosed to have diverticulitis/ inflammatory bowel disease/ stomach ulcer	☐	☐	☐

After reading the relevant information (leaflets/patient's packs), methods of administration/ course of therapy and discussing my options for treatment; Please read the following statement and tick to confirm you agree that:

- I have been informed about my treatment options, as well as its benefits and possible risks. ☐
- I am clear about which benefits and risks matter most to me. ☐
- I am fully aware of my choices and have been given the chance to be involved in the decision. ☐
- I feel I had enough support and advice enabling me to make a choice. ☐
- I am aware of the nature of my disease and feel satisfied with my decision. ☐

Therefore, I have decided, I would prefer to receive my biologic therapy as intravenous infusions administered in the hospital / Subcutaneous injections <u>self-administered</u> (……………………………..) at my home (please delete as appropriate).

Signature:…………………………………………………………………… **Date: / /201**

Fig. 18.4 Prebiologic therapy screening questionnaire (From Ref. [141], with permission)

To be completed by the Treating Rheumatology nurse / Rheumatologist

Biologic Naïve □	**Biologic Therapy Switch** □

Disease Activity Measures	
Rheumatoid Arthritis: □	
/ / 201	**RA: DAS- 28 Score:**
/ / 201	**RA: DAS-28 Score:**
Ankylosing Spondylitis: □	**HLA-B27: Pos.** □ **Neg.** □
Past NSAID Therapy:	
/ / 201	**BASDAI: BASFI: BASG: Spinal Pain: / 10 ASDAS:**
/ / 201	**BASDAI: BASFI: BASG: Spinal Pain: / 10 ASDAS:**
Psoriatic Arthritis: □	**HLA-B27: Pos.** □ **Neg.** □
/ /201	**TJC: /78 SJC: /76 PGA: /100 PhGA: /100** | **PASI: /72** | **BSA: %**

Pre-Biologic Screening			
Body Wt.: Kg	**Height:** cm	**BMI:**	**BP:** / mm/Hg
Chest X-ray:			**Date:** / / 201
T-spot (IGRA) test result: Non-reactive: □	Reactive: □		Indeterminate: □
Repeat T-spot test result (in Indeterminate cases):	Reactive: □		Non- Reactive: □
Rheumatoid factor: Pos.: □ Neg.: □ Titer: IU/ml		**Anti-CCP:** Pos.: □ Neg.: □ Titer:	
ANA: Positive: □ Negative: □ Titer:		**ENA:**	
LFT: Normal:□ **Abn.:** □	Kid. Fn.: Normal:□ Abn.: □	ESR: mm/h	CRP: mg/dl
Lipid Profile result: Cholesterol: Tg.: HDL: LDL: Chol/HDL:			
Hepatitis B status:		**Hepatitis C status:**	
Immunoglobulin: IgG IgM: IgA: Date: / / 201			
Tocilizumab can affect the efficacy of atorvastatin; calcium channel blockers (high BP); theophylline (asthma); warfarin; phenytoin (epilepsy); ciclosporin; and anti-anxiety medicines such as benzodiazepines.			

The patient was reviewed in the pre-biologic therapy clinic on / / 201

And it has been agreed with ……………………………… to start biologic therapy in the form of:………………………………

Information leaflet/ patient's pack were given to the patient, treatment course explained & treatment will start once funding is approved.

Signature:……………………………………………… Date: / / 201

Rheumatology 2011; 50 S3): 99

Fig. 18.4 (continued)

Patient-Reported Comorbidity

As comorbidity is an important independent predictor of in-hospital mortality, which can influence patient outcomes and is routinely used in risk adjustment, it has been highly recommended to screen inflammatory arthritis patients whether acute (such as gouty arthritis) or chronic (such as RA, SpA or SLE) for comorbid conditions. Comorbidity information can be collected from either medical records or administrative data sources. However, this approach can be limited by (1) quality of documentation [79, 80], (2) limited availability of recent documentation, and (3) under-reporting of preadmission conditions judged by clinicians to be less pertinent to patients' admitting diagnoses [81–83]. Medical record notes may also frequently contain elements of both patient self-report and earlier professional documentation, sometimes offering a hybrid source of original data [84]. These limitations have led to increased interest in using patient self-report to calculate composite comorbidity levels [84–87].

Research has shown that many patients can accurately report their current [45–47] and past medical conditions [88–90], including comorbidities. However, data are limited regarding how well a self-report comorbidity score predicts functional capacity or quality of life health outcomes. The few global self-report comorbidity measures have been far less widely used and validated than administrative or medical record-derived measures [91, 92]. While self-report measures are subject to missing data due to incomplete filling of forms, the main challenge with any self-report measure is to translate medical language to plain language that patients can understand without assistance from a health professional. The most frequently used measure was developed by Katz et al. [79]. The self-administered comorbidity questionnaire was designed to be an equivalent self-report analogue of the Charlson index. Silliman et al. [93] designed a "quasi" self-report study using time to death as the outcome of interest but only used the self-administered comorbidity questionnaire measure with only 303 breast cancer patients. Other self-report measures are generally disease specific rather than general measures. A recent study [94] compared the reporting and level of agreement of comorbidities ascertained from rheumatologists, patients and health administrative data among patients with RA. 1787 patients were included in that study. The prevalence of cancer, diabetes, and hypertension reported by rheumatologists was lower than those reported by both patients and administrative data. Patients reported more cancers than rheumatologists and administrative data, which was illustrated in the lower sensitivity of administrative data in detecting cancers. There was substantial agreement between each of the three comorbidities ascertained from each data source (kappas ranging from 0.53 to 0.79).

PROMs and Comorbidity

Historically, assessment of healthcare quality has been quantified using disease-specific measures, such as targeted laboratory values or preventable hospitalisations [95–98]. A more stringent and patient-centred standard, however, is to assess quality with the person, rather than the disease, as the unit of analysis [99–101].

Doing so requires the use of patient-centred measures that express the net influence of all health conditions and their treatments on outcomes that are meaningful to patients. One example of such a measure is patient-reported outcomes that cross disease-specific boundaries (such as general health status or physical functioning) [102]. Assessing quality based on outcomes that matter to patients requires additional attention to measurement processes using these outcomes [103–106]. Using patient-reported outcomes is particularly relevant when assessing process, content, and quality of health outcomes for persons with multiple interacting medical conditions as well as for assessing multidimensional care interventions, such as implementations of the patient-centred medical home [107, 108].

Over the past years, patient-reported outcome measures (PROMs) booked its place as a valid tool to monitor the patients' status in the standard outpatient rheumatology setting. Over time, the role of PROMs expanded from mere assessment of disease activity parameters to playing an active role in the diagnosis, assessment of disease activity scores, identification and monitoring of comorbidities, adherence to therapy, and patient self-management [109]. As PROMs progressed from the generic phase into a disease-specific era, this helped in transforming the patient-centred care concept into reality. The multidimensional, chronic, debilitating, autoimmune nature of inflammatory arthritic condition affects the patients both directly and indirectly in almost all organ systems, from cardiovascular disorders and infections to increased risk of falling and osteoporotic fractures, depression, sexual dysfunction, and gastrointestinal ulcers. Guidelines [78, 110, 111] have highlighted that it is the rheumatologists' responsibility to assess for these risks when treating the patient.

The potential role of PROMs in the assessment of these comorbidities in arthritic patients is a good example of the evolving nature of PROMs. Recent PROM questionnaires allow the treating clinician to assess for arthritis-associated comorbidities at each visit. In its early stages, arthritic patients may not have significant comorbidities that warrant instant or long-term management. However, as the disease progresses and becomes more active, the patient can be prone to sustain one or more of these comorbidities. Screening for these symptoms is highly recommended on a regular basis for every patient at every clinic visit. This approach would facilitate on-the-spot assessment for cardiovascular risk, falls risk and osteoporosis, as well as depression [112–115]. By incorporating such parameters, PROMs attained its multidimensional nature, which takes into account not only how a person functions physically, mentally and socially but also incorporates comorbidity assessment, work ability, quality of life, disease activity and an evaluative component for self-helplessness/ motivation that assesses a person's satisfaction with his or her current health status [112, 116].

e-PROMs and e-Comorbidity

Advances in technology led to a heightened interest in exploring the use of this technology in the standard rheumatology practice. This led to rapid developments in the health system toward accredited health and care apps as well as digital information services. Using rapidly advancing technologies and online sources, patients will be able to log on and view their own health records via a portal. There will be unified real-time digital data flows between healthcare professionals and careers to support individuals' health and management. As the patients will be able to control their mobile care records, they will be able to add their own records from wearable devices. Online softwares and apps are already available for the patients to record their e-patient-reported outcome measures or functional disability.

Recent studies were published to assess the use of electronic patient-reported outcome measures (e-PROMs) in rheumatoid arthritis as well as SLE patients [117, 118]. Results revealed that e-PROMs could be administered through tablets, computers, and smart phones. It was feasible to sum the patient's disease activity parameters, and based on the scores calculated, clinical relevant actions tailored to the patient's status could be taken which would reflect on the disease control and target achieved. Another recent study [119, 120] was carried out to assess the validity of an electronically comorbidity assessment strategy to identify comorbid conditions among RA and PsA patients in standard practice and to evaluate the impact of e-comorbidity assessment on the patients' care and adherence to therapy. Results revealed that the sensitivity for identifying comorbidities using the electronic approach ranged from a minimum of 94% for atlanto-axial subluxation to a maximum of 100% for cardiovascular risk. The patients' adherence to antirheumatic therapy was significantly ($p < 0.1$) higher in the studied group, whereas stopping DMARDs for intolerability was significantly ($p < 0.01$) higher in the control group. Number of procedure/screening tests for comorbidity risk assessment was significantly higher in the e-comorbidity group ($P < 0.001$). In conclusion, the study reported that e-comorbidity assessment offered a specific and dynamic approach tailored to the patient's needs over the 2-year study period, which is applicable in standard practice. Patient-reported e-comorbidity outperformed the standard medical recording systems and can have a role in healthcare management and research. Reclassifying RA patients according to their comorbidity risk would have a positive impact on their adherence to therapy, early assessment of comorbidities with subsequent preventive or treatment decisions. The results of these studies paved the way for a project called "rheumote" [118] aiming at providing electronic patient-reported outcome measure service for patients with RA, ankylosing spondylitis, psoriatic arthritis, SLE, fibromyalgia and osteoarthritis in different languages.

Comorbidity Self-Management Tailored to the Patient's Need

While patient educational opportunities for primary prevention of arthritis are limited, a large variety of organised programmes have been developed to help patients deal with their disease and its associated comorbidities. These were planned according to the commonly accepted principles of education, psychology and psychotherapy, applied consistently by personnel with some kind of training and were able to produce desirable changes in knowledge, behaviour as well as health outcome in arthritis patients. The most common types of educational intervention in the treatment of arthritis are self-management programmes and cognitive-behavioural therapy. Both approaches emphasise learning new skills helpful in managing one's disease [121]. Self-management programmes are broadly focused on using information, problem-solving and coping skills for symptom management. Their aim is not only to achieve more than the provision of information to increase knowledge but also to change health behaviour and health status, teaching patients to identify and solve problems, set goals and plan actions [122]. Recent study looked into integrating the PROMs and medical education in one-on-one discussions, which provided a major opportunity for arthritis patient education. Viewing the PROMs scores before and after treatment in parallel with targeted patient education led to a significant greater reduction of disease activity parameters, DAS-28 score, comorbidities as well as improvement of the patients' adherence to antirheumatic therapy.

Modification of shared lifestyle risk factors such as smoking and promoting physical inactivity and body weight are all pivotal steps to reduce both the prevalence and severity of inflammatory arthritis-associated comorbidities (e.g. cardiovascular disease) and to reduce overall mortality [123–125]. In addition to the study outcomes reporting that cigarette smoking significantly increases the risk of developing RA [126, 127], a meta-analysis of observational studies revealed that the OR to be diagnosed with RA in males with 20 or more pack-years of smoking was 2.3 (95% CI: 1.6–3.4) [123]. Although the exact mechanism behind this effect remains uncertain, the process of citrullination is considered to be an important factor for the development of RA in the anti-citrullinated protein antibody (ACPA)-positive patients [127]. Whether (cessation of) smoking influences the disease course in patients with RA remains controversial. There is no clear association between smoking and HAQ, DAS28, CRP or the erythrocyte sedimentation rate (ESR) [123, 128, 129]. However, there is a strong statistical association between smoking and lung cancer as well as cardiovascular disease. In a meta-analysis that combined the radiographic data of six cohorts, it was concluded that smoking was not an independent risk factor for radiological progression in RA but that the effect was mediated via ACPA [130].

Regular exercise training in patients with inflammatory as well as noninflammatory arthritis is associated with improvement of and functional ability (e.g. aerobic fitness and muscle strength) without exacerbating disease activity, maintaining a healthy body weight and alleviating the persons' mood [131–134]. Studies that address the association between body weight and disease activity show conflicting results, and a high body mass index (BMI) has been correlated with both higher [135–137] and lower RA disease activity [138]. On the other hand, there is a significant relation between high body weight, diabetes mellitus, cardiovascular risk and metabolic syndrome. The European League Against Rheumatism (EULAR) has formulated recommendations about the need and timing of cardiovascular risk assessment in patients with RA [86]. In general, cardiovascular risk assessment should be performed regularly, at least annually [110]. However, currently, no RA-specific management model is available for risk assessment and management of cardiovascular disease. According to the EULAR recommendations, cardiovascular risk prediction charts (e.g. Framingham Risk Score) should be multiplied by a factor of 1.5 in case two out of three of the following criteria are present: (1) disease duration >10 years, (2) presence of rheumatoid factor or ACPA and (3) presence of extra-articular manifestations [139].

Building on what we know, comorbidity will book its place in modern approaches of management of patients living with both inflammatory and noninflammatory arthritis. Bearing in mind the variable nature of comorbidities and its progression over time, patient-reported outcome measures are the best tool to screen as well as document the patient's current comorbidity status at every patient visit. Electronic patient outcome apps will be the next step, to fill the gap between the rapidly growing technology and the current standard clinical practice. Patient management as well as education regarding their comorbidity status will be part of the standard rheumatology practice.

References

1. Methodology Committee of the Patient-Centered Outcomes Research Institute (PCORI). Methodological standards and patient-centeredness in comparative effectiveness research: the PCORI perspective. JAMA. 2012;307:1636–40.
2. Kjeken I, Dagfinrud H, Mowinckel P, et al. Rheumatology care: involvement in medical decisions, received information, satisfaction with care, and unmet health care needs in patients with rheumatoid arthritis and ankylosing spondylitis. Arthritis Rheum. 2006;55:394–401.
3. El Miedany Y, El Gaafary M, Palmer D. Assessment of the utility of visual feedback in the treatment of early rheumatoid arthritis patients: a pilot study. Rheumatol Int. 2012;32(10):3061–8.
4. Feinstein A. The pre/therapeutic classification of co/morbidity in chronic disease. J Chronic Dis. 1970;23:455–69.
5. Gabriel SE, Crowson CS, O'Fallon WM. Comorbidity in arthritis. J Rheumatol. 1999;26:2475–9.
6. Michaud K, Wolfe F. Comorbidities in rheumatoid arthritis. Best Pract Res Clin Rheumatol. 2007;21:885–906.
7. Norton S, et al. A study of baseline prevalence and cumulative incidence of comorbidity and extra-articular manifestations in RA and their impact on outcome. Rheumatology (Oxford). 2012;52:99–110.
8. Allebeck P, Ahlbom A, Allander E. Increased mortality among persons with rheumatoid arthritis, but where RA does not appear on death certificate. Eleven-year follow-up of an epidemiological study. Scand J Rheumatol. 1981;10:301–6.
9. Berkanovic E, Hurwicz ML. Rheumatoid arthritis and comorbidity. J Rheumatol. 1990;17:888–92.
10. Goodson NJ, et al. Mortality in early inflammatory polyarthritis: cardiovascular mortality is increased in seropositive patients. Arthritis Rheum. 2002;46:2010–9.
11. Zulling L, Bosworth H, Jeffreys A, Corsino L, et al. The association of comorbid conditions with patient-reported outcomes in Veterans with hip and knee osteoarthritis. Clin Rheumatol. 2015;34(8):1435–41.
12. van den Akker M. Comorbidity or multimorbidity: what's in a name? Eur J Gen Pract. 1996;2:65–70.
13. Dougados M, Soubrier M, Antunez A, Balint P, Balsa A, Buch MH, et al. Prevalence of comorbidities in rheumatoid arthritis and evaluation of their monitoring: results of an international, cross-sectional study (COMORA). Ann Rheum Dis. 2014;73:62–8.
14. Dougados M, Soubrier M, Perrodeau E, Gossec L, Fayet F, Gilson M, et al. Impact of a nurse-led programme on comorbidity management and impact of a patient self-assessment of disease activity on the management of rheumatoid arthritis: results of a prospective, multicentre, randomised, controlled trial (COMEDRA). Ann Rheum Dis. 2015;74:1725–33.

15. Tugwell P, Bombardier C. A methodologic framework for developing and selecting end-points in clinical trials. J Rheumatol. 1982;9:758–62.
16. Bombardier C, Tugwell P. A methodological framework to develop and select indices for clinical trials: statistical and judgmental approaches. J Rheumatol. 1982;9:753–7.
17. El Miedany Y. Adopting patient-centered care in standard practice: PROMs moving toward disease-specific era. Clin Exp Rheumatol. 2014;32(Suppl. 85):S40–6.
18. Project Europe 2030. http://espas.eu/orbis/sites/default/files/generated/document/en/Project%20Europe%202030.pdf. Accessed 30 Dec 2015.
19. Ranganath VK, Maranian P, Elashoff DA, Woodworth T, Khanna D, Hahn T, et al. Comorbidities are associated with poorer outcomes in community patients with rheumatoid arthritis. Rheumatology (Oxford). 2013;52:1809–17.
20. Arnold MB, Bykerk VP, Boire G, Haraoui BP, Hitchon C, Thorne C, CATCH Investigators, et al. Are there differences between young- and older-onset early inflammatory arthritis and do these impact outcomes? An analysis from the CATCH cohort. Rheumatology (Oxford). 2014;53(6):1075–86.
21. Zink A, Strangfeld A, Schneider M, Herzer P, Hierse F, Stoyanova-Scholz M, et al. Effectiveness of tumor necrosis factor inhibitors in rheumatoid arthritis in an observational cohort study: comparison of patients according to their eligibility for major randomized clinical trials. Arthritis Rheum. 2006;54:3399–407.
22. Burmester GR, Ferraccioli G, Flipo RM, Monteagudo-Sáez I, Unnebrink K, Kary S, et al. Clinical remission and/or minimal disease activity in patients receiving adalimumab treatment in a multinational, open-label, twelve-week study. Arthritis Rheum. 2008;59:32–41.
23. Sokka T, Hetland ML, Mäkinen H, Kautiainen H, Hørslev-Petersen K, Luukkainen RK, et al. Questionnaires in Standard Monitoring of Patients with Rheumatoid Arthritis Group. Remission and rheumatoid arthritis: data on patients receiving usual care in twenty-four countries. Arthritis Rheum. 2008;58:2642–51.
24. Krishnan E, Häkkinen A, Sokka T, Hannonen P. Impact of age and comorbidities on the criteria for remission and response in rheumatoid arthritis. Ann Rheum Dis. 2005;64:1350–2.
25. Barnett K, Mercer SW, Norbury M, Watt G, Wyke S, Guthrie B, et al. Epidemiology of multimorbidity and implications for health care, research, and medical education: a cross-sectional study. Lancet. 2012;380:37–43.
26. Loza E, Lajas C, Andreu JL, Balsa A, González-Álvaro I, Illera O, et al. Consensus statement on a framework for the management of comorbidity and extra-articular manifestations in rheumatoid arthritis. Rheumatol Int. 2015;35:445–58.
27. Konrat C, Boutron I, Trinquart L, Auleley GR, Ricordeau P, Ravaud P. Underrepresentation of elderly people in randomised controlled trials. The example of trials of 4 widely prescribed drugs. PLoS One. 2012;7:e33559.
28. De Groot V, Beckerman H, Lankhorst GJ, Bouter LM. How to measure comorbidity. A critical review of available methods. J Clin Epidemiol. 2003;56:221–9.
29. El Miedany Y. Co-morbidity index in rheumatoid arthritis: time to think. Clin Rheumatol. 2015;34:1995–2000.
30. Mold J, Blake G, Becker L. Goal-oriented medical care. Fam Med. 1991;23:46–51
31. Burmester GR, Ferraccioli G, Flipo RM, et al. Clinical remission and/or minimal disease activity in patients receiving adalimumab treatment in a multinational, open label, twelve-week study. Arthritis Rheum. 2008;59:3241.
32. Sokka T, Makinen H, Hannonen P, et al. Most people over age 50 in the general population do not meet ACR remission criteria or OMERACT minimal disease activity criteria for rheumatoid arthritis. Rheumatology. 2007;46:1020–3.
33. Michaud K, Wolfe F. Patterns of comorbidity in rheumatic disorders [abstract]. Arthritis Rheum. 2007;54:S339.
34. Radner H, Smolen JS, Aletaha D. Impact of comorbidity on physical function in patients with rheumatoid arthritis. Ann Rheum Dis. 2010;69:536–41.

35. Radner H, Smolen JS, Aletaha D. Comorbidity affects all domains of physical function and quality of life in patients with rheumatoid arthritis. Rheumatology. 2011;50:381–8.
36. Verbrugge LM, Lepkowski JM, Imanaka Y. Comorbidity and its impact on disability. Milbank Q. 1989;67:450–84.
37. Verbrugge LM, Lepkowski JM, Konkol LL. Levels of disability among U.S. adults with arthritis. J Gerontol. 1991;46:S71–83.
38. Michaud K, Wallenstein G, Wolfe F. Treatment and non-treatment predictors of health assessment questionnaire disability progression in rheumatoid arthritis: a longitudinal study of 18,485 patients. Arthritis Care Res. 2011;63:366–72.
39. Holla JF, van der Leeden M, Knol DL, Roorda LD, van der Esch M, et al. The association of body mass index and depressed mood with knee pain and activity limitations in knee osteoarthritis: results from the Amsterdam osteoarthritis cohort. BMC Musculoskelet Disord. 2013;14(1):296.
40. Singh JA, Lewallen DG. Time trends in the characteristics of patients undergoing primary total knee arthroplasty. Arthritis Care Res. 2013;66(6):897–906.
41. Martin KR, Kuh D, Harris TB, Guralnik JM, Coggon D, Wills AK. Body mass index, occupational activity, and leisure-time physical activity: an exploration of risk factors and modifiers for knee osteoarthritis in the 1946 British birth cohort. BMC Musculoskelet Disord. 2013;14:219.
42. Perruccio AV, Davis AM, Hogg-Johnson S, Badley EM. Importance of self-rated health and mental well-being in predicting health outcomes following total joint replacement surgery for osteoarthritis. Arthritis Care Res. 2011;63(7):973–81.
43. Perruccio AV, Katz JN, Losina E. Health burden in chronic disease: multimorbidity is associated with self-rated health more than medical comorbidity alone. J Clin Epidemiol. 2012;65(1):100–6.
44. Cleveland RJ, Luong ML, Knight JB, Schoster B, Renner JB, Jordan JM, Callahan LF. Independent associations of socioeconomic factors with disability and pain in adults with knee osteoarthritis. BMC Musculoskelet Disord. 2013;14:297.
45. Charles-Schoeman C, Fleischmann R, Davignon J, Schwartz H, et al. Potential mechanisms leading to the abnormal lipid profile in patients with rheumatoid arthritis versus healthy volunteers and reversal by tofacitinib. Arthritis Rheumatol. 2015;67(3):616–25.
46. Ronda N, Greco D, Adorni MP, Zimetti F, Favari E, Hjeltnes G, et al. Newly identified anti-atherosclerotic activity of methotrexate and adalimumab: complementary effects on lipoprotein function and macrophage cholesterol metabolism. Arthritis Rheumatol. 2015;67:1155–64.
47. Roubille C, Richer V, Starnino T, McCourt C, McFarlane A, Fleming P, et al. The effects of tumour necrosis factor inhibitors, methotrexate, non-steroidal anti-inflammatory drugs and corticosteroids on cardiovascular events in rheumatoid arthritis, psoriasis and psoriatic arthritis: a systematic review and meta-analysis. Ann Rheum Dis. 2015;74:480–9.
48. Sakthiswary R, Das S. The effects of TNF α antagonist therapy on bone metabolism in rheumatoid arthritis: a systematic review. Curr Drug Targets. 2013;14:1552–7.
49. Van der Goes MC, Jacobs JW, Jurgens MS, Bakker MF, van der Veen MJ, van der Werf JH, et al. Are changes in bone mineral density different between groups of early rheumatoid arthritis patients treated according to a tight control strategy with or without prednisone if osteoporosis prophylaxis is applied? Osteoporos Int. 2013;24:1429–36.
50. Toussirot É. Effects of TNFα inhibitors on adiposity and other cardiovascular risk factors: implications for the cardiovascular prognosis in patients with rheumatoid arthritis. Expert Opin Drug Saf. 2015;14:525–32.
51. Engvall IL, Tengstrand B, Brismar K, Hafström I. Infliximab therapy increases body fat mass in early rheumatoid arthritis independently of changes in disease activity and levels of leptin and adiponectin: a randomised study over 21 months. Arthritis Res Ther. 2010;12:R197.
52. Metsios GS, Stavropoulos-Kalinoglou A, Douglas KM, Koutedakis Y, Nevill AM, Panoulas VF, et al. Blockade of tumour necrosis factor-alpha in rheumatoid arthritis: effects on components of rheumatoid cachexia. Rheumatology (Oxford). 2007;46:1824–7.

53. Marcora SM, Chester KR, Mittal G, Lemmey AB, Maddison PJ. Randomized phase 2 trial of anti-tumor necrosis factor therapy for cachexia in patients with early rheumatoid arthritis. Am J Clin Nutr. 2006;84:1463–72.
54. Serelis J, Kontogianni MD, Katsiougiannis S, Bletsa M, Tektonidou MG, Skopouli FN. Effect of anti-TNF treatment on body composition and serum adiponectin levels of women with rheumatoid arthritis. Clin Rheumatol. 2008;27:795–7.
55. Abbott R, Whear R, Nikolaou V, Bethel A, Coon JT, Stein K, et al. Tumour necrosis factor-α inhibitor therapy in chronic physical illness: a systematic review and meta-analysis of the effect on depression and anxiety. J Psychosom Res. 2015;79:175–84.
56. Kekow J, Moots R, Khandker R, Melin J, Freundlich B, Singh A. Improvements in patient-reported outcomes, symptoms of depression and anxiety, and their association with clinical remission among patients with moderate-to-severe active early rheumatoid arthritis. Rheumatology (Oxford). 2011;50:401–9.
57. McCarey DW, McInnes IB, Madhok R, Hampson R, Scherbakov O, Ford I, et al. Trial of Atorvastatin in Rheumatoid Arthritis (TARA): double-blind, randomised placebo-controlled trial. Lancet. 2004;363:2015–21.
58. Schoenfeld SR, Lu L, Rai SK, Seeger JD, Zhang Y, Choi HK. Statin use and mortality in rheumatoid arthritis: a general population-based cohort study. Ann Rheum Dis. 2015; doi:10.1136/annrheumdis-2015-207714.
59. El Miedany Y, Palmer D, Youssef S, El Gaafary M. Psychometric outcome measures in early vs late ankylosing spondylitis patients. Ann Rheum Dis. 2010;69(Suppl 3):435.
60. Oldroyd J, Schachna L, Buchbinder R, Staples M, et al. Ankylosing spondylitis patients commencing biologic therapy have high baseline levels of comorbidity: a report from the Australian Rheumatology Association database. Int J Rheumatol. 2009. Article ID 268569; doi:10.1155/2009/268569.
61. Ferrari-Lacraz S, Ferrari S. Do RANKL inhibitors (denosumab) affect inflammation and immunity? Osteoporos Int. 2011;22:435–46.
62. Cohen SB, Dore RK, Lane NE, et al. Denosumab Rheumatoid Arthritis Study Group. Denosumab treatment effects on structural damage, bone mineral density, and bone turnover in rheumatoid arthritis: a twelve-month, multicenter, randomized, double-blind, placebo-controlled, phase II clinical trial. Arthritis Rheum. 2008;58:1299–309.
63. Sacre S, Medghalchi M, Gregory B, Brennan F, Williams R. Fluoxetine and citalopram exhibit potent antiinflammatory activity in human and murine models of rheumatoid arthritis and inhibit toll-like receptors. Arthritis Rheum. 2010;62:683–93.
64. Bawa FL, Mercer SW, Atherton RJ, Clague F, Keen A, Scott NW, et al. Does mindfulness improve outcomes in patients with chronic pain? Systematic review and meta-analysis. Br J Gen Pract. 2015;65(635):e387–400.
65. Richards BL, Whittle SL, Buchbinder R. Antidepressants for pain management in rheumatoid arthritis. Cochrane Database Syst Rev. 2011:CD008920.
66. Richards BL, Whittle SL, van der Heijde DM, Buchbinder R. The efficacy and safety of antidepressants in inflammatory arthritis: a Cochrane systematic review. J Rheumatol Suppl. 2012;90:21–7.
67. Faselis C, Doumas M, Papademetriou V. Common secondary causes of resistant hypertension and rational for treatment. Int J Hypertens. 2011;2011:236239.
68. FitzGerald GA. COX-2 and beyond: approaches to prostaglandin inhibition in human disease. Nat Rev Drug Discov. 2003;2(11):879–90.
69. Lanas A, Garcia-Tell G, Armada B, Oteo-Alvaro A. Prescription patterns and appropriateness of NSAID therapy according to gastrointestinal risk and cardiovascular history in patients with diagnoses of osteoarthritis. BMC Med. 2011;9:38.
70. Galesić K, Jelaković B. Nonsteroidal antirheumatics and hypertension. Lijec Vjesn. 2011;133(3–4):101–6.
71. Francois H, Coffman TM. Prostanoids and blood pressure: which way is up? J Clin Invest. 2004;114(6):757–9.

72. Lanza FL, Chan FK, Quigley EM. Practice Parameters Committee of the American College of Gastroenterology. Guidelines for prevention of NSAID-related ulcer complications. Am J Gastroenterol. 2009;104(3):728–38.
73. Wasko MC, Kay J, Hsia EC, Rahman MU. Diabetes mellitus and insulin resistance in patients with rheumatoid arthritis: risk reduction in a chronic inflammatory disease. Arthritis Care Res (Hoboken). 2011;63(4):512–21.
74. Antohe JL, Bili A, Sartorius JA, et al. Diabetes mellitus risk in rheumatoid arthritis: reduced incidence with anti-tumor necrosis factor α therapy. Arthritis Care Res (Hoboken). 2012;64(2):215–21.
75. Situnayake RD, Kitas G. Dyslipidemia and rheumatoid arthritis. Ann Rheum Dis. 1997;56(6):341–2.
76. Ettinger WH, Klinefelter HF, Kwiterovitch PO. Effect of short-term, low-dose corticosteroids on plasma lipoprotein lipids. Atherosclerosis. 1987;63(2–3):167–72.
77. Visser K, Katchamart W, Loza E, et al. Multinational evidence-based recommendations for the use of methotrexate in rheumatic disorders with a focus on rheumatoid arthritis: integrating systematic literature research and expert opinion of a broad international panel of rheumatologists in the 3E initiative. Ann Rheum Dis. 2009;68(7):1086–93.
78. Singh JA, Furst DE, Bharat A, et al. 2012 update of the 2008 American College of Rheumatology recommendations for the use of disease-modifying anti-rheumatic drugs and biologic agents in the treatment of rheumatoid arthritis. Arthritis Care Res (Hoboken). 2012;64(5):625–39.
79. Katz JN, Chang LC, Sangha O, Fossel AH, Bates DW. Can comorbidity be measured by questionnaire rather than medical record review? Med Care. 1996;34(1):73–84.
80. Skinner KM, Miller DR, Lincoln E, Lee A, Kazis LE. Concordance between respondent self-reports and medical records for chronic conditions: experience from the Veterans Health Study. J Ambul Care Manage. 2005;28(2):102–10.
81. Tisnado DM, Adams JL, Liu H, Damberg CL, Chen WP, Hu FA, Carlisle DM, Mangione CM, Kahn KL. What is the concordance between the medical record and patient self-report as data sources for ambulatory care? Med Care. 2006;44(2):132–40.
82. Sangha O, Stucki G, Liang MH, Fossel AH, Katz JN. The self-administered comorbidity questionnaire: a new method to assess comorbidity for clinical and health services research. Arthritis Rheum. 2003;49(2):156–63.
83. Byles JE, D'Este C, Parkinson L, O'Connell R, Treloar C. Single index of multimorbidity did not predict multiple outcomes. J Clin Epidemiol. 2005;58(10):997–1005.
84. Susser SR, McCusker J, Belzile E. Comorbidity information in older patients at an emergency visit: self-report vs. administrative data had poor agreement but similar predictive validity. J Clin Epidemiol. 2008;61(5):511–5.
85. Horton M, Rudick RA, Hara-Cleaver C, Marrie RA. Validation of a self-report comorbidity questionnaire for multiple sclerosis. Neuroepidemiology. 2010;35(2):83–90.
86. Streibelt M, Schmidt C, Brunger M, Spyra K. Comorbidity from the patient perspective – does it work? Validity of a questionnaire on self-estimation of comorbidity (SCQ-D). Orthopade. 2012;41(4):303–10.
87. Mechanic D. The experience and reporting of common physical complaints. J Health Soc Behav. 1980;21(2):146–55.
88. Motl RW, Fernhall B, McAuley E, Cutter G. Physical activity and self-reported cardiovascular comorbidities in persons with multiple sclerosis: evidence from a cross-sectional analysis. Neuroepidemiology. 2011;36(3):183–91.
89. Linet MS, Harlow SD, McLaughlin JK, McCaffrey LD. A comparison of interview data and medical records for previous medical conditions and surgery. J Clin Epidemiol. 1989;42(12):1207–13.
90. Colditz GA, Martin P, Stampfer MJ, Willett WC, Sampson L, Rosner B, Hennekens CH, Speizer FE. Validation of questionnaire information on risk factors and disease outcomes in a prospective cohort study of women. Am J Epidemiol. 1986;123(5):894–900.

91. Fiest KM, Currie SR, Williams JV, Wang J. Chronic conditions and major depression in community-dwelling older adults. J Affect Disord. 2011;131(1–3):172–8.
92. Greenfield S, Sullivan L, Dukes KA, Silliman R, D'Agostino R, Kaplan SH. Development and testing of a new measure of case mix for use in office practice. Med Care. 1995;33(4 Suppl):AS47–55.
93. Silliman RA, Lash TL. Comparison of interview-based and medical-record based indices of comorbidity among breast cancer patients. Med Care. 1999;37(4):339–49.
94. Widdifield J, Bernatsky S, Paterson M, Abrahamowicz M et al. Comparisons of reporting and level of agreement of comorbidities ascertained from rheumatologists, patients and health administrative data: a data linkage study among patients with rheumatoid arthritis. Ann Rheum Dis. 2015 (EULAR 2015: 4798).
95. Nolan T, Berwick DM. All-or-none measurement raises the bar on performance. JAMA. 2006;295(10):1168–70.
96. Shekelle PG, MacLean CH, Morton SC, Wenger NS. Assessing care of vulnerable elders: methods for developing quality indicators. Ann Intern Med. 2001;135(8 Pt 2):647–52.
97. Elixhauser A, Pancholi M, Clancy CM. Using the AHRQ quality indicators to improve health care quality. Jt Comm J Qual Patient Saf. 2005;31(9):533–8.
98. Shortell SM, Gillies R, Siddique J, et al. Improving chronic illness care: a longitudinal cohort analysis of large physician organizations. Med Care. 2009;47(9):932–9.
99. Berwick DM. Measuring physicians' quality and performance: a drift on Lake Wobegon. JAMA. 2009;302(22):2485–6.
100. Werner RM, Greenfield S, Fung C, Turner BJ. Measuring quality of care in patients with multiple clinical conditions: summary of a conference conducted by the Society of General Internal Medicine. J Gen Intern Med. 2007;22(8):1206–11.
101. Glasgow RE, Peeples M, Skovlund SE. Where is the patient in diabetes performance measures? The case for including patient-centered and self-management measures. Diabetes Care. 2008;31(5):1046–50.
102. Stewart AL, Greenfield S, Hays RD, et al. Functional status and well-being of patients with chronic conditions. Results from the Medical Outcomes Study. JAMA. 1989;262(7):907–13.
103. Mandelblatt JS, Bierman AS, Gold K, et al. Constructs of burden of illness in older patients with breast cancer: a comparison of measurement methods. Health Serv Res. 2001;36(6 Pt 1):1085–107. Corrected in Health Serv Res. 2007;42(5):2088
104. Perruccio AV, Katz JN, Losina E. Health burden in chronic disease: multimorbidity is associated with self-rated health more than medical comorbidity alone. J Clin Epidemiol. 2012;65(1):100–6.
105. Fortin M, Lapointe L, Hudon C, Vanasse A, Ntetu AL, Maltais D. Multimorbidity and quality of life in primary care: a systematic review. Health Qual Life Outcomes. 2004;2:51.
106. Safford MM, Allison JJ, Kiefe CI. Patient complexity: more than comorbidity. The vector model of complexity. J Gen Intern Med. 2007;22(Suppl 3):382–90.
107. Rosen AK, Reid R, Broemeling AM, Rakovski CC. Applying a risk adjustment framework to primary care: can we improve on existing measures? Ann Fam Med. 2003;1(1):44–51.
108. Peek CJ, Baird MA, Coleman E. Primary care for patient complexity, not only disease. Fam Syst Health. 2009;27(4):287–302.
109. El Miedany Y. PROMs in inflammatory arthritis: moving from static to dynamic. Clin Rheumatol. 2013;32:735–42.
110. Smolen J, Landewé R, Breedveld F, et al. EULAR recommendations for the management of rheumatoid arthritis with synthetic and biological disease-modifying antirheumatic drugs. Ann Rheum Dis. 2010; doi:10.1136/ard.2009.126532.
111. The Management of Rheumatoid Arthritis in Adults. NICE, London. 2009. www.nice.org.uk/CG79. Accessed 16 June 2015.
112. Pincus T, Callahan LF, Sale WG, Brooks AL, Payne LE, Vaughn WK. Severe functional declines, work disability, and increased mortiality in seventy-five rheumatoid arthritis patients studied over nine years. Arthritis Rheum. 1984;27:864–72.

113. El Miedany Y, El Gaafary M, Youssef S, Palmer D. Answering the difficult question: how to identify rheumatoid arthritis patients at higher risk of cardiovascular disease in the standard practice? Ann Rheum Dis. 2009;68(SIII):554.
114. El Miedany Y, Palmer D, El Gaafary M. Further analysis of helplessness measurement in inflammatory arthritis/spondyloarthritis: the development of the modified rheumatology attitude index. Rheumatology (Oxford). 2010;49(S1):162.
115. El Miedany Y, Palmer D, Toth M. Assessment of falls risk in patients with rheumatoid arthritis in the standard rheumatology practice: mission possible. Rheumatology (Oxford). 2009;48(Suppl 1):i128.
116. Palmer D, El Miedany Y. Self-helplessness in arthritis: an important but overlooked index. Br J Nurs. 2010;19(15):965–71.
117. El Miedany Y, El Gaafary M, Youssef S, Bahlas S, Almedany S, Ahmed I, Palmer D. Toward electronic health recording: evaluation of electronic patient-reported outcome measures system for remote monitoring of early rheumatoid arthritis. J Rheumatol. 2016. pii: jrheum.151421.
118. El Miedany Y, Bahlas S, El Gaafary M, Youssef S, Ahmed I. Electronic patient reported outcome measures in systemic lupus erythematosus: a potential disease modifying impact on the management of disease activity flares and damage accrual. Arthritis Rheumatol. 2015;67(S10):1994.
119. El Miedany Y, El Gaafary M, Youssef S, Bahlas S, Ahmed I, Hegazi M. Rheumatoid arthritis comorbidity index: development and validation of a new specific tool for classifying prognostic comorbidity in rheumatoid arthritis patients. Ann Rheum Dis. 2016;75(Suppl 2):154.
120. El Miedany Y, El Gaafary M, Youssef S, Bahlas S, Ahmed I, Hegazi M. Psoriatic arthritis comorbidity index: development and validation of a new specific tool for classifying prognostic comorbidity in psoriatic arthritis patients. Ann Rheum Dis. 2016;75(Suppl 2):89.
121. Daltroy LH, Liang MH. Advances in patient education in rheumatic disease. Ann Rheum Dis. 1991;50(Suppl 3):415–7.
122. Lorig K. Partnership between expert patients and physicians. Lancet. 2002;359(9309):814–5.
123. Roubille C, Richer V, Starnino T, McCourt C, McFarlane A, Fleming P, et al. Evidence-based recommendations for the management of comorbidities in rheumatoid arthritis, psoriasis, and psoriatic arthritis: expert opinion of the Canadian dermatology-rheumatology comorbidity initiative. J Rheumatol. 2015;42:1767–80.
124. Leitzmann MF, Park Y, Blair A, Ballard-Barbash R, Mouw T, Hollenbeck AR, Schatzkin A. Physical activity recommendations and decreased risk of mortality. Arch Intern Med. 2007;167:2453–60.
125. Berrington de Gonzalez A, Hartge P, Cerhan JR, et al. Body-mass index and mortality among 1.46 million white adults. N Engl J Med. 2010;363:2211–9.
126. Sugiyama D, Nishimura K, Tamaki K, Tsuji G, Nakazawa T, Morinobu A, Kumagai S. Impact of smoking as a risk factor for developing rheumatoid arthritis: a meta-analysis of observational studies. Ann Rheum Dis. 2010;69:70–81.
127. Källberg H, Ding B, Padyukov L, Bengtsson C, Rönnelid J, Klareskog L, et al. EIRA Study Group. Smoking is a major preventable risk factor for rheumatoid arthritis: estimations of risks after various exposures to cigarette smoke. Ann Rheum Dis. 2011;70:508–11.
128. Mattey DL, Hutchinson D, Dawes PT, Nixon NB, Clarke S, Fisher J, et al. Smoking and disease severity in rheumatoid arthritis: association with polymorphism at the glutathione S-transferase M1 locus. Arthritis Rheum. 2002;46(3):640–6.
129. Finckh A, Dehler S, Costenbader KH, Gabay C, Swiss Clinical Quality Management Project for RA. Cigarette smoking and radiographic progression in rheumatoid arthritis. Ann Rheum Dis. 2007;66:1066–71.
130. De Rooy DP, van Nies JA, Kapetanovic MC, Kristjansdottir H, Andersson ML, Forslind K, et al. Smoking as a risk factor for the radiological severity of rheumatoid arthritis: a study on six cohorts. Ann Rheum Dis. 2014;73:1384–7.

131. Metsios GS, Stavropoulos-Kalinoglou A, Veldhuijzen van Zanten JJ, Treharne GJ, Panoulas VF, et al. Rheumatoid arthritis, cardiovascular disease and physical exercise: a systematic review. Rheumatology (Oxford). 2008;47:239–48.
132. Hurkmans E, van der Giesen FJ, Vliet Vlieland TP, Schoones J, Van den Ende EC. Dynamic exercise programs (aerobic capacity and/or muscle strength training) in patients with rheumatoid arthritis. Cochrane Database Syst Rev. 2009:CD006853.
133. Plasqui G. The role of physical activity in rheumatoid arthritis. Physiol Behav. 2008;94:270–5.
134. Cooney JK, Law RJ, Matschke V, Lemmey AB, Moore JP, Ahmad Y, et al. Benefits of exercise in rheumatoid arthritis. J Aging Res. 2011;2011:681640.
135. Veldhuijzen van Zanten JJ, Rouse PC, Hale ED, Ntoumanis N, Metsios GS, Duda JL, et al. Perceived barriers, facilitators and benefits for regular physical activity and exercise in patients with rheumatoid arthritis: a review of the literature. Sports Med. 2015;45:1401–12.
136. Ajeganova S, Andersson ML, Hafström I, BARFOT Study Group. Association of obesity with worse disease severity in rheumatoid arthritis as well as with comorbidities: a long-term followup from disease onset. Arthritis Care Res (Hoboken). 2013;65:78–87.
137. Papadakis JA, Sidiropoulos PI, Karvounaris SA, Vrentzos GE, Spanakis EK, Ganotakis ES, Kritikos HD, et al. Metabolic syndrome is common among middle-to-older aged Mediterranean patients with rheumatoid arthritis and correlates with disease activity: a retrospective, cross-sectional, controlled, study. Ann Rheum Dis. 2007;66:28–33.
138. Van der Helm-van Mil AH, van der Kooij SM, Allaart CF, Toes RE, Huizinga TW. A high body mass index has a protective effect on the amount of joint destruction in small joints in early rheumatoid arthritis. Ann Rheum Dis. 2008;67:769–74.
139. Peters MJ, Symmons DP, McCarey D, Dijkmans BA, Nicola P, Kvien TK, et al. EULAR evidence-based recommendations for cardiovascular risk management in patients with rheumatoid arthritis and other forms of inflammatory arthritis. Ann Rheum Dis. 2010;69 325–31.
140. El Miedany YM, Palmer D, El Gaafary M. Validity of a non-steroidal anti-inflammatory risk assessment questionnaire (NARAQ) for standard clinical practice. Rheumatology (Oxford). 2006;45(suppl 1):i59.
141. El Miedany Y, El Gaafary M, Youssef SS, et al. Incorporating patient reported outcome measures in clinical practice: development and validation of a questionnaire for inflammatory arthritis. Clin Exp Rheumatol. 2010;28:734–44.

Chapter 19
e-Comorbidity and Information Technology

Yasser El Miedany

Background

In 1991, the Institute of Medicine (USA) issued a report concluding that computer-based patient record was an "essential technology" for health care and in 1997 called for the widespread adoption of a computer-based patient record over the next 10 years [1]. In 2001, the Institute of Medicine's report, "Crossing the Quality Chasm: A New Health System for the 21st Century," targeted six areas of health care which required significant improvement: safety, efficacy, timeliness, efficiency, equality, and patient-centeredness [3]. The report outlined why and how health information technology can be implemented to achieve all six aims.

Medicine is an information-rich enterprise. A greater and more seamless flow of information within a digital health-care infrastructure, such as that created by electronic health records (eHR), can transform the way health care is delivered. With eHRs, information is available whenever and wherever it is needed; consequently, this improves the providers' ability to make well-informed treatment decisions quickly and safely. Initially, in rheumatology, information technology was implemented to monitor patients' disease activity; however, recent studies showed its value also to monitor patients' comorbidity as well as motivation [4–6]. The benefits of electronic health records (eHRs) are numerous and greatly outweigh the cost of implementation (Fig. 19.1). Its positive impact was not only confined to the patients or health-care physicians but extended to include also the physician-patient relationship as well as setting up treatment protocols tailored to the patient's needs. It also helped to monitor their comorbidities, functional abilities, as well as quality of lives [7]. This paved the

Y. El Miedany, MD, FRCP (✉)
King's College, London, UK

Rheumatology and Rehabilitation, Ain Shams University, Cairo, Egypt

Department of Rheumatology, Darent Valley Hospital, Dartford, Kent, UK
e-mail: yasser_elmiedany@yahoo.com

Y. El Miedany (ed.), *Comorbidity in Rheumatic Diseases*,
DOI 10.1007/978-3-319-59963-2_19

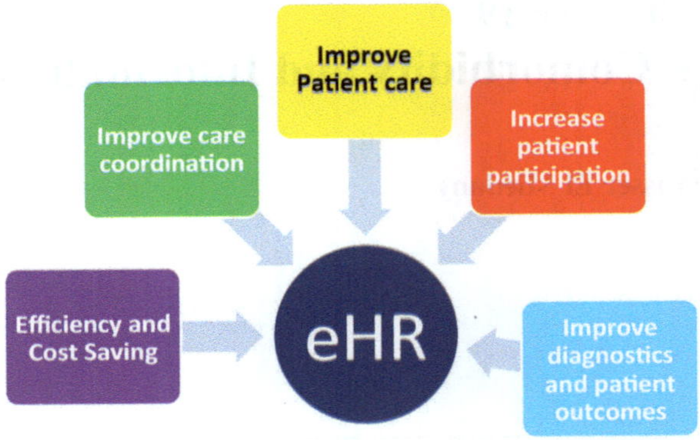

Fig. 19.1 Benefits of electronic health record (eHR)

way to a new trend in medicine which is applicable to rheumatology. This chapter will address the latest developments regarding the use of modern technology in the standard rheumatology practice, its impact on the delivery of direct health care, services tailored to the patient, as well as real-time monitoring of the disease vital signs and comorbidity. It will not focus on what technology will be like in the future, but rather, what will rheumatologists be like.

Electronic Health Care

Several new terms have been introduced to the modern medicine literature. Terms such as electronic medical, health, and personal records have been commonly used over the past years; however, the reader usually gets confused with their definitions and what are the differences among them. An electronic medical record (eMR) contains the standard medical and clinical data gathered in one provider's office. Therefore, an electronic medical record is a digital version of a paper chart that contains all of a patient's medical history from one practice [8]. An electronic medical record is mostly used by providers for diagnosis and treatment. However, the information stored in eMRs is not easily shared with providers outside of a practice. A patient's record might even have to be printed out and delivered by mail to specialists and other members of the care team. In contrast, electronic health records (eHRs) go beyond the data collected in the provider's office and include a more comprehensive patient history. Therefore, eHRs are designed to contain and share information from all providers involved in a patient's care. eHR data can be created, managed, and consulted by authorized providers and staff from across more than one health-care organization. Unlike electronic medical records, eHRs also permit the patients' health record to move with them—to other health-care providers, specialists, hospitals, nursing homes, and even across geographical regions [9].

Electronic personal health record, (ePHR) is an online document with information about the person's health (including also the health of family members) that the person has to keep up to date for easy reference. Using the person's ePHR

Table 19.1 Models of electronic data recording

Electronic medical record (eMR)	Electronic health record (eHR)	Electronic personalized record (ePR)
An eMR is more beneficial than paper records because it allows providers to	An eHR is a real-time, patient-centered record, which brings together in one place everything about a patient's health	An online document with information about the person's health
Track data over time	Improve patient care	Friendly and very easy to use
Identify patients who are due for preventive visits and screenings	Improve care coordination	Information about the person's, and his family's, health in one folder
Monitor how patients measure up to certain parameters, such as vaccinations and blood pressure/sugar readings	Improve diagnostics and patient outcomes	Enables tracking of the person's as well as his/her family's health information, such as the date of the immunizations, last physical exam
Improve overall quality of care in a practice	Enhance patient participation	Can be available on mobile/smart gadgets
	Improve centers efficiencies and cost savings	Give the person the opportunity to take a more active role in managing his/her health care

enables tracking of his/her family's health information, such as the date of the children's immunizations, last physical exam, allergies, or a list of family medicines, major illnesses, and operations. Many ePHRs are easy to use and may be provided free from health providers, the government, or private companies (who tend to charge a monthly or annual fee for this service). More recently, apps have been developed to do the same role. The availability of the ePHR on the Web enabled the person to get into and manage his/her health information from anywhere. Empowering the people to collect, view, manage, and share their health information electronically will in turn give the person the opportunity to take a more active role in managing his/her health care [10]. Table 19.1 includes a comparison of the three major health-care systems and their positive impact on the patients' management.

Telehealth and telemedicine have also been recently included in the electronic patient management dictionary. While both terms refer to the use of telecommunications and information technology to provide health-care services at a distance, i.e., remote health care; telemedicine is considered a subset of telehealth. Key differences in definitions related to whether the patient care is delivered in real time or asynchronously. Telemedicine refers to direct patient care or clinical services through a "Two-way, real-time interactive communication between the patient and the physician or practitioner at the distant site." In contrast, telehealth is used to refer to remote health care that does not always involve clinical services. Examples of health-care services delivered via telehealth include direct patient care, education, health administration, and public health interventions. Services may be delivered asynchronously or synchronously (real time) [8].

Toward Electronic Health-Care Service

Implementing recent technology for patients' management and care has become a mandatory development for modern health-care service. Not only it has a constructive impact on the patients' management, but it also has a positive reflection on disease prevention. Outside the traditional care, new technologies transformed the care provided in standard practice in general and rheumatology in particular. This includes the following items.

Patient-Centered Care

"Patient partnership" can be considered as the logo for this era in medical care. Similar to any evolving project, the scope has crept over years, starting with patient information leaflets handed to the patients at the end of the consultation [11]; to patient-reported outcome measures, which are completed by the patient before their clinical assessment in the outpatient clinics [12]; and lastly to patient education and self-management protocols set up and tailored based on the patient's needs [13]. One of the criticisms of the traditional population-based treatment regimens, used to be implemented in standard practice, is that interventions, usually calibrated against a baseline average, are derived from generalizations regardless of the patient's unique medical status. This approach is notorious for under- or over-compensating the needs of an individual. With modern eHRs, information can now be displayed automatically and provide the treating health-care professionals with relevant care and treatment guidelines that are adapted for an individual patient. Moreover, a standardized yet data-driven algorithm assures that the individual's care plan is evidence-based and logical. As instructions and protocols get constantly updated, this would enable coordinated and consistent care tailored to the unique patient's needs. There is also significant evidence that combining eHRs with clinical decision support systems will revolutionize health care and transform collected data into actionable information.

Prediction of Outcomes/Prognosis

Adopting eHRs fully in standard medical care is not the only challenge facing the implementation of electronic health-care infrastructure. Handling the data collected is by itself is another challenge. In fact, data collected in eHRs have much greater potential than what is currently being utilized for. When these systems are enabled to connect multiple sources of information, they are better equipped to generate predictive algorithms regarding a patient's treatment response. This will transform the shape of medicine and how people are managed in the future.

Earlier research [14, 15] tested this approach in diabetes care (eHRs were combined with clinical algorithms); results revealed that eHR was superior to current practice. The combined approach of personal data with prognosis prediction surpassed the efficacy of previous methods and offered better interpretation of patient information and improved care guidelines.

Recently CVS Health (CVS) and IBM announced a partnership [16], designed to better predict deteriorating health using the colossal predictive analytical power of IBM's Watson computer to provide personalized care to CVS customers. The joint venture will enable CVS to better identify consumers who may be at risk for negative health outcomes and then deliver tailored services to them, which in turn is expected to increase the odds of improving their well-being. The move to add predictive elements, based on personalized patient health data, will likely be quickly imitated by competitors and is only the beginning of increasing the use of artificial intelligence to improve population health.

Shared Care

Another great opportunity offered by digital health technology is the opportunity for increased patient engagement. Patients can now view, download, and access their health information, as well as make informed decisions about their treatment options. In 2013, 30% of surveyed physicians routinely used capabilities for secure messaging with patients, and 24% routinely provided patients with the ability to view online, download, or transmit their health records [17]. This number is expected to grow in the coming years and further increase patient-doctor collaboration.

New strategies are being deployed all the time to increase patient engagement through technology. *Mercy*, a health organization, has launched a chronic diseases outreach program, in which it paired technology with its health coaches [18]. Mercy Health Coaches are licensed, registered nurses who work with primary care doctors to provide one-on-one care to help patients set and achieve health improvement goals. They use technology to help motivate patients to take personal initiative and get more involved in their own care. This agrees with a recent study carried out including arthritis patients. The study revealed that measuring patients' motivation reflects their proactivity, engagement, and activation to self-manage their disease which is of value both at the individual level (e.g., tailoring management and interventions) and at the educational program evaluation (e.g., monitor efficacy in enhancing activation) [4]. In this sense, technology alone is not the answer. Human connection helps shift attitude and supports positive behavior change, while technology amplifies this effect. Human interaction will likely continue to be an important factor and remain a determinant regarding the success of health outcomes, even as the evolution of technology helps us improve in ways that accelerate and scale progress toward better well-being.

Patient Empowerment

Providing patients online access to their electronic personal health record (ePHR) offers a new perspective on patient empowerment [19]. In several research works [20–25], including studies on subjects living with rheumatic diseases, patients were keen on having access of their ePHR, independent of age, race, or education level. Patients reported that such approach is expected to enhance involvement in their treatment and that it would give them the feeling of ownership of their own medical information [25]. However, despite potential benefits and patients' positive feedback, studies among health professionals in several areas show that professionals are more cautious toward providing patients home access to their health record [20, 26, 27]. While health professionals have acknowledged benefits, such as increased patient knowledge and empowerment, or improved doctor-patient communication, many concerns were raised particularly about confused patients, frequency of patients' contact, and subsequent increased workload [20, 28]. As a result, the service of providing patients home access to their medical data remains, so far, scarcely implemented [27, 29].

In the field of rheumatology, patient home access to their ePHR seems particularly useful, since patient self-management and patient empowerment are considered highly important. Moreover, rheumatology care providers often have a long-term treatment relationship with their patients, in which cooperation plays an important role [30, 31].

Interoperability in Exchanging Health Information

Interoperability is the ability of systems and organizations to work together. In the context of health care, interoperability refers to the ability of health information systems (e.g., electronic health records, patient registries) to connect with other systems to share, interpret, and present clinical data in such a way that the users can understand and interpret. Another way of thinking about interoperability is that it allows health information to follow the patient anywhere in the health-care system [32, 33].

The objective is that full interoperability in health information exchange improves the safety, quality, efficiency, and cost of health care by facilitating communication between patients, their health-care providers, and public health entities.

Interoperability can be achieved at three varying levels (Fig. 19.2):

- *Basic level (foundational interoperability)*: This simply allows health information exchange from one information system to another but does not require the ability for the receiving system to interpret the data.

Example A primary care physician (PCP) diagnoses a patient with inflammatory arthritis and refers the patient to the rheumatologist for further evaluation and treatment.

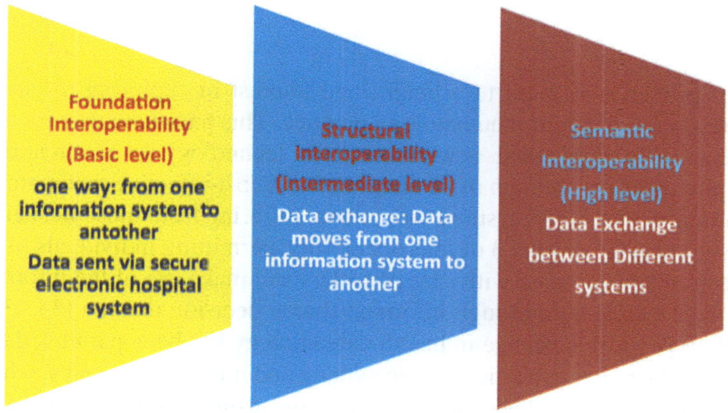

Fig. 19.2 Interoperability in exchanging health information

In addition to the referral letter, the PCP sends a PDF of the patient's X-ray report and most recent blood test results to the rheumatologist's office via secure electronic hospital system. An admin staff member at the hospital/rheumatologist's office can upload the PDF into the eHR. In this instance of foundational interoperability, health information was exchanged, but the receiving system (rheumatologist's eHR) cannot interpret the data in any way.

- *Intermediate level (structural interoperability)*: This entails data exchange to enable uniform movement of health-care data from one information system to another. The clinical or operational purpose and meaning of the data is preserved in the exchange process.

Example The PCP sends the lab data, for a rheumatoid arthritis patient who had abnormal liver function test results, to the rheumatologist's eHR using a messaging standard which labels the information as "lab results." The rheumatologist's eHR automatically deposits the information in the "lab results" section of the patient's record. This is structural interoperability because the receiving system (rheumatologist's eHR) correctly identified the type of incoming information.

- *High level (semantic interoperability)*: This is the ability of participating information systems to automatically interpret, organize, and use the exchanged information. Semantic interoperability requires standardized structuring and codification of data, such that data can be exchanged meaningfully and accurately between information systems used by different health-care facilities. This level of interoperability allows for data exchange which is capable of supporting clinical decision support, care coordination, public health reporting, and research.

Example Although they are made by different vendors, the eHRs of the PCP and the rheumatologist view the lab results in the same way. The results are fully integrated into both systems. When the rheumatologist orders another set of labs to monitor the patient's liver status, the eHR organizes the new results and old results into comparison tables and flow charts.

e-Rheumatology

Advances in technology led to a heightened interest in exploring the use of this technology in the standard rheumatology practice. This paved the way for a strategy transformation to implement new information technology into standard clinical practice aiming at the creation of an integrated and cost-effective rheumatology service. Optimal health IT ecosystem, for patients suffering from musculoskeletal conditions, should achieve level 3 of interoperability, permitting individuals to securely share electronic health data with care providers and make use of the information to manage their own health through informed shared decision making [34, 35]. Over the past few years, this change in health-care strategy has been paralleled by a new trend among the patients, particularly the young and middle age groups, who tend to gather information about their medical conditions using electronic communication tools; hence they have been called "e-patients." A national survey carried out by Pew Research Internet project [36], and published in 2013, revealed that one in three American adults have gone online to inquire about a medical condition. The results depicted also that 8 out of 10 Internet users noted that their last health-related search started with a search engine—a figure that has not changed since Pew last asked that question in 2000. In a study carried by Berland et al. [37] to evaluate health information available through search engines and Web sites, results revealed that accessing health information using search engines and simple search terms is not efficient. Coverage of key information on Web sites is poor and inconsistent, although the accuracy of the information provided is generally good. High reading levels are required to comprehend Web-based health information [67].

On another front, digital approaches which connect rheumatologists to general practitioners or doctors with patients have evolved rapidly over the past few years. e-clinics have been set up by some rheumatologists to answer emails sent by general practitioners inquiring about their cases [38, 39]. Similarly, other online services have been launched to help patients access their doctors' advice. HealthTap [40] has been set up to help patients share photos or test results and get immediate answers, prescriptions, and referrals to help them feel better anywhere. This service is provided 24/7, via the Web or mobile device, securely and privately. Another Web site "Ringadoc" [41] triage calls from the patients to doctors via video conference. Such approach would serve as a hot clinic and would be of value for patients suffering from inflammatory arthritis sustaining a flare up of their disease. Quick advice regarding the management of the acute flare may fix the problem and enable the patient to continue his/her activities of daily living, holiday as well as work [42]. Twitter has also helped in sharing recent advances in rheumatology conferences. Attendees can tweet live during the lectures as to what they consider as the most interesting speakers' messages for their followers. By adding the meeting hashtag at the end of each tweet, any individual on Twitter can read all the messages sent during the conference (e.g., "#ACR16" and "#EULAR2016" were used in 2016 for the annual meetings of the ACR and EULAR, respectively) [43]. Similarly, a community devoted to rheumatologists was launched on Google Plus under the name of

"Rheumatology World" [44]. Cleveland and Mayo Clinic apps [45] have been promoted as tools to help doctors stay connected, understand, and communicate for better care.

Electronic Disease Activity Monitoring

As electronic health recording started to have its place in standard rheumatology practice, direct provision of patient-reported outcomes via standardized electronic questionnaires (ePROMs) was suggested as a tool to improve the efficiency, completeness, and accuracy of data collection. This overall approach is consistent with a broader movement in the health-care delivery toward patient-centered approach, quality of care provided, as well as the functioning of electronic health recording. This was paralleled by the introduction of disease-specific PROM tools, in addition to the available non-specific instruments [46].

For several years, a key barrier to the use ePROMs in standard clinical care was the difficulty of transforming the paper-based questionnaires into an instantly accessible application [45]. With the rapid expansion of Internet-connected gadgets and mobile devices, it became possible to develop online systems with a broad range of implementations both at home and in the clinical setting. A recent study [46] was carried out to assess the use of ePROMs in RA patients. Results revealed that ePROMs could be administered through tablets, computers, and smartphones. It was feasible to sum the patient's disease activity parameters, and based on the scores calculated, clinical relevant actions tailored to the patient's status could be taken which would reflect on the disease control and target achieved. Another recent study [47] was carried out to assess the value of ePROMs in the assessment and management of SLE disease activity flares observed over a 24-month period; its association with adherence to therapy as well as organ damage adjusted for potential confounding factors. Results revealed that ePROMs have a potential disease-modifying effect as it facilitated close monitoring of disease activity with an option of management escalation whenever indicated. Disease activity as measured by SLEDAI over a 24-month observation period predicted the risk of subsequent organ damage independently of other known risk factors. Though there are no earlier data published about ePROMs in rheumatic diseases, studies done in oncology [48] revealed that these smart electronic systems supported multiple clinical activities, including assessment of symptoms and toxicities related to chemotherapy and radiation, post-operative surveillance, and symptom management during palliative care.

A study [49] highlighted that integrating electronic data recording made visual feedback possible in the standard rheumatology clinical practice. This was a randomized controlled study aiming at the assessment of how ubiquitous computing technology can improve the patients' compliance and adherence to therapy. Viewing the disease activity parameters as well as patient-reported outcome measures on the e-personal health recording system leads to a significant greater reduction in disease activity parameters as well as improvement of the patients' adherence to antirheumatic therapy. Furthermore, stopping the DMARDs therapy because of intolerance was significantly less. The study concluded that sharing the outcomes recorded on the e-personal health record had a potential disease-modifying value. Therefore the use of health information technology and electronic prescribing provides a significant opportunity to measure and improve medication adherence at the point of care and to identify nonadherence as well. Furthermore, medication compromise may be another significant outcome of the e-health-recording use as it provides a mean for the individual's health-care team to retrieve information about their management across the care continuum—particularly during transitions of care, hospital admissions, and hospital discharges [50].

e-Comorbidity

Shortened life expectancy in patients with inflammatory arthritis conditions has been linked to the persistence of disease activity as well as associated comorbidities. This highlighted the importance of screening and management of associated comorbidity(ies) as a requirement for proper patient management. Understanding the burden of comorbidity and its impact on rheumatic disease helped to identify the role it plays in the patient's prognosis and premature mortality risk. Recent studies [51, 52] carried out on rheumatoid as well as psoriatic arthritis patients revealed that separate patterns of comorbidity have been identified in patients with different rheumatic diseases. These patterns include the type of comorbid variables reported and their associations with age and disease duration. Electronic comorbidity (e-comorbidity) assessment has the potential of being specific and dynamic approach tailored to the patient's needs. A study published in the American College of Rheumatology conference (2016) [53] was carried out to assess the validity of an electronically comorbidity assessment strategy to identify comorbid conditions among RA and PsA patients in standard practice and to evaluate the impact of e-comorbidity assessment on the patients' care and adherence to therapy.

The study included a cohort of 448 RA and 437 PsA subjects with varying disease duration who met the RA ACR/EULAR criteria and psoriatic arthritis CASPAR criteria. Electronic patient-reported comorbidity questionnaire according to rheumatoid arthritis comorbidity index (RACI) [1] and psoriatic arthritis comorbidity index (PsACI) [2] was implemented as part of electronic patient-reported outcome measures tool. The sensitivity, specificity, and positive and negative predictive values of the electronic data entry and calculated comorbidity risk were compared to ICD-10 medical record (reference standard) and rheumatology clinic visits outcomes. A control group of 241 RA patients and 252 PsA patients who continued their clinical management per standard protocols were also assessed and monitored for 2 years as a control group. Primary endpoint was no inferiority of outcomes of the electronic and standard formats. Secondary endpoint was the patients' adherence to their medications and actions taken to assess and manage the comorbidity risk. Results of the study revealed that the sensitivity for identifying comorbidities using the electronic approach ranged from a minimum of 94% for atlanto-axial subluxation to a maximum of 100% for cardiovascular risk. Sensitivities for extracting comorbidities using ICD-10 codes ranged from a minimum of 8% for anxiety to 100% for tumors, whereas sensitivities for extracting comorbidities using clinic outcomes data ranged from a minimum of 4% for falls risk to 100% for diabetes and tumors. The median positive predictive value (PPV) and negative predictive value (NPV) were 97.7% and 99.6% for the e-comorbidity tool Vs 61.8% and 97.4% for the ICD-10 codes, respectively. The patients' adherence to antirheumatic therapy was significantly higher in the studied group, whereas stopping DMARDs for intolerability was significantly higher in the control group. The number of procedure/screening tests for comorbidity risk assessment was significantly higher in the e-comorbidity group. The study concluded that patient reported e-comorbidity outperformed the standard medical recording systems and can have a role in healthcare management and research. Reclassifying RA patients according to their comorbidity risk would have a positive impact on their adherence to therapy, early assessment of comorbidities with subsequent preventive or treatment decisions.

e-Shared Decision Making

Providing care for a patient results in the meeting of two value systems: the physician's and the patient's, which represents the core of patient-centered care. The characteristic nature of inflammatory arthritic conditions and the variable treatment options made rheumatology a uniquely suited speciality to implement shared decision making successfully. Shared decision making is based on explaining the different options available without bias, and therefore decision aids have been designed to help people make decisions about difficult health-care choices. While shared decision-making leaflets are still in its early stages, studies have already started on using the Web, emails, or tablets to facilitate the e-shared decision making [34]. The electronic shared decision enables the patient engagement as it gives the patient the time to read and make decision in preparation for their visit to the clinic which would enable embedding the shared decision making in the day-to-day clinical practice. Furthermore, it ensures that the decision agreed is a good decision. A good decision is one that is approached systematically, is based on reliable, evidence-based information, and with time allowed to consider all the options carefully [26]. However, in real-life practice, the challenge may arise when the patient opt for avoiding the responsibility of making a decision and ask the doctor for his view. Such challenge can be handled through proper presentation of the data tailored to the patients' level, using graphs and figures rather than texts. In general, e-shared decision making represents a cultural change in behavior and practice as it will assist in changing the environment of medical paternalism to a more inclusive approach based on the Health Act "No decision about me without me" [22]. This would have a positive impact on reduction in complaints and litigation as well as enhanced recovery.

m-Health

Mobile health (m-health) has booked its place in the modern medicine. Basically it is based on the use of mobile technology as a health-care delivery method. This varies from text message to interactive pillboxes as well as wearable digital devices such as Fitbit Flex, Fitbit one, Nike, Garmin, and Jawbone. m-Health is distinctive, in that it uses a global technology, mobile phones, which are currently utilized widely all over the world. The use of m-health intermediations has the potential of changing the patient's behavior through closer and frequent interaction with the person at a convenient time for him/her [27]. Text messaging has been used to remind patients of their appointments in the hospital as well as a tool for disease management. In a recent review, ten research studies evaluated the use of mobile technology to improve treatment adherence [28]. Specifically for hypertension, a review of randomized clinical trials revealed that the patient adherence to therapy improved after adopting reminder systems [29]. Interactive voice response (IVR) tele-monitoring technology [30, 31] has been shown to improve adherence to therapy in patients suffering from chronic diseases. Basically it is a computer-based telephone system that initiates/receives calls, provides information, and collects data from users. Patients often respond to these automated systems to book clinic appointments and/or get a repeat prescription. Earlier studies [31, 32] revealed improvements in adherence to therapy and intermediate outcomes in patients suffering from chronic medical conditions such as diastolic blood pressure and diabetes mellitus (hemoglobin A_1C). Rheumatology wise, m-health can have several applications for patients with rheumatic diseases. An example is the sensors which can be fitted into the patient's shoes and analyze continuously the patient's gait. This technology can be helpful in setting up a customized rehabilitation programs for osteoarthritis patients. Another example is computer-based algorithms which can facilitate the work for a diagnosis in some conditions which have well-established clinical and laboratory criteria, such as early rheumatoid arthritis or SLE [33].

e-Talk: Apps

The role of apps for both the rheumatologists as well as patients suffering from rheumatic diseases is advancing at a speed which could not be expected. As management of rheumatic diseases got controlled by guidelines and checklists, and greater attention is paid to quality and safety, the utility of such apps will gain stronger ground in standard clinical practice. Examples for apps for rheumatologists include:

1. Rheumatoid Arthritis Vital Education (RAVE) mobile app: This app automatically calculates and reports each patient's classification score according to the 2010 ACR/EULAR classification criteria. Users get a single-screen overview for each patient, with key lab results, their prescribed medications, reported adverse effects, and notes. The chart can be printed or e-mailed directly from the app.

2. Doximity: This app gives the doctors gain to physician-only online social communities in which doctors in different of specialties can discuss medical issues and get feedback on cases.
3. ACR: The app includes news, study abstracts, articles, and other publications such as the journals *Arthritis & Rheumatology*, *Arthritis Care & Research*, as well as *The Rheumatologist* [21].

Furthermore, an app has been released recently for ultrasonography (the SonoAccess app) which gives access to a library of clinical videos, case studies, clinical image galleries, and reference guides available to any medical professional or student. Similarly, variable apps have been released for the use of rheumatoid arthritis patients. Examples are myRA, Track + react, Rheuma Track RA, my Pain Diary, and Rheuma helper. Other apps have been also released for physical activity and exercise such as Cody, Fitstar, Fitness, Argus, Human, and Map My Fitness. A major problem with health-related apps is the ethical as well as patient privacy components. Also, once downloaded, they keep working as originally designed unless users take active steps to update or remove them. Therefore, the onus is on the users, not primarily on the developers, to stay informed and update frequently. A malfunctioning app that remains active until the user remembers to update obviously has the potential to create serious problems. So far, there have not been any standardized regulations and no approval process or "Good App Seal of Approval" exists, though developers can seek approval for applications voluntarily [21].

Electronic Prescribing

Electronic prescribing or e-prescribing (eRx) is a way for the treating doctor and other health-care providers to send the prescriptions they issue to the pharmacy electronically. Instead of writing out a prescription and having the patient taking it to the local drugstore, the treating doctor orders the patient's medication through the office computer, which then generates a secure electronic prescription to the pharmacy.

Electronic prescribing helps to:

- Avoid mistakes due to the doctor's handwriting or pharmacist's misreading of the prescription abbreviations.
- Avoid harmful drug interactions by letting the doctor know that the drugs being ordered may interact with a medication the patient is already taking.
- Enable the treating doctor to see what medications are on the patient's current health plan's drug formulary to make sure the drug being ordered is covered.

"E-prescribing" is a computer-based electronic filling, generation, as well as transmission of a prescription which would replace the paper prescriptions. E-prescribing allows a physician, nurse practitioner, or physician assistant to electronically transmit a new prescription or renewal authorization to a community surgery or pharmacy [20]. E-prescribing is a potent system allowing the health-care professionals manage their patients' medications safely and efficiently. In comparison with paper prescribing, e-prescribing improves patients' adherence to therapy as well as safety, enhances accuracy and efficiency of prescribing medications, and lessens costs of health care through avoiding medications' adverse events and swapping of less expensive medication substitutes [21]. Medication errors were identified by the Institute of Medicine as the commonest category of medical error in health care, approximating that this causes several thousand deaths per year [22]. Therefore, daily methotrexate prescriptions can be a never event. E-prescribing also plays a substantial role in efforts to minimize the incidence of drug diversion by forewarning pharmacists and providers of duplicative prescriptions for controlled substances [23].

On the other hand, limitations and challenges which may deter the implementation of e-prescribing include:

Financial: The cost incurred in purchasing, uploading, supporting, and maintaining the system is considered one of the greatest application hurdles which may be beyond the means of most small clinical practices.

Service switchover: Transitioning from paper to e-prescribing is a challenge by itself in particular in busy practices. Pharmacists also will need to adjust workflow and surge their awareness of new types of errors associated with e-prescribing.

Choosing the right hardware podium and software applications: This can be a challenge in particular in small and busy settings [21].

Erroneous alerts: The inability to efficiently implement clinical decision support systems due to the flawed triggering of pop-up alerts with ill-defined software is another big limitation.

Privacy and security: As with other e-health applications, privacy of the patients' information saved in electronic format may lead to the possibility of errors, such as unintentional disclosure of confidential health information through inadequate security policies.

Downtime: Either due to network-related glitches or software technical problems.

Considerations regarding the procedures should such situations arise should be discussed) [24, 25].

Wearable and Portable Sensors for Personal Telehealth

A paradigm shift in the management of inflammatory as well as noninflammatory arthritic conditions, toward self-management strategies, has been advocated to reduce the patient and societal burden of such diseases [54, 55]. Guidelines recommend regular monitoring of the disease activity, in addition to educational and exercise programs to mitigate symptoms and disease progression. However, the effectiveness of these protocols is highly dependent on supervision and compliance, which is often poor [56]. Recent advancements in health-related measuring technologies has offered new opportunities for delivery of such management approaches outside the clinical setting, allowing remote monitoring and feedback of key measures to both health professionals and patients [57, 58]. These portable devices could potentially enable patients to become more active in the management of their condition and fulfil their interest in personalized health information while also aligning with the current focus on patient self-management [57] as well as the need for more accurate objective measures of patients' functions [59]. These devices are designed to record quantitative data in a mobile environment, embedded in the user's clothing or fitted as an accessory [60]. Numerous devices have been developed to date aimed at monitoring patient disease activity status as well as ambulatory performance, but their uptake and acceptance in clinical environments remains poor [61–63]. The uptake of these technologies is influenced by their intended use, perceived usefulness, ease of learning, success in early experimentation, right fit to a specific clinical context, as well as user needs [63–65]. Therein lies a problem. The development of these technologies has been largely driven by engineering requirements [62]. Consequently, less attention has been devoted to users' preferences [61, 62]. Recent research conducted to address this gap in knowledge has focused on examining patients' preferences for wearable technologies. By contrast, comparatively scarce attention has been given to health professionals' views of these devices [66]. Therefore, relatively little is known among doctors about how these devices might work in the context of clinical practice. Health professionals, like patients, represent a key user group. Unlike patients, however, they possess knowledge and insight of clinical practice, which would be critical in identifying realistic implementation strategies. Moreover, health professionals could assist with promoting acceptability among patient groups. Several studies showed the usefulness of using such devices for the management of patients suffering from inflammatory as well as degenerative joint disease. However, concerns were raised regarding patient confidentiality and who might have access to the patients' data. Organization bodies are discussing recommendations for using such high-tech tools on a wider base.

The Dark Side of Digital Health

There is a thin line between being well informed and becoming a cyberchondriac.

Online self-diagnosing is becoming routine for Internet users who are increasingly aware of the vast amount of available online health resources and want to feel in control of their bodies and well-being. Instead of waiting for an appointment, having to discuss their symptoms with a doctor and occasionally pleading for additional diagnostic tests, potential patients now perform extensive searches of the Web and juxtapose different diagnoses with their symptoms until they discover the one that seems to fit best.

The Internet makes health-related information almost universally accessible. It helps educate people about their health and enables them to make informed decisions about their treatment options. There are examples of people diagnosing themselves correctly after years of misdiagnosis. A recent example is the unfortunate story of Bronte Doyne [68]. Bronte was told by her doctors to stop self-diagnosing and ultimately died of a condition she had identified, but a condition that went unnoticed by the physicians treating her until it was too late.

On the other hand, Googling the medical symptoms does not necessarily end in a resolution and can in many cases bring out unnecessary anxieties, transforming former hypochondriacs into present-day cyberchondriacs. Some can even get addicted to constantly searching for health information online, examining themselves, and looking for reassurance, as well as demanding tests and screenings that might not be appropriate.

Escalation of Innocuous Symptoms

Common symptomatology can prompt some users to start exploring rare and serious conditions that came up during their online searches. A large-scale survey completed in 2008 [69] showed that Web search engines have the potential to escalate medical concerns of people who have little or no medical training. The study showed that escalation was influenced by the amount and distribution of medical content viewed by users, the use of alarming terminology on the sites they visited, and the person's predisposition to becoming anxious. In contrast, there are some people who can indeed diagnose themselves correctly, especially if what they are experiencing is very specific and atypical. For instance, in cases like Bronte's, this was discussed in the last paragraph. Interestingly, an outlier can sometimes get ignored or overlooked and treated by the medical team as a common medical condition when it is not.

Conclusion

The evolution of information technology reached a turning point in medicine and is gradually maturing. Information and communication technologies have already made a massive move into medical practice, not only in selected areas of "high-tech" medicine or surgery but also in the standard day-to-day practice. Health information tools can facilitate population health management, enable the patients to monitor their disease and functional ability, and stay communicated with their treating health-care professional. However, technology alone is not sufficient for improving the health of a group of patients. Critical elements for success include committed leadership, training of health-care providers in population health principles, supportive reimbursement models, workflow redesign, and harmonious care coordination teams and processes. The degree to which health information tools work seamlessly together will also influence the effectiveness of population health programs. This trend is likely to continue and bring new aspects for patients' diagnosis and management.

References

1. Institute of Medicine. The computer-based patient record: an essential technology for health care. Washington, DC: National Academy Press; 1997.
2. Weiner M, Biondich P. The influence of information technology on patient-physician relationships. J Gen Intern Med. 2006;21(Suppl 1):S35–9.
3. Institute of Medicine. Crossing the quality chasm: a new health care system for the 21st century. Washington, DC: National Academy Press; 2001.
4. El Miedany Y, El Gaafary M, Youssef S, Palmer D. Development of the patient motivation questionnaire: conceptualizing and measuring motivation in patients with inflammatory arthritis. Ann Rheum Dis. 2016;75(Suppl2):469.
5. El Miedany Y, Shams K. The electronic recording of outcome measures in inflammatory arthritis: is there a room for the second generation. Ann Rheum Dis. 2009;68(Suppl3):737.
6. El Miedany Y. e-rheumatology: are we ready. Clin Rheumatol. 2015;34(5):831–7.
7. El Miedany Y, El Gaafary M, Youssef S, Palmer D. Electronic patient reported outcome measures (e-PROMS) for early arthritis in standard clinical practice: a pilot study. Ann Rheum Dis. 2015;74(Suppl 2):65.
8. Text of the Telehealth Modernization Act of 2013. Accessed 25 June 2014. https://www.govtrack.us/congress/bills/113/hr3750/text.
9. American Telemedicine Association. What is telemedicine? Accessed 24 June 2014. https://s3.amazonaws.com/rdcms-himss/files/production/public/HIMSSorg/Content/files/Line%2016%20- %20What%20Is%20Telemedicine.pdf.
10. Doarn CR, et al. Federal efforts to define and advance telehealth – a work in progress. Telemed J E Health. 2014;20(5):409–18. Accessed 25 June 2014
11. National Collaborating Centre for Chronic Conditions. Rheumatoid arthritis: national clinical guideline for management and treatment in adults. London: Royal College of Physicians; 2009.
12. Palmer D, El Miedany Y. PROMs: a novel approach to arthritis self-management. Br J Nurs. 2012;21(10):601–5.
13. Palmer D, El Miedany Y. EROMIA in inflammatory arthritis: the next step in standard practice. Br J Nurs. 2010;19(1):42–6.
14. Varroud-Vial M. Improving diabetes management with electronic medical records. Diabetes Metab. 2011;37(Suppl 4):S48–52.
15. Meng X, Yang J-J. Visual analysis for type 2 diabetes mellitus – based on electronic medical records, Chapter Smart Health Volume 8549 of the series Lecture notes in computer science. Cham: Springer; 2014. p. 160–70.
16. Jaspen B. CVA and IBM's Watson cloud pursue ways to predict patient health. Forbes.com. 2015. http://www.forbes.com/sites/brucejapsen/2015/07/30/cvs-and-ibms-watson-partner-to-predict-patient-health-needs/#431d14c68ac9.
17. Furukawa M, King J, Patel V, Hsiao CJ, Adler-Milstein J, Jha A. Despite substantial progress in EHR adoption, health information exchange and patient engagement remain low in office settings. Health Aff. 2014;33:1672–9. doi:10.1377/hlthaff.2014.0445. http://content.healthaffairs.org/content/early/2014/08/05/hlthaff.2014.0445
18. Mercy Health Coach Program. https://www.mercydesmoines.org/healthcoach.

19. Demiris G, Afrin LB, Speedie S, et al. Patient-centered applications: use of information technology to promote disease management and wellness. A white paper by the AMIA knowledge in motion working group. J Am Med Inform Assoc. 2008;15:8–13.
20. Ross SE, Todd J, Moore LA, et al. Expectations of patients and physicians regarding patient-accessible medical records. J Med Internet Res. 2005;7:e13.
21. Ferreira A, Correia A, Silva A, et al. Why facilitate patient access to medical records. Med Care Compunetics. 2007;4:77–90.
22. Honeyman A, Cox B, Fisher B. Potential impacts of patient access to their electronic health records. Inform Prim Care. 2005;13:55–60.
23. Van der Vaart R, Drossaert CHC, Taal E, et al. Patient preferences for a hospital based rheumatology Interactive Health Communication Application, and factors associated with these preferences. Rheumatology. 2011;50:1618–26.
24. Van der Vaart R, Drossaert CHC, Taal E, et al. Experiences and preferences of patients with rheumatic diseases regarding an interactive health communication application. In: Proceedings of the 2nd eTELEMED international conference on ehealth, telemedicine, and social medicine, Saint Martin; 2010 Feb, p. 64–71. doi:10.1109/eTELEMED.2010.16.
25. Richter JG, Becker A, Koch T, et al. Changing attitudes towards online electronic health records and online patient documentation in rheumatology outpatients. Clin Exp Rheumatol. 2010;28:261–4.
26. Masys D, Baker D, Butros A, et al. Giving patients access to their medical records via the internet: the PCASSO experience. J Am Med Inform Assoc. 2002;9:181–91.
27. Reti SR, Feldman HJ, Ross SE, et al. Improving personal health records for patient-centered care. J Am Med Inform Assoc. 2010;17:192–5.
28. Earnest M, Ross SE, Wittevrongel L, et al. Use of a patient-accessible electronic medical record in a practice for congestive heart failure: patient and physician experiences. J Am Med Inform Assoc. 2004;11:410.
29. Winkelman WJ, Leonard KJ. Overcoming structural constraints to patient utilization of electronic medical records: a critical review and proposal for an evaluation framework. J Am Med Inform Assoc. 2004;11:151–5.
30. Leonard K, Wiljer D, Casselman M. An innovative information paradigm for consumers with chronic conditions: the value proposition. J Inf Tech Health Care. 2008;6:274–82.
31. El Miedany Y. Joint fitness programme for arthritic patients – the value of patient-reported outcome measures in designing a tailored approach to patient education. Eur Musculoskelet Rev. 2012.; https://www.touchmusculoskeletal.com
32. Fridsma D. Interoperability vs health information exchange: setting the record straight. Accessed 11 June 2014. https://www.healthit.gov/buzz-blog/meaningful-use/interoperability-health-information-exchange-settingrecord- straight/.
33. Healthcare Information and Management Systems Society. What is interoperability? Accessed 8 June 2014. http://www.himss.org/library/interoperability-standards/what-is-interoperability.
34. El Miedany Y, El Gaafary M, Sayed S, Palmer D, Ahmed A. Implementing shared decision making in clinical practice: outcomes of new shared decision making aid for chronic inflammatory arthritis patients. J Pat Care. 2016;2(2):117–23.
35. Palmer D, El Miedany Y. Shared decision making for patients living with inflammatory arthritis. Br J Nurs. 2016;25(1):31–5.
36. Pew Research Internet Project. http://www.pewinternet.org/2013/01/15/health-online-2013/.
37. Berland GK, Elliott MN, Morales LS, et al. Health information on the Internet: accessibility, quality, and readability in English and Spanish. JAMA. 2001;285(20):2612–21.
38. Tang H, Kwoon J. Googling for a diagnosis-use of Google as a diagnostic aid: Internet based study. BMJ. 2006; doi:10.1136/bmj.39003.640567.AE.
39. Albert D, Merrihew K, Pletcher S. Tele-rheumatology: the future is now [abstract]. Arthritis Rheum. 2012;64(Suppl 10):2053. doi:10.1002/art.39785.
40. Health Tap Inc. [US]. https://www.healthtap.com/.
41. Ringadoc. https://www.ringadoc.com/.

42. Berenbaum F. The social (media) side to rheumatology. Nat Rev Rheumatol. 2014;10:314–31.
43. John Hopkins Kimmel Cancer in Baltimore. Doctors often use social media on the job: survey. 2013. http://health.usnews.com/health-news/news/articles/2013/01/01/docs-often-use-social-media-on-the-job-survey.
44. Google+. Rheumatology world [online]. 2015. https://plus.google.com/communities/108852894746535117171.
45. Mayo clinic App. 2015. http://www.mayoclinic.org/apps/mayo-clinic.
46. El Miedany Y, El Gaafary M, Youssef S, Bahlas S, Almedany S, Ahmed I, Palmer D. Toward electronic health recording: evaluation of electronic patient-reported outcome measures system for remote monitoring of early rheumatoid arthritis. J Rheumatol. 2016;43(12):2106–12.
47. El Miedany Y, El Gaafary M, El Aroussy M, Bahlas S, Hegazi M, Palmer D, Youssef S. Toward electronic health recording: evaluation of electronic patient reported outcome measures (e-PROMs) system for remote monitoring of early systemic lupus patients. Clin Rheumatol. 2017; doi:10.1007/s10067-017- 3675-9.
48. Fox S, Fallows D. Health searches and email have become more commonplace, but there is room for improvement in searches and overall Internet access. 2003. http://www.pewinternet.org/files/old-media//Files/Reports/2003/PIP_Health_Report_July_2003.pdf.pdf.
49. El Miedany Y, El Gaafary M, Palmer D. Assessment of the utility of visual feedback in the treatment of early rheumatoid arthritis patients: a pilot study. Rheumatol Int. 2012;32:3061–8.
50. Bosworth HB, Granger BB, Mendys P. Medication adherence: a call for action. Am Heart J. 2011;162(3):412–24.
51. El Miedany Y, El Gaafary M, Youssef S, Bahlas S, Ahmed I, Hegazi M Rheumatoid arthritis comorbidity index: development and validation of a new specific tool for classifying prognostic comorbidity in rheumatoid arthritis patients. Ann Rheum Dis. 2016;75(Suppl2):154.
52. El Miedany Y, El Gaafary M, Youssef S, Bahlas S, Ahmed I, Hegazi M. Psoriatic arthritis Comorbidity Index: development and validation of a new specific tool for classifying prognostic comorbidity in psoriatic arthritis patients. Ann Rheum Dis. 2016;75(Suppl2):89.
53. El Miedany YM, El Gaafary M, Youssef S, Bahlas S, Hegazi M, Ahmed I. E-comorbidity: evaluation of the validity of electronic comorbidity assessment in identifying comorbid conditions among patients with rheumatoid and psoriatic arthritis. Arthritis Rheumatol. 2016; 68 (suppl 10).
54. Hunter DJ. Lower extremity osteoarthritis management needs a paradigm shift. Br J Sports Med. 2011;45:283–8.
55. National Institute for Health and Clinical Excellence. Osteoarthritis: care and management in adults, Clinical guideline CG177. London: NICE; 2014. https://www.nice.org.uk/guidance/cg177
56. Bennell KL, Kyriakides M, Hodges PW, et al. Effects of two physiotherapy booster sessions on outcomes with home exercise in people with knee osteoarthritis: a randomized controlled trial. Arthritis Care Res (Hoboken). 2014;66:1680–7.
57. Swan M. Emerging patient-driven health care models: an examination of health social networks, consumer personalized medicine and quantified self-tracking. Int J Environ Res Public Health. 2009;6:492–525.
58. Bonato P. Wearable sensors and systems. From enabling technology to clinical applications. IEEE Eng Med Biol Mag. 2010;29:25–36.
59. Muro-de-la-Herran A, Garcia-Zapirain B, Mendez-Zorrilla A. Gait analysis methods: an overview of wearable and non-wearable systems, highlighting clinical applications. Sensors (Basel). 2014;14:3362–94.
60. Lukowicz P, Kirstein T, Troster G. Wearable systems for health care applications. Methods Inf Med. 2004;43:232–8.
61. Shull PB, Jirattigalachote W, Hunt MA, et al. Quantified self and human movement: a review on the clinical impact of wearable sensing and feedback for gait analysis and intervention. Gait Posture. 2014;40:11–9.
62. Bergmann JHM, McGregor AH. Body-worn sensor design: what do patients and clinicians want? Ann Biomed Eng. 2011;39:2299–312.

63. Appelboom G, Camacho E, Abraham ME, et al. Smart wearable body sensors for patient self-assessment and monitoring. Arch Public Health. 2014;72:28.
64. Singh A, Klapper A, Jia J, et al. Motivating people with chronic pain to do physical activity: opportunities for technology design. In: ACM proceedings of the 33rd ACM conference on human factors in computing systems, New York; 2014, p. 2803–12.
65. Renaud K, van Biljon J. Predicting technology acceptance and adoption by the elderly: a qualitative study. In: Proceedings of the 2008 annual research conference of the South African Institute of Computer Scientists and Information Technologists on IT research in developing countries: riding the wave of technology, Wilderness; 2008, p. 210–19.
66. Papi E, Belsi A, McGregor AH. A knee monitoring device and the preferences of patients living with osteoarthritis: a qualitative study. BMJ Open. 2015;5:e007980.
67. Vize R. Google search vs doctor diagnosis – always an imperfect balance. https://www.theguardian.com/healthcare-network/2015/jun/19/google-search-doctor-diagnosis-imperfect-balance-bronte-doyne-cancer.
68. White R, Horvitz E. Cyberchondria: studies of the escalation of medical concerns in web search. Microsoft research. 2008. https://www.microsoft.com/en-us/research/wp-content/uploads/2016/02/TR-2008-178.pdf.
69. Elkin PL, Liebow M, Bauer BA, Chaliki S, Wahner-Roedler D, Bundrick J, Lee M, Brown SH, Froehling D, Bailey K, Famiglietti K, Kim R, Hoffer E, Feldman M, Barnett GO. The introduction of a diagnostic decision support system (DXplain™) into the workflow of a teaching hospital service can decrease the cost of service for diagnostically challenging Diagnostic Related Groups (DRGs). Int J Med Inform. 2010;79(11):772–7.

Index

Y. El Miedany (ed.), *Comorbidity in Rheumatic Diseases*,
DOI 10.1007/978-3-319-59963-2

S

MIX
Papier aus verantwortungsvollen Quellen
Paper from responsible sources
FSC® C105338

If you have any concerns about our products,
you can contact us on
ProductSafety@springernature.com

In case Publisher is established outside the EU,
the EU authorized representative is:
Springer Nature Customer Service Center GmbH
Europaplatz 3, 69115 Heidelberg, Germany

Printed by Libri Plureos GmbH
in Hamburg, Germany